MODERN MEDICAL LANGUAGE

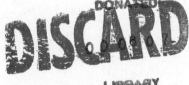

MODERN MEDICAL LANGUAGE

C. EDWARD COLLINS
Northern Alberta Institute of Technology

JUANITA J. DAVIES
Northern Alberta Institute of Technology

WEST PUBLISHING COMPANY
Minneapolis/St. Paul   New York   Los Angeles   San Francisco

For three special friends: Julie, Len, and Art

This book is dedicated with love to my husband Jim and to my children Lisa and Georgia

---

Production Credits
Copyedit: *Michele Scheid*
Composition: *University Graphics, Inc.*
Interior Design and Page Layout: *Maureen McCutcheon Design*
Art: *Radiant Illustration and Design; University Graphics, Inc.*
Proofread: *June Gomez*
Cover photo: © Peter Angelo Simon/Phototake

Photo credits follow the index.

West's Commitment to the Environment
In 1906, West Publishing Company began recycling materials left over from the production of books. This began a tradition of efficient and responsible use of resources. Today, 100% of our legal bound volumes are printed on acid-free, recycled paper consisting of 50% new paper pulp and 50% paper that has undergone a de-inking process. We also use vegetable-based inks to print all of our books. West recycles nearly 22,650,000 pounds of scrap paper annually—the equivalent of 187,500 trees. Since the 1960s, West has devised ways to capture and recycle waste inks, solvents, oils, and vapors created in the printing process. We also recycle plastics of all kinds, wood, glass, corrugated cardboard, and batteries, and have eliminated the use of polystyrene book packaging. We at West are proud of the longevity and the scope of our commitment to our environment.

West pocket parts and advance sheets are printed on recyclable paper and can be collected and recycled with newspapers. Staples do not have to be removed. Bound volumes can be recycled after removing the covers.

Production, Press, Printing and Binding by West Publishing Company.

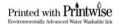

Printed with Printwise
Environmentally Advanced Water Washable Ink

The information in this book is presented solely for educational purposes and is not intended to be relied upon in place of advice from qualified professionals. For further information in the subjects discussed, West Publishing recommends that readers contact the various sources mentioned in the text or other appropriate professionals. West Publishing does not represent or warrant the safety, effectiveness, completeness or accuracy of the information contained in this book, and readers assume all risks associated with their use of such information.

British Library Cataloguing-in-Publication Data. A catalogue record for this book is available from the British Library.

ISBN 0–314–06702–7

BRIEF CONTENTS

CONTENTS

CHAPTER 11

The Digestive System   280

CHAPTER 12

The Endocrine System   328

CHAPTER 16

The Urinary and Male Reproductive Systems   466

CHAPTER 17

The Female Reproductive System, Human Genetics, and Obstetrics   504

Acquiring a Medical Vocabulary

In acquiring a medical vocabulary, most students follow a path that diverges sharply from that of an infant's natural, unsystematic approach to learning a language. The first major difference is that the word precedes (or perhaps supersedes altogether) the experience. Most people add technical words to their vocabularies in this way. For example, a person learning auto repair would no doubt learn the meanings of the words piston, valve, and cylinder before being exposed to the actual techniques of engine overhaul. Likewise, students in the health care field learn words first by seeing them written, by hearing them on audiotape, or by exposure through other learning aids. The second difference is that most successful medical terminology students take an analytical approach, learning each word's origin and its simplified meaning before going on to a more advanced understanding of terms and their interconnections.

The quickest and surest way to acquire medical language is to treat it as a technical subject.

1. Study medical terms systematically, learning their origins, memorizing their definitions, and listening to the sounds they make.

2. Realize that knowing the meanings of medical terms is only a first step in becoming a proficient user of a medical vocabulary. As you progress, you will become more and more aware of the subtleties of human anatomy and physiology and of the corresponding language structures in which medical terms must be cast.

The Parts of the Book

This book takes a pedagogical approach that rests on the principles of systematic language acquisition. Part I introduces students to the origins of medical terms. Deriving chiefly from Greek and Latin, medical terms can be learned in the context of word

elements adopted from these languages. Although etymological study does impart an elementary word sense, it does not lead one inevitably to an in-depth understanding of the terms studied.

Part II provides the next logical step by offering background information related to anatomical systems, along with pertinent illustrations and the terms related to each system. Most chapters in Part II contain one or more concept maps, which are outlines in illustration form. The concept map differs from an ordinary outline in that its topics and subtopics are arranged in a spatial presentation. For example, the integumentary system is divided into structure and function. The subdivisions of these two blocks are connected by arrows, both within and between topic areas, thus making the relationships apparent.

Part III follows with overviews of special medical areas, again including illustrations and using the terms to be learned within the context of the discussion of each specialty. Parts II and III make continuous reference to the etymological analyses techniques presented in Part I.

Special Features

Graphics   The graphic features of this text have been chosen to make maximum use of visual learning techniques.

1. **All illustrations appear with the terms to be learned** rather than as a disconnected set of "plates."

2. **Anatomical art appears in full color,** as it does in much more expensive books on anatomy and physiology.

3. **Much of the information is presented in tables** so that the student may quickly assimilate parallel relationships.

4. Beginning with Chapter 5, **tables repeat and summarize** preceding text material. Thus, they may be used for initial learning or as a review. The Term Analysis tables (Chapters

5–18) are particularly useful this way. Even chapter openers often have tables, called "Word Elements Prominent."

5. To add to their usefulness, **tables are color-coded.**

Tan	General
Green	Term Analysis with Pronunciation
Blue	Abnormal Conditions; Physical Examination, Diagnosis, and Treatment
Red	Abbreviations

Exercises and Exercise Answers

1. **Traditional exercises,** including definitions, matching, and word-building.
2. **In-context medical document exercises,** including hospital summary records, in which students are asked to define underlined words.
3. **Crossword puzzles.**
4. **Answers to all the exercises,** permitting **self evaluation** of progress.

Dictionary of Medical Terms A Dictionary of Medical Terms is included at the back of the book for **quick reference.** It includes terms beyond those covered in the text, and may allow postponing the purchase of a separate medical dictionary for a future term.

The Supporting Package

Various supporting materials are available for students and instructors.

For the student:
1. **Activity cards,** sometimes called flash cards (ISBN 0-314-08925-x). These can be shrink-wrapped with the text.
2. **Audio cassette tape,** pronunciation only. This can be shrink-wrapped with the text.
3. **Audio cassette tapes including spellings, meanings, and activities.** Ask your West sales representative about availability. Usually the school would put these on reserve.
4. **Interactive software.** Ask your West sales representative about availability.

For the instructor:
1. An **Instructor's Manual** includes teaching suggestions, lecture outlines, additional exercises, and "Word Find" puzzles.
2. **Transparency Masters** and **Acetates** include illustrations from the text and other sources.
3. A **Test Bank** contains 1850 terms (50–110 per chapter), primarily in multiple-choice format.
4. WESTEST 3.1 is **Computerized Testing Software** for IBM and Macintosh.
5. **Microsoft PowerPoint** affords state-of-the-art presentation options that combine graphics, animation, and sound from a disk containing more than 1200 illustrations.

Acknowledgments

The authors are deeply indebted to the many people who helped in this book's writing and production. First of all, we wish to thank the staff of West College Publishing: acquisitions editor Christopher Conty for his boundless energy, enthusiasm, and faith in the project; developmental editor Elizabeth Riedel for her astute observations and analyses throughout the review process; and project editors Amy Gabriel and Holly Henjum for their diligent and exceptionally skillful editing of the manuscript.

We wish to thank Dr. Carl Waddle and MaryAnn Woods for preparing the Instructor's Manual; Janet Taylor for writing the Dictionary of Terms; Melisse Gross for preparing the Activity Cards and the Audio Cassette Tapes; Kasey Summer for creating the Test Bank; Nancy Akery for inserting the pronunciations appearing throughout the book; Lisa Resau for creating the Word-Find Puzzles; Marge Warren for preparing the Powerpoint software; Clifford M. Renk and David L. Heiserman for preparing the interactive software; Lorene Collins for researching and writing most of the material for Chapters 11, 12, 15, 16, and 20; Glen Heggie for supplying information for the Nuclear Medicine Section in Chapter 18; and the following people for checking the technical accuracy of the manuscript: Peggy Camp, RN, MSN, Association of Operating Room Nurses, Inc., Denver, Colorado; Richard P. Lafleur, M.D., Mark B. Richard, M.D., and Edmund S. Schiavoni, Jr., M.D., Southern New Hampshire Internal Medicine Associates, Derry, New Hampshire; and Brian Stainken,

M.D., Albany Medical Center Hospital, Albany, New York.

We would also like to acknowledge the help of Dr. Barbara Thomas and Hugh Read of the Society for Technical Communication; Eleanor Smoley, Karen Israelson, and medical records staff members at the University of Alberta Hospital; Dr. Gary Chornell; Marjorie Phillips, R.N.; Maryann James; Dr. Marc Moreau; and Doris Graham.

We owe a very special thanks to the following reviewers, whose experience and pedagogical knowledge helped immeasurably in a multitude of editorial decisions: Nancy Akery, M.T., Baylor College of Medicine, TX; Marie T. Conde, City College of San Francisco, CA; Melisse Gross, Vancouver Community College, BC; Steven Forshier, Pima Medical Institute, AZ; Craig Hart, Apollo Center, OH; S. Clare Haskin, Fanshawe College of Applied Arts & Technology, ON; Sondra Sue Hein, Saddleback College, CA; Wendy C. Holder, Belleville Area College, Il; Lisa Resau, Essex Community College, MD; Kimberly H. Rubesne, Median School of Allied Health Careers, PA; Alice Serey, Indian River Community College, FL; Mary C. St. Cin, Chattanooga State Tech. Community College, TN; Kasey C. Summer, Ultrasound Diagnostic School, GA; Janet L. Taylor, Maric College of Medical Careers, CA; Antonio C. Wallace, Ultrasound Diagnostic School, GA; Margaret T. Warren, Rockland Community College, NY; and MaryAnn Woods, Fresno City College, CA.

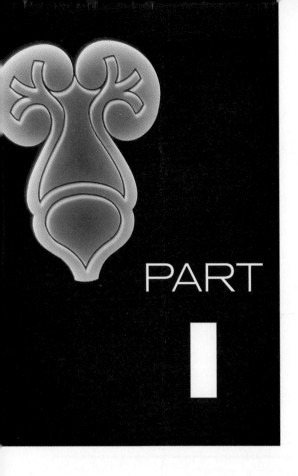

PART

I

WORD ELEMENTS

1

CONSTRUCTION OF MEDICAL TERMS

CHAPTER OBJECTIVES

Upon successful completion of this chapter, the student will be able to do the following:

1. Distinguish the suffixes, prefixes, and roots of example terms.
2. Form plurals of singular medical terms.
3. Form singulars of plural medical terms.

INTRODUCTION

Words are curious things. Some semanticists (students of the meanings of words) hold that words are unimportant in themselves. They state that an object might have been called anything and that the choice of the word makes no difference in how we view a given object of reality or in the effect the object has on our lives. Poets disagree, however, and hold that the sounds words make are important. They believe that sounds convey a deeper meaning than is possible in the simple act of identifying objects. Cultural historians and some linguists also disagree with the semanticists' view, declaring that language is rich in allusions and that it is far more than a random collection of sounds.

As you proceed with the study of medical terminology, you will find that nearly all medical terms have their origins in Greek or Latin and that your knowledge of a given medical term's origins will help you to understand its meaning.

▶ 1.1 COMPONENT PARTS OF WORDS IN GENERAL

Words of all kinds can be broken up into smaller units, a process that helps us to understand them. These units are called **roots**, **prefixes**, and **suffixes**. You may remember from a spelling class that a root is the main part of a word. You may also remember that a prefix is something added to the beginning of a word to change its meaning in some way, and a suffix is added to the end of a word to change its form or meaning. To see how this works, let's look at an example. Take the word **septic** from the Latin **septicus** meaning putrid. When we add the prefix **anti-** from the Greek (against) to the root word septic, we form a new word **antiseptic**, which means either "something that acts against germs" (noun) or "acting against germs" (adjective).

If we now take the word antiseptic and add the suffix **-ize** to it, we get the word **antisepticize**, which is the process of ridding an object of germs.

(prefix)	(root)	(suffix)
anti-	septic	-ize

We have converted our noun/adjective **antiseptic** to the verb **antisepticize** by adding a very common suffix derived from the Greek verbal suffix **-izein** (the function of the Greek suffix **-izein** is exactly the same as that of the English suffix **-ize**—it converts an adjective to a verb). You will use this technique constantly in your acquisition of a medical vocabulary. It is important to note, though, that you should not use this method to coin new words, but rather to decipher words with which you may be unfamiliar. The example given illustrates the point nicely, since we would most likely use *sterilize* rather than *anticepticize* to refer to the process of ridding an object of germs. However, *anticepticize* is an English word, and if we were to run across it, we could undertand its meaning simply by recalling the meanings of its parts.

▶ 1.2 COMPONENT PARTS OF MEDICAL TERMS

The components of a medical term are exactly the same as those of any other complex word. The root is the main part of the word, to which prefixes and suffixes may be added. In one respect, each complex medical term is a kind of shorthand that represents an English phrase. Let us consider an example of a familiar term, *appendicitis*. Appendicitis is a one-word term that is shorthand for the phrase, *inflammation of the appendix*. When we look at medical terms this way, we see that the central part of the phrase is often represented by the suffix (-itis) and not the root (appendix). Thus, when we decipher a term, we sometimes have to begin with the suffix, at least until we become so familiar with the deciphering process that we do it automatically. Tables 1–1 and 1–2 show some examples of suffixes and roots.

In Table 1–1 and throughout this book, suffixes appearing alone are preceded by a hyphen, and prefixes appearing alone are shown with a hyphen at the end. Writing these elements this way helps you distinguish between them.

TABLE 1–1

Suffixes and Their Meanings

SUFFIX	MEANING
-itis	inflammation
-pathy	disease process
-logy	study of

The slash (/) in the first column of Table 1–2 indicates that the final letter or letters may be omitted to accommodate suffixes beginning with a vowel. You will notice, however, that some roots are difficult or impossible to pronounce without the final letter and would be hard to remember without their accompanying vowels.

TABLE 1–2

Roots and Their Meanings

ROOT	MEANING
gastr/o	stomach
hepat/o	liver
aden/o	gland
card/i/o	heart

Table 1–3 gives the suffixes and roots shown in Tables 1–1 and 1–2 in all their possible combinations.

TABLE 1–3

Suffixes and Roots Combined

COMBINATION	PRONUNCIATION	MEANING
gastritis	găs-trī′-tĭs	inflammation of the stomach
hepatitis	hĕp″-ă-tī′-tĭs	inflammation of the liver
adenitis	ăd″-ĕ-nī′-tis	inflammation of a gland
carditis	kăr-dī′-tĭs	inflammation of the heart
gastropathy	găs-trŏp′-ă-thē	disease of the stomach
hepatopathy	hĕp″-ă-tŏp′-ă-thē	disease of the liver
adenopathy	ăd″-ĕ-nŏp′-ă-thē	disease of a gland
cardiopathy	kăr″-dē-ŏp′-ă-thĕ	disease of the heart
gastrology	găs-trŏl′-ō-jē	study of the stomach
hepatology	hĕp″-ă-tŏl-ō-jē	study of the liver
adenology	ăd″-ĕ-nŏl′-ō-jē	study of the glands
cardiology	kăr-dē-ŏl′-ō-jē	study of the heart

In several of the terms listed in Table 1–3, we omitted the vowel or vowels following the slash. (The vowel at the end of most roots is an **o**.) Thus, "gastroitis," which is difficult to pronounce, becomes **gastritis**. In the word **gastropathy**, on the other hand, the vowel o is retained in order to have a pronounceable word; the final vowel is kept for any suffix that begins with a consonant. In carditis, both the i and the **o** are omitted. When two roots are joined, both roots are usually retained in their entirety (vowels included), as in **gastroenterology**. Although the first **o** is not necessary for pronunciation, it is nevertheless retained to signal that two roots are being joined. The second **o** in that term, which *is* necessary for pronunciation, is retained for that reason. The root **enter/o** refers to the intestine. Thus **gastroenterology** means "the study of the stomach and intestine."

The prefix, the final piece in the puzzle, is added to the beginnings of some terms to change their meanings in some way. Table 1–4 gives a few examples.

TABLE 1–4

Prefixes and Their Meanings

PREFIX	MEANING
sub-	below
trans-	across; through
peri-	surrounding

Table 1–5 gives some examples of terms using these three prefixes, along with several more roots and suffixes.

TABLE 1–5

Examples Containing All Three Word Elements: Suffixes, Roots, and Prefixes

TERM WITH PREFIX UNDERSCORED	NEW ROOT	NEW SUFFIX
subcutaneous	cutane/o (skin)	-ous (pertaining to)
transvesical	vesic/o (bladder)	-al (pertaining to)
pericardial	card/i/o (heart)	-al (pertaining to)

Note: In the term pericardial we retained the **i** and dropped the **o** from the root **card/i/o**. You have already learned two other terms using the same root: **carditis**, in which we drop both vowels, and **cardiology**, in which we retain both vowels.

As you can see from the foregoing examples in Table 1–5, the best way to figure out a medical term is to define its suffix first, its prefix second, and its main part, the root, last. This order leads to a proper definition.

It is important to note that many terms do not contain all three elements. Table 1–6 gives the definitions of our three terms.

TABLE 1–6

Definitions

TERM	PRONUNCIATION	DEFINITION
subcutaneous	sŭb″-kū-tā′-nē-ŭs	pertaining to that which is beneath the skin
transvesical	trăns-vĕs′-ĭ-kăl	pertaining to that passing through the bladder
pericardial	pĕr-ĭ-kăr′-dē-ăl	pertaining to that which surrounds the heart

Chapters 2, 3, and 4 deal with suffixes, roots, and prefixes.

1.3 FORMING PLURALS OF MEDICAL TERMS

To form the plural of singular words ending in **is,** change the **i** to an **e,** as shown in the following examples:

singular	plural
diagnosis	diagnoses
pelvis	pelves
neurosis	neuroses

To form the plural of many singular words ending in **us,** change the **us** to an **i,** as shown in the following examples:

singular	plural
bronchus	bronchi
bacillus	bacilli
calculus	calculi
embolus	emboli

A few exceptions are to be found. For example, the plural of virus is viruses, and the plural of sinus is sinuses.

The plural of singular words ending in **a** is formed by adding an **e** to the word, as shown in the following examples:

singular	plural
vena cava	venae cavae
sclera	sclerae
scapula	scapulae

To form the plural of singular words ending in **um,** change the **um** to an **a,** as shown in the following examples:

singular	plural
acetabulum	acetabula
capitulum	capitula
septum	septa
diverticulum	diverticula

To form the plural of singular words ending in **ix** or **ex,** change the ending to **ices,** as shown in the following examples:

singular	plural
calix	calices
cervix	cervices
index	indices
varix	varices

Singular words ending in **oma** are made plural by the addition of an **s** or by an additional **ta,** as shown in the following examples:

singular	plural
adenoma	adenomata or adenomas
carcinoma	carcinomata or carcinomas
fibroma	fibromata or fibromas

To form the plural of singular words ending in **nx**, change the **nx** to an **nges**, as shown in the following examples:

singular	plural
larynx	larynges
phalanx	phalanges

To form the plural of singular words ending in **on**, change the **on** to an **a** or simply add an **s**, as shown in the following example:

singular	plural
ganglion	ganglia or ganglions

To form the plural of singular words ending in **ax**, change the **ax** to **aces**, as shown in the following example:

singular	plural
thorax	thoraces

▶ **EXERCISE 1–1**

Fill in the Blanks

Briefly answer the following questions.

Answers to the exercises in Chapter 1 are found in Appendix A.

The Component Parts of Medical Terms

1. The main part of a medical term is the _____ .

2. The component part placed at the beginning of a medical term that contains all three component parts is the _____ .

3. The suffix in the term **subcutaneous** is _____ .

4. The suffix **-al** means _____ .

5. The prefix **peri-** means _____ .

▶ **EXERCISE 1–2**

True or False

Circle the correct response.

True or False

1. In the term **hepatitis**, the final vowel is dropped from the root. T F

2. The best way to define a medical term is to begin with the prefix. T F

3. The root **card/i/o** refers to the heart. T F

4. Most medical terms have their origins in Greek, Latin, or both. T F

5. The suffix **-pathy** means "study of." T F

▶ **EXERCISE 1–3**

Word Building

Give the plural form of the following singular terms.

Forming Plurals and Singular Terms

1. naris   _____   6. virus   _____
2. psychosis   _____   7. maxilla   _____
3. fundus   _____   8. diverticulum _____
4. fungus   _____   9. fornix   _____
5. glomerulus _____   10. carcinoma   _____

Give the singular form of the following plural terms.

11. diagnoses _____

12. malleoli _____

13. sinuses _____

14. os coxae _____

15. meati _____

16. petechiae _____

17. acetabula _____

18. menisci _____

19. ganglia _____

20. thoraces _____

_____

_____

_____

_____

_____

_____

_____

_____

_____

_____

_____

_____

_____

_____

_____

_____

_____

_____

_____

_____

_____

_____

CHAPTER

2 MEDICAL SUFFIXES

CHAPTER OBJECTIVES

Upon successful completion of this chapter, the student will be able to do the following:

1. Spell and give the meaning for suffixes.
2. Define and spell the medical terms that use the suffixes in this chapter.
3. Distinguish suffixes that signify pathological conditions from those that signify diagnostic and surgical procedures.
4. Identify suffixes used to convert medical nouns to adjectives.

INTRODUCTION

Medical terms, like all other English words, function in sentences as parts of speech, namely as nouns, verbs, or adjectives. Suffixes are often used to establish the part of speech that a medical term can be. You may remember the example given in Chapter 1 of the noun/adjective *antiseptic* being changed to a verb by the addition of the suffix **-ize**.

The suffix of a medical term may also indicate a pathological condition or a procedure, either diagnostic or surgical.

2.1 SUFFIXES USED TO INDICATE PATHOLOGICAL CONDITIONS

See Tables 2–1 and 2–2.

TABLE 2–1

Suffixes Used to Indicate
Pathological Conditions,
-algia to -phobia

SUFFIX	MEANING	EXAMPLE
-algia	pain	cephalalgia; cephalgia (sĕf-ă-lăl′-jē-ă; sĕf-ăl′-jē-ă)
-cele	hernia	adipocele (ăd′-ĭ-pō-sēl″)
-dynia	pain	arthrodynia (ăr″-thrō-dīn′-ē-ă)
-ectasis	dilation; stretching	bronchiectasis (brŏng″-kē-ĕk′-tă-sĭs)
-emesis	vomiting	hematemesis (hĕm-ăt-ĕm′-ĕ-sĭs)
-emia	blood condition	ischemia (ĭs-kē′-mē-ă)
-iasis	abnormal condition	cholecystolithiasis (kō″-lē-sĭs″-tō-lĭ-thī′-ă-sĭs)
-itis	inflammation	arthritis (ăr-thrī′-tĭs)
-lith	stone; calculus	cholelith (kō′-lĕ-lĭth)
-lysis	destruction; separation; breakdown	hemolysis (hē-mŏl′-ĭ-sĭs)
-malacia	softening	osteomalacia (ŏs″-tē-ō-măl-ā′-shē-ă)
-megaly	enlargement	cardiomegaly (kăr″-dē-ō-mĕg′-ă-lē)
-oma	tumor; growth; neoplasm	hepatoma (hĕp″-ă-tō′-mă)
-osis	abnormal condition or increase	dermatosis (dĕr″-mă-tō′-sĭs)
-pathy	disease; disease process	encephalopathy (ĕn-sĕf″-ă-lŏp′-ă-thē)
-penia	decrease; deficiency	leukocytopenia (loo″-kō-sī″-tō-pē′-nē-ă)
-phobia	irrational fear	acrophobia (ăk″-rō-fō′-bē-ă)

Complete Exercise 2–1, Review of the Suffixes (-algia to -phobia), found at the end of the chapter.

SUFFIX	MEANING	EXAMPLE(S)
-plegia	paralysis	quadriplegia (kwod″-rĭ-plē′-jē-ă)
-ptosis	downward displacement; dropping; prolapse; sagging	blepharoptosis (blĕf″-ă-rō-to′-sĭs)
-ptysis	spitting	hemoptysis (hē-mŏp′-tĭ-sĭs)
-rrhage; -rrhagia	bursting forth	hemorrhage (hĕm′-ă-rĭj)
-rrhea	flow; discharge	leukorrhea (loo-″kō-rē′-ă)
-rrhexis	rupture	splenorrhexis (splē-nor-ĕks′-ĭs)
-sclerosis	hardening	arteriosclerosis (ăr-tē″-rē-ō-sklĕ-rō′-sĭs)
-stenosis	narrowing; stricture	arteriostenosis (ar-tē″-rē-ō-stĕ-nō′-sĭs)
-y	disease process	syndactyly (sĭn-dăk′-tĭ-lē)

Complete Exercise 2–2, Review of the Suffixes (-plegia to -y), found at the end of the chapter.

▶ 2.2 SUFFIXES USED TO INDICATE DIAGNOSTIC AND SURGICAL PROCEDURES

See Tables 2–3, 2–4, and 2–5.

SUFFIX	MEANING	EXAMPLE
-centesis	surgical puncture to remove fluid	abdominocentesis (ăb-dŏm″-ĭ-nō-sĕn-tē′-sĭs)
-desis	binding; surgical fusion	arthrodesis (ar″-thrō-dē′-sĭs)
-ectomy	excision; surgical removal	mastectomy (măs-tĕk′-tŏ-mē)
-graphy	process of recording; producing images; x-rays	radiography (rā-dē-ŏg′-ră-fē)
-gram	record; writing; x-ray film	radiogram (rā′-dē-ō-grăm)
-graph	instrument used to record; instrument used to produce x-rays	radiograph (rā′-dē-ō-grăf)

TABLE 2–4

SUFFIX	MEANING	EXAMPLE
-meter	measure	pelvimeter (pĕl-vĭm′-ĕ-ter)
-opsy	to view	biopsy (bī′-ŏp-sē)
-pexy	surgical fixation	gastropexy (găs′-trō-pĕk″-sē)
-plasty	surgical reconstruction; surgical repair	arthroplasty (ăr′-thrō-plăs″-tē)
-rrhaphy	suture	splenorrhaphy (splē-nōr′-ă-fē)
-scope	instrument used to visually examine (a body cavity or organ)	bronchoscope (brŏng′-kō-skōp)
-scopy	process of visually examining (a body cavity or organ) by means of an instrument	bronchoscopy (brŏng-kŏs′-kō-pē)

TABLE 2–5

SUFFIX	MEANING	EXAMPLE
-stasis	stopping; controlling	hemostasis (hē″mō-stā′-sĭs)
-stomy	new opening	tracheostomy (trā″-kē-ŏs′-tō-mē)
-tome	instrument used to cut into or incise	craniotome (krā′-nē-ō-tōm)
-tomy	incise; incision; process of cutting into	arthrotomy (ăr-thrŏt′-ō-mē)

Summary of the Suffixes -Graphy, -Gram, and -Graph

1. **-Graphy** is the process of writing or recording. Remember that "y" means process.
2. **-Gram** is the written record. When you write, you produce a record (in most cases, -gram refers to an x-ray film or its written record).
3. **-Graph** is the instrument used to produce the record.

continued

The root **radi/o** is used to mean x-ray of any of the internal body structures. To specify the organ being x-rayed, radi/o is changed to the root of the organ being studied. For example: **cardiography** instead of **radiography**.

Exceptions: Monitoring the electrical activity of the heart or brain (electrocardiography and electroencephalography, respectively) does not involve x-rays.

Summary of the Suffixes -Scopy and -Scope

1. **-Scopy** is the process of visually examining with the use of an instrument.
2. **-Scope** is the instrument used to visually examine.

Complete Exercise 2–3, Review of the Suffixes Indicating Diagnostic and Surgical Procedures, found at the end of this chapter.

 ## 2.3 GENERAL SUFFIXES

See Table 2–6.

TABLE 2–6

General Suffixes

SUFFIX	MEANING	EXAMPLE
-blast	immature; growing thing	erythroblast (ĕ-rĭth′-rō-blăst)
-cyte	cell	leukocyte (loo′-kō-sīt)
-er; -ist; -or; -ian	specialist; one who specializes	practitioner (prăk-tĭsh′-ŭn-ĕr)
		ophthalmologist (ŏf-thăl-mŏl′-ō-jĭst)
		donor (dō′-ner)
		physician (fĭ-zĭsh′-ŭn)
-logy	study of; process of study	hepatology (hĕp″-ă-tŏl′-ō-jē)
-phagia	to eat; swallow	aphagia (ă-fā′-jē-ă)
-plasia	formation; development	hyperplasia (hī″-pĕr-plā′-ze-ă)
-pnea	breathing	apnea (āp′-nē-ă)

TABLE 2—6

SUFFIX	MEANING	EXAMPLE
-trophy	development; growth; nutrition	hypertrophy (hī-pĕr′-trŏ-fē)
-uria	urine; urination	anuria (ăn-ū′-rē-ă)

◢ 2.4 SUFFIXES USED TO CREATE MEDICAL ADJECTIVES

See Table 2–7.

TABLE 2—7

Suffixes Used to Create Medical Adjectives

SUFFIX	MEANING	EXAMPLE
-genic	producing	carcinogenic (kăr″-sǐ-nō-jĕn′-ǐk)
-genous	produced by; produced from	endogenous (ĕn-dŏj′-ĕ-nŭs)
-oid	resembling	lithoid (lǐth′-oyd)
-ole; -ule	small	bronchiole (brŏng′-kē-ōl)
		venule (vĕn′-ūl)
-ac; -al; -ar; -ary; -eal; -ic; -ior; -ose; -ous; -ic	pertaining to	cardiac (kar′-dē-ăk)
		renal (rē′-nŭl)
		tonsillar (tŏn′-sǐ-lăr)
		mammary (măm′-ă-rē)
		pharyngeal (făr-ǐn′-jē-ăl)
		gastric (găs′-trǐk)
		anterior (ăn-tēr′-ē-ŏr)
		adipose (ăd′-ǐ-pōs)
		venous (vē′-nus)
		necrotic (nĕk′-rō′-tǐc)

Note: Although there are some exceptions, the suffixes meaning "pertaining to" are not generally interchangeable with a given root. For example, one can create the adjectives renal and cardiac, **but not** renac, renar, renary, cardiar, cardieal, cardious, or cardiose.

Complete Exercise 2–4, Review of the Suffixes (-blast to -tic), found at the end of the chapter.

Review of the Suffixes Indicating Pathological Conditions (-algia to -phobia)

1. -algia _____
2. -cele _____
3. -dynia _____
4. -ectasis _____
5. -emia _____
6. -iasis _____
7. -itis _____
8. -lith _____
9. -lysis _____
10. -megaly _____
11. -oma _____
12. -osis _____
13. -pathy _____
14. -penia _____
15. -phobia _____

Review of the Suffixes Indicating Pathological Conditions (-plegia to -y)

Directions

Define the following suffixes.

1. -y _____
2. -plegia _____
3. -ptosis _____
4. -rrhagia _____
5. -rrhea _____
6. -rrhexis _____

Write the suffix for the following.

7. hardening _____   11. stricture _____
8. narrowing _____   12. prolapse _____
9. rupture _____   13. bursting forth _____
10. condition _____   14. discharge _____

Review of the Suffixes Indicating Diagnostic and Surgical Procedures (-centesis to -tomy)

Definitions

Define the following suffixes.

1. -centesis _____
2. -gram _____

3. -graph _____

4. -graphy _____

5. -desis _____

6. -meter _____

Write the suffix for the following.

7. to view _____

8. surgical fixation _____

9. surgical puncture _____

10. surgical repair _____

11. instrument used to measure _____

12. instrument used to cut _____

13. suture _____

14. instrument used to visually examine _____

15. process of visually examining _____

16. stopping _____

▶EXERCISE 2–4   Review of the Suffixes -blast to -genic

Definitions

Define the following suffixes.

1. -blast _____

2. -cyte _____

3. -logy _____

4. -phagia _____

5. -ist _____

6. -genic _____

Write the suffix for the following.

7. produced by _____

8. resembling _____

9. formation; development _____

10. breathing _____

11. pertaining to (give ten suffixes) _____

_____

_____

_____

_____

Matching Suffixes with Meanings

Match the suffixes in Column A with their meanings in Column B.

Column A		Column B
1. -algia	_____	A. disease
2. -ectasis	_____	B. deficiency
3. -megaly	_____	C. rupture
4. -osis	_____	D. suture
5. -pathy	_____	E. pain
6. -rrhea	_____	F. abnormal condition
7. -rrhexis	_____	G. flow
8. -rrhagia	_____	H. enlargement
9. -rrhaphy	_____	I. bleeding
10. -penia	_____	J. dilation
11. -plasia	_____	K. hardening
12. -trophy	_____	L. study of
13. -phagia	_____	M. blood condition
14. -sclerosis	_____	N. stone
15. -stenosis	_____	O. formation
16. -ist	_____	P. narrowing
17. -logy	_____	Q. nutrition
18. -emia	_____	R. specialist
19. -lith	_____	S. to eat
20. -lysis	_____	T. destruction

Selecting a Suffix

Give the suffix(es) for the following.

1. pain _____

2. inflammation _____

3. hernia _____

4. tumor _____

5. resembling _____

6. irrational fear _____

7. vomiting _____

8. paralysis _____

9. measure _____

10. drooping _____

11. instrument used to cut _____

12. binding; fusion _____

13. instrument used to look into
    a body cavity or organ _____

14. record _____

15. to view _____

16. surgical reconstruction _____

17. surgical removal _____

18. surgical fixation _____

19. surgical puncture to remove fluid _____

20. new opening _____

1-2

Write the meaning of each of the following suffixes.

21. -iasis _____   31. -scopy _____

22. -gram _____   32. -logy _____

23. -plasia _____   33. -tomy _____

24. -rrhaphy _____   34. -genic _____

25. -graphy _____   35. -tome _____

26. -stomy _____   36. -lith _____

27. -graph _____   37. -pnea _____

28. -phagia _____   38. -lysis _____

29. -rrhexis _____   39. -ptysis _____

30. -stasis _____   40. -emia _____

Place a check mark beside each suffix that means "pertaining to."

41. -sis _____   49. -or _____

42. -ar _____   50. -ose _____

43. -ium _____   51. -ism _____

44. -ac _____   52. -ia _____

45. -er _____   53. -tic _____

46. -iac _____   54. -um _____

47. -al _____   55. -ous _____

48. -ary _____

▶ **EXERCISE 2–7**

Identifying and Defining Suffixes

Parts of Words

Underline and define each suffix in the following words.

1. cardiopathy _____

2. gastralgia _____

3. cystocele _____

4. otodynia _____

5. nephrectasis _____

6. ischemia _____

7. nephrolith _____

8. hepatosplenomegaly _____

9. osteoma _____

10. hyperplasia _____

11. hemostasis _____

12. dysuria _____

13. carcinogenic _____

14. lithoid _____

15. endogenous _____

16. dermatosclerosis _____

17. arthritis _____

18. electrolysis _____

19. leukocytosis _____

20. leukopenia _____

21. quadriplegia _____

22. leukorrhea _____

23. arteriostenosis _____

24. blepharoptosis _____

25. odontorrhagia _____

26. hypochondriasis _____

27. hypertrophy _____

28. abdominocentesis _____

29. spondylodesis _____

▶ **EXERCISE 2–8**

Choosing the Correct Suffix

Word Building

Add the appropriate adjectival suffix meaning "pertaining to" to each of the roots that follows. Since the proper choice is a matter of remembering specific terms, you may wish to look up those terms of which you are not certain. After you have finished the exercise, look up all the terms to confirm your choices. Don't forget to include or omit vowels as required.

1. card/i/o _____   6. gastr/o _____

2. ren/o _____   7. anter/o _____

3. tonsill/o _____   8. adip/o _____

4. mamm/o _____   9. ven/o _____

5. pharyng/o _____   10. necr/o _____

I–2

_____

_____

_____

_____

_____

_____

_____

_____

_____

_____

_____

_____

_____

_____

_____

_____

_____

_____

_____

CHAPTER

3 MEDICAL TERM ROOTS

CHAPTER ORGANIZATION

This chapter has been designed to help the student learn some common medical word roots.

3.1 External Anatomy
3.2 Internal Anatomy

CHAPTER OBJECTIVES

Upon completion of this chapter, the student will be able to do the following:

1. Give meanings for roots.
2. Define and pronounce terms containing roots.
3. Build medical terms.

INTRODUCTION

Before going on to specific body systems, most students benefit from a study of common medical word roots. Roots appear often in a variety of medical terms, and for that reason, this book devotes an entire chapter to them. These key word elements are divided into two categories: those pertaining to external anatomy and those pertaining to internal anatomy.

▷ 3.1 EXTERNAL ANATOMY

See Table 3–1.

TABLE 3–1

Roots Pertaining to
External Anatomy

ROOT	MEANING	EXAMPLE
abdomin/o	abdomen	abdominal (ăb-dŏm′-ĭ-năl)
axill/o	armpit	axillary (ăk′-sĭ-lār-ē)
cephal/o	head	cephalic (sĕ-făl′-ĭk)
cervic/o	neck	cervical (sĕr′-vĭ-kăl)
crani/o	skull	cranial (krā′-nē-ăl)
cutane/o	skin	cutaneous (kū-tā′-nē-ŭs)
derm/o; dermat/o	skin	dermatitis (dĕr″-mă-tī′-tĭs)
mamm/o	breast	mammography (măm-ŏg′-ră-fē)
mast/o	breast	mastitis (măs-tī′-tĭs)
nas/o	nose	nasal (nā′-zl)
ophthalm/o	eye	ophthalmoscope (ŏf-thăl′-mō-skōp)
or/o	mouth	oral (ōr′-ăl)
ot/o	ear	otitis (ō-tī′-tĭs)
rhin/o	nose	rhinitis (rī-nī′-tĭs)
thorac/o	chest	thoracic (thō-răs′-ĭk)

Complete Exercise 3–1, Review of Roots Pertaining to External Anatomy, found at the end of the chapter.

See Tables 3–2 and 3–3.

TABLE 3–2

Roots Pertaining to
Internal Anatomy (A–G)

ROOT	MEANING	EXAMPLE
aden/o	gland	adenoma (ăd″-ĕ-nō′-mă)
angi/o	vessel	angiogram (ăn′-jē-ō-grăm)
arteri/o	artery	arterial (ăr-tē′-rē-ăl)
arthr/o	joint	arthralgia (ăr-thrăl′-jē-ă)
card/i/o	heart	cardiac (kăr′-dē-ăk)
cerebr/o	brain	cerebral (sĕr′-ĕ-brăl *or* sĕ-rē′-brăl)
chondr/o	cartilage	chondromalacia (kŏn″-drō-măl-ā′-shē-ă)
col/o	colon; large intestine	colic (kŏl′-ĭk)
cost/o	rib	costal (kŏs′-tăl)
cyst/o	urinary bladder	cystoplegia (sĭs″-tō-plē′-jē-ă)
cyt/o	cell	cytology (sī-tŏl′-ō-jē)
electr/o	electricity	electrocardiogram (ē-lek″-trō-kăr′-dē-ō-grăm)
encephal/o	brain	encephalomyelopathy (ĕn-sĕf″-ă-lō-mī″-ĕl-ŏp′-ă-thē)
enter/o	small intestine	enteritis (ĕn″-tĕr-ī′-tĭs)
gastr/o	stomach	gastralgia (găs-trăl′-jē-ă)
gloss/o; lingu/o	tongue	hypoglossal (hī″-pō-glŏs′-ăl) sublingual (sŭb-lĭng′-gwăl)

Complete Exercise 3–2, Review of Roots Pertaining to Internal Anatomy (A–G), at the end of the chapter.

TABLE 3–3

Roots Pertaining to
Internal Anatomy (H–Z)

ROOT	MEANING	EXAMPLE
hem/o; hemat/o	blood	hematoma (hē″-mă-tō′-mă)
		hemolysis (hē-mŏl′-ĭ-sĭs)
hepat/o	liver	hepatitis (hĕp″-ă-tī′-tĭs)
hist/o	tissue	histology (hĭs-tŏl′-ō-jē)
hyster/o	uterus	hysterectomy (hĭs-tĕr-ĕk′-tō-mē)
myel/o **Note:** When the root word is alone, the usual meaning is spinal cord.	spinal cord; bone marrow	myelitis (mī-ĕ-lī′-tĭs)
my/o; muscul/o	muscle	myoma (mī-ō′-mă)
		muscular (mŭs′-kū-lăr)
nephr/o	kidney	nephritis (nĕf-rī′-tĭs)
neur/o	nerve	neural (nū′-răl)
oophor/o	ovary	oophorectomy (ō″-ŏf-ō-rĕk′-tō-mē)
oste/o	bone	osteitis (ŏs-tē-ī′-tĭs)
phleb/o	vein	phlebitis (flē-bī′-tĭs)
pneumon/o; pulmon/o	lung	pneumonectomy (nū″-mŏn-ĕk′-tō-mē)
		pulmonary (pŭl′-mō-nĕ-rē)
ren/o	kidney	renal (rē′-năl)
spin/o	spine; spinal column; backbone	spinal (spī′-năl)
testicul/o	testicles	testicular (tĕs-tĭk′-ū-lăr)
ven/o	vein	venous (vē′-nŭs)
vertebr/o	vertebra	vertebral (vĕr′-tĕ-brăl)

TABLE 3-3

Roots Pertaining to
Internal Anatomy (H–Z)
(concluded)

ROOT	MEANING	EXAMPLE
viscer/o; organ/o	organ	visceral (vǐs′-ěr-ǎl) organomegaly (or-″gǎ-nō-měg′-ǎ-lē)

Note: A common question is: when does myel/o mean spinal cord and when does it mean bone marrow?
1. When myel/o is used with the suffixes: -cele, -algia, -graphy, or -malacia it means **spinal cord**.
2. When myel/o is used with the suffixes: -blast, -cyte, or -genous it means **bone marrow**.
3. When myel/o is used with the suffix -itis, it can mean **both** spinal cord and bone marrow.

Complete Exercise 3–3, Review of Roots Pertaining to Internal Anatomy (H–Z), at the end of the chapter.

▶**EXERCISE 3-1**

Review of Roots Pertaining to External Anatomy

Fill in the Blank

Fill in the blank(s) for the following questions.

Answers to Chapter 3 exercises are found in Appendix A.

1. Two roots for breast are _____ and _____ .
2. Two roots for skin are _____ and _____ .
3. The root for neck is spelled _____ .
4. Build the medical term meaning headache. _____
5. The root for chest is _____ .
6. Define: cutaneous _____
   nasal _____
7. The root for eye is _____ .

▶**EXERCISE 3-2**

Review of Roots Pertaining to Internal Anatomy (A–G)

Definitions

Differentiate between the following roots.

1. angi/o and arteri/o _____

2. arthr/o and oste/o _____
   _____

3. cyst/o and cyt/o _____

4. enter/o and col/o _____

5. gastr/o and abdomin/o _____
   _____

Give the root for the following.

6. heart _____   10. cell _____

7. large intestine _____   11. small intestine _____

8. rib _____   12. stomach _____

9. bladder _____   13. tongue _____

▶EXERCISE 3–3   Review of Roots Pertaining to Internal Anatomy (H–Z)

Definitions

Differentiate between the following roots.

1. hem/o and hepat/o _____
_____

2. hist/o and hyster/o _____
_____

3. my/o and myel/o _____
_____

Give the root for the following words.

4. kidney _____   7. vein (give two) _____

5. bone _____   _____

6. nerve _____   8. lung (give two) _____
_____

9. ovaries _____

Define the following terms.

10. hematoma _____

11. myelogram _____

12. vertebral _____

13. visceral _____

14. hematuria _____

▶EXERCISE 3–4   Definition of Roots in Chapter 3

Definitions

Define the roots in the space provided.

1. abdomin/o _____

2. cephal/o _____

3. cervic/o _____

4. crani/o _____

5. cutane/o _____

6. dermat/o _____

7. mamm/o _____

8. mast/o _____

9. nas/o _____

10. rhin/o _____

11. or/o _____

12. ot/o _____

13. thorac/o _____

14. aden/o _____

15. angi/o _____

16. arteri/o _____

17. arthr/o _____

18. card/i/o _____

19. cerebr/o _____

20. chondr/o _____

21. col/o _____

22. cost/o _____

23. cyst/o _____

24. cyt/o _____

25. enter/o _____

26. gastr/o _____

27. gloss/o _____

28. hem/o _____

29. hepat/o _____

30. hist/o _____

31. hyster/o _____

32. myel/o _____

33. nephr/o _____

34. neur/o _____

35. oophor/o _____

36. oste/o _____

37. phleb/o _____

38. pneumon/o _____

39. ren/o _____

40. spin/o _____

41. testicul/o _____

42. ven/o _____

43. vertebr/o _____

44. viscer/o _____

Give roots for the following words.

45. nose _____
46. chest _____
47. abdomen _____
48. skin _____
49. gland _____
50. artery _____
51. brain _____
52. large intestine _____
53. cell _____

54. nerve _____
55. blood _____
56. tissue _____
57. bone _____
58. lung _____
59. spinal column _____
60. spinal cord _____
61. vein _____
62. vertebra _____

Define the following terms.

63. craniotomy _____
64. craniotome _____
65. otorrhea _____
66. ophthalmoscope _____
67. ophthalmoscopy _____
68. rhinitis _____
69. thoracic _____
70. cutaneous _____
71. angitis _____
72. angioma _____
73. cardiac _____
74. arthrodynia _____
75. colitis _____
76. mammography _____
77. arthralgia _____
78. oral _____
79. dermal _____
80. cerebral _____
81. thoracentesis _____
82. costal _____
83. mastitis _____
84. adenopathy _____
85. cystoscopy _____
86. ophthalmorrhagia _____
87. ophthalmorrhea _____

1–3

Circle the roots in the following terms and define each.

88. erythropenia _____

89. gastritis _____

90. hematoma _____

91. histology _____

92. leukocyte _____

93. neuropathy _____

94. oophorectomy _____

95. osteocyte _____

96. venous _____

97. myelogram _____

▶EXERCISE 3–5

Matching

Match each root in Column A with its meaning in Column B.

Matching Roots with Meanings

Column A		Column B
1. crani/o	_____	A. neck
2. cutane/o	_____	B. heart
3. ophthalm/o	_____	C. vein
4. cervic/o	_____	D. small intestine
5. mast/o	_____	E. breast
6. card/i/o	_____	F. stomach
7. pneumon/o	_____	G. uterus
8. phleb/o	_____	H. organ
9. gastr/o	_____	I. vessel
10. nephr/o	_____	J. skin
11. enter/o	_____	K. bone
12. hyster/o	_____	L. kidney
13. cyst/o	_____	M. skull
14. oste/o	_____	N. eye
15. angi/o	_____	O. bladder
16. viscer/o	_____	P. lung

▶EXERCISE 3–6

Word Building

Build medical terms for the following.

Building Terms

1. inflammation of the kidney _____

2. study of the heart _____

3. pertaining to the neck _____

4. pertaining to the abdomen _____

5. tumor of a gland _____

6. process of recording (taking an x-ray of) a vessel _____

7. pertaining to an artery _____

8. inflammation of a joint _____

9. inflammation of the ear _____

10. softening of the cartilage _____

11. headache _____

12. excision of the breast _____

13. incision of the chest _____

14. inflammation of the skin _____

15. record of a vessel _____

16. hernia of the spinal cord _____

17. process of visually examining the eye _____

18. pertaining to the colon _____

19. pertaining to the ribs and vertebra _____

20. surgical puncture of the chest _____

21. process of visually examining the joint _____

22. study of cells _____

23. pertaining to the nose _____

24. inflammation of the small intestines _____

▶EXERCISE 3-7

Spelling

Spelling

Place a check mark beside any misspelled word in the following list. Correctly spell those you checked off.

1. enteroseal ☐ _____

2. neuropathy ☐ _____

3. gastralgia ☐ _____

4. hypoglosal ☐ _____

5. hemolisis ☐ _____

6. hysterectomy ☐ _____

7. opthalmoscope ☐ _____

8. nephritis ☐ _____

9. mylogram ☐ _____

10. vertabral ☐ _____

CHAPTER

4 MEDICAL PREFIXES

CHAPTER OBJECTIVES

Upon successful completion of this chapter, the student will be able to do the following:

1. Give meanings for prefixes
2. Distinguish prefixes that signify direction and position from those that signify negation or number.
3. Match prefixes that are synonymous with one another.
4. Identify prefixes that are opposite in meaning.

INTRODUCTION

As stated in Chapter 1, a medical term often acts as a shortened version of an English phrase. Most of the time, the prefix of a term takes the place of the adverb in the phrase; adverbs answer questions such as when, where, how, how many, why, or which direction? Prefixes can be classified for study based on their adverbial characteristics.

In some medical prefixes, the final consonant of the prefix is changed before a root starting with a consonant. Often the final consonant will change to the first letter of the following component part. For example: the prefix **con-** (meaning with) becomes **col-** in the term collateral; **in-** becomes **ir-** in the terms irradiation and irreducible; **in-** becomes **im-** in immature (see tables 4-1 and 4-2).

See Table 4-1.

TABLE 4—1

Prefixes Denoting
Direction and Position
(When, Where, How
Situated?)

PREFIX	MEANING	EXAMPLE
ab-	away from	abduction (ăb-dŭk′-shŭn)
ad-	toward	adduction (ă-dŭk′-shŭn)
ante-	before	antenatal (ăn-tē-nā′-tŭl)
Note: Both ante and before have the letter e in the word. Compare with anti- in Table 4-2.		
circum-	around	circumduction (sur″-kŭm-dŭk′-shŭn)
con-	with; together	convergent (kŏn-ver′-jĭnt)
(becomes co- before vowels or h)		coarticulation (kō″-ăr-tĭ-kū-lā′-shŭn) cohesion (kō-hē-zhŭn)
(becomes col- before l)		collateral (kō-lăt′-er-ŭl)
(becomes com- before m or p)		comminuted (kŏm-ĭ-noot′-ĕd) complication (kŏm″-plĭ-kā′-shŭn)
(becomes cor- before r)		corrosive (kor-ō′-sĭv)
dia-	through; complete	dialysis (dī-a′-lĭ-sĭs)
ecto-	outside	ectogenous (ĕk-tŏj′-ĕ-nŭs)
endo-; en-	within	endoscope (ĕn′-dō-skōp) encephalalgia (ĕn-sĕf″-ăl-ăl′-jă)
epi-	upon; on; above	epicardium (ĕp″-ĭ-kar′-dē-um)
eso-	within	esotropia (ĕs″-ō-trō′-pē-ă)

I—4

TABLE 4—1

Prefixes Denoting
Direction and Position
(When, Where, How
Situated?) (concluded)

PREFIX	MEANING	EXAMPLE
ex-; exo-	away from	excise (ĕk′-sīz) exotropia (ĕk″-sō-trō′-pē-ă)
hyper-	above; excessive	hyperplasia (hī-per-plā′-zhă)
hypo-	below; deficient	hypogastric (hī-pō-găs′-trĭk)
in- (becomes ir- before r)	in; into	incision (ĭn-sĭ′-zhŭn) irradiation (ĭr-ā″-dē-ā′-shŭn)
infra-	below; beneath	infracostal (ĭn-fră-kŏs′-tŭl)
inter-	between	intercellular (ĭn-ter-sĕl′-ū-ler)
intra-	within	intracranial (ĭn-tră-krā′-nē-ăl)
meta-; ultra-	beyond	metaplasia; (mĕt-ă-plā′-zhă) ultrasound (ŭl′-tră-sound)
per-	through	perfusion (per-fū′-zhŭn)
peri-	around	perineuritis (per″-ē-noo-rī′-tĭs)
post-	after	postpartum (pōst-par′-tŭm)
pre-	before; in front of	prenatal (prē-nā′-tăl)
pro-	before	prognosis (prŏg-nō′-sĭs)
sub-	under	sublingual (sŭb-lĭng′-gwăl)
trans-	across	transection (trăn-sĕk′-shŭn)

4.2 PREFIXES OF NEGATION

See Table 4-2.

TABLE 4–2

Negative Prefixes (Which Direction, How, How Much?)

PREFIX	MEANING	EXAMPLE
anti- **Note:** An "i" appears in both anti- and against.	against	antiarthritic (ăn″-tē-ar-thrĭ′-tĭc)
a-; an-	no; not	atoxic (ā-tŏk′-sĭk) anuria (ăn-ū′-rē-ă)
contra-	against	contralateral (kŏn″-tră-lăt′-er-ăl)
in- (becomes ir- before r) (becomes im- before m, b, and p)	not	indigestible (ĭn-dĭ-jĕs′-tĭ-bl) irreducible (ĭr-rē-doo′-sĭ-bl) immature (ĭm-ă-choor′) imbalance (ĭm-bă′-lĕns) impotence (ĭm′-pŏ-tĕns)
ana-	apart; backward; up	anaplasia (ăn-ă-plā′-zhă)
auto-	self	autolysis (au-tŏl′-ĭ-sĭs)
bio-	life	biology (bī-ŏl′-ŏ-jē)
brady-	slow	bradypnea (brăd-ĕ-nē′-ă)
dys-	bad; difficult; painful	dysplasia (dĭs-plā-zhă)
macro-	large	macrocyte (măk′-rō-sīt)
mal-	bad	malaise (măl-āz′)
micro-	small	microencephaly (mī″-krō-ĕn-sĕf′-ă-lē)
neo-	new	neonatal (nē-ō-nā′-tăl)

1—4

TABLE 4–2

PREFIX	MEANING	EXAMPLE
pan-	all	pancarditis (păn-kar-dī′-tĭs)
syn-	joined	synarthrotic (sĭn-ar-thrŏ′-tĭc)
(becomes sym- before b, m, and p)		symbiotic (sĭm-bē-ŏt′-ĭk) symmetry (sĭm′-ĕ-trē) symphysis (sĭm′-fĭ-sĭs)
tachy-	rapid	tachycardia (tăk″-ĭ-kar′-dē-ă)

▶ 4.3 PREFIXES DENOTING NUMBER

See Table 4-3.

TABLE 4–3

**Prefixes Denoting
Number (How Many?)**

PREFIX	MEANING	EXAMPLE
bi-; di-	two	bilateral (bī-lăt′-er-ăl) diplegia (dī-plē′-jă)
hemi-; semi-	half	hemihepatectomy (hĕm″-ē-hĕp-ă-tĕk′-tŏ-mē) semicomatose (sĕm-ē-kō′-mă-tōs)
mono-; uni-	one	monocyte (mŏn′-ō-sīt) unilateral (ū-nĭ-lăt′-er-ăl)
multi-; poly-	many	multiform (mŭl′-tĭ-form) polyadenoma (pŏl-ĭ-ăd-ĕ-nō′-mă)
quadri-	four	quadriplegia (kwăd-rĭ-plē′-jă)
tri-	three	triceps (trī′-sĕps)

Matching Prefixes and Meanings

Match each item in column A with the meaning in column B that most closely corresponds to it.

Column A		Column B
1. ab-	_____	A. around
2. ad-	_____	B. beyond
3. ante-	_____	C. toward
4. circum-	_____	D. with
5. con-	_____	E. away from
6. dia-	_____	F. outside
7. ecto-	_____	G. upon
8. endo-	_____	H. through
9. epi-	_____	I. within
10. meta-	_____	J. before

Match each of the prefixes in column A with its opposite in column B.

Column A		Column B
11. ab-	_____	A. ad-
12. ante-	_____	B. ana-
13. con-	_____	C. brady-
14. ecto-	_____	D. endo-
15. tachy-	_____	E. hypo-
16. hyper-	_____	F. micro-
17. macro-	_____	G. post-

The Meaning of a Given Prefix

Give meanings for the following prefixes.

1. bi-	_____	6. endo-	_____
2. hemi-	_____	7. in-	_____
3. hypo-	_____	8. auto-	_____
4. ecto-	_____	9. ana-	_____
5. peri-	_____	10. mal-	_____

11. three   _____

12. against   _____

13. with   _____

14. around   _____

15. slow   _____

16. fast   _____

17. under   _____

18. toward   _____

19. away from   _____

20. many   _____

▶ EXERCISE 4–3

Parts of Words

Underline the prefix.

Prefixes Within Terms

1. immature

2. contralateral

3. antenatal

4. abduction

5. tachycardia

6. synarthrotic

7. pancarditis

8. monocyte

9. indigestible

10. microencephaly

_____

_____

_____

_____

_____

_____

_____

_____

_____

_____

_____

_____

_____

_____

_____

_____

_____

_____

_____

_____

_____

_____

_____

_____

1—4

5 AN OVERVIEW OF ANATOMICAL TERMS

CHAPTER OBJECTIVES

Upon successful completion of this chapter, the student will be able to do the following:

1. Define anatomy and physiology.
2. Describe the levels of organization into which the body is arranged.
3. List the body systems and the principal organs within each system.
4. Define and give examples of homeostasis and metabolism.
5. Define the anatomical position.
6. List and define the correct terminology used for direction, anatomical planes, abdominal regions and abdominal quadrants.
7. Analyze, pronounce, define, and spell terms related to the body as a whole

INTRODUCTION

Anatomy, a branch of biology, includes the study of plant, animal, and human structures. Human anatomy is the study of the structure of the human body. In studying anatomy, we discover how small structures come together to form ever larger units of anatomical definition. For example, the heart is made up of different types of tissue, such as muscle tissue, connective tissue, and epithelial tissue. The heart has upper and lower chambers, valves, and its own internal nervous system. Physiology, on the other hand, is the study of bodily function. The two subjects are linked, of course, since one could not study physiology without reference to anatomy and, to some extent, vice versa. Again using the example of the heart, we can see that the heart's physiological nature, or function, is to pump blood to all body tissues.

The subjects of anatomy and physiology go back more than 2,000 years. Division of the subject into gross anatomy (study with the naked eye), histology (study of tissue), and cytology (study of cells) occurred with the development of the microscope. By the middle of the eighteenth century, it was known that all tissues are composed of cells.

5.1 LEVELS OF ORGANIZATION

One may regard the body as a series of units of increasing size. The smallest units of life, cells, unite to become tissues, tissues make up organs, organs come together as major parts of body systems, and systems compose the human body as a whole. See Figure 5–1, the structural levels of the human body.

FIGURE 5–1 Levels of Organization

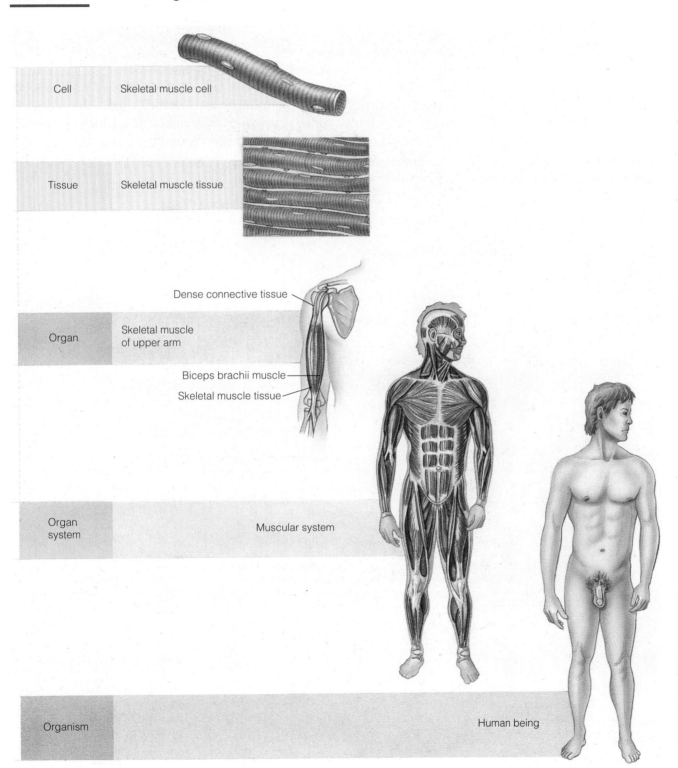

Cell — Skeletal muscle cell

Tissue — Skeletal muscle tissue

Dense connective tissue

Organ — Skeletal muscle of upper arm

Biceps brachii muscle
Skeletal muscle tissue

Organ system — Muscular system

Organism — Human being

Cellular Level

Cells are differentiated; that is, each class of cell is capable of performing its own function, which varies from that of other cells.

Although cells perform different functions, they are generally the same from an anatomical standpoint. All cells, no matter what their function, are surrounded by a **plasma (cell) membrane,** which acts as a barrier between extracellular and intracellular material, keeping substances within the cell inside and substances outside the cell outside. However, the plasma membrane is also semipermeable, which means that it allows certain substances to pass through while blocking others.

All cells have a **cytoplasm.** The cytoplasm (the protoplasm within a cell) is located between the plasma membrane and the **nucleus.** The cytoplasm contains **organelles** (little organs), which carry out all the necessary functions of the cell. Such organelles include the **mitochondria,** which supply the cell with its energy; the **lysosomes,** which attack bacteria; **ribosomes,** which synthesize protein; the **endoplasmic reticulum,** which transports the protein to where it is needed within the cell; and the **Golgi apparatus,** which collects and stores the cell's synthetic products (see Figure 5–2).

FIGURE 5–2 Component Parts of the Cell

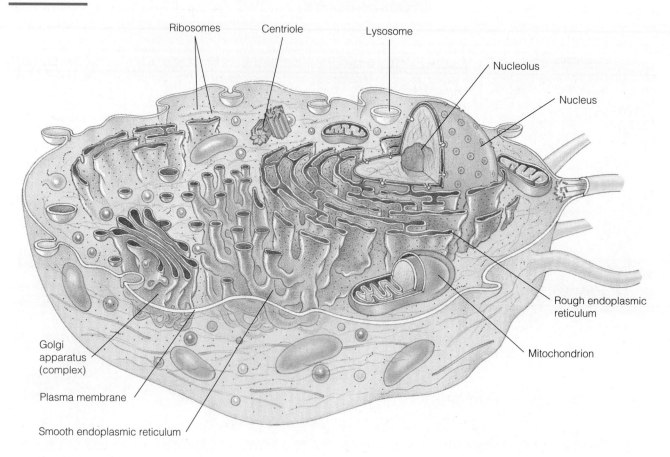

The final component of the cell is the nucleus. Usually located in the center of the cytoplasm, the nucleus consists of a **nuclear membrane,** which separates the cytoplasm from the contents of the nucleus; the **karyoplasm,** which is the protoplasm of the nucleus; and a **nucleolus,** which literally means "a small nucleus." The nucleus contains **deoxyribonucleic acid (DNA),** which is responsible for transmitting hereditary characteristics, and **ribonucleic acid (RNA),** which is necessary for protein synthesis. Growth, repair, and reproduction are the functions generally attributed to the nucleus.

Tissue Level

Cells of similar function are grouped together to form the next level of complexity, the tissue level. The major tissues formed from these cells are epithelial, connective, nerve, and muscle. Each tissue type performs a specific function or functions as described below.

Epithelial Tissue   Epithelial tissue covers the internal and external surfaces of the body. The internal surface is called the **mucous membrane,** and the external surface is known as the skin. Epithelial tissue has several functions, depending on where it is located. For example, the epithelial tissue making up the **skin** serves as **protection,** while some of the epithelial tissue found in the **digestive tract** functions in **absorption,** and the tissue making up the **glands secrete** chemical substances.

Connective Tissue   Connective tissue is the most extensive tissue in the body. It functions to support and shape the body structures; it attaches organs together and holds them in place. The common types of connective tissue are **tendons, ligaments, blood, bone, cartilage, fat,** and **blood cells.**

Muscle Tissue   Muscle tissue takes its name from its location in the body; for example, in the heart it is called **cardiac** muscle tissue, within organs such as the stomach and intestines it is called **visceral** or **smooth** muscle tissue, and that associated with bones is called **skeletal** muscle tissue. All muscles, no matter what their location, create movement of some kind. Muscle cells are not spherical but long and slender. For this reason, muscle cells are often referred to as **fibers.** For a muscle to move, the fibers (muscle cells) have to shorten or contract, decreasing the length of the fiber.

Nerve Tissue   The tissues making up the nervous system receive stimuli (excitement) from inside or outside the body. The nervous system allows the body to respond to this stimuli by transmitting impulses to and from the brain and spinal cord.

Organ Level

Within the body, cells make up tissues, and tissues of similar structure make up organs. For example, bone cells make up bone tissue, which make up bone. Other organs include **blood cells, muscle, nerves, heart, lungs,** and **intestines.** Each organ, however, is not composed of one type of tissue but a mixture of different tissues. For example, the intestines are made up of muscle, epithelial, nervous, and connective tissue, with each tissue type performing its specialized function.

1–5

FIGURE 5–3 Body Systems and Their Organs

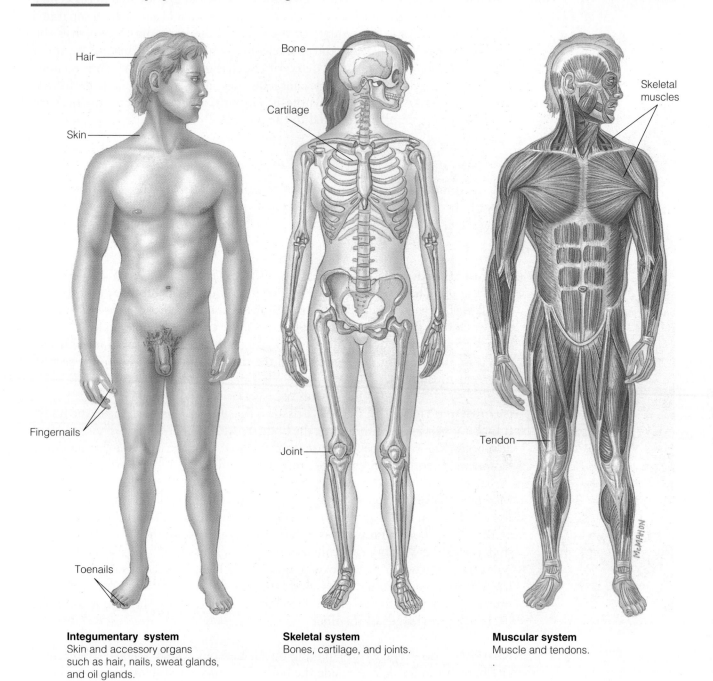

Integumentary system
Skin and accessory organs
such as hair, nails, sweat glands,
and oil glands.

Skeletal system
Bones, cartilage, and joints.

Muscular system
Muscle and tendons.

System Level

Organs do not work independently but are grouped together by function. All the similar organs are grouped into twelve systems that together make up the body as a whole. See Figure 5–3 for each body system and the organs.

FIGURE 5–3 **Body Systems and Their Organs** (continued)

Brain

Spinal
cord

Nerves

Pineal
gland

Parathyroid
glands

Thymus
gland

Hypothalamus

Pituitary
gland

Thyroid
gland

Adrenal
glands

Pancreas
(islets)

Ovaries

Testes

Arteries

Heart

Veins

Nervous system Brain, spinal
cord, and nerves.

Endocrine system Pituitary, thyroid,
parathyroid, thymus, adrenal, and
pineal glands, as well as portions
of hypothalamus, pancreas, liver,
kidneys, skin, heart, digestive tract,
ovaries, testes, and placenta. Also
included are hormonal secretions
from each gland.

Circulatory system Heart, arteries,
veins, capillaries and blood.

I–5

FIGURE 5–3 **Body Systems and Their Organs** (continued)

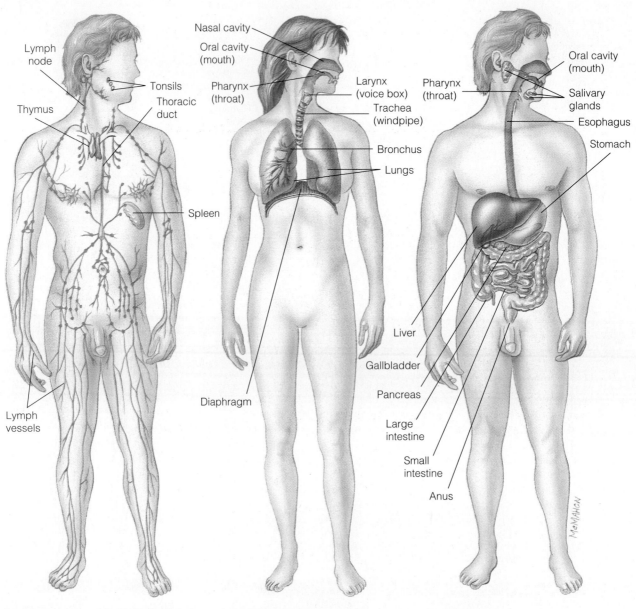

Lymphatic and immune systems
Thymus, bone marrow, spleen,
tonsils, lymph nodes, lymph capillaries,
lymph vessels, lymphocytes, and lymph.
.

Respiratory system Lungs,
nasal cavity, pharynx, larynx,
trachea, bronchi, and bronchioles.
.

Digestive system Mouth,
pharynx, esophagus, stomach,
small intestine, large intestine,
salivary glands, pancreas,
gallbladder, and liver.

FIGURE 5–3 **Body Systems and Their Organs** (concluded)

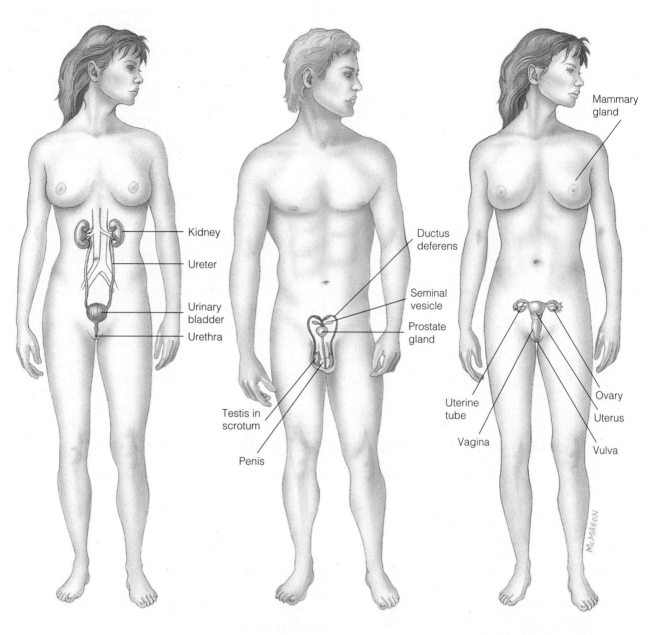

Urinary system Kidneys, ureters, urinary bladder, urethra.

Reproductive systems Male: testes, epididymides, vas deferens, ejaculatory ducts, penis, seminal vesicles, prostate gland, and bulbourethral glands.

Reproductive systems Female: ovaries, uterine tubes, uterus, vagina, external genitalia, and mammary glands.
.

Twelve systems make up the human organism. These systems contain organs that work together to maintain **homeostasis,** a term describing the body's ability to respond to external and internal stimuli while the body remains relatively stable. For example, our normal body temperature is approximately 98.6 degrees F (37.0 degrees C). Our body maintains this temperature despite fluctuations in atmospheric temperature. Whether the air temperature is 95 degrees F (35 degrees C), or a chilly 50 degrees F (10 degrees C), the body's temperature remains stable. The body is able to maintain its temperature through processes that allow it to give off heat in hot conditions and conserve heat in cold.

Other examples of homeostasis include the body's ability to maintain stable blood sugar levels, blood oxygen levels, and kidney and digestive functions. These are just a few examples of homeostasis. Survival depends on stable chemical processes within the body.

The name given to all these chemical processes is **metabolism.** Metabolism comprises two phases: a breaking-up process (**catabolism**) and a building-up process (**anabolism**). The body's ability to use food is a well-known example of metabolism. Food is taken in and broken down (the catabolic phase) into smaller units that can be absorbed. These same units are then utilized in the building up (anabolic phase) of new substances and in tissue repair. In summary, homeostasis and metabolism are essential life processes.

A good understanding of the body systems and the organs that make them up is essential before one attempts to analyze the etymology of the various terms. For that reason, it is suggested that you study the common organs of each system and their roots (Table 5–1) and complete Exercise 5.1 before continuing.

▶ 5.2 COMMON ANATOMICAL ROOTS OF EACH BODY SYSTEM

Table 5–1 lists the core anatomical roots and their definitions.

TABLE 5–1 Common Anatomical Roots

ROOT	MEANING	ROOT	MEANING
Body as a Whole		**Skeletal System**	
axill/o	armpit	arthr/o	joints
cephal/o	head	chondr/o	cartilage
cervic/o	neck	crani/o	skull
cyt/o	cell	cost/o	rib
Integumentary System		myel/o	bone marrow; spinal cord (see nervous system)
adip/o; lip/o; steat/o	fat	oste/o	bone
cili/o; pil/o	hair	vertebr/o	vertebra
derm/o; dermat/o	skin		
onych/o; ungu/o	nail		

TABLE 5—1   Common Anatomical Roots (continued)

ROOT	MEANING
Muscular System	
my/o; muscul/o	muscles
Nervous System, Eyes, Ears	
blephar/o	eyelid
cerebr/o; encephal/o	brain
myel/o	spinal cord
neur/o	nerve
ophthalm/o; ocul/o	eye
ot/o	ear
Digestive System	
cheil/o	lips
cholecyst/o	gallbladder
col/o	large intestines
enter/o	small intestines
esophag/o	esophagus
gastr/o	stomach
gingiv/o	gums
gloss/o; lingu/o	tongue
hepat/o	liver
lapar/o	abdominal wall
odont/o	teeth
or/o; stomat/o	mouth
pancreat/o	pancreas
pharyng/o	throat; pharynx (also part of the respiratory system)
Endocrine System	
aden/o	gland
adren/o	adrenal gland
parathyroid/o	parathyroid gland
pituitar/o	pituitary gland
thyroid/o	thyroid gland

ROOT	MEANING
Circulatory System	
angi/o; vascul/o; vas/o	vessel
arteri/o	artery
card/i/o	heart
hem/o; hemat/o	blood
ven/o; phleb/o	vein
Respiratory System	
alveol/o	air sacs; alveolus
bronch/o; bronchi/o	bronchus
bronchiol/o	small bronchial tubes
laryng/o	voice box; larynx
nas/o; rhin/o	nose
pharyng/o	throat; pharynx (also part of the digestive tract)
pneum/o; pneumon/o	lungs
thorac/o	chest
trache/o	windpipe; trachea
Lymphatic and Immune Systems	
adenoid/o	adenoids
lymph/o	lymph (clear, watery fluid)
lymphaden/o	lymph glands
lymphangi/o	lymph vessels
splen/o	spleen
tonsill/o	tonsils
Urinary System	
cyst/o	urinary bladder
ren/o; nephr/o (ren/o usually is in anatomical terms; nephr/o in pathological terms)	kidneys

I–5

TABLE 5–1 Common Anatomical Roots (concluded)

ROOT	MEANING	ROOT	MEANING
Urinary System (continued)		*Female Reproductive System*	
ureter/o	ureters	colp/o; vagin/o	vagina
urethr/o	urethra	mast/o; mamm/o	breast
Male Reproductive System		oophor/o; ovari/o	ovary
balan/o	glans penis	salping/o	fallopian tubes; uterine tubes
epididym/o	epididymis		
orchid/o; testo; testicul/o	testicle	thel/o	nipple
		uter/o; hyster/o; metr/o	uterus
phall/o	penis		
prostat/o	prostate gland	vulv/o	vulva; external genitalia
vas/o	vas deferens		

▶ 5.3 ANATOMICAL ARRANGEMENT OF BODY PARTS

We find order in many articles that we use on a daily basis. For example, a backpack contains many separate pouches. We may use the main pouch to carry books, clothing, or food, and the smaller pouches to carry pencils, pens, bus passes, and other personal items. The body is like a backpack in that respect, but instead of pouches it has cavities (hollow spaces), and instead of personal belongings the cavities contain organs.

Cavities of the Body and Organ Arrangement

The body has two main cavities: the **dorsal** (back) cavity and the **ventral** (front) cavity. The dorsal cavity is further divided into the **cranial cavity,** which contains the brain, and the **spinal cavity,** which contains the spine. See Figure 5–4. The ventral cavity is also subdivided into smaller cavities. The **thoracic cavity** contains the lungs, heart, aorta, esophagus, and trachea. (A subdivision of the thoracic cavity is the **mediastinum,** which is located in the middle of the thoracic cavity between the lungs. It contains the heart, aorta, trachea, and esophagus.) The **abdominal cavity** is home to the stomach, intestines, liver, pancreas, gallbladder, and spleen. The **pelvic cavity** holds the urinary (excluding the kidneys and ureters) and reproductive organs. The latter two cavities are also known collectively as the **abdominopelvic cavity.** The thoracic and abdominal cavities are separated by the **diaphragm,** a respiratory muscle.

FIGURE 5–4

**Major Body Cavities and
Their Subdivisions**

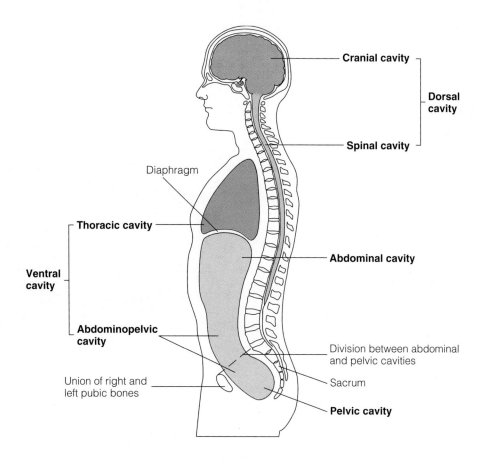

Cranial cavity

Dorsal cavity

Spinal cavity

Diaphragm

Thoracic cavity

Abdominal cavity

Ventral cavity

Abdominopelvic cavity

Division between abdominal and pelvic cavities

Union of right and left pubic bones

Sacrum

Pelvic cavity

Also within the thoracic and abdominal cavities are three cavities that do not contain organs but fluid. They are the **pleural** and **pericardial cavities** (within the thoracic cavity) and the **peritoneal cavity** (within the abdominal cavity). The pleural cavity surrounds the lungs, the pericardial cavity surrounds the heart, and the peritoneal cavity surrounds the abdominopelvic cavity. The fluid is called pleural fluid, pericardial fluid, and peritoneal fluid, respectively. See Figure 5–5 and Table 5–2.

▷▷ 5.4 DIRECTIONAL TERMINOLOGY

We use north, south, east, and west to give directions. We might say in response to a query from a stranger, for example, that the shopping mall is two blocks east of the campus. When communicating with one another, medical professionals need to identify structures with a great deal more precision than such casual directions might afford. Thus, medical workers use specific directional terminology to ensure a high degree of specificity when describing locality of structures or disease. This specific terminology is defined below.

Anatomical Position

Like the earth with its geographical directions, the human body has characteristics that make precise discussion of it possible. Unlike the earth, however, the body can assume many positions and face many directions. For that reason, one position, the **anatomical position**, is used as a reference for directional discussion of anatomy. This position has the patient standing erect, head facing the front, feet forward, and the arms by the side with the palms facing forward.

FIGURE 5-5 **Right and Left Pleural Cavities** Notice that the pleural cavities do not contain the lungs, but rather surround each lung.

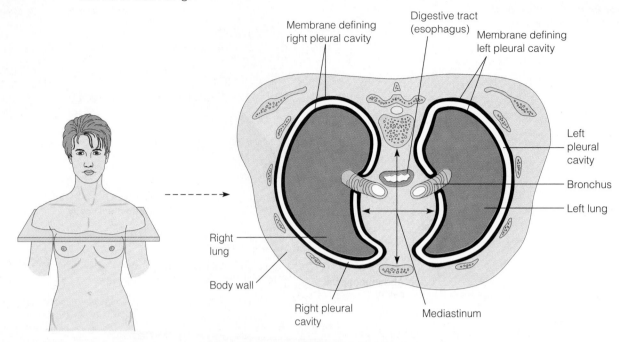

This position must be constantly kept in mind when describing the relationship of one body part to another.

Directional Terms

Directional terms are used to describe precisely the relationship of one body part to another. These terms are listed in Table 5–3. See also Figures 5–6 and 5–7. Also see Table 5–4.

TABLE 5-2 **Summary of Major Body Cavities, Their Subdivisions and Organs**

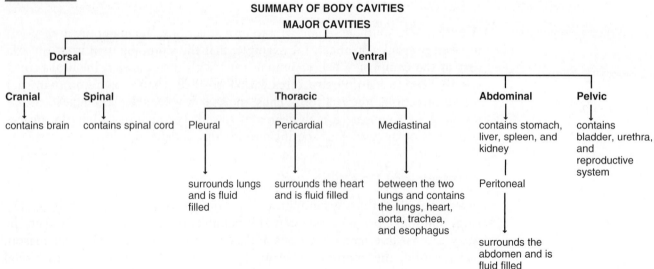

Note: The three cavities, the mediastinal, pleural, and pericardial, are subdivisions of the thoracic cavity, which is a subdivision of the ventral cavity.

TABLE 5–3

Contrasting Directional
Terms

DIRECTION	DESCRIPTION AND EXAMPLES
superior; cranial	above, toward the head **Example:** The head is superior to the neck.
inferior; caudal	below; toward the tail **Example:** The neck is inferior to the head.
anterior; ventral	toward the front surface of the body; belly side of the body **Example:** The thoracic cavity is anterior to the spinal cavity.
posterior; dorsal	toward the back surface of the body **Example:** The spinal cavity is posterior to the thoracic cavity.
medial	toward the midline of the body (The midline is an imaginary line drawn down the center of the body from the tip of the head to the feet.) **Example:** The big toe is medial to the small toe.
lateral	away from the midline **Example:** The small toe is lateral to the big toe; the ear is lateral to the nose.
proximal	toward the point of origin or nearest the point of attachment to the trunk In relation to the arms and legs, the proximal portion of either is the part closest to the attachment to the trunk. **Example:** The elbow is proximal to the wrist, and the wrist is proximal to the fingers.
distal	farthest away from the point of origin or farthest away from the attachment to the trunk In relation to the digestive system, the proximal portion is the part closest to the point of origin, that is, the mouth. The distal portion is the part farthest from the point of origin. **Example:** The intestines are distal to the stomach, and the stomach is distal to the esophagus. **Example:** The stomach is proximal to the intestines but distal to the esophagus.
superficial	near or toward the surface of the body **Example:** The skin is superficial to underlying organs.
deep	away from the surface of the body **Example:** Internal organs are deep to the skin.
peripheral	away from the center **Example:** Peripheral nerves are those away from the brain and spinal cord. Peripheral blood vessels are those in the extremities.

I–5

TABLE 5–3

Contrasting Directional Terms (concluded)

DIRECTION	DESCRIPTION AND EXAMPLES
supine	lying on the back, face up When the term relates to the arms, the palms are facing up. **Note:** To help you remember this term, notice that supine has "up" as part of the word.
prone	lying on the abdomen, face down Related to the arms, the palms are facing down.

FIGURE 5–6 Directional Terms Relating to Anatomical Position

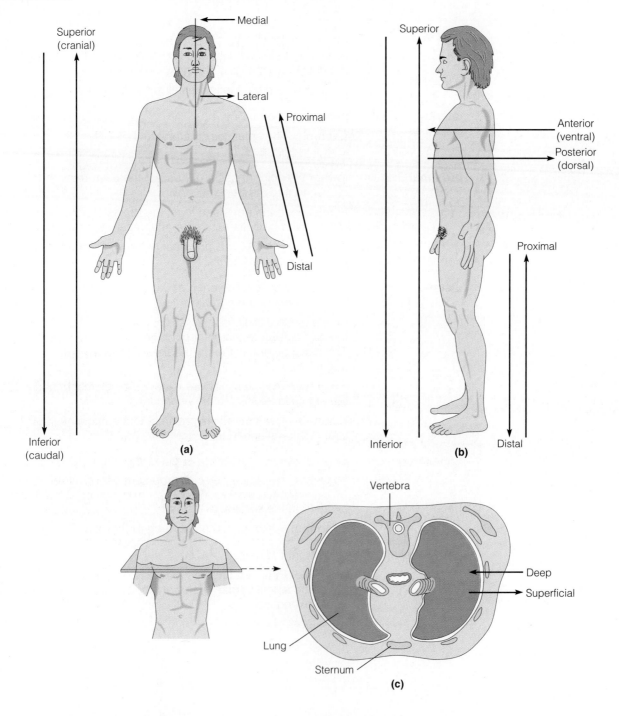

FIGURE 5–7

Planes of the Body

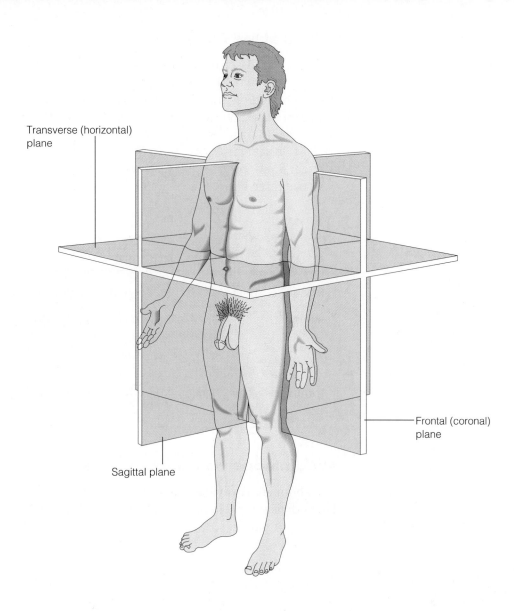

Transverse (horizontal) plane

Frontal (coronal) plane

Sagittal plane

TABLE 5–4

Special Directional Terminology for the Feet and Hands

DIRECTION	DESCRIPTION
plantar; volar **Note:** volar = concave or hollow space	sole of the foot; posterior surface of foot
dorsum	the anterior or upper surface of the foot
	It should be noted that dorsum generally refers to the back or posterior aspect. However, related to the foot, dorsum refers to the anterior surface.
palmar; volar	palm of the hand; anterior surface of the hand in the anatomical position

I–5

Planes of the Body

Planes can be described as imaginary cuts through the body or as flat surfaces revealing internal structures. By viewing different planes, one can see the same internal structures from different perspectives. Imagine a grapefruit. If you cut along one plane, you will see grapefruit segments. If you then cut the grapefruit in a plane at right angles to the first, you will see a grapefruit that has to be peeled to be eaten. Although in both cases the inside of the grapefruit is visible, different views of its internal structures are revealed.

The three body planes are described in Table 5–5.

TABLE 5–5

Body Planes

PLANE	VIEW PROVIDED
frontal; coronal	divides the body or structure into front and back
sagittal	divides the body or structure into right and left unequal portions **Note:** If the sagittal plane divides the body into equal right and left portions, the plane is referred to as **midsagittal.**
transverse	divides the body or structure into superior and inferior parts, which may be unequal

Abdominopelvic Regions and Quadrants

The abdomen is divided into regions (Figure 5–8) or quadrants (Figure 5–9). These divisions facilitate the identification of abdominopelvic organs and the location of pain.

FIGURE 5–8

Abdominopelvic Regions

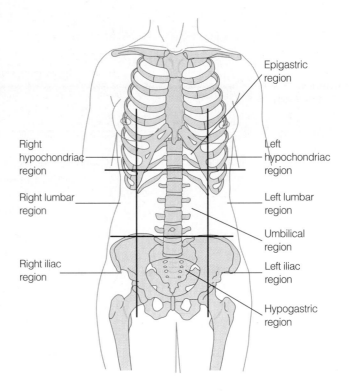

FIGURE 5—9

Abdominopelvic
Quadrants

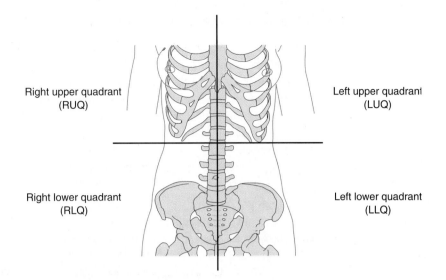

Right upper quadrant (RUQ)

Left upper quadrant (LUQ)

Right lower quadrant (RLQ)

Left lower quadrant (LLQ)

Divisions of the Back

There are 33 individual bones known as vertebrae that make up the vertebral column or backbone. (An illustration showing the vertebral column is shown in Figure 7–8.) The vertebrae are grouped together from superior to inferior as shown in Table 5–6.

TABLE 5—6

Vertebrae Grouping

NAME	ABBREVIATION	LOCATION
cervical	C1-C7	7 vertebrae located in the neck region
thoracic also known as **dorsal** and **thoracodorsal**	T1-T12 D1-D12	12 vertebrae located in the chest region, attached to the ribs
lumbar	L1-L5	5 vertebrae located in the lower back
sacrum	S1-S5	5 vertebrae that are fused together to make one bone
coccyx	(no abbreviation)	4 vertebrae fused together to form the tailbone

1—5

▶ 5.5 Analysis and Definition of Terms Used in the Body as a Whole

Sections 5.5 and 5.6 list terms used in the body. To use this table as a review, cover the center and right-hand columns in each section. Using the pronunciation guide in the left-hand column, pronounce each term, and then define it using the analysis techniques you learned in chapters 1 through 4. Check your answers by uncovering the other columns.

TERM	ANALYSIS	DEFINITION
anabolism ă-năb′-ŏ-lĭzm	-ism = process ana- = up bol/o = throw	process of building up complex substances from less complex substances **Note:** An example is the combining of amino acids to form protein.
anatomy ă-năt′-ō-mē	-tomy = to cut; incise; incision; process of cutting ana- = up	the science that deals with the study of the structure of the human body **Note:** Anatomy literally means to "cut up" because anatomy is based upon the dissection of body parts. Notice that a prefix and a suffix combine to form the word anatomy.
anterior ăn-tĭr′-ē-er	-ior = pertaining to anter/o = front	pertaining to the front of the body or the front of an organ
axillary ăks′-ĭ-ler-ē	-ary = pertaining to axill/o = armpit	pertaining to the armpit
catabolism kăt-ă′-bō-lĭzm	-ism = process cata- = down bol/o = throw	metabolic process in which complex substances are broken into simpler substances **Note:** An example of catabolism is complex proteins broken down into simpler amino acids.
caudal kau′-dl	-al = pertaining to caud/o = tail	pertaining to the tail; toward the tail
cervical ser′-vĭ-kl	-al = pertaining to cervic/o = neck of the body; neck of the uterus	pertaining to the neck of the body
coccygeal kŏks-ĭ′-jē-ăl	-eal = pertaining to coccyg/o = tailbone	pertaining to the tailbone or coccyx
cranial krā′-nē-ăl	-al = pertaining to crani/o = skull	pertaining to the skull
cytoplasm sī-′tō-plăzm	-plasm = development; formation cyt/o = cell	portion of the cell within the cell membrane excluding the nucleus
diagnosis dī-ăg-nō′-sĭs	-gnosis = knowledge dia- = through; complete	one disease is differentiated from another disease after complete knowledge is obtained of the disease through a study of the signs, symptoms, laboratory, x-ray, and other diagnostic procedures
dorsal dor′-săl	-al = pertaining to dors/o = back	pertaining to the back **Note:** An exception is the dorsum of the foot; in this instance dorsum refers to the upper surface of the foot.

(continued)

TERM	ANALYSIS	DEFINITION
epigastric ĕp-ĭ-găs′-trĭk	-ic = pertaining to epi- on; upon; above gastr/o = stomach	pertaining to upon the stomach **Note:** Refers to an abdominal region located on or upon the stomach (see Figure 5–8).
epithelial ĕp-ĭ-thē′-lē-ăl	-al = pertaining to epitheli/o = epithelium	pertaining to the epithelium, which is the internal and external coverings of the body **Note:** Epithelium literally means "upon a nipple," where nipple refers to the nipplelike shape of the dermis upon which the epithelium sits (see Figure 6–1).
etiology ē-tē-ŏl′-ō-jē	-logy = study of et/i = cause	the study of the cause of disease
histiocyte hĭs′-tē-ō-sīt	-cyte = cell histi/o = tissue	cells that make up tissue; tissue cell
histology hĭs-tŏl′-ă-jē	-logy = study of hist/o = tissue	study of tissues **Note:** The root meaning tissue can be spelled hist/o or histi/o.
homeostasis hō-mē-ō-stā′-sĭs	-stasis = stopping; controlling home/o = same	a normal state of balanced and stable internal environment, which can vary slightly to accommodate external changes
idiopathic ĭd′-ē-ō-păth′-ĭc	-ic = pertaining to idi/o = self-produced path/o = disease	disease that occurs without an apparent, outside cause
iliac ĭl′-ē-ăk	-ac = pertaining to ili/o = hip	pertaining to the hip
inferior ĭn-fē′-rĭ-or	-ior = pertaining to infer/o = below; downward	pertaining to below or in a downward position; a structure below another structure
inguinal ĭng′-gwĭ-năl	-al = pertaining to inguin/o = groin	pertaining to the groin
lateral lăt′-er-ăl	-al = pertaining to later/o = side	pertaining to the side
lumbar lŭm′-bar	-ar = pertaining to lumb/o = loins; lower back	pertaining to the loins or lower back
medial mē-dē-ăl	-al = pertaining to medi/o = middle	pertaining to the middle
metabolism mĕ-tăb′-ō-lĭzm	-ism = process meta- = beyond; change bol/o = throw	the chemical changes that occur in the body, including catabolism and anabolism
nucleoplasm nū′-klē-ō-plăzm	-plasm = development; formation nucle/o = nucleus	substances within the nucleus such as carbohydrates, proteins, and fats
pathology pă-thŏl′-ō-jē	-logy = study of path/o = disease	study of disease
pelvic pĕl′-vĭc	-ic = pertaining to pelv/o = pelvis	pertaining to the pelvis

(continued)

I–5

TERM	ANALYSIS	DEFINITION
pericardial pĕ-rĭ-kar′-dē-ăl	-al = pertaining to peri- = around card/i/o = heart	pertaining to a region around the heart
peritoneal pĕr″-ĭ-tō-nē′-ăl	-al = pertaining to peri- = around tone/o = stretch	pertaining to the membrane lining the abdominopelvic cavity. **Note:** The peritoneal membrane stretches around the abdominopelvic cavity.
phrenic frĕ′-nĭk	-ic = pertaining to phren/o = diaphragm	pertaining to the diaphragm
pleural ploo′-răl	-al = pertaining to pleur/o = pleura	pertaining to the pleura **Note:** The pleura is the membrane covering the lung and lining the thoracic cavity (see Figure 5–5).
posterior pŏs-tē′-rē-ōr	-ior = pertaining to poster/o = back	pertaining to the back of the body or an organ or to that located behind an organ or structure
prognosis prŏg-nō′-sĭs	-gnosis = knowledge pro- = before	prediction or forecast of the outcome of the disease
proximal prŏks′-ĭ-măl	-al = pertaining to proxim/o = near; close	pertaining to that which is close to a point of reference
sacral sā′-krŭl	-al = pertaining to sacr/o = sacrum	pertaining to the sacrum
spinal spī′-nŭl	-al = pertaining to spin/o = spinal column, backbone, vertebral column	pertaining to the spinal column
superior sū-pē′-rĭ-ōr	-ior = pertaining to super/o = above; toward the head	pertaining to a structure or organ situated either above another or toward the head
syndrome sĭn′-drōm	-drome = to run syn- = together	signs and symptoms occurring (running) together and indicating a particular condition or disease
thoracic thor-ă′-sĭk	-ic = pertaining to thorac/o = chest	pertaining to the chest
ventral vĕn′-trŭl	-al = pertaining to ventr/o = front	pertaining to the front of the body or organ
visceral vĭs′-er-ŭl	-al = pertaining to viscer/o = organs of the body	pertaining to the organs of the body

TERM	ANALYSIS	DEFINITION
adenoma ăd-ĕ-nō′-ma	-oma = tumor; mass aden/o = gland	tumor of a gland
adenoidectomy ă-dĕn-oyd-ĕk-tō-mē	-ectomy = surgical removal; excision adenoid/o = adenoids	excision of the adenoids
alveolar ăl-vē′-ŏ-ler	-ar = pertaining to alveol/o = alveolus; air sacs	pertaining to the alveolus
blepharopexy blĕf-ă-rŏp′-ĕks-ē	-pexy = surgical fixation blephar/o = eyelid	surgical fixation of the eyelid
bronchitis brong-kī′-tĭs	-itis = inflammation bronch/o = bronchus	inflammation of the bronchus
carcinoma kar-sĭ-nō′-mă	-oma = tumor; mass carcin/o = cancerous; cancer	malignant cancerous tumor of epithelial tissue
cheilitis kĭ-lī′-tĭs	-itis = inflammation cheil/o = lips	inflammation of the lips
cholecystitis kō″-lĕ-sĭs-tī′-tĭs	-itis = inflammation cholecyst/o = gallbladder	inflammation of the gallbladder
cholecystolithiasis kō″-lĕ-sĭs-tō-lĭ-thī′-ă-sĭs	-iasis = abnormal condition cholecyst/o = gallbladder lith/o = stone	condition of stones in the gallbladder
encephalocele ĕn-sĕf′-ă-lō-sēl″	-cele = hernia encephal/o = brain	hernia of the brain in which brain tissue protrudes through an opening in the skull
encephalopathy ĕn-sĕf-ă-lŏp′-ă-thē	-pathy = disease process encephal/o = brain	any disease process of the brain
epididymitis ĕp″-ĭ-dĭd″-ĭ-mī′-tis	-itis = inflammation epididym/o = epididymis	inflammation of the epididymis
esophageal ĕ-sŏf-ĕ-jē′-ăl	-eal = pertaining to esophag/o = esophagus	pertaining to the esophagus
gingivitis jĭn-jĭ-vī′-tĭs	-itis = inflammation gingiv/o = gums	inflammation of the gums
hypoglossal hī-pō-glŏs′-ăl	-al = pertaining to hypo- = under gloss/o = tongue	pertaining to under the tongue

(continued)

I—5

TERM	ANALYSIS	DEFINITION
hysterectomy hĭs-ter-ĕk′-tō-mē	-ectomy = surgical excision; removal hyster/o = uterus	excision of the uterus
laryngitis lar-ĭn-jī′-tĭs	-itis = inflammation laryng/o = larynx; voicebox	inflammation of the voice box or larynx
lymphadenitis lĭm-făd-ĕ-nī′-tĭs	-itis = inflammation lymph/o = lymph aden/o = gland	inflammation of the lymph gland
lymphadenopathy lĭm-făd-ĕn-ŏp′-ă-thē	-pathy = disease process lymphaden/o = lymph glands	disease process of the lymph glands; enlarged lymph glands
lymphangiogram lĭm-făn′-jē-ō-grăm	-gram = record lymph/o = lymph angi/o = vessel	record of a lymph vessel
lymphocyte lĭm′-fō-sīt	-cyte = cell lymph/o = lymph	lymph cell (a type of cell found in the lymphatic tissue)
lymphoma lĭm-fō′-mă	-oma = tumor; mass lymph/o = lymph	tumor of the lymph
myelitis mī-ĕ-lī′-tĭs	-itis = inflammation myel/o = spinal cord	inflammation of the spinal cord
myoma mī-ō′-mă	my/o = muscle -oma = tumor; mass	tumor of the muscle
myosarcoma mī-ō-sār-kō′-mă	-oma = tumor; mass sarc/o = flesh; connective tissue my/o = muscle	malignant tumor of muscle tissue (muscle tissue is a type of connective tissue)
odontalgia ō-dŏn-tăl′-jē-ă	-algia = pain odont/o = tooth	pain in the tooth; toothache
onychomalacia ŏn-ē-kō-mă-lā′-shă	-malacia = softening onych/o = nail	softening of the nail
oophorectomy ō-ŏf-ă-rĕk′-tō-mē	-ectomy = surgical removal; excision oophor/o = ovaries	surgical removal of the ovaries
orchidopexy or′-kĭd-ō-pĕk″-sē	-pexy = surgical fixation orchid/o = testicle; testis	surgical fixation of the testicle
pancreatectomy păn-krē-ă-tĕk′-tō-mē	-ectomy = surgical removal; excision pancreat/o = pancreas	excision of the pancreas

(continued)

TERM	ANALYSIS	DEFINITION
pharyngitis fă-rĭn-jī′-tĭs	-itis = inflammation pharyng/o = pharynx; throat	inflammation of the pharynx
prostatectomy prŏs-tă-tĕk′-tŏ-mē	-ectomy = surgical removal; excision prostat/o = prostate	surgical removal of the prostate
salpingitis săl-pĭn-jī′-tĭs	-itis = inflammation salping/o = fallopian tube; uterine tube	inflammation of the fallopian tubes
sarcoma sar-kō′-mă	-oma = tumor; mass sarc/o = connective tissue; flesh	malignant tumor of connective tissue such as bone, muscle, lymph, cartilage **Note:** Compare sarcoma with carcinoma, which is a malignant tumor of epithelial tissue.
splenorrhagia splĕ-nō-rā′-jă	-rrhagia = bursting forth splen/o = spleen	bursting forth of blood from the spleen
spondylitis spŏn-dĭ-lī′-tĭs	-itis = inflammation spondyl/o = vertebra	inflammation of the vertebra **Note:** Spondyl/o is most often used to denote pathological conditions.
stomatitis stō-mă-tī′-tĭs	-itis = inflammation stomat/o = mouth	inflammation of the mouth
sublingual sŭb-lĭng′-gwăl	-al = pertaining to sub- = under lingu/o = tongue	pertaining to below the tongue
tendinitis tĕn-dĭ-nī′-tĭs	-itis = inflammation tendin/o = tendon	inflammation of a tendon
thelitis thĕ-lī′-tĭs	-itis = inflammation thel/o = nipple	inflammation of the nipple
tonsillectomy tŏn-sĭ-lĕk′-tŏ-mē	-ectomy = surgical removal; excision tonsill/o = tonsils	excision of the tonsils
tracheostomy trā-kē-ŏs′-tŏ-mē	-stomy = new opening trache/o = trachea; windpipe	new opening into the windpipe, trachea **Note:** This new opening can be permanent or temporary.
tracheotomy trā-kē-ŏt′-ŏ-mē	-tomy = to cut into; incision; incise; process of cutting trache/o = trachea; windpipe	to cut into the windpipe or trachea
ureteral ū-rē′-tĕr-ăl	-al = pertaining to ureter/o = ureter	pertaining to the ureter

(continued)

I-5

TERM	ANALYSIS	DEFINITION
urethral ū-rē′-thrăl	-al = pertaining to urethr/o = urethra	pertaining to the urethra
uteropexy ū′-ter-ō-pĕks″-ē	-pexy = surgical fixation uter/o = uterus	surgical fixation of the uterus
vaginitis vă-jĭ-nī′-tĭs	-itis = inflammation vagin/o = vagina	inflammation of the vagina
vasectomy vă-sĕk′-tō-mē	-ectomy = surgical removal; excision vas/o = vas deferens (vessel for the passage of sperm)	surgical removal of the vas deferens **Note:** Vasectomy is a common sterilization technique.
vertebritis ver-tĕ-brī′-tĭs	-itis = inflammation vertebr/o = vertebra	inflammation of the vertebra
vulvovaginitis vŭl-vō-vă-jĭ-nī′-tĭs	-itis = inflammation vulv/o = vulva vagin/o = vagina	inflammation of the vulva and vagina

5.7 PATHOLOGY

Pathology is the branch of medicine concerned with disease. This study goes beyond a mere definition of individual diseases, however. For example, the study of pneumonia encompasses definition, causes, types, developmental process, disease course, possible complications, and predisposing factors. The word "disease" means literally "not at ease." In other words, the term disease can be applied to any abnormal condition of the body. A health care practitioner who suspects that a patient has a disease or who wishes to confirm that no disease is present proceeds through several discrete steps, the first of which may be a physical examination.

5.8 PHYSICAL EXAMINATION, DIAGNOSIS, AND TREATMENT

Health care practitioners examining patients may use any or all of the following techniques: **inspection, palpation, percussion,** and **auscultation (IPPA);** these techniques are discussed below. During an exam, the health care practitioner looks for signs and symptoms of disease. The examination often results in a **diagnosis** (identification of disease or condition) and a suggested method of treatment, which may in turn depend on the cause or causes (**etiology**) of the symptoms. Having established the diagnosis, etiology, and subsequent treatment, the health care practitioner then arrives at a **prognosis** (prediction of a probable outcome).

When the physical examination does not produce a diagnosis, it may be followed by diagnostic tests, such as laboratory, x-ray, or other clinical procedures.

Inspection

Inspection consists of a careful visual examination of the body. Observations include abnormalities to the skin surface (such as cuts), the shape of the abdomen (flat or round), any discoloration to the skin, and any bone or muscle abnormality.

Palpation

Palpation means "touching" (palpate is the verb). The health care practitioner touches the patient with the hands and fingers to determine any abnormality of the body surface or underlying tissue. Such abnormalities might include unusual masses, high or low pulse rate, or pain produced by palpation.

Percussion

Percussion means "to tap." The health care practitioner sharply strikes the body with the tips of the fingers to detect any abnormality of sound in the underlying organs. For example, a normal lung resonates (vibrate) when tapped because it is filled with air and not congested with fluid or occupied by abnormal masses. When fluid or abnormal masses are in the lung, the sound change reflects the abnormality.

Auscultation

Auscultation means "to listen." The health care practitioner listens to the sounds of the body with a stethoscope. Auscultation is useful in determining abnormal breath sounds, heart sounds, blood pressure, and bowel sounds.

Diagnosis

A diagnosis consists of distinguishing one disease from another or in confirming that no disease is present. The diagnosis may or may not include diagnostic tests. **Syndrome** refers to a collection of symptoms that indicate a distinctive disease or condition. This word has entered the modern lexicon, and unfortunately, many people outside the medical profession use it incorrectly.

Etiology

Etiology is the study of the causes of disease. For example, some types of pneumonia are caused by bacteria, the common cold is caused by a virus, a heart attack is caused by a lack of blood supply to the heart muscle, and so on. Sometimes, the etiology of a disease is unknown. For example, the etiology of Crohn's disease, a chronic inflammation of the intestines, is unknown. The term **idiopathic** is used to indicate disease of unknown origin.

Signs and Symptoms

A **sign** is an abnormality observed by the medical professional during the physical examination. Examples include tenderness, masses, abnormal heart sounds, or abnormal pulse rate. These are objective signs and are usually recorded in a medical document under the heading physical examination.

Symptoms are abnormalities made known by the patient to the health care practitioner, such as abdominal pain, numbness, difficulty in moving, and so on. These symptoms are subjective and are usually recorded in medical documents as patient complaints. The difference, then, between a sign and a symptom is that a sign is the health care practitioner's assessment made during the physical examination and a symptom is the patient's complaint.

Treatment

Treatment is the method used to cure the disease or to relieve its signs and symptoms. In the example of pneumonia, the treatment may be a regimen of antibiotics. In general, treatment is characterized as surgical or medical. Surgical treatment involves an operation usually performed under anesthesia. Medical treatment includes the use of drugs, x-rays, and therapies to cure a disease or to alleviate its signs and symptoms and does not involve an operation.

Prognosis

Once the diagnosis, etiology, and treatment modalities are confirmed, a **prognosis** can be made. The prognosis is a prediction or an "educated guess" about how the disease will affect the patient or, stated another way, about the consequences of the disease. Again referring to the example of pneumonia, the prognosis would likely be good—meaning that the chance of the patient's recovery is good—if the patient is relatively healthy and is given the proper treatment. However, if the pneumonia is a complication of a more serious condition and the patient is in a weakened state, the prognosis might be poor, meaning that the chances of recovery are not good.

Review of Body Systems

Matching

Study the organs that are included in each of the body systems shown in Figure 5-3, and then place the correct letter from column B that corresponds to each body system next to each organ it contains in column A.

Answers to the exercises are found in Appendix A.

Column A		Column B
1. joints _____		A. integumentary system (skin)
2. brain _____		B. skeletal system
3. esophagus _____		C. muscular system
4. cartilage _____		D. nervous system
5. uterus _____		E. endocrine system
6. lymph glands _____		F. circulatory system
7. lymph _____		G. lymphatic system
8. stomach _____		H. respiratory system
9. ovaries _____		I. digestive system (gastrointestinal)
10. pancreas _____		J. urinary system
11. hair _____		K. reproductive system
12. uterine tubes _____		
13. vulva _____		
14. mouth _____		
15. liver _____		
16. trachea _____		
17. urethra _____		
18. vas deferens _____		
19. penis _____		
20. bronchus _____		
21. gallbladder _____		
22. pituitary _____		
23. larynx _____		

24. lymph vessels _____

25. thyroid _____

26. spinal cord _____

27. muscle _____

28. nails _____

29. pharynx _____

30. prostate _____

31. adrenals _____

32. spleen _____

33. parathyroid _____

34. tonsils _____

35. ureters _____

36. bladder _____

▶EXERCISE 5–2   **Practice Quiz**

Short Answer

Briefly answer the following
questions.

1. Define "anatomy" in one sentence. _____
   _____

2. Define "physiology" in one sentence. _____
   _____

3. What is the fundamental composition of the cell? _____
   _____

4. Name the four types of tissue. _____
   _____

5. What term do we use to refer to the body's ability to remain relatively
   stable while responding to internal and external stimuli? _____
   _____

6. What general term describes the body's chemical processes? _____
   _____

7. Name the two main cavities of the body. _____

_____

8. In which of the two main body cavities would one find the brain and the spine? _____

_____

9. What term describes the position of the body we use for a directional discussion of anatomical phenomena? _____

_____

10. Name the three body planes. _____

_____

11. Name the four techniques a physician may use in a physical examination.

_____

_____

Matching Terms with Meanings

Matching

Match the term in Column A with its meaning in Column B.

Column A		Column B
1. adenoidectomy	_____	A. pertaining to the tailbone
2. blepharopexy	_____	B. inflammation of the lips
3. bronchitis	_____	C. excision of the adenoids
4. cheilitis	_____	D. pertaining to the skull
5. cholecystitis	_____	E. pertaining to below the tongue
6. coccygeal	_____	F. disease of the brain
7. cranial	_____	G. inflammation of the bronchus
8. encephalopathy	_____	H. pertaining to the esophagus
9. esophageal	_____	I. inflammation of the gallbladder
10. sublingual	_____	J. surgical fixation of the eyelid

Choose a term for a body cavity from Column B and place it next to the organ it houses in Column A.

Column A		Column B
11. stomach	_____	cranial
12. heart	_____	spinal
13. lungs	_____	thoracic
14. spine	_____	abdominopelvic
15. brain	_____	
16. intestines	_____	

1–5

17. aorta   _____

18. spleen   _____

19. liver   _____

Match the term in Column A with its definition in Column B.

Column A		Column B
20. superior	_____	A. away from the center
21. lateral	_____	B. lying on the abdomen, face down
22. supine	_____	C. away from the surface of the body
23. inferior	_____	D. lying on the back, face up
24. proximal	_____	E. anterior surface of the hand in the anatomical position
25. prone	_____	F. upper surface of the foot
26. anterior	_____	G. below
27. superficial	_____	H. above
28. dorsum	_____	I. close to a point of reference
29. posterior	_____	J. toward the surface of the body
30. peripheral	_____	K. front
31. palmar	_____	L. away from the midline
32. medial	_____	M. back
33. deep	_____	N. posterior surface of the foot
34. plantar	_____	O. toward the midline

▶ **EXERCISE 5–4**

Spelling Practice

Spelling

Place a check mark beside all misspelled words in the list that follows. Correctly spell those that you checked off.

1. adenoidectomy ☐ _____

2. axxillary ☐ _____

3. balintitis ☐ _____

4. anatamy ☐ _____

5. bronchioectasis ☐ _____

6. cirvisitis ☐ _____

7. cholecystolithiasis ☐ _____

8. cocygeal ☐ _____

9. encephalocele ☐ _____

10. epodidimitis ☐ _____

11. femural ☐ _____

12. fibilar ☐ _____

13. gingivitis ☐ _____

14. hypoglossal ☐ _____

15. laringitis ☐ _____

I–5

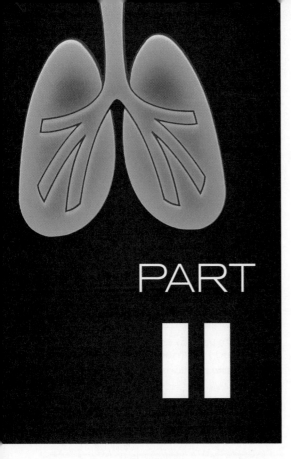

PART

II

BODY SYSTEMS

6 THE INTEGUMENTARY SYSTEM

CHAPTER ORGANIZATION

This chapter is about the anatomy and physiology of the integumentary system.

CHAPTER OBJECTIVES

Upon successful completion of the chapter, the student will be able to do the following:

1. Name and describe the anatomical structures of the integumentary system including the accessory organs.
2. List and describe the functions of the integumentary system including the accessory organs.
3. Describe the role of melanin and carotene in skin pigmentation.
4. Pronounce, analyze, define, and spell medical terms used in the integumentary system.
5. Define terms relating to the physical examination and symptomatology of the integumentary system.
6. Define selected diseases of the integumentary system.
7. Define terms relating to diagnosis and treatment in integumentary pathology.
8. Define abbreviations common to the integumentary system.

WORD ELEMENTS PROMINENT IN THIS CHAPTER

WORD ELEMENT	ELEMENT TYPE	MEANING	WORD ELEMENT	ELEMENT TYPE	MEANING
acanth/o	root	thorny	epi-	prefix	upon
-blast	suffix	a growing thing; immature	eschar/o	root	scab
			follicul/o	root	follicle
cyan/o	root	blue	-graft	suffix	transplant
-cyte	suffix	cell	hidr/o	root	sweat
derm/o; dermat/o	root	skin	ichthy/o	root	fish

WORD ELEMENT	ELEMENT TYPE	MEANING	WORD ELEMENT	ELEMENT TYPE	MEANING
kerat/o	root	horn-like	-phyte	suffix	plant
melan/o	root	black	pil/o	root	hair
onych/o	root	nail	sudor/i	root	sweat
papill/o	root	small elevation	xer/o	root	dry

6.1 ANATOMY OF THE INTEGUMENTARY SYSTEM

The Latin word *integumentum* means "covering." The integumentary system includes those structures that act as coverings of the body, such as the skin, and associated structures, such as hair, nails, and glands.

Skin

The skin, the largest organ in the body, has two separate layers: the **epidermis** and the **dermis** (see Figure 6–1). The epidermis is made up of epithelial tissue and is the outermost layer. The dermis, which is made up of connective tissue,

FIGURE 6–1 The Skin

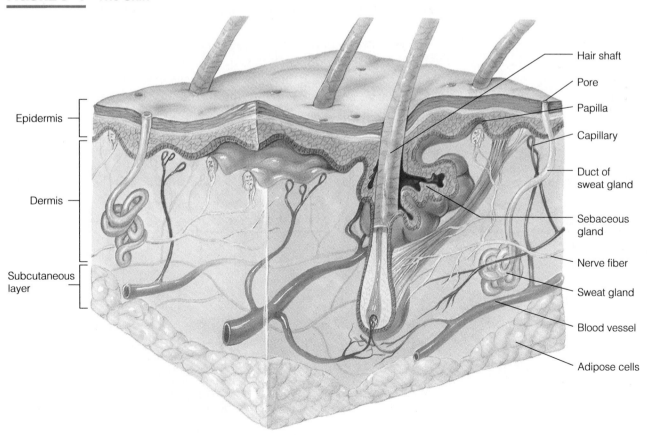

Epidermis

Dermis

Subcutaneous layer

Hair shaft
Pore
Papilla
Capillary
Duct of sweat gland
Sebaceous gland
Nerve fiber
Sweat gland
Blood vessel
Adipose cells

lies beneath the epidermis. The **subcutaneous tissue** (superficial fascia) is also made up of connective tissue and lies beneath the dermis, but it is not considered to be a layer of the skin. In the following pages, each of these layers is discussed according to cell type, tissue type, general characteristics, and functions.

General Characteristics of the Epidermis   **Epithelial cells** cover the body's surfaces and line its cavities. Along with epithelial cells are specialized cells called **melanocytes** and **keratinocytes.** Melanocytes produce a skin pigment called **melanin,** which darkens the skin. The darkness of the skin is directly proportional to the activity of melanocytes.

Keratinocytes, the other specialized cells of the epidermis, produce **keratin,** a protein that infiltrates dead skin cells and makes the skin tough, waterproof, and resistant to bacteria. Skin cells infiltrated with keratin are said to be **keratinized.**

The epidermis is arranged in five layers, or **strata** (see Figure 6–2). Some of the general characteristics of each of these layers are given in Table 6–1. Another general characteristic of the epidermis is **avascularity,** which means it contains no blood vessels. Therefore, abraded or scraped epidermis does not bleed. With no blood vessels of its own, the epidermis receives its oxygen and nutrients from the blood supply in the dermis.

In summary, the cellular activity of the epidermis is as follows: the epithelial cells are constantly dying and being replaced; cells germinate from the basal cell layer of the epidermis, rise to the upper layers, die, and become infiltrated with keratin. This process is continuous, the life span of skin cells being approximately 28 days.

General Characteristics of the Dermis   The dermis is also called the **corium.** The dermis, a nonlayered structure of the skin located beneath the epidermis, is connective tissue that contains blood vessels, nerves, glands, and hair follicles.

The cell types of the dermis are **fibroblasts, macrophages, mast cells,** and **plasma cells.** Fibroblasts produce **collagen,** a protein providing strength and stability. Macrophages are white blood cells responsible for phagocytosis. Mast cells produce **heparin,** an anticoagulant, and **histamine,** a substance important in inflammatory reactions. Plasma cells produce **antibodies.**

FIGURE 6–2   **Epidermal Layers** (a) Photograph of epidermal layers. (b) Schematic drawing of epidermal layers.

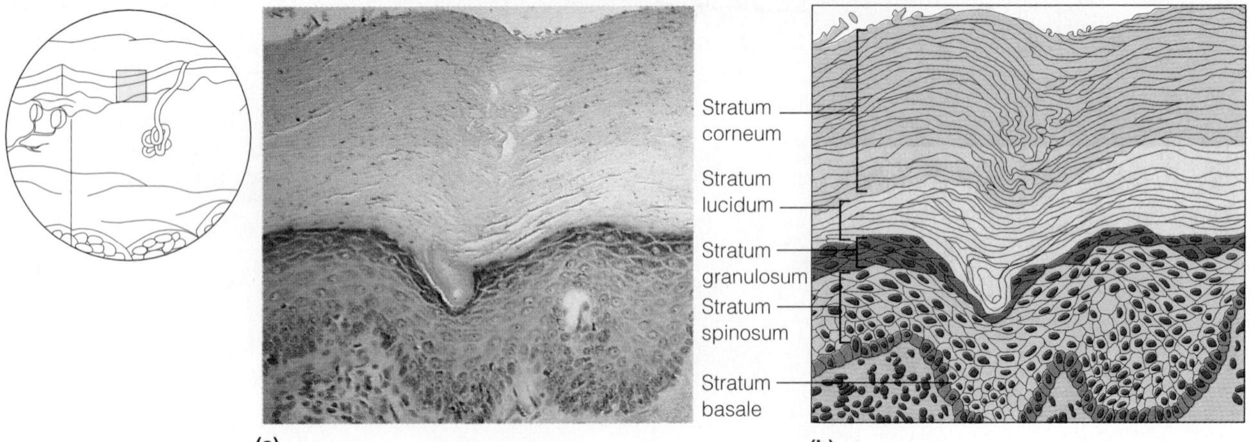

Stratum corneum
Stratum lucidum
Stratum granulosum
Stratum spinosum
Stratum basale

(a)   (b)

TABLE 6—1

The Epidermis

II–6

STRATA	DESCRIPTION
stratum basale/basal cell layer (the deepest layer)	This layer is responsible for regeneration. New cells move upward, and as they move farther away from their nutrition source, they die and are sloughed off.
stratum spinosum/prickle cell layer (second layer from the bottom)	This layer is the actively growing layer. The stratum spinosum and stratum basale are often called collectively the **stratum germinativum** (jer″-mi-na-ti′-vum), as they frequently undergo cellular division.
stratum granulosum (third layer from the bottom)	The cells die in this layer.
stratum lucidum (fourth layer from the bottom)	This layer consists of dead or dying cells and is found only in the soles of the feet and palms of the hands. Named after the transparent compound **eleidin** (ĕ-lē′-ĭ-dĭn), a substance believed to be formed in the granulosum layer from keratin, it is thin and transparent.
stratum corneum (outermost layer)	This layer, which is also called the horny layer, consists of scalelike dead cells that have been filled with **keratin.** Keratin gives the stratum corneum its hard, tough, and water-resistant character. Keratinized cells are constantly sloughed off (shed) and replaced.

Subcutaneous Tissue   The **subcutaneous tissue** is composed of connective tissue and deposits of adipose (fatty) tissue. This layer, also called superficial fascia, connects the dermis to the underlying organs and muscles. It also serves as a kind of padding or shock absorber and acts as an insulator for the deeper tissues against extreme temperature changes.

▶ 6.2 PHYSIOLOGY OF THE INTEGUMENTARY SYSTEM

While the epidermis acts as a barrier against water and bacteria, the dermis functions are thermoregulation, nutritive supply, skin sensation, and glandular secretions.

As a **thermoregulator,** the skin controls heat loss. When the body needs to dissipate heat, the blood vessels in the skin dilate, allowing more blood to come to the surface, where it can be cooled. Conversely, when the body needs more heat, the blood vessels constrict to keep heat within the deep structures. This phenomenon is an example of homeostasis (see Chapter 5).

To supply nutrients to the skin, the dermis again uses the blood vessels. Interruption of the blood supply to skin cells kills skin tissue. For example, **decubitus ulcers** (decubitus means "lying down") sometimes occur when a patient must lie in one position for an extended period of time. Circulation to pressure points, such as the elbows, shoulders, and buttocks, is cut off, and this loss of circulation kills the tissue in these body regions. The dead tissue (**necrotic** tissue) sheds, leaving an open and relatively deep sore. Decubitus ulcers are commonly called bedsores.

The dermis contains sensory receptors, which receive stimuli from the external and internal environment and send nervous impulses to the spinal cord and brain. The dermis also contains glands that secrete substances to the surface of the skin.

A summary of the anatomy and physiology of the skin is given in Table 6–2. General burn terminology is contained in Table 6–3.

TABLE 6–2   The Anatomy and Physiology of the Skin

SKIN LAYER	Location	Cell Types	ANATOMY Tissue	Layers	Other Attributes	PHYSIOLOGY
Epidermis	outer, most superficial layer	Epithelial cells, melanocytes, and keratinocytes	epithelial	5 strata	avascular no nerves	Resistant to water and bacteria
Dermis	below the epidermis	fibroblasts, macrophages, mast cells, and plasma cells	connective	not layered	contains blood vessels, nerves, glands, and hair follicles	provides thermoregulation, nutrition, sensation, and glandular secretions
Subcutaneous Tissue	below the dermis	fibroblasts, macrophages, mast cells, plasma cells, and fat cells	connective	not layered	contains mostly fatty deposits	connects the dermis to underlying organs and muscles; provides padding, shock absorption, and insulation

Note: The subcutaneous layer is not actually a layer of the skin, but is part of the anatomy of the integumentary system.

TABLE 6–3   General Burn Terminology

TERM	MEANING
First, second, and third degree burn	**First degree burn** or **superficial burn** damages only the outler layer of the epidermis. Characterized by a redness of the skin and no scarring. Example: sunburn. **Second degree burn** or **partial thickness burn** damages a portion of the epidermis and a portion of the dermis is affected. There is the occurrence of large blisters. Regeneration can occur if no infection ensues. **Third degree burn** or **full-thickness burn** involves the epidermis and dermis and can extend into the subcutaneous tissues, bone, and muscle. Since the burn does not heal spontaneously, skin grafting is necessary. **Fourth degree burn** chars the skin and involves the epidermis, dermis, subcutaneous tissue, muscle, bone, and underlying structures.

TABLE 6—3 General Burn Terminology (concluded)

TERM	MEANING
eschar	permanently damaged skin; the first skin that can be peeled off following a burn
escharotomy	incision into the eschar, to relieve the tightness of the burned skin
Hubbard tank	large tank filled with water The burn is immersed into the water, making the skin soft and pliable for easy removal of the burned skin
hypertrophic scar	exaggerated scars in areas of trauma as a result of a healing process that produces excessive collagen. A **keloid scar** is similar to a hypertrophic scar.
Jobst garment	a piece of elastic material stretched over the burn site to prevent hypertrophic scarring
major burn	third degree burn on 20% or more of the body
meshed graft	partial thickness (epidermis and portion of the dermis) skin graft in which many tiny holes have been made to allow for drainage of excess fluid and to permit the graft to stretch and contour to the body shape
Ringer's lactate solution	a saline replacement fluid given to patients when they have lost a significant amount of body fluid

▷ 6.3 ACCESSORY ORGANS

The accessory organs in the integumentary system are the **hair, nails,** and **glands.**

Hair

Hair develops at the base of a **hair follicle** from epidermal cells. A hair follicle is a tube that surrounds the root of a hair. The epidermal cells that make up the hair divide, grow, push upward, and become keratinized, thereby forming the shaft of the hair (Figure 6–3). The amount of melanin in the epidermis determines hair color. As a person ages, the body stops producing melanin, and the hair loses its color and turns gray.

FIGURE 6—3

Hair and Related Structures

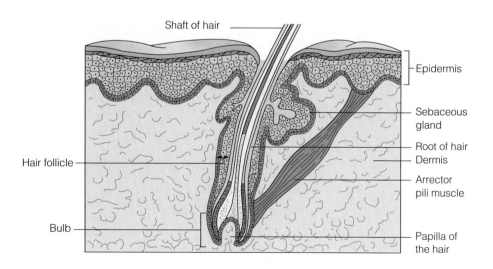

Shaft of hair
Epidermis
Sebaceous gland
Root of hair
Dermis
Hair follicle
Arrector pili muscle
Bulb
Papilla of the hair

Nails

Nails are protective coverings on the ends of fingers and toes. Nail cells are keratinized epithelial cells. At the base of each nail is the white, half-moon shaped **lunula** (luna is the Latin word for moon). It is from the lunula that the nail grows. Other anatomical structures are the **nail bed** and **eponychium** (or cuticle). The nail bed is the tissue on which the nail lies, and the eponychium is located on the base of the nail (Figure 6–4).

FIGURE 6–4 **The Nail** (a) Posterior view of finger. (b) Fingernail and underlying structures.

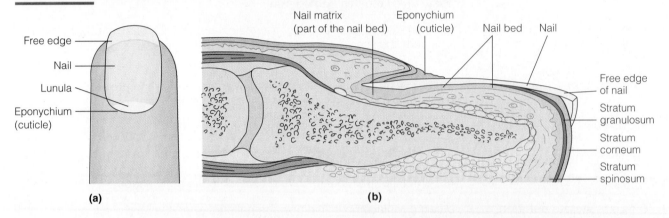

(a)

(b)

Glands

Sebaceous glands secrete an oily substance called **sebum** onto the surface of the skin and along the hair shaft (Figure 6–5). The gland secretes through ducts that open directly onto the epidermis. The function of sebum is to keep hair pliable and the skin soft and waterproof.

FIGURE 6–5

Sebaceous and Sudoriferous Glands
(a) Schematic drawing of the sebaceous sudoriferous glands.
(b) Photograph of sebaceous and suderiferous glands.

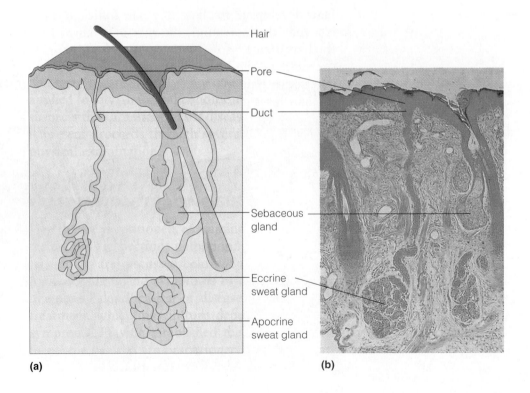

(a)

(b)

Sudoriferous (sweat) glands secrete sweat through pores. There are two types of sweat glands: **eccrine** and **apocrine.** The eccrine glands respond to heat and exercise, and the apocrine glands respond to emotional stress. The sweat glands play a role in thermoregulation. When the body overheats, the glands secrete sweat that evaporates on the surface of the skin, helping to cool the body.

Ceruminous glands secrete a waxy substance called **cerumen.** Cerumen is secreted within the external ear and protects the ear from bacterial invasion. A buildup of cerumen can cause a temporary hearing impairment, however.

Skin Pigmentation

Skin coloring is a result of two pigments found in the skin: **melanin,** a brown pigment, and **carotene,** a yellow one. The capillary blood found in the dermis also affects skin color.

Melanin is endogenous, meaning it is produced by an internal source, in this case in the epidermis by melanocytes. The amount of melanin produced depends upon both heredity and environment. For instance, some individuals, who do not inherit the ability to produce melanin, have a condition known as **albinism** (Figure 6–6). This condition is characterized by a lack of pigment in the skin, hair, and eyes.

Ultraviolet (UV) light, a component of sunlight, darkens the skin because it increases the production of melanin from melanocytes. The increased amounts of melanin then block out UV rays. In some people, the sun increases the activity of melanocytes, simultaneously increasing the amount of melanin and producing a suntan, which then protects the skin from UV light. In other people, the sun has little effect on melanocytes, and these people sunburn easily. The pituitary gland can also influence melanocytic activity.

Carotene is exogenous, meaning that it comes from an external source, namely, from the ingestion of yellow vegetables, such as carrots and squash.

FIGURE 6–6

Albinism

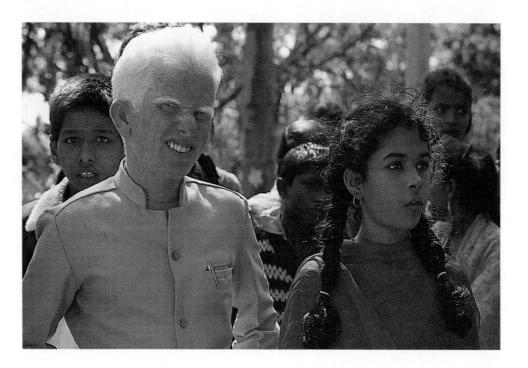

Concept Maps

Everyone understands outlines. A concept map is an outline too, but with an important difference. The conventional outline starts with the first major concept relating to a particular topic, details the specifics relating to that concept, moves on to the next major concept, and so on until the topic is complete. Such an outline can be difficult to complete on a single page, unless significant detail is left out. However, with the concept map, even large topics can be comprehensively outlined on one page. This allows the student to get an overview of a topic without sacrificing any detail.

A concept map always begins by breaking up a topic into its major components. For example, the integumentary system could be divided into "structure" and "function," with each of these further divided into their respective components. Arrows or connecting lines are used to join related divisions, so that relationships are readily apparent. Where it is necessary to show relationships among items on the same level, this can be done by additional arrows or connecting lines. When this is done, it is often helpful to include a brief description of the nature of the relationship being outlined. For example, in a concept map of the structure of the integumentary system, the sebaceous glands and sebum can be joined by a connecting line that is accompanied by the descriptive word "secrete." As well, sebum and hair can be joined by a connecting line that is accompanied by the term "softens."

While at first concept maps may seem difficult to follow, with a little work students will find that they are powerful tools for understanding and remembering. They add a visual dimension that is missing in conventional outlines, and summarize great amounts of information in a small space. This makes them a great study tool.

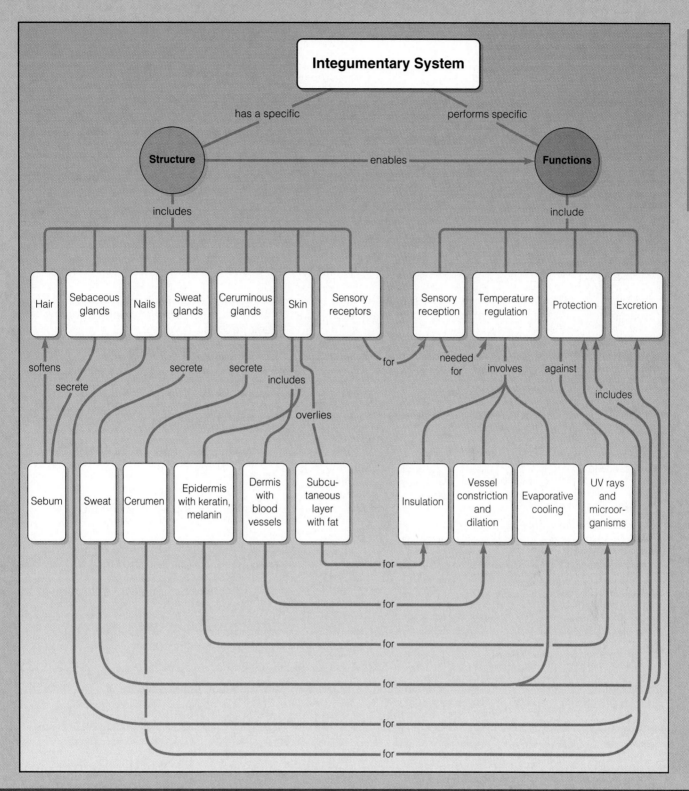

TERM WITH PRONUNCIATION	ANALYSIS	DEFINITION
acantholysis ă-kăn-thŏl′-ĭ-sĭs	-lysis = breakdown acanth/o = thorny or spiny	breakdown of the spiny layer of the skin
acanthosis ăk″-ăn-thō′-sĭs	-osis = abnormal condition acanth/o = thorny or spiny	abnormal thickening of the thorny or spiny layer of the skin (stratum spinosum)
adipocele ăd′-ĭ-pō-sēl	-cele = hernia adip/o - fat	hernia containing fat
adipose ăd′-ĭ-pōs	-ose - pertaining to adip/o = fat	pertaining to fat
allograft ăl′-ō-grăft	-graft - transplant all/o = referring to another	transplant of tissue between individuals of the same species but of different genetic backgrounds
anhidrosis ăn″-hī-drō′-sĭs	-osis = abnormal condition a(n)- = lack of; no; not hidr/o = sweat	lack of sweat
autograft aw′-tō-grăft	-graft = transplant auto- = self	transplant of tissue from one part of the patient's body to another
avascular ă-văs′-kū-lăr	-ar = pertaining to a(n)- = lack of; no; not vascul/o = vessel	pertaining to an absence of blood vessels
carotenemia kăr″-ō-tĕ-nē′-mē-ă	-emia = blood condition caroten/o = carrot	excess amounts of carotene in the blood
carotenoderma kar-ŏt′-ĕn-ō-dĕr″-mă	-derma = skin caroten/o = carrot	yellowness of the skin due to increased amounts of carotene in the blood
ceruminous sĕ-roo′-mĭ-nŭs	-ous = pertaining to cerumin/o = wax	pertaining to cerumen, a waxy substance
cyanosis sī-ă-nō′-sĭs sī-ăn-ō′-sĭs	-osis = abnormal condition cyan/o = blue	abnormal condition exhibited by a bluish discoloration of the skin
dermatitis dĕr″-mă-tī′-tĭs	-itis = inflammation dermat/o = skin	inflammation of the skin
dermatology dĕr″-mă-tŏl′-ō-jē	-logy = study of dermat/o = skin	study of skin
dermatome dĕr′-mă-tōm	-tome = instrument dermat/o = skin	instrument to cut the skin
dermatomycosis dĕr″-mă-tō-mī-kō′-sĭs	-osis = abnormal condition dermat/o = skin myc/o = fungus	fungal infection of the skin
dermatophyte dĕr′-mă-tō-fīt	-phyte = plant dermat/o = skin	a fungal parasite that infects the skin (the condition resulting is called "dermatophytosis")
dermatophytosis dĕr″-mă-tō-fī-tō′-sĭs	-osis = abnormal condition dermat/o = skin phyt/o = plant	fungal infection of the skin

TERM WITH PRONUNCIATION	ANALYSIS	DEFINITION
diaphoresis dī″-ă-fō-rē′-sĭs	-sis = state of diaphor/e = profuse sweating	state of profuse sweating
discoid dĭs′-koid	-oid = resembling disc/o = disk	resembling a disk
epidermis ĕp″-ĭ-dĕr′-mĭs	-dermis = skin epi- = upon; above	upon the dermis (the outermost skin layer)
epithelium ĕp″-ĭ-thē′-lē-ŭm	-um = structure eptheli/o = covering	the structure covering outer and inner body surfaces
eponychium ĕp″-ō-nĭk′-ē-ŭm	-ium = structure epi- = upon; above onych/o = nail	portion of epidermis extending from the edge of the proximal nail onto the nail itself; also known as the cuticle
erythematous er″-ĭ-thĕm′-ă-tŭs	-ous = pertaining to erythemat/o = red	pertaining to redness
fibroblast fī′-brō-blăst	-blast = immature; a growing thing fibr/o = fiber	immature fibrous cell that eventually makes up connective tissue
filiform fĭl′-ĭ-form	-form = shape fil/i = thread	shaped like a thread
follicular fō-lĭk′-ū-lăr	-ar = pertaining to follicul/o = follicle; small sac	pertaining to a follicle or small sac
hemangioma hē-măn″-jĭ-ō′-mă	-oma = tumor; mass hem/o = blood angi/o = vessel	benign tumor or mass composed of blood vessels
hyperhidrosis hī″-pĕr-hī-drō′-sĭs	-osis = abnormal condition hyper- = increase; excessive; above normal hidr/o = sweat	excessive sweating
hyperkeratosis hī″-pĕr-kĕr″-ă-tō′-sĭs	-osis = abnormal condition hyper- = increase; excessive; above normal kerat/o = hard; hornlike	abnormal condition characterized by hard or hornlike overgrowth of epithelial tissue
ichthyosis ĭk″-thē-ō′-sĭs	-osis = abnormal condition ichthy/o = fish	dry and scaly skin; fishlike skin
keratinocyte kĕ-răt′-ĭ-nō-sīt	-cyte = cell kerat/o = hornlike	cell that produces keratin
keratosis kĕr-ă-tō′-sĭs	-osis = abnormal condition kerat/o = hornlike	abnormal condition characterized by hard or horny overgrowth of epithelial tissue
lipoma lī-pō′-mă	-oma = tumor or mass lip/o = fat	tumor or mass containing fat
melanocyte měl′-ăn-ō-sīt	-cyte = cell melan/o = black	cell that produces melanin

TERM WITH PRONUNCIATION	ANALYSIS	DEFINITION
melanoma měl″-ă-nō′-mă	-oma = tumor; mass melan/o = black	benign or malignant tumor of the melanocytes
necrotic nĕ-krŏt′-ĭc	-tic = pertaining to necr/o = death	pertaining to death (of tissues)
onychomycosis ŏn″-ĭ-kō-mī-kō′-sĭs	-osis = abnormal condition onych/o = nail myc/o = fungus	fungal condition of a nail
papilloma păp-ĭ-lō′-mă	-oma = tumor or mass papill/o = a small elevation; nipplelike	benign epithelial tumor
paronychia păr-ō-nĭk′-ē-ă	-ia = state of; condition para = beside; near onych/o = nail	inflammation of the tissue surrounding the nail **Note:** The suffix -itis meaning inflammation is not used in this medical term.
periungual pĕr″-ē-ŭńǵ-gwăl	-al = pertaining to peri- = around ungu/o = nail	pertaining to the area around the nail
pilosebaceous pī″-lō-sĕ-bā′-shŭs	-ous = pertaining to pil/o = hair seb/o = sebum (oily secretion of the sebaceous glands)	pertaining to hair follicles and sebaceous glands
pyoderma pī-ō-dĕr′-mă	-derma = skin py/o = pus	any pus-producing disease of the skin
pyogenic pī-ō-jĕn′-ĭk	-genic = producing py/o = pus	pus producing
seborrhea sĕb-or-ē′-ă	-rrhea = discharge seb/o = sebum	increased discharge of sebum from the sebaceous glands
steatoma stē″-ă-tō′-mă	-oma = tumor; mass steat/o = fat	fatty tumor of the sebaceous gland
sudoriferous sū-dor-ĭf′-ĕr-ŭs	-ferous = bearing; producing sudor/i = sweat	producing sweat
xenograft zĕn′-ō-grăft	-graft = transplant xen/o = strange	the transplantation of tissue from an organism of a different species **Note:** This transplant is also called a "heterograft."
xeroderma zē″-rō-dĕr′-mă	-derma = skin xer/o = dry	dry skin

Skin conditions can develop from a variety of causes, categorized as infectious, inflammatory, erythematous, dyschromic, and idiopathic. Additional conditions include those caused by tumors, burns, and disorders of the hair follicles.

Infectious Skin Diseases

Common causes of infectious skin diseases include bacteria, viruses, funguses, and parasites.

Bacterial Skin Infections

TERM	MEANING
carbuncle	an infection of the skin and subcutaneous tissue, resulting in a cluster of pustules Caused by *staphylococcus*. Occuring most frequently in males and at the back of the neck. Predisposing factors include poor hygiene, feeble patients, and diabetes. If the condition is persistent and troublesome, it is called **carbunculosis.**
erysipelas	a surface cellulitis of the skin, particularly the dermis and subcutaneous tissue. Caused by *streptococcus*.
furuncle	an inflammation of the hair follicle, commonly known as a boil. Caused by *staphylococcus* Common locations include the back of the neck and face. Called **furunculosis** if persistent and troublesome.
impetigo	superficial but highly contagious skin lesions, seen mainly in children Caused by *staphylococcus* or *streptococcus*. Characteristic lesions are pustules and vesicles usually around the mouth area.

Viral Skin Infections

TERM	MEANING
herpes simplex (cold sore)	an infection of the skin and mucous membrane caused by the microorganism **herpes simplex type I (HSV–1);** transmitted through respiratory and oral secretions, the disease manifests itself in vesicular lesions around the mouth, lips, or eyes The type 1 virus should not be confused with **Herpes simplex type II (HSV-2),** which is transmitted through sexual contact. Treatment of herpes type I is with idoxuridine (IDU) or acyclovir.
warts (verucca)	contagious **papilloma** caused by the human papilloma virus (HPV) **Note:** A wart can be flat or long and narrow, in which case it is called **filiform.** If it is attached to underlying tissue by a stem, it is called **pedunculated.** **Verucca vulgaris** (the common wart) occurs mostly in children and young adults, appearing on the fingers, elbows, or face. Warts are contagious, and most are nonmalignant. **Plantar warts** occur on the bottom of the foot, either singly or in pinpoint-sized clusters called mosaic warts. **Venereal warts,** also called **condyloma acuminatum,** are found on the penis, rectum, and female genitalia. This condition is transmitted through sexual contact.

TERM	MEANING
warts (verucca) (*continued*)	**Seborrheic keratosis** (seborrheic warts) usually occur in elderly patients. They are often described as having a "stuck-on" appearance. Treatment includes destruction by the application of salicyclic and lactic acid directly onto the affected area; cryotherapy (freezing with liquid nitrogen); and electrocautery, which destroys tissue using an electric current.

Fungal Skin Infections

TERM	MEANING
tinea barbae	fungal infection of the beard
tinea capitis	fungal infection of the scalp (from caput, Latin for head) also known as ringworm
tinea corporis	fungal infection of the body (from corpus, Latin for body)
tinea cruris	fungal infection commonly seen in males involving the groin and skin between the anus and testicles (also known as jock itch)
tinea pedis	fungal infection of the foot; athlete's foot
tinea unguium (most commonly known as onchyomycosis)	fungal infection of the nail

Note: Fungal infections of the skin are also known as **dermatophytosis** or **dermatomycosis.** Fungal infections occur when the skin is invaded by the **dermatophyte. Tinea** (Latin for moth or worm) or ringworm are the terms commonly used to describe various fungal infections.

Parasitic Skin Infections

scabies	infestation by the itch mite **Note:** Scabies, transmitted by skin-to-skin contact, is also known simply as "the itch."
Lyme's disease	an inflammatory disorder caused by the microorganism Borrelia burgdorferi, which was first discovered in Lyme, Connecticut, in the mid 1970s **Note:** This tick-transmitted microorganism enters the skin at the site of a tick bite and appears as a red macular or papular lesion called erythema chronicum migrans (ECM). This initial symptom may be followed by neurological, cardiac, and joint dysfunctions.
pediculosis	infestation by lice usually resident in the hair **Note:** Pediculosis is transmitted easily from person to person and is often seen in schoolchildren.

Inflammatory Skin Disorders

TERM	MEANING
dermatitis	inflammation of the skin of which there are several types including: **atopic dermatitis,** a chronic inflammation that is allergic in nature. Although the cause is obscure, it tends to occur in families with a history of allergic disorders such as hay fever and asthma. Usually appears between the ages of 1 month to 2 years and may last up to 4 years before it subsides. **contact dermatitis** is an inflammation due to chemical substances that come in contact with the skin such as detergents, cosmetics, or medications. **Photodermatitis** is a type of contact dermatitis caused by exposure to UV light on chemicals applied to the skin such as sunscreen, certain drugs, and cosmetics. **seborrheic dermatitis** is characterized by greasy scales, usually on the scalp, trunk, and face; known as dandruff in its most benign form. In neonates, seborrheic dermatitis is known as "**cradle cap.**"

Erythematous Disorders

TERM	MEANING
erythema multiforme	an inflammation of the skin where the lesions are of multiple forms or shapes, such as macules, papules, pustules, vesicles, and wheals
acne	infection and inflammation of sebaceous glands primarily affecting adolescents and young adults characterized by keratin-plugged pilosebaceous follicles that turn black when open to the air, hence the term **blackhead** **Note:** Factors causing acne are increased hormone and sebum production.
discoid lupus erythematosus (DLE)	disease of unknown origin involving skin eruptions of the face, scalp, neck, and arms causing disfigurement and scarring **Note:** Discoid lupus erythematosus may progress to systemic lupus erythematosus (SLE), which affects not only the skin but multiple organs and can be fatal. The classic lesion of DLE is the **butterfly rash,** where skin eruptions occur on the cheeks and across the bridge of the nose, forming a butterfly appearance.

Dyschromia

TERM	MEANING
dyschromia	abnormal color of the skin There are a variety of dyschromias including: **vitiligo** or **leukoderma,** which is the depigmentation of the skin showing up as a white patch or patches on the epidermis; **café au lait spots,** tan spots on the skin similar in color to coffee with milk

Abnormal skin conditions can arise without apparent cause.

Idiopathic Skin Conditions

TERM	MEANING
pityriasis rosea	characterized by macules, papules, and lesions with silvery scales **Note:** Although the cause of this condition is unknown, it is believed to be noncontagious. It can affect people of any age, but is usually seen in adolescents and young adults.
psoriasis	one of the most common skin conditions, believed to be genetically based although the exact cause is unknown Psoriasis can be triggered by the environment, cold weather, emotional stress, hormonal changes, or pregnancy. Silvery scales, papules, and plaques are the characteristic lesions. Treatment includes **topical applications,** exposure to UV light (the **Goeckerman regimen,** which uses tar baths with UV light), and psoralens (sor'-ah-lens) ultraviolet light A **(PUVA)** (see under treatment).

Disorders of the Hair Follicles

Listed below are the terms used to describe abnormal skin conditions that can result from blocked pores and hair follicles.

TERM	MEANING
hirsutism	excessive hair growth This condition is idiopathic or secondary. Secondary hirsutism may result from pituitary dysfunction or as a side effect of the use of hormones in menopausal women.
alopecia 	medical term for baldness In males, the condition is called **male-pattern baldness** because it is genetically transferred. It relates to the production of an enzyme that causes hair follicles to stop making hair. The condition can also occur in women, but the hair usually thins significantly without falling out completely. **Toxic alopecia** is caused by disease. **Drug-induced** is caused by toxic chemicals, such as in chemotherapy. **Alopecia areata** refers to temporary bald patches.

Benign and Malignant Neoplasms

A **neoplasm** is an abnormal growth characterized by uncontrolled cell multiplication. Neoplasms of the skin, which may be benign or malignant, are listed below.

TERM	MEANING
nevus	a usually benign lesion of the skin commonly known as a birthmark (nevus is Latin for birthmark) **Note:** Although many birthmarks are congenital, some, such as the **vascular spider nevi,** can be acquired (see below). There are many different types of nevi, including moles. The **pigmented hair nevus** is a mole containing hair. Other types of nevi are the **hemangiomas,** a collection of blood vessels near the surface of the skin giving a raised, red appearance. Sometimes referred to as **strawberry nevi, vascular spider nevi,** and **nevi flammeus.**
basal cell carcinoma	most common type of malignant tumor of epithelial tissue, usually occurring on areas of the skin exposed to the sun, although other areas can be affected Metastasis is rare, and although there can be extensive destruction of the localized tissue, the condition is seldom fatal.
squamous cell carcinoma	a malignant condition of the squamous or flat, scalelike cells of epithelial tissue Metastasis can occur.
malignant melanoma	a malignant tumor of the melanocytes Although once rare, malignant melanoma is becoming relatively common. The condition is associated with overexposure to the sun, and if it is detected early, the cure rate is high. If the condition remains undiagnosed, however, metastasis can occur with fatal results.

Physical Examination

During a physical examination, the physician will inspect and palpate (feel) the skin to determine any abnormality of skin color, texture, elasticity, and lesions (blemishes).

Physical Examination of the Skin

COLOR	MEDICAL TERM	CAUSES
redness	erythema	inflammation; anxiety
blue	cyanosis	lack of oxygen
purple	ecchymosis; petechia	bleeding into the skin
yellow	jaundice; icterus	liver pathology
white, pale	pallor	shock; anemia; blood loss

TEXTURE	MEDICAL TERM	DEFINITION
rough and hard; callused	keratosis; squamous	growth of the horny layer of the epidermis
puffy	edematous	accumulation of excess fluid into tissue spaces **Note:** Variations in the degree of edema can be described by edema +, edema ++, edema +++, edema ++++, where each additional + indicates an increased degree of edema. Pitting edema is characterized by an indentation left on the skin following light pressure.
scaly	squamous	scalelike flakes of skin
	desquamation; exfoliation	the shedding of skin; the peeling of the skin in layers

---

Other Terms Signifying Skin Damage

TERM	MEANING
pruritus	itching
weeping	oozing fluid

Symptomatology

Mobility and Turgor   **Mobility** is the readiness with which the skin can be lifted, and **turgor** is the readiness with which the skin returns to its normal position. In the elderly, turgor is sometimes diminished.

Skin Lesions   A **skin lesion** is an abnormality resulting from disease or injury (trauma). Any deviation from the normal appearance of the skin can be called a lesion. Various names are used to describe lesions. Distinguishing the various kinds of skin lesions is important, since they characterize specific diseases.

Lesions are categorized as **primary** or **secondary.** Primary lesions are defects that occur during the early stages of skin disease. Secondary lesions occur as a result of changes to the primary lesion. The tables below describe the various kinds of lesion.

Primary Skin Lesions

TERM	MEANING
cyst	a closed, hollow space or cavity filled with a variety of material that can be solid, semisolid, or liquid Example: **Pilonidal cyst**—a swelling containing hair; located on the sacral area of the back. The hair is enclosed within a sac lined by a membrane. The membrane forms the hollow cavity, and the hair is the solid material that occupies the space.
macule	discolored, unelevated area of the skin Examples: birthmarks, German measles. A lesion of this type greater than 1 cm is called a **patch.**
papule	solid, elevated area of skin A larger, deeper, and more solid lesion is called a **nodule.** Example: acne
polyp	swelling arising from the mucous membrane and extending into the body cavity Also known as **papilloma,** a polyp is a benign tumor of epithelial tissue. It may be precancerous. Two types of polyps are **sessile** and **pedunculated.** The difference between the two is the way the polyp is attached to the underlying tissue. A pedunculated polyp is attached by a small foot or stem (ped/o means foot). A sessile polyp has a broad-base attachment. Polyps are most often found in the nose, rectum, and uterus.

TERM	MEANING
purpura 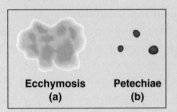 Ecchymosis (a) Petechiae (b)	small purple hemorrhagic lesions caused by bleeding into the skin Examples: **ecchymosis** a bruise; **petechia** a small pinpoint hemorrhage
pustule 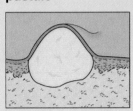	small, elevated area of skin that contains pus Examples: acne, abscesses
wheal 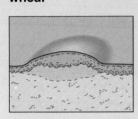	raised, circular area of skin usually pale in the center, surrounded by an erythematous coloration Does not contain fluid or pus but is a solid mass. Examples: mosquito bite, urticaria (hives)
vesicle 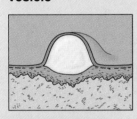	elevated area of skin containing clear fluid A lesion of this type larger than 1 cm is called a **bulla** Example: blister
maculopapular	a combination of macular and papular lesions
maculovesicular	a combination of macular and vesicular lesions
papulopustular	a combination of papular and pustular lesions
papulosquamous	a combination of papular and scaly lesions

TERM	MEANING
atrophy 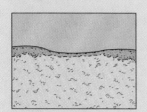	wasting away of the skin, characterized by thinning and loss of the normal skin creases This skin condition, signified by a transluscent look, is sometimes seen in persons of advanced years.
cicatrix 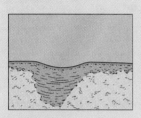	a scar
crust 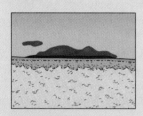	the outer layer or covering that forms over a wound during healing
erosion 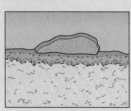	destruction or breakdown of the superficial epidermis Example: blisters that break producing an erosion as seen in some bacterial skin infections If the erosion is produced by scratching or abrasion it is called an **excoriation.**
fissure 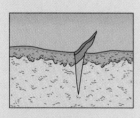	a deep cracklike sore Example: athlete's foot
lichenification 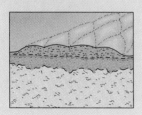	seen in chronic dermatitis where severe itching and scratching results in skin that looks like lichen on a tree (natural skin creases are accentuated)

Secondary Skin Lesions (*concluded*)

TERM	MEANING
scale 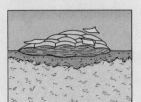	flat flakes of dried, or squamous, skin Examples: dandruff, psoriasis

Lesions Caused by Trauma

TERM	MEANING
contusion	wound in which the skin is not broken
dehiscence	breaking open of a wound, especially following surgery such as abdominal surgery
incision	wound made with a surgical instrument, such as a knife; usually has straight, even edges
laceration	wound with torn, uneven edges
nonpenetrating	injury to the structures beneath the skin but no puncture of the skin itself
open	skin is broken, and there is direct communication to the underlying structures
penetrating/puncture	penetration of the underlying tissue caused by a sharp, long object
perforation	penetration of the underlying tissue and an organ or cavity caused by a sharp, long object

Diagnosis and Treatment

Listed are five of the most common procedures for determining the causes underlying various skin conditions.

Diagnostic Terminology	
TERM	**MEANING**
biopsy	removal of tissue for examination This procedure aids in the diagnosis of conditions from simple dermatoses to malignant neoplasms.
culture and smear and sensitivity	methods of identifying bacteria and determining treatment. A sample is taken from the patient and put in an environment that fosters growth. The microorganism multiplies and thus is readily identified. Then its sensitivity to various antibiotics is observed, so that the most effective one can be prescribed. Cultures are taken from the skin, throat, blood, eye, ear, nose, skin, stool, urine, spinal fluid, etc.
immunofluorescent (IF) tests	study of a specimen stained with a fluorescent dye that highlights any tissue abnormality; may be used in biopsies of scalp
patch test	identifies the allergen (substances producing an allergy) in atopic dermatitis The suspect allergen is placed on the skin under an adhesive patch. If the patient is allergic, an erythematous area will appear. Patch tests are also carried out in diagnostic tests for tuberculosis. See Chapter 14. The Respiratory System.
Wood's light examination	used to identify various skin disorders such as tinea When the suspect sample of skin is examined under ultraviolet light, it turns green or orange-red, depending on the species.

Terminology Relating to Therapy

Many forms of therapy are available to physicians who treat skin disorders. Among those available are the ones listed below.

Medical Treatment	
TERM	**MEANING**
Goeckerman's regimen	regimen of tar and ultraviolet light as a treatment for psoriasis
psoralen ultraviolet A (PUVA)	psoralen ultraviolet A, used in conjunction with methoxsalen, a drug used for repigmentation in such cases as psoriasis and vitiligo

Medical Treatment (*continued*)

TERM	MEANING
topical medications	medications that are rubbed onto a localized area of affected skin for symptomatic relief Topical preparations include: **anti-infectives** used to stop bacterial growth such as impetigo, carbuncles, and furuncles **antifungals** to treat fungal infections such as tinea capitis, tinea barbae, and tinea pedis **antipruritics** to relieve itching associated with contact dermatitis and insect bites **keratolytics** to control dry scaly skin such as psoriasis and dandruff **emollients** soften and soothe the skin in such conditions as sunburn and diaper rash **scabicides** and **pediculicides** used to kill scabies and lice

Surgical Treatment

TERM	MEANING
cryotherapy	surgical destruction of tissue by freezing Liquid nitrogen, which boils at −321 degrees F, is often used in attaining the low temperatures necessary for cryotherapy.
electrodesiccation and **curettage**	use of electricity to kill tissue and the removal of the dead tissue by scraping This procedure is used on warts and basal cell carcinoma.
electrolysis	destruction of tissue by an electric current Electrolysis is used to destroy hair follicles, thus removing body hair.
laser therapy	a beam of light used to remove skin lesions such as hemangiomas and papillomas
liposuction	used to withdraw (aspirate) unwanted fat from the subcutaneous tissue Complications include infection, bruising, necrosis, and scarring. **Note:** This surgical procedure involves the introduction of a tube into the subcutaneous layer. The tube is attached to a strong suction apparatus that sucks out unwanted fat, contouring the body, and making it more aesthetically pleasing. Although most liposuction is done for cosmetic reasons, it can also be performed for the removal of lipomas.

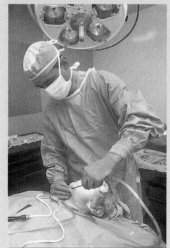

Surgical Treatment (concluded)

TERM	MEANING
skin grafting	skin grafting is necessary when the skin will not heal spontaneously, as in a full-thickness burn Types include: autograft, allograft (heterograft), and xenograft.
surgical debridement	the removal of any unwanted tissue (calluses or corns) or cleansing a contaminated site (burns, etc.)
surgical excision	surgical removal of lesions, such as moles, lipomas, or warts
Mohs' surgery	the layered removal of a malignant growth Layered removal involves extracting the tumor in thin horizontal layers. Each layer is frozen, sliced thinly, and examined under a microscope to determine the extent of the cancer. Successive layers are removed until microscopic examination reveals no further cancerous cells.

▶ 6.7 ABBREVIATIONS

ABBREVIATION	MEANING	ABBREVIATION	MEANING
bx	biopsy	**HPV**	human papilloma virus
C	centigrade	**HSV–1**	herpes simplex virus type 1
decub	decubitus	**HSV–2**	herpes simplex virus type 2
DLE	discoid lupus erythematosus	**IF**	immunofluorescent
ECM	erythema chronicum migrans	**LE**	lupus erythematous
EM	erythema multiforme	**PUVA**	psoralens ultraviolet light A
F	Fahrenheit	**SLE**	systemic lupus erythematosus
		UV	ultraviolet

Practice Quiz

Short Answer

Answers to all exercise questions in chapter 6 appear in Appendix A.

1. Name the five epidermal layers of the skin. _____
   _____
   _____

2. Name the layer of the epidermis responsible for regeneration. _____
   _____

3. The corneum stratum is also known as the _____
   layer.

4. If there are no blood vessels in the epidermal layer, how does the epidermis
   receive oxygen? _____
   _____

5. What kind of tissue is found in the epidermis? the dermis? the subcutaneous
   layer? _____
   _____

6. Name four functions of the dermis. _____
   _____

7. List three functions of the subcutaneous tissue. _____
   _____

8. State the location of the lunula and nail bed. _____

9. Eccrine glands secrete in response to _____ and apocrine
   glands secrete in response to _____ .

10. List three glands found in the dermis, their secretions, and the function of
    each secretion. _____
    _____
    _____

► **EXERCISE 6–2**

Vocabulary Study

Definitions

Write definitions for the
following terms.

1. albinism _____

2. apocrine glands _____

3. carotene _____

4. cerumen _____

5. ceruminous glands _____

6. collagen _____

7. corium _____

8. decubitus ulcers _____

9. dermis _____

10. eccrine glands _____

11. eleidin _____

12. epidermis _____

13. epithelial cell _____

14. eponychium _____

15. fibroblast _____

16. hair follicle _____

17. heparin _____

18. histamine _____

19. hyperkeratosis _____

20. keratin _____

21. lunula _____

22. macrophage _____

23. mast cell _____

24. melanin _____

25. necrotic tissue   _____

26. plasma cell   _____

27. pyogenic   _____

28. sebaceous glands   _____

29. stratum basale   _____

30. stratum germinativum   _____

31. stratum granulosum   _____

32. stratum lucidum   _____

33. stratum spinosum   _____

34. subcutaneous tissue   _____

35. sweat glands   _____

▶ EXERCISE 6–3

Matching

Match the term in Column A with its meaning in Column B.

Matching Terms with Meanings

Column A	Column B
1. erythema _____	A. discolored, unelevated area of skin
2. petechiae _____	B. wasting away of the skin
3. macule _____	C. elevated area of skin containing solid material
4. polyp _____	D. redness
5. vesicle _____	E. the breaking open of a surgical incision
6. papule _____	F. growth arising from the mucous membrane and extending into the body cavity
7. excoriation _____	G. a blister
8. atrophy _____	H. destruction of the skin by scratching
9. dehiscence _____	I. broken skin with underlying structures in communication with air
10. open wound _____	J. ecchymosis

Match the term in Column A with its definition in Column B.

Column A

11. cyanosis _____
12. fissure _____
13. squamous _____
14. incision _____
15. wheal _____
16. crust _____
17. icterus _____
18. laceration _____
19. dermis _____
20. cicatrix _____
21. ecchymosis _____
22. hemangioma _____

Column B

A. a blue discoloration of the skin

B. a yellow discoloration of the skin

C. a scar

D. a cracklike wound

E. a wound with uneven edges

F. a wound with a straight edge

G. a red, circular skin lesion with a pale center

H. benign tumor composed of blood vessels

I. a scab

J. bleeding into the skin

K. corium

L. scaly

Match the term in Column A with its definition in Column B.

Column A

23. desquamation _____
24. pruritus _____
25. edema _____
26. Wood's light _____
27. patch test _____

Column B

A. excessive accumulation of fluid in tissues

B. the procedure carried out to identify the allergen in allergic dermatitis

C. shedding of skin symptomatic of some types of skin disorders

D. itching

E. procedure for diagnosing tinea

▶**EXERCISE 6–4**

Identifying Terms for Skin Conditions and Therapeutic Procedures

Multiple Choice

Underline the correct answer.

1. A group of boils is known as a (carbuncle, furuncle).

2. The shedding of necrotic tissue is called (exfoliation, ulcer).

3. Dermatitis that is caused by an allergy is called (atopic, seborrheic).

4. A fungal infection of the scalp is called (tinea capitis, tinea corporis).

5. (Pediculosis, Psoriasis) is a papulosquamous disorder characterized by silvery, scaly lesions.

6. (Alopecia, Hirsutism) is the term used to refer to excessive hair growth, usually in women.

7. Cold sore is caused by the virus (HSV 1, HSV 2).

8. (Condylomata acuminata, Plantar warts) are located on the sole of the foot.

9. (Nevus, Wart) is a term used to refer to a birthmark.

10. The therapeutic destruction of tissue by an electric current is called (electrolysis, debridement).

11. The destruction of tissue by freezing is called (debridement, cryotherapy).

12. (Mohs' surgery, electrolysis) is a treatment for malignant melanoma.

13. (Cryotherapy, Curettage) is the scraping away of extraneous material.

14. (Debridement, Mohs' surgery) refers to the removal of necrotic tissue and foreign material accumulated in an injury site.

15. (Mohs' surgery, PUVA) is a treatment for psoriasis.

▶EXERCISE 6–5

Spelling

Place a check mark beside all misspelled words in the list that follows. Correctly spell those that you checked off.

Spelling Practice

1. caratin ☐ _____

2. germinatvum ☐ _____

3. collangenous ☐ _____

4. integumentary ☐ _____

5. seruminous ☐ _____

6. erythema ☐ _____

7. echymosis ☐ _____

8. vesicle ☐ _____

9. dehisence ☐ _____

10. immunofluorescent ☐ _____

11. impetago ☐ _____

12. pitiriasis ☐ _____

13. soriasis ☐ _____

14. hirsutism ☐ _____

15. verruca ☐ _____

16. curettage ☐ _____

17. electrodesiccation ☐ _____

18. keloid ☐ _____

19. pruritus ☐ _____

20. lichenification ☐ _____

Use of Medical Terms in Context

Medical Terms in Context

Define the terms in boldface type as they are used in context.

UNIVERSITY HOSPITAL ✚

SUMMARY RECORD

A 75-year-old farmer was referred to Dr. S. for management of **malignant melanoma** located on his chest area. On admission, he gives a history of a **pigmented** lesion on his anterior chest for the last 20 years. However, over the last several months prior to admission, this lesion became **nodular** and in the past several weeks prior to admission it also was **symptomatic,** with episodic **hemorrhaging.**

There was no family history of melanoma and on past history Mr. S. suffered only from **arthritis.** He did not have any other significant medical history.

PHYSICAL EXAMINATION:

On examination on admission, his blood pressure was 160/90. Head and neck exam revealed that the **pharynx** was clear and the neck did not reveal any **lymphadenopathy.** He did not have any **axillary** or **inguinal** lymphadenopathy. Chest exam was clear and **cardiovascular** exam was normal. **Abdominal** exam revealed that the abdomen was soft, and there was no **visceromegaly.**

On skin examination, the patient had scattered **seborrheic keratosis** and a few **dysplastic nevi** located over his trunk. On examination of the skin of the chest, a large pigmented lesion measuring 5 cm in diameter is present, and this lesion was a nodule and there appeared to be some areas of old blood. The color of the lesion was black and blue.

DISCHARGE DIAGNOSIS: MALIGNANT MELANOMA

SIGNATURE OF DOCTOR IN CHARGE _____

Define the terms in the space provided.

1. malignant melanoma _____

2. pigmented _____

3. nodular _____

4. symptomatic _____

5. hemorrhaging _____

6. arthritis _____

7. pharynx _____

8. lymphadenopathy _____

9. axillary _____

10. inguinal _____

11. cardiovascular _____

12. abdominal _____

13. visceromegaly _____

14. seborrheic keratosis _____

15. dysplastic nevi _____

UNIVERSITY HOSPITAL

SUMMARY RECORD

ADMISSION DATE: April 14, 19-

DISCHARGE DATE: April 28, 19-

REASON FOR ADMISSION: This 32-year-old male was outside burning a bush when he poured some gasoline on the fire and the fire came toward him, burning both hands and his face. On presentation to the local hospital, he had no **respiratory** complications and was transferred here with a **diagnosis** of 27% burns to the hands and face.

PAST HISTORY: Unremarkable

PHYSICAL EXAMINATION: He was not distressed, blood pressure was 110/70, pulse 80 and regular. Examination of the face revealed **deep partial thickness** burns to his face including his right ear and more **superficial** burns over the lower face and neck. Chest exam revealed good air entry **bilaterally.** His right hand had deep partial and full thickness burns with skin **sloughing** and blistering. His left hand had more superficial burns with some blistering as well. Our impression here was that he had burns to both hands and face totalling approximately 5% body surface area.

INVESTIGATION: Routine laboratory work done. **Swabs** of his wounds revealed some **streptococcus.** Negative for **staphylococcus.** The patient was brought into hospital and treated with pain killers and dressing changes. After a couple of days, his burns had progressed to their full extent, and he was brought to the operating room for **debridement** and **split thickness skin graft.** The burns to his left hand and face were left to heal with just dressing changes.

The patient was discharged on April 28th in good condition.

DIAGNOSIS:

  5% BODY SURFACE AREA BURNS INCLUDING

  BILATERAL HANDS AND FACE.

OPERATION PERFORMED: SPLIT THICKNESS BURN GRAFTING TO RIGHT HAND.

SIGNATURE OF DOCTOR IN CHARGE _____

Define the terms in the space provided.

16. respiratory _____

17. diagnosis _____

18. deep partial thickness _____

19. superficial _____

20. bilaterally _____

21. sloughing _____

22. swabs _____

23. streptococcus _____

24. staphylococcus _____

25. debridement _____

26. split thickness skin graft _____

►EXERCISE 6-7

Crossword Puzzle

The Integumentary System

Across

1 Arising from outside the organism
3 Pertaining to fat
4 Dry and scaly skin
5 Abnormal condition of the spiny layer of skin
9 Yellow skin
11 Lack of sweat
12 The outermost layer of skin
13 Thread-shaped
14 Study of the skin
15 Bloodless

Down

2 Incision of eschar to relieve the tightness of a burned area
3 Breakdown of the spiny layer of the skin
6 Tissue transplant between individuals of the same species but of different genetic backgrounds
7 Bluish discoloration of the skin
8 Pertaining to cerumen
9 Excessive carotene in the blood
10 Profuse sweating

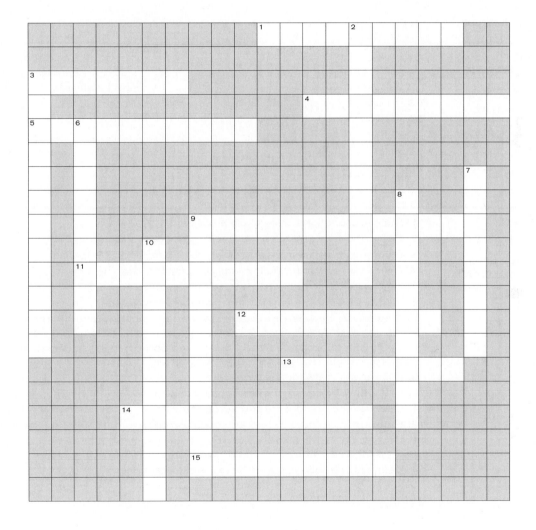

7 THE SKELETAL SYSTEM

CHAPTER OBJECTIVES

After completing this chapter, the student will be able to do the following:

1. State five functions of the skeletal system.
2. Define the terms that describe the microscopic structures of bone.
3. Differentiate between osteocytes, osteoblasts, and osteoclasts.
4. Define the terms relating to macroscopic structures of bone.
5. Define the terms relating to bone classification.
6. Identify and distinguish between bone marking types.
7. Differentiate between the axial and appendicular skeletons and name the bones included in each.
8. Describe and locate the major bones and bone markings of the skull, vertebrae, thoracic cage, pectoral girdle, pelvic girdle, and upper and lower extremities.
9. Differentiate between the three categories of joints.
10. Compare and contrast different types of joint movements.
11. Describe the anatomical structures of the knee.
12. Pronounce, analyze, define, and spell common terms of the skeletal system.
13. List and define terms describing the physical examination, abnormal conditions, and diagnostic and therapeutic procedures common to the skeletal system.
14. Define abbreviations common to the skeletal system.

WORD ELEMENT	ELEMENT TYPE	DEFINITION	WORD ELEMENT	ELEMENT TYPE	DEFINITION
arthr/o; articul/o	root	joint	olecran/o	root	olecranon; elbow
brachi/o	root	arm	ost/e/o; osse/o	root	bone
calcane/o	root	heel	pector/o	root	chest
carp/o	root	wrist	pelv/o	root	pelvic bone
cervic/o	root	neck	phalang/o	root	one of the bones making up the fingers or toes
chondr/o	root	cartilage			
clavicul/o	root	clavicle; collar bone	rachi/o	root	spine
coccyg/o	root	coccyx; tailbone	radi/o	root	radius
			sacr/o	root	sacrum
cost/o	root	rib	scapul/o	root	scapula; shoulder blade
crani/o	root	skull	synovi/o	root	synovium (synovial membrane) tendon sheath; synovia (synovial fluid)
dactyl/o	root	finger or toe			
ethm/o	root	sieve; ethmoid bone			
femor/o	root	femur; thigh bone			
fibul/o	root	fibula; small bone of the lower leg	tars/o	root	tarsals
			tempor/o	root	temporal bone
humer/o	root	humerus; upper arm	thorac/o	root	chest
			tibi/o	root	tibia; shinbone
ili/o	root	ilium; hip	uln/o	root	ulna
lumb/o	root	loin; lower back	vertebr/o; spondyl/o	root	vertebra
mandibul/o	root	lower jaw			
myel/o	root	bone marrow	xiph/o	root	sword; xiphoid process
occipit/o	root	occiput; back part of the skull			

⬦ 7.1 GENERAL ANATOMY AND PHYSIOLOGY OF BONE

The skeletal system consists of 206 bones and the joints. The skeletal system has five main functions: support, protection, movement, mineral storage, and the formation and development of blood cells.

The skeleton acts as a support by forming the body's framework onto which everything else is attached, while at the same time protecting the underlying soft-tissue structures; for example, the skull protects the brain, the rib cage protects the heart and lungs, and so on.

Bones combine with muscles, tendons, and ligaments to allow movement at the joints. They store calcium and phosphorus, releasing these minerals into the blood when the concentration of blood calcium and phosphorus is low and take up these minerals when the concentration of calcium and phosphorus is higher than the normal value. This example of homeostasis controls the extracellular fluid levels of calcium and phosphorus. Red blood cells (RBC) and white blood cells (WBC) are both produced in the red bone marrow.

Microscopic Bone Structure

Bone cells include **osteoblasts, osteocytes,** and **osteoclasts. Osteoblasts** are immature bone cells responsible for the formation of new bone. This formation is called **ossification** or **osteogenesis. Osteocytes** are mature bone cells, and **osteoclasts** are bone cells that break down and reabsorb bone.

Osteoblasts secrete collagen, the main intercellular substance found in all types of connective tissue. However, deposits of inorganic salts, such as calcium carbonate and calcium phosphate, cause the collagen in bone to **calcify** and become hard, forming a special connective tissue called **osseous** tissue. Osteoblasts are most active during the growth periods of early life and adolescence. When osteoblasts become part of an adult's bone structure, they are called osteocytes. They continue building bone during adulthood.

The skeletal structure constantly adjusts to accommodate changes in the size, weight, and strength of muscles; the shifting relationship of bones to one another; and the resulting stresses on the body. Osteoblasts and osteocytes respond to the changes in the skeletal structure by forming new bone, while osteoclasts take on the opposite function, that of disintegrating bone tissue. Together, bone cells form a part of the body's homeostatic system, remodeling bones to suit the body's changing structural needs.

Macroscopic Bone Structure

All bones contain **spongy** or **cancellous** bone, which, as one of its names suggests, looks like a sponge with many spaces. All bones also contain **compact** bone, which is dense and hard. The differences between these two types of bone are evident in a chicken's thigh bone. It has a bulbous top and bottom which feels spongy because it contains spaces within the tissue (cancellous). The shaft of that same bone, however, is dense and unyielding (compact).

Bone Classification

Bones are classified according to their shapes: long, short, flat, and irregular. See Figure 7–1.

The long bones include the **humerus** (upper arm), the **femur** (thigh), and the **tibia** (shinbone). Examples of short bones are found in the wrist and ankle. Flat bones include the **skull,** the **sternum** (breast bone), **ribs,** and **shoulder.** Irregular bones are those of mixed shapes, such as the **vertebrae,** bones of the **ear,** and the **patella.**

Long bones have seven distinct parts: the **diaphysis** (dī-ăf′-ĭ-sĭs), **endosteum** (ĕn-dŏs′-tē-ŭm), **epiphysis** (ĕ-pĭf′ĭ-sĭs), **articular cartilage** (ăr-tĭk′-ū-lăr kăr′-tĭ-lĭj), **epiphyseal** (ĕp″-ĭ-fĭz′-ē-ăl) **plate** or cartilage, **periosteum** (pĕr-ē-ŏs′-tē-ŭm), and **medullary** (mĕd′-ū-lăr-ē) **cavity.** See Figure 7–2. Diaphysis refers to the long shaft of the bone, which contains compact bone and a thin layer of spongy bone. The diaphysis provides strong support without itself being heavy.

FIGURE 7–1

Bone Classification

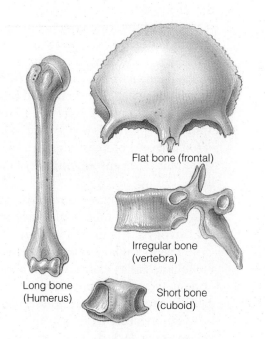

Flat bone (frontal)

Irregular bone
(vertebra)

Long bone
(Humerus)

Short bone
(cuboid)

FIGURE 7–2

Structure of Long Bones (a) Diaphysis, epiphysis, and medullary cavity. (b) Compact bone surrounding yellow bone
marrow in the medullary cavity. (c) Spongy bone and compact bone in the epiphysis.

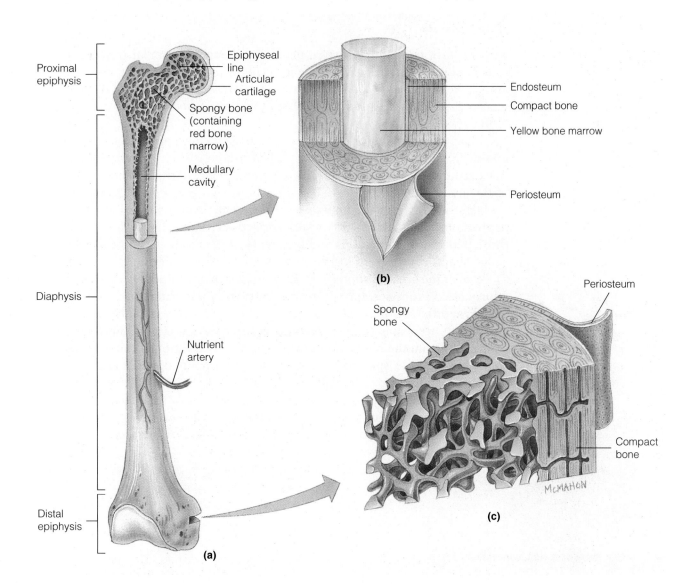

Proximal
epiphysis

Epiphyseal
line

Articular
cartilage

Spongy bone
(containing
red bone
marrow)

Medullary
cavity

Diaphysis

Nutrient
artery

Distal
epiphysis

Endosteum

Compact bone

Yellow bone marrow

Periosteum

(b)

Periosteum

Spongy
bone

Compact
bone

MCMAHON

(c)

(a)

The endosteum is the long bone's inner lining, which functions in osteogenesis, the production of new bone. The epiphysis (the bulbous proximal and distal segments of the long bone) contains mostly spongy bone. It provides for muscle attachment and stability at the joint.

Articular cartilage covers the epiphysis on the joint surfaces where two bones meet. It is the "gristle," the white, tough cartilage sitting on top of the epiphysis, which acts as a padding.

The epiphyseal plate is a cartilaginous line between the epiphysis and diaphysis at both ends of the long bone. Growth occurs at this line as new cartilage is formed and old cartilage is replaced by bone. Once growth stops, the epiphyseal plate stops producing cartilage, becomes bone, and is called the **epiphyseal line.**

The periosteum surrounds the diaphysis. It holds muscles firmly in place as the periosteal fingers interlace with the muscle fibers. It contains osteoblasts (or osteocytes) and the blood vessels necessary for bone growth and repair.

The medullary cavity is the hollow center of the diaphysis. In children, the medullary cavity contains red bone marrow, and in adults, it contains yellow bone marrow. In the early years of life, red bone marrow is needed for blood cell production (**hematopoiesis**). As one gets older and the need for blood cell production decreases, fat replaces the red marrow and gives the marrow its yellow color. Adults normally retain red marrow in the skull, sternum, and ribs. Some conditions may also cause yellow marrow in adults to convert to red marrow for the resumption of hematopoiesis.

Bone Markings

A bone marking is simply that: a mark on a bone. It is similar in some respects to a familiar landmark. When giving general directions to our house, for example, we might say we live near a well-known shopping center. Likewise, bone markings serve as descriptive addresses for the location of muscles, nerves, and blood vessels.

There are two major categories of bone markings: **projections** or **processes** and **depressions**. A projection is a part of a bone rising above the level of the bone around it. A depression is the opposite, a part of the bone below the level of the area around it.

Just as different landmarks have different names, so do projections and depressions. There are two types of projections: those that fit into a joint and those that attach to tendons and ligaments. Projections that fit into a joint are called **heads, condyles,** or **facets.** Although all of these bone markings rise above the level of the areas around them, they differ in shape. Both heads and condyles are rounded processes, but a facet has a smooth, flat surface.

Five different projections attach tendons and ligaments. These projections are named according to their shapes. A **trochanter** is a very large process or protrusion from the bone, a **tuberosity** is a slight elevation, a **tubercle** is a small rounded process, a **spinous process** is sharp and pointed, and a **crest** is a sharp projection appearing as a ridge.

Four types of depressions are named according to their shapes. A **fossa** is a hollow space, a **sinus** is a cavity within a bone, a **foramen** is a hole through which blood vessels and nerves pass, and a **meatus** is a long, tube-shaped depression. Table 7–1 gives a list of bone markings.

TABLE 7–1

Bone Markings

Projections:

PROJECTIONS THAT FIT INTO A JOINT

BONE MARKING	DESCRIPTION	EXAMPLE
head	rounded process	head of femur
condyle	rounded process	proximal tibia
facet	smooth, flat surface	rib

PROJECTIONS THAT ACT AS AN ATTACHMENT FOR TENDONS AND LIGAMENTS

BONE MARKING	DESCRIPTION	EXAMPLE
trochanter	very large process	greater and lesser trochanter of femur
tuberosity	slight elevation	deltoid tuberosity of humerus
tubercle	small rounded process	greater and lesser tubercle of the humerus
spinous process	sharp, pointed process	vertebra
crest	ridge	ilium

Depressions

BONE MARKING	DESCRIPTION	EXAMPLE
fossa	hollow space	iliac fossa
sinus	cavity or space in a bone	frontal sinus
foramen	a hole for the passage of blood vessels and nerves	foramen magnum of the occipital bone
meatus	a long, tube-shaped depression	external auditory meatus of the ear

▷ 7.2 SKELETON

The skeleton is divided in two major parts: the **axial** and **appendicular skeletons**. See Figure 7–3. The axial skeleton, which consists of the **skull, hyoid bone, vertebral column,** and **thoracic cage,** occupies the central area of the body and attaches to the appendicular skeleton. The appendicular skeleton includes the **pectoral girdle, upper extremities, pelvic girdle,** and **lower limbs.**

FIGURE 7–3 **The Human Skeletal System** (a) Anterior view. (b) Posterior view.

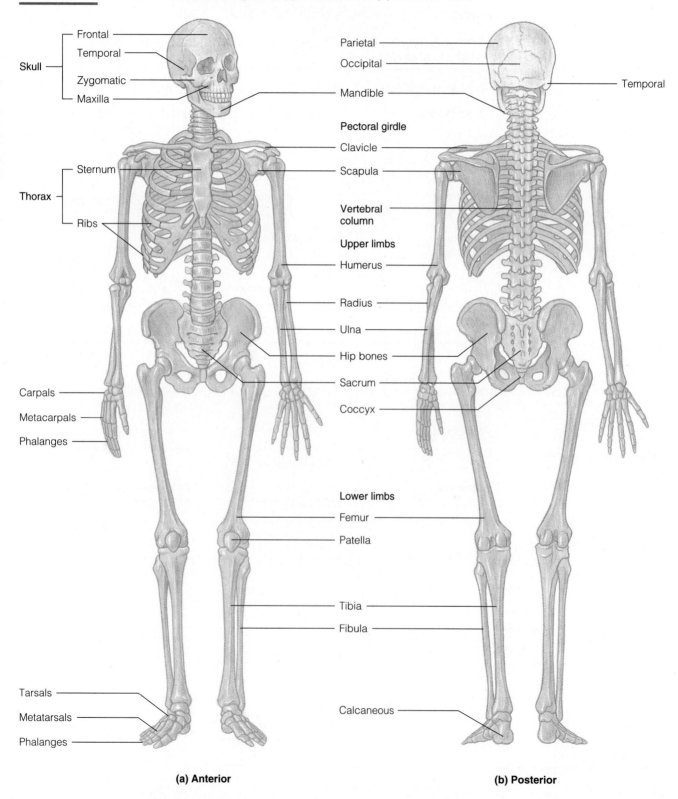

(a) Anterior (b) Posterior

Axial Skeleton

Skull   The skull consists of the cranial bones and the facial bones.

Cranial Bones   The **cranial bones** protect the brain. There are eight cranial bones, four of which are paired. The paired **parietal** bones form the top of the skull, and the two **temporal** bones are thin bones, commonly known as the temples, located on either side of the cranium. The **frontal** bone forms the forehead and the superior segments of the orbits in which the eyes sit, and the **occipital** bone is located at the back of the skull above the neck. See Figure 7–4.

The **sphenoid** bone, which resembles wings of a bat, contains the **sella turcica,** a slight depression that houses the pituitary gland.

Paranasal sinuses, hollow spaces within the skull bones, are lined with mucous membrane. They are named after the bones in which they lie, and so

FIGURE 7–4   **The Cranial Bones**

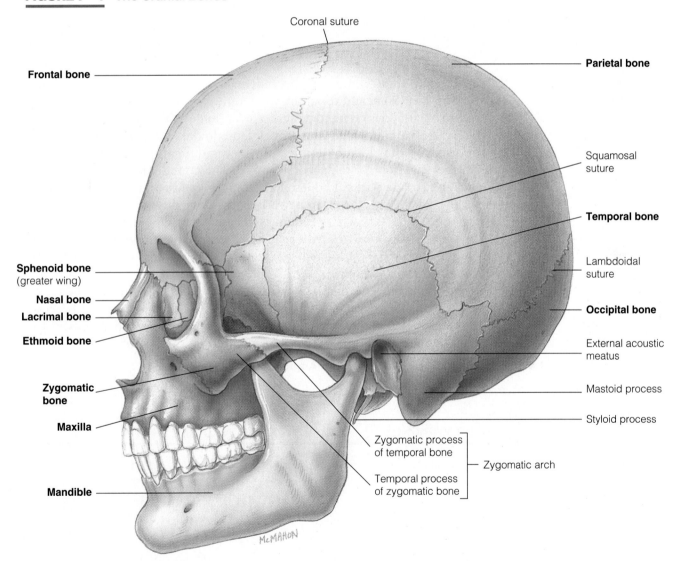

Coronal suture

Parietal bone

Frontal bone

Squamosal suture

Temporal bone

Lambdoidal suture

Sphenoid bone
(greater wing)

Occipital bone

Nasal bone

Lacrimal bone

External acoustic meatus

Ethmoid bone

Mastoid process

Zygomatic bone

Styloid process

Maxilla

Zygomatic process of temporal bone

Temporal process of zygomatic bone

Zygomatic arch

Mandible

McMAHON

FIGURE 7–5

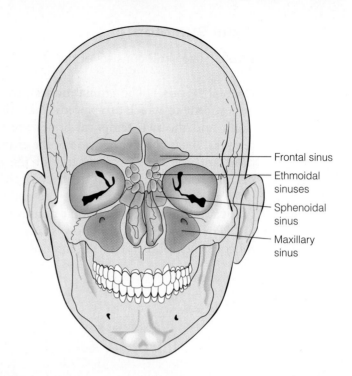

Frontal sinus

Ethmoidal sinuses

Sphenoidal sinus

Maxillary sinus

they are called frontal, ethmoid, sphenoid, and maxillary sinuses. They function mainly to lighten bone and to aid in phonation (see Figure 7–5).

The cranial bones come together to form immovable joints called **sutures,** of which there are four: **sagittal, coronal, lambdoidal,** and **squamosal.** The parietal bones are joined at the midline at the sagittal suture. The frontal bone joins the parietal bone at the coronal suture. The lambdoidal stuture joins the occipital bone to the parietal bones. The temporal bones unite with the parietal bone at the squamosal suture. In newborns, the cranial bones have not united, leaving "soft spots" known as **fontanels.** These soft membranous areas allow the skull bones to move toward each other, narrowing the head as it passes through the birth canal during delivery. The fontanels eventually close between the ages of 12 and 18 months.

The **foramen magnum,** a bone marking, is a large hole for the passage of nerves into the spinal cord. Other bone markings include the **mastoid process, styloid process, zygomatic arch, frontal sinuses,** and the **ethmoidal sinuses.** Table 7–2 lists the cranial bones, major bone markings, and sutures.

TABLE 7–2 Cranial Bones with Major Bone Markings and Adjacent Sutures

MAJOR CRANIAL BONE	BONE MARKINGS	ADJACENT SUTURES
frontal	frontal sinuses	coronal
parietal (two)		sagittal, coronal, lambdoidal, and squamosal
occipital	foramen magnum	lambdoidal
temporal (two)	mastoid process, styloid process, and zygomatic process	squamosal and lambdoidal
sphenoid	sphenoid sinuses and sella turcica	coronal and squamosal
ethmoid	ethmoid sinuses	coronal

Facial Bones   The facial bones include the **inferior nasal conchae**, the **superior nasal conchae**, the **middle nasal conchae**, the **mandible**, the **maxillae**, the **nasal**, the **palatine**, the **vomer**, the **lacrimal** and the **zygomatic** bones. See Figure 7–6.

The inferior nasal conchae, also known as **turbinates,** are located on the lateral walls of each nasal cavity. Two other conchae, the superior and middle nasal conchae, are considered part of the ethmoid bone. The mandible, the lower jaw bone, is the only movable facial bone. The mandible unites with the temporal bone at the **temporomandibular joint (TMJ).**

FIGURE 7–6   **The Facial Bones**

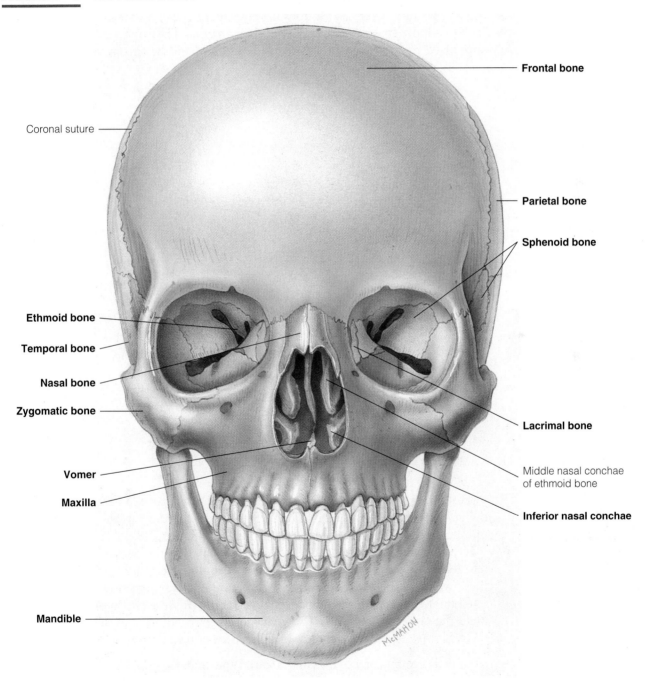

- Frontal bone
- Coronal suture
- Parietal bone
- Sphenoid bone
- Ethmoid bone
- Temporal bone
- Nasal bone
- Zygomatic bone
- Lacrimal bone
- Vomer
- Maxilla
- Middle nasal conchae of ethmoid bone
- Inferior nasal conchae
- Mandible

McMAHON

The maxillae are paired bones that form the upper jaw, the orbits, the nasal cavities, and the roof of the mouth. The maxillae contain the maxillary sinuses. The paired nasal bones form the bridge of the nose. The two palatine bones form the posterior aspect of the roof of the mouth, called the hard palate. The vomer bone makes up the inferior segment of the nasal septum.

The paired zygomatic bones are commonly referred to as the cheekbones. Each one has a temporal process extending posteriorly to meet the zygomatic process of the temporal bone. The union of these two processes forms the **zygomatic arch,** shown in Figure 7–4.

Hyoid Bone The **hyoid bone** is a u-shaped bone located in the neck between the larynx and lower jaw. It does not articulate with any other bone but rather lends support to several muscles and ligaments. The tongue, for example, is supported by the hyoid bone. It is the only bone in the throat. See Figure 7–7.

FIGURE 7–7

The Hyoid Bone and Adjacent Structures

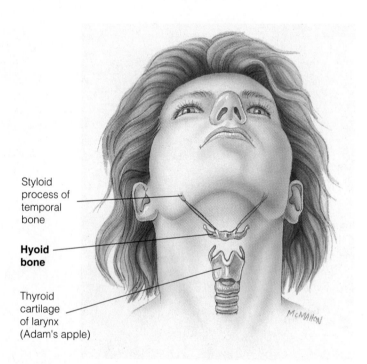

Styloid process of temporal bone

Hyoid bone

Thyroid cartilage of larynx (Adam's apple)

Vertebrae A **vertebra** is an individual bone. Thirty-three vertebrae make up the spinal column. The vertebrae are grouped according to their location and numbered sequentially within each group. See Figure 7–8.

Seven **cervical vertebrae** (C1–C7) are located in the neck, 12 **thoracic vertebrae** (T1–T12) are located in the chest, 5 **lumbar vertebrae** (L1–L5) reside in the lower back below the lumbar region, and 5 **sacral vertebrae** (fused to form one bone), along with the 4 **coccygeal vertebrae** (fused to form one bone), complete the vertebral column. The coccygeal vertebrae are commonly known as the tailbone. Together, the vertebrae have several functions:

1. Form a protective casing around the spinal cord
2. Support the head
3. Provide for movement of the trunk
4. Serve as an attachment of the ribs

FIGURE 7–8

The Vertebral Column

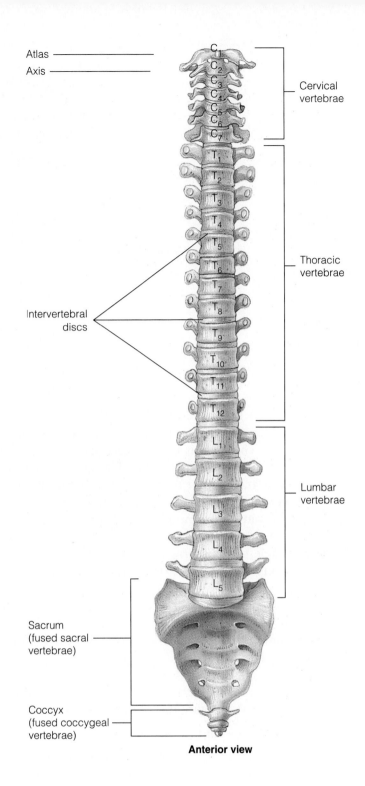

Atlas

Axis

Cervical
vertebrae

Thoracic
vertebrae

Intervertebral
discs

Lumbar
vertebrae

Sacrum
(fused sacral
vertebrae)

Coccyx
(fused coccygeal
vertebrae)

Anterior view

II–7

FIGURE 7–9

**Characteristics of a
Typical Vertebra**

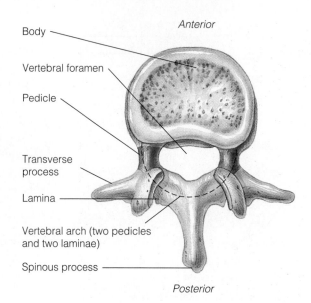

Body

Vertebral foramen

Pedicle

Transverse
process

Lamina

Vertebral arch (two pedicles
and two laminae)

Spinous process

Anterior

Posterior

Superior view

A typical vertebra, illustrated in Figure 7–9, has the following anatomical parts: a **body,** two **pedicles,** and two **laminae.**

The body is the anterior, oval part of the vertebra, and the two pedicles extend posteriorly from it. The two laminae extend from the pedicles. The pedicles and laminae together form the posterior segment of the vertebra called the vertebral arch. The vertebral arch (also called the neural arch) and the body of the vertebra form a hole referred to as the **vertebral foramen,** through which the spinal cord passes along the entire length of the spinal column. Finally, a single **spinous process** extends posteriorly from the vertebral arch, and two **transverse processes** extend laterally, one from each side of each vertebra.

Some vertebrae do not contain all the anatomical features just described. For example, C1 has no body and is no larger than a normal vertebral foramen. It has two facets that support the skull. For this reason, C1 is also called **atlas,** for the character in Greek mythology who supported the world on his shoulders. See Figure 7–10.

The second cervical bone, C2, is sometimes called the **axis.** It has a **dens** (a toothlike structure) also known as the **odontoid process.** This process allows the head to rotate on its axis. Two other atypical vertebrae are the **sacrum** and **coccyx.**

FIGURE 7—10

Atypical Vertebra (a) C1
(atlas). (b) C2 (axis).

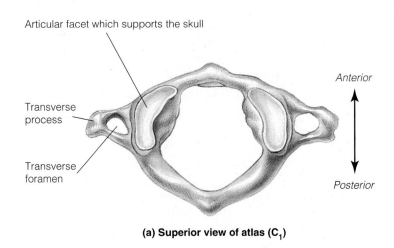

Articular facet which supports the skull

Transverse
process

Transverse
foramen

Anterior

Posterior

(a) Superior view of atlas (C₁)

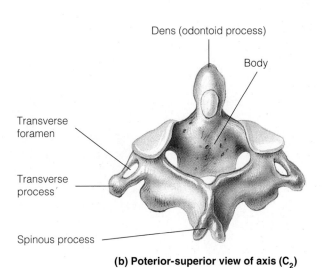

Dens (odontoid process)

Body

Transverse
foramen

Transverse
process

Spinous process

(b) Poterior-superior view of axis (C₂)

Intervertebral Discs   Situated between the vertebral bodies, **intervertebral, fibrocartilaginous discs** absorb the shock of daily movements such as running
and walking. Each intervertebral disc is filled with a gelatinous material, **nucleus
pulposus,** surrounded by a fibrocartilaginous ring called **annulus fibrosus.** At
times, the nucleus pulposus becomes displaced, which may put pressure on a
nearby nerve. This painful condition is commonly known as a slipped disc or,
properly, a **herniated disc.**

Intervertebral Foramina   Literally meaning a hole between the vertebrae, the
intervertebral foramina provides a passage for spinal nerves to the periphery of
the body. Unlike a typical bone marking, these foramina are not actual holes
within a bone, but are natural openings formed by the placement of one vertebra
above the other.

Thoracic Cage The thoracic cage includes the sternum, costal cartilage, ribs, and thoracic vertebrae to which the ribs are attached. See Figure 7–11.

The sternum is a flat bone located in the center, anterior segment of the thoracic cage. It has three parts, the **manubrium,** the **body,** and the **xiphoid process.** The manubrium and body are attached to the ribs through the costal cartilage. The xiphoid process attaches to several abdominal muscles. See Figure 7–12.

Costal cartilage is the tough, fibrous connective tissue connecting the sternum to the ribs anteriorly. The ribs, 12 pairs in total, are described as true ribs or false ribs. The true ribs, the first 7 pairs (starting from the top), are attached directly to the sternum through the costal cartilage. The false ribs comprise 3 pairs that attach to the sternum through the costal cartilage of pair number 7

FIGURE 7–11

Thoracic Cage, Anterior View

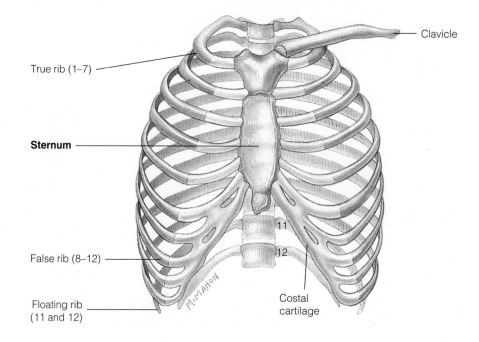

Clavicle

True rib (1–7)

Sternum

False rib (8–12)

Floating rib (11 and 12)

11

12

Costal cartilage

FIGURE 7–12

The Sternum, Anterior View

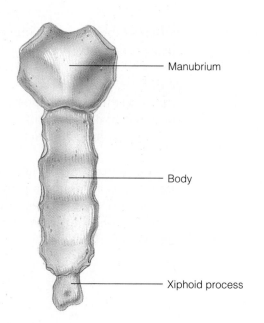

Manubrium

Body

Xiphoid process

and 2 pairs that do not attach to the sternum at all. Because these last 2 pairs are free-standing, they are called floating ribs. Posteriorly, the 12 pairs of ribs attach to the 12 thoracic vertebrae.

Appendicular Skeleton

Pectoral Girdle   The **pectoral** (shoulder) girdle to which the upper extremities are attached includes the **clavicle** (collarbone) and **scapula** (shoulder blade). The scapula is composed of a pair of flat, triangular-shaped bones located on the top posterior of the ribs, covering the second to the seventh pair. Bone markings of the scapula include the **spinous process,** a sharply pointed prominence; the **acromion process,** the lateral tip of the shoulder; the **coracoid process** for muscle attachment; and the **glenoid cavity** (fossa) for attachment of the arm. See Figure 7–13.

FIGURE 7–13   Scapula (a) Anterior view. (b) Posterior view.

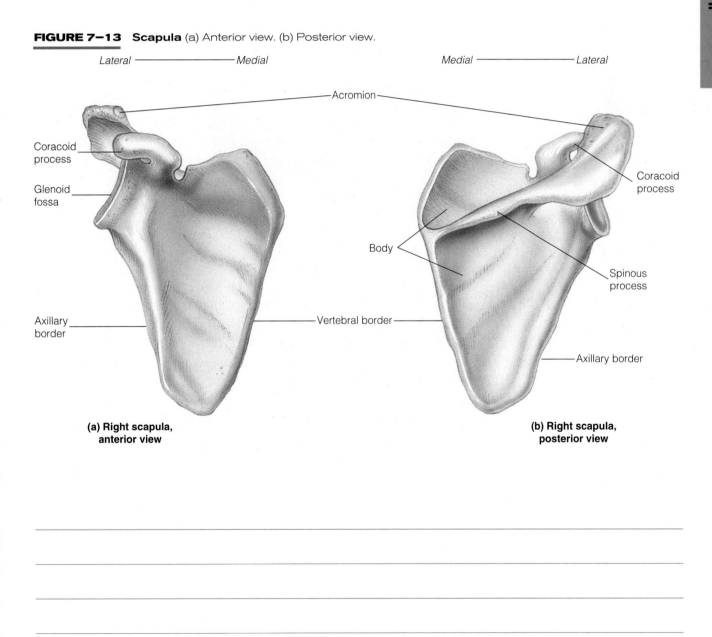

(a) Right scapula, anterior view

(b) Right scapula, posterior view

Pelvic Girdle The pelvic girdle protects the pelvic organs and includes the two hip bones, which are also called the **innominate bones.** This latter name seems peculiar when one considers that "innominate" means unnamed. Another name for the hip bone is the **coxal bone,** or **os coxa.**

Each of the hip bones contains three segments: the **ilium,** the **pubis,** and the **ischium.** These three segments, unjoined in young children, become fused in the adult.

Bone markings include the **iliac crest, anterior superior iliac spine (ASIS), anterior inferior iliac spine (AIIS), acetabulum, iliac fossa, ischial tuberosity, ischial spine,** and **obturator foramen.** See Figure 7–14.

FIGURE 7–14 Right Hip Bone

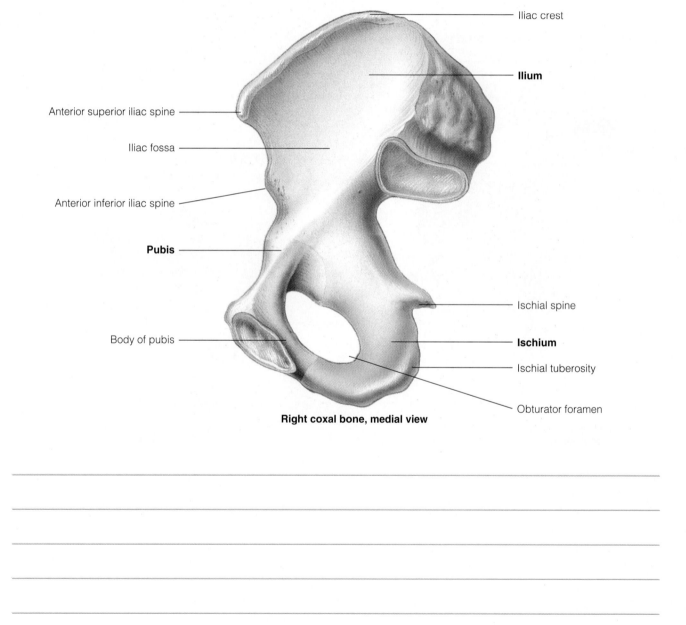

Iliac crest

Ilium

Anterior superior iliac spine

Iliac fossa

Anterior inferior iliac spine

Pubis

Ischial spine

Body of pubis

Ischium

Ischial tuberosity

Obturator foramen

Right coxal bone, medial view

Upper Extremities (Arms and Hands) The upper extremities include the **humerus, ulna, radius, carpals, metacarpals,** and **phalanges.**

The **humerus** is the long, upper bone of the arm between the shoulder and the elbow. The **epiphysis,** head of the humerus, attaches to the glenoid cavity of the scapula to form a freely movable joint.

The **ulna** is the medial bone of the forearm. Located between the elbow and the wrist, it contains the **olecranon process** (the elbow). The **radius** is the smaller lateral bone of the forearm. The name *radius* is easily remembered because this bone rotates around the ulna. See Figure 7–15.

FIGURE 7–15 **Right Radius and Ulna** (a) Anterior view. (b) Posterior view.

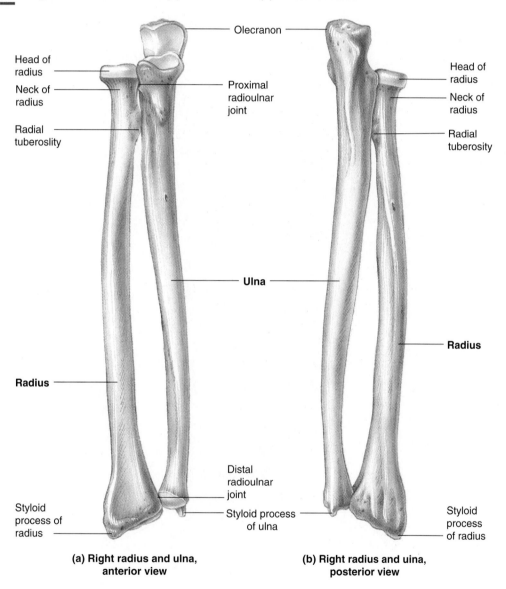

Head of radius
Neck of radius
Radial tuberoslity
Radius
Styloid process of radius

Olecranon
Proximal radioulnar joint
Ulna
Distal radioulnar joint
Styloid process of ulna

Head of radius
Neck of radius
Radial tuberosity
Radius
Styloid process of radius

(a) Right radius and ulna, anterior view

(b) Right radius and uina, posterior view

II–7

The **carpals** are the eight wrist bones, which are arranged in two rows. From lateral to medial, the proximal row (toward the arm) includes the **scaphoid, lunate, triquetral,** and **pisiform.** The distal row (toward the fingers) includes the **trapezium, trapezoid, capitate,** and **hamate** (see Figure 7–16).

The **metacarpals** make up the hand. Figure 7–16 shows the Roman numerals that indicate each of the metacarpals. Number I indicates the metacarpal extending toward the thumb, while V refers to the metacarpal extending toward the little finger.

The **phalanges** make up the fingers. Each finger has three phalanges: proximal, medial, and distal. The thumb has two phalanges: proximal and distal. Each of the phalanges is connected at a joint called the **interphalangeal (IP) joint.**

FIGURE 7–16   Bones of the Wrist and Hand

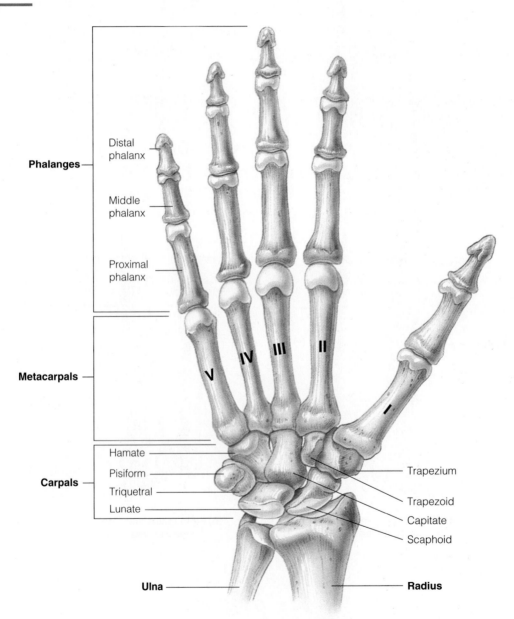

Lower Extremities (Legs and Feet) The **lower extremities** are composed of the **femur, patella, tibia, fibula, tarsals, metatarsals,** and **phalanges.**

The **femur** (thigh bone) is the longest bone in the body and includes the head, neck, **greater** and **lesser trochanters,** and the **medial** and **lateral condyles.** See Figure 7–17.

Articulation (connection) of the femur with the tibia forms the **knee joint,** which is protected by the **patella** or kneecap. The patella is a **sesamoid** (floating) bone held in place by tendons and ligaments.

FIGURE 7–17

The Femur (a) Anterior view. (b) Posterior view.

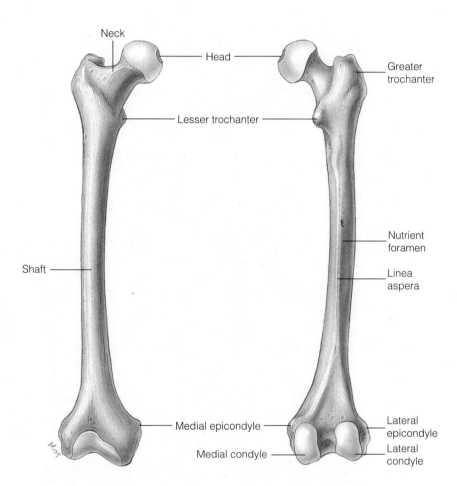

Neck

Head

Greater trochanter

Lesser trochanter

Shaft

Nutrient foramen

Linea aspera

Medial epicondyle

Medial condyle

Lateral epicondyle

Lateral condyle

(a) Right femur, anterior view   **(b) Right femur, posterior view**

7–7

The **tibia** is the larger of the two bones making up the lower leg. It includes the **medial** and **lateral condyles** at its proximal end and the **medial malleolus** at its distal end. The prominence on the anterior tibia, just below the knee, is called the **tibial tuberosity.** See Figure 7–18.

The **fibula** is the long, slender bone located alongside the tibia. It includes the **lateral malleolus,** which articulates with the ankle bone called the **talus.**

The seven bones called the **tarsals** include the **calcaneus, talus, navicular, cuboid, first cuneiform, second cuneiform,** and **third cuneiform.** See Figure 7–19.

The **metatarsals** are located just beyond the tarsals in the same way that the metacarpals of the hand are located beyond the carpals. Figure 7–20 shows the Roman numerals that indicate each of the metatarsals. Number I indicates the metatarsal extending towards the big toe, while number V refers to the metatarsal extending toward the little toe.

Three **phalanges** (proximal, medial, and distal) connect with each other to make up each toe, except for the big toe, which has only two phalanges, proximal and distal.

FIGURE 7–18   **The Tibia and Fibula** (a) Anterior view. (b) Posterior view.

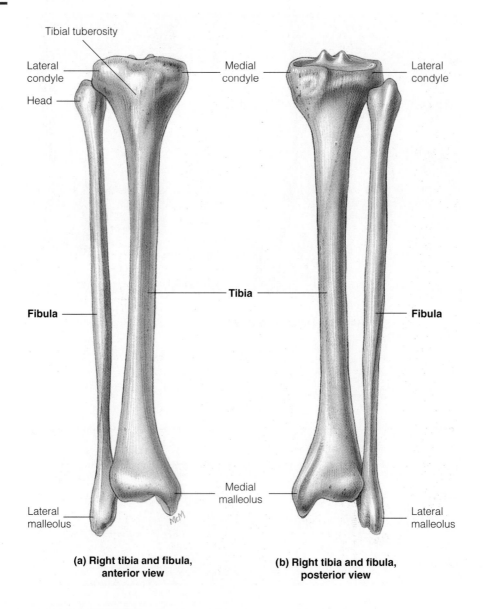

Tibial tuberosity

Lateral condyle

Head

Medial condyle

Lateral condyle

Fibula

Tibia

Fibula

Lateral malleolus

Medial malleolus

Lateral malleolus

(a) Right tibia and fibula, anterior view

(b) Right tibia and fibula, posterior view

FIGURE 7–19

**Right Ankle and Foot,
Lateral View**

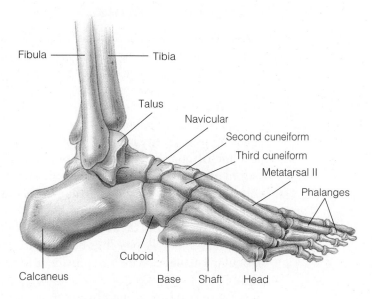

Right ankle and foot, lateral view

Fibula — Tibia

Talus

Navicular

Second cuneiform

Third cuneiform

Metatarsal II

Phalanges

Cuboid

Calcaneus

Base Shaft Head

FIGURE 7–20

**Right Ankle and Foot,
Superior View**

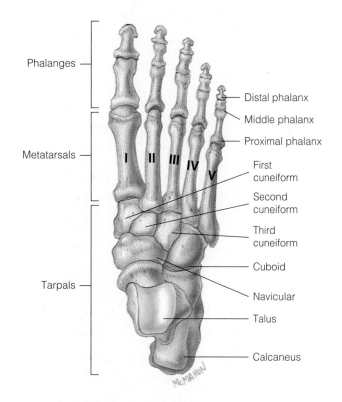

Right ankle and foot, superior view

Phalanges

Distal phalanx

Middle phalanx

Proximal phalanx

Metatarsals

I II III IV V

First cuneiform

Second cuneiform

Third cuneiform

Cuboid

Navicular

Tarpals

Talus

Calcaneus

Categories of Joints

A joint is the place where bones unite. We are familiar with movable joints such as the shoulder joint or knee joint, but joints can also be stationary, as those between the bones of the skull. Joints may be classified in a number of different ways. We will consider the three main structural categories: **fibrous, cartilaginous,** and **synovial.**

Fibrous joints, such as the sutures of the skull, permit no movement because no joint cavity is present and because the bones are bound by only a small amount of connective tissue. Some cartilaginous joints, such as those found within the spinal vertebrae, permit slight movement, although they likewise contain no joint cavity. In cartilaginous joints, the bones are bound together by means of cartilage.

Synovial joints contain a joint cavity and are **diarthrotic,** i.e., freely movable. Movement is possible because the ends of the bones are covered with **articular cartilage,** which fits inside a joint cavity filled with **synovial fluid** (see Figure 7–21). Between the articulating cartilage of the bones is a **joint cavity** lined with a **synovial membrane** that secretes a synovial fluid into the joint. A **fibrous joint capsule** encases the joint.

The **bursae,** although they are not parts of synovial joints, are found near joints to aid in movement. Bursae are closed cavities lined with synovial membrane and filled with synovial fluid. These soft sacs prevent friction between muscles and bones, tendons and bones, skin and bones, and tendons and ligaments.

FIGURE 7–21

A Synovial Joint

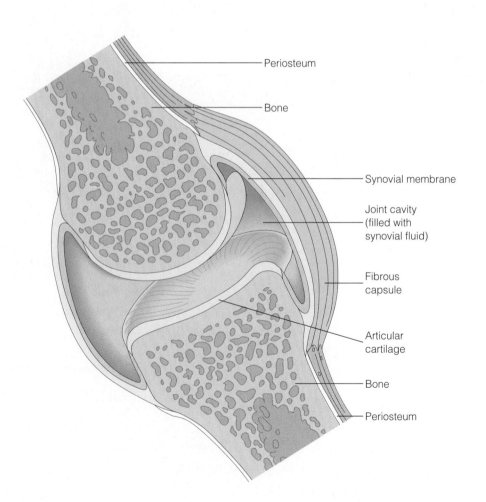

- Periosteum
- Bone
- Synovial membrane
- Joint cavity (filled with synovial fluid)
- Fibrous capsule
- Articular cartilage
- Bone
- Periosteum

Names of Joints

Joints are named for the bones or processes forming the union. For example, the joint between the acromion process of the scapula and clavicle is called the **acromioclavicular joint,** and the joint between the sternum and clavicle is called the **sternoclavicular joint.**

Joint Movement

The terms that refer to the movements that joints can make are defined in Table 7-3. See also Figure 7–22.

TABLE 7–3

Terms Signifying the Types of Joint Movement

TERM	DEFINITION
flexion	decreasing the angle between two bones at a joint
extension	increasing the angle between two bones at a joint; return from flexion
hyperextension	overextending the joint or extending it beyond the anatomical position
abduction	movement away from the medial line of the body, usually involving the upper or lower extremities
adduction	movement toward the medial line of the body, usually involving the upper or lower extremities
circumduction	movement of a joint in a circular manner
supination	movement, usually of the palm of the hand forward, as in the anatomical position; or movement of the body lying on a table so that the ventral cavity is facing up
pronation	movement, usually of the palm of the hand backward; or movement of the body lying on a table so that the ventral cavity is facing down
inversion	movement of the tarsals so that the sole of the foot is facing toward the midline
eversion	movement of the tarsals so that the sole of the foot is facing away from the midline
elevation	movement that raises a part; moving the shoulders up
depression	movement that lowers a part; moving the shoulders down
protraction	movement of a part forward; moving the lower jaw forward
retraction	movement of a part back; moving the lower jaw back
plantar flexion	flexing the foot toward the sole
dorsiflexion	flexing the foot dorsally (opposite of plantar flexion)

FIGURE 7–22 Movements at Synovial Joints

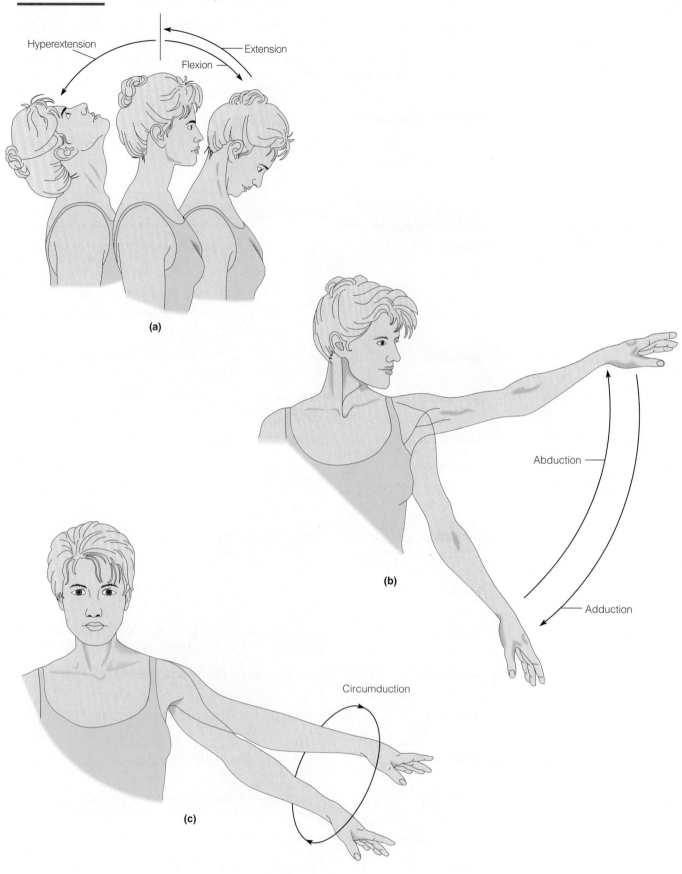

(a)

(b)

(c)

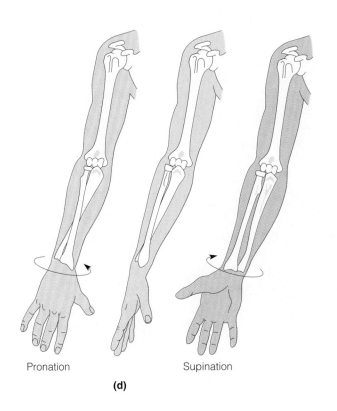

Pronation   Supination

(d)

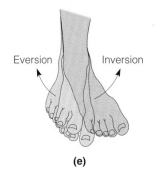

Eversion   Inversion

(e)

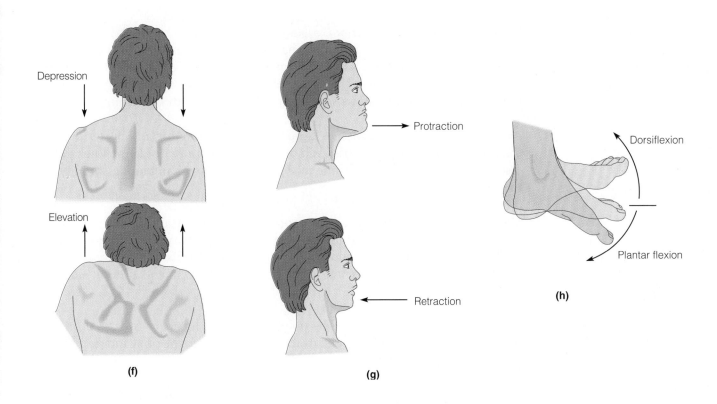

Depression

Elevation

(f)

Protraction

Retraction

(g)

Dorsiflexion

Plantar flexion

(h)

FIGURE 7–23 Ligaments and Cartilages of the Right Knee Joint

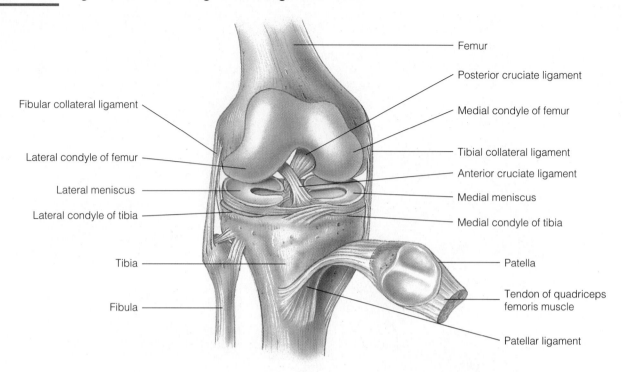

Femur

Posterior cruciate ligament

Medial condyle of femur

Tibial collateral ligament

Anterior cruciate ligament

Medial meniscus

Medial condyle of tibia

Patella

Tendon of quadriceps femoris muscle

Patellar ligament

Fibular collateral ligament

Lateral condyle of femur

Lateral meniscus

Lateral condyle of tibia

Tibia

Fibula

Knee   The knee joint (Figure 7-23) is the largest joint stabilized by cartilage and ligaments from within and surrounding the joint. The following structures help to secure the knee joint.

Medial and Lateral Semilunar Cartilages or Menisci   The medial and lateral semilunar cartilage or menisci are c-shaped, cartilaginous structures that sit on top of the tibial condyles. They prevent friction between the two articulating bones, the femur and tibia. They also help to deepen the articulating surface of the tibia, providing a shallow socket for articulation with the femur.

Anterior and Posterior Cruciate Ligaments   The anterior and posterior cruciate (crossing) ligaments cross each other, forming an X inside the knee joint. These ligaments secure the femur to the tibia, thereby maintaining stability of the joint when it rotates.

Medial and Lateral Collateral Ligaments   The medial and lateral collateral ligaments are located on the medial and lateral aspects of the knee joint. The medial collateral ligament connects the femur with the tibia. The lateral collateral ligament connects the femur to the fibula. These ligaments prevent side-to-side movement.

Oblique Popliteal Ligament   The oblique popliteal ligament is located on the posterior aspect of the knee joint, attaching the femur to the tibia and stabilizing the posterior knee joint.

Arcuate Popliteal Ligament   The arcuate popliteal ligament is also located behind the knee joint. It attaches to the femur and fibula. Like the oblique popliteal ligament, it stabilizes the posterior knee joint.

Patella   The patella is commonly known as the kneecap. Not to be confused with the knee joint, the patella is the bone that protects the knee joint. The knee joint is the union between the femur and tibia and has the same characteristics as any synovial joint. The patella is held in place by tendons and ligaments.

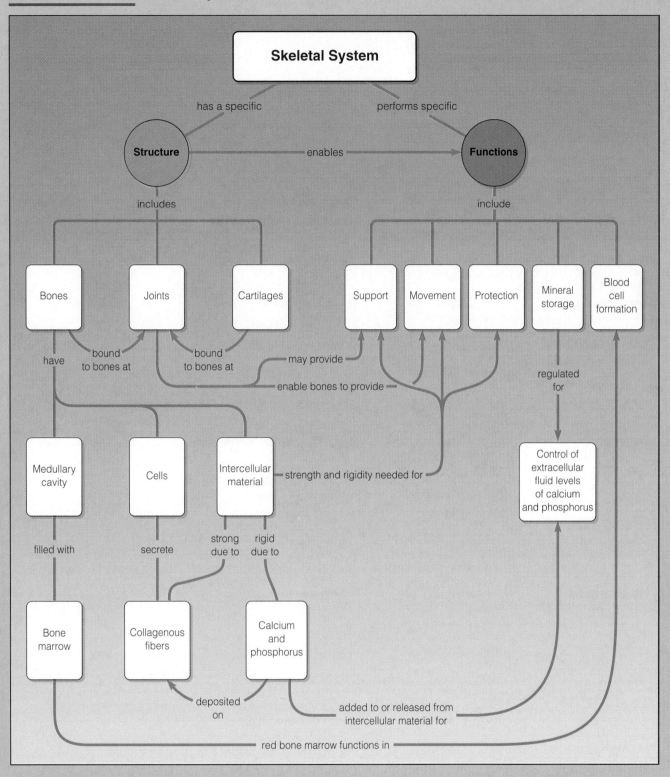

Skeletal System Terminology

TERM WITH PRONUNCIATION	ANALYSIS	DEFINITION
acetabular ăs″-ĕ-tăb′-ū-lăr	-ar = pertaining to acetabul/o = acetabulum (hip socket)	pertaining to the hip socket
brachial brā′-kī-ăl	-al = pertaining to brachi/o = arm	pertaining to the arm
calcaneal kăl-kā′-nĕ-ăl	-al = pertaining to calcane/o = heel	pertaining to the heel
carpal kăr′-păl	-al = pertaining to carp/o = wrist	pertaining to the wrist
cervical cĕr′-vĭ-kăl	-al = pertaining to cervic/o = neck	pertaining to the neck
chondrosarcoma kŏn-drō-săr-kō′-mă	-oma = tumor or mass chondr/o = cartilage sarc/o = flesh	malignant tumor of cartilage
clavicular klă-vĭk′-ū-lăr	-ar = pertaining to clavicul/o = collarbone	pertaining to the collarbone
coccygeal kŏk-sĭj′-ē-ăl	-eal = pertaining to coccyg/o = coccyx (tailbone)	pertaining to the tailbone
costal kŏs′-tăl	-al = pertaining to cost/o = rib	pertaining to the rib
costochondral kŏs″-tō-kŏn′-drăl	-al = pertaining to cost/o = rib chondr/o = cartilage	pertaining to the rib and cartilage
costovertebral kŏs″-tō-vĕr′-tĕ-brăl	-al = pertaining to cost/o = rib vertebr/o = vertebra	pertaining to the rib and vertebra
craniotomy krā-nē-ŏt′-ō-mē	-tomy = process of cutting crani/o = skull	incision into the skull
ethmoid ĕth′-moyd	-oid = resembling ethm/o = sieve	sievelike; resembling a sieve; refers to the ethmoid bone of the cranium
femoral fĕm′-or-ăl	-al = pertaining to femor/o = femur (thighbone)	pertaining to the thighbone
fibular fĭb′-ū-lăr	-ar = pertaining to fibul/o = fibula (lateral bone of the lower leg)	pertaining to the fibula **Note:** Fibula is Latin for clasp or pin. The fibula is pinned on like a brooch to the tibia.
frontal frŏn′-tăl	-al = pertaining to front/o = frontal bone	pertaining to the frontal bone

TERM WITH PRONUNCIATION	ANALYSIS	DEFINITION
glenoid glē′-noyd	-oid = resembling glen/o = socket; pit	resembling a socket or pit; refers to the glenoid cavity, a deep socket articulating with the head of the humerus
humeral hū′-měr-ăl	-al = pertaining to humer/o = humerus (upper arm)	pertaining to the upper arm
iliac ĭl′-ē-ăk	-ac = pertaining to ili/o = hip	pertaining to the hip
interphalangeal ĭn″-těr-fă-lăn′-jē-ăl	-eal = pertaining to inter- = between phalang/o = phalanx (one of the bones making up the fingers or toes)	pertaining to between the phalanges
ischial ĭs′-kē-ăl	-al = pertaining to ischi/o = ischium (posterior portion of the hip bone)	pertaining to the ischium
laminectomy lăm″-ĭ-něk′-tō-mē	-ectomy = excision; removal lamin/o = lamina (portion of the vertebra)	removal of the lamina
lumbar lŭm′-băr	-ar = pertaining to lumb/o = lower back; loins	pertaining to the lower back or loins
malleolar măl-ē′-ō-lăr	-ar = pertaining to malleol/o = malleolus (bony projection on the distal aspect of the fibula and tibia)	pertaining to the malleolus
mandibular măn-dĭb′-ū-lăr	-ar = pertaining to mandibul/o = lower jaw	pertaining to the lower jaw
maxillary măk′-sĭ-lěr″-ē	-ary = pertaining to maxill/o = upper jaw	pertaining to the upper jaw
myeloma mī-ě- lō′-mă	-oma = tumor or mass myel/o = bone marrow	tumor of bone marrow
occipital ŏk-sĭp′-ĭ-tăl	-al = pertaining to occipit/o = occiput (back part of the head)	pertaining to the occiput
olecranal ō-lěk′-răn-ăl	-al = pertaining to olecran/o = olecranon (elbow)	pertaining to the elbow
osteoblast ŏs′-tē-ō-blăst	-blast = immature oste/o-bone	immature bone cell
osteochondritis ŏs″-tē-ō-kŏn-drī′-tĭs	-itis = inflammation oste/o = bone chondr/o = cartilage	inflammation of bone and cartilage

TERM WITH PRONUNCIATION	ANALYSIS	DEFINITION
osteocyte ŏs′-tē -ō-sīt″	-cyte = cell oste/o = bone	bone cell
parietal pă-rī′-ĕ-tăl	-al = pertaining to pariet/o = parietal bone; wall	pertaining to the parietal bone
patellar pă-tĕl′-ăr	-ar = pertaining to patell/o = patella (kneecap)	pertaining to the kneecap
pectoral pĕk′-tō-răl	-al = pertaining to pector/o = chest	pertaining to the chest
pelvic pĕl′-vĭk	-ic = pertaining to pelv/o = pelvis	pertaining to the pelvis
phalangeal fă-lăn′-jē-ăl	-eal = pertaining to phalang/o = phalanx	pertaining to the phalanges
popliteal pŏp″-lĭt-ē′-ăl	-eal = pertaining to poplit/o = posterior surface of the knee	pertaining to the posterior surface of the knee
pubic pū′-bĭk	-ic = pertaining to pub/o = pubis	pertaining to the pubis
rachitis rā-kī′-tĭs	-itis = inflammation rach/o = spine	inflammation of the spine
radial rā′-dē-ăl	-al = pertaining to radi/o = radius (lateral bone of the lower arm)	pertaining to the radius
sacral sā′-krăl	-al = pertaining to sacr/o = sacrum	pertaining to the sacrum
scapular skăp′-ū-lăr	-ar = pertaining to scapul/o = scapula (shoulder blade)	pertaining to the shoulder blade
sphenoid sfē′-noyd	-oid = resembling sphen/o = sphenoid bone; wedge	pertaining to the sphenoid bone, which is wedge shaped
spondylosis spŏn″-dĭ-lō′-sĭs	-osis = abnormal condition spondyl/o = vertebra	immobility of a vertebral joint
sternal stĕr′-năl	-al = pertaining to stern/o = sternum (breastbone)	pertaining to the breastbone
syndactylism sĭn-dăk′-tĭl-ĭzm	-ism = process syn- = together; with dactyl/o = fingers; toes	webbed fingers or toes
tarsal tăr′-săl	-al = pertaining to tars/o = tarsals (ankle)	pertaining to the tarsals, bones located between the leg and foot; ankle

Skeletal System Terminology *(continued)*

TERM WITH PRONUNCIATION	ANALYSIS	DEFINITION
temporal tĕm′-por-ăl	-al = pertaining to tempor/o = temporal bone; temples	pertaining to the temporal bones
thoracic thō-răs′-ĭk	-ic = pertaining to thorac/o = chest	pertaining to the chest
tibial tĭb′-ē-ăl	-al = pertaining to tibi/o = tibia (shin)	pertaining to the shin
ulnar ŭl′-năr	-ar = pertaining to uln/o = ulna (medial bone of the lower arm)	pertaining to the ulna
vertebral vĕr′-tĕ-brăl	-al = pertaining to vertebr/o = vertebra	pertaining to the vertebra
xiphoid zĭf′-oyd	-oid = resembling xiph/o = sword	resembling a sword; refers to the xiphoid process of the sternum
zygomatic zī″-gō-măt′-ĭk	-ic = pertaining to zygomat/o = cheekbone	pertaining to the cheekbone

Joint Terminology

TERM WITH PRONUNCIATION	ANALYSIS	DEFINITION
acromioclavicular ă-krō″-mē-ŏ-klă-vĭk′-ū-lăr	-ar = pertaining to acromi/o = acromion process clavicul/o = collarbone	pertaining to (the joint between) the acromion process and the collarbone
ankylosis ăng″-kĭ-lō′-sĭs	-osis = abnormal condition ankyl/o = bent; crooked	joint fusion and immobility due to disease or injury **Note:** An example is **ankylosing spondylitis,** which is the fusion and subsequent immobility of the vertebrae due to disease.
arthralgia ăr-thrăl′-jē-ă	-algia = pain arthr/o = joint	joint pain
arthritis ăr-thrī′-tĭs	-itis = inflammation arthr/o = joint	inflammation of a joint
arthrodesis ăr-thrō-dē′-sĭs	-desis = surgical fusion; binding arthr/o = joint	surgical fusion of a joint rendering the joint immobile
arthropathy ăr-thrŏp′-ă-thē	-pathy = disease arthr/o = joint	diseased joint
arthroplasty ăr′-thrō-plăs″-tē	-plasty = surgical reconstruction arthr/o = joint	surgical repair of a joint
arthroscopy ăr-thrŏs′-kō-pē	-scopy = process of visual examination arthr/o = joint	process of visually examining a joint by means of an arthroscope

II–7

Joint Terminology (continued)

TERM WITH PRONUNCIATION	ANALYSIS	DEFINITION
arthrotomy ăr-thrŏt′-ō-mē	-tomy = to cut; incise arthr/o = joint	incision into a joint
articular ăr-tĭk′-ū-lăr	-ar = pertaining to articul/o = joint	pertaining to a joint
bursitis bŭr-sī′-tĭs	-itis = inflammation burs/o = bursa; fluid-filled sac	inflammation of the bursa
glenohumeral glĕ″-nō-hū′-mĕr-ăl	-al = pertaining to glen/o = socket; pit humer/o = humerus (upper arm)	pertaining to (the joint between) the glenoid cavity and the humerus
hemarthrosis hĕm-ăr-thrō′-sĭs	-osis = abnormal condition hem/o = blood arthr/o = joint	blood in a joint
hydrarthrosis hī″-drăr-thrō′-sĭs	-osis = abnormal condition hydr/o = water arthr/o = joint	accumulation of water (fluid) in a joint
osteoarthritis ŏs″-tē-ō-ăr-thrī′-tĭs	-itis = inflammation oste/o = bone arthr/o = joint	inflammation of the bone and joints
periarthritis pĕr″-ē-ăr-thrī′-tĭs	-itis = inflammation peri- = around arthr/o = joint	inflammation around a joint
sacroiliac sā″-krō-ĭl′-ē-ăk	-ac = pertaining to sacr/o = sacrum ili/o = hip	pertaining to the sacrum and hip; also iliosacral
sternoclavicular stĕr″-nō-klă-vĭk′-ū-lăr	-ar = pertaining to stern/o = sternum (breastbone) clavicul/o = collarbone	pertaining to (the joint between) the breastbone and collarbone
synovectomy sĭn″-ō-vĕk′-tō-mē	-ectomy = excision; removal synov/i/o = synovium (synovial membrane); tendon sheath	removal of the synovial membrane or tendon sheath **Note:** Synov/i/o has two meanings: synovia, which means synovial fluid, and synovium, which means synovial membrane.
synovial sĭn-ō′-vē-ăl	-al = pertaining to synov/i/o = synovia (synovial fluid)	pertaining to synovial fluid
synovitis sĭn″-ō-vī′-tĭs	-itis = inflammation synov/i/o = synovium (synovial membrane)	inflammation of the synovial membrane
temporomandibular tĕm″-pō-rō-măn-dĭb′-ū-lăr	-ar = pertaining to tempor/o = temporal bone mandibul/o = lower jaw	pertaining to the temporal bone and lower jaw

Arthropathies

CONDITION	DESCRIPTION
arthritis	inflammation of a joint **Note:** The term arthritis is applied to rheumatoid (see below) as well as to osteoarthritis (see below); however, it is only the rheumatoid type that shows all the signs of inflammation.

rheumatoid arthritis (RA)
 	
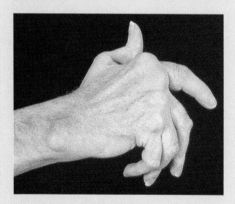
	Rheumatoid arthritis involves connective tissue throughout the entire body but mainly involves the synovium in the joint.
	    Rheumatoid arthritis is considered an autoimmune disease (abnormal response against one's own body). In the disease process, the body does not recognize its own natural antibodies as "self." Because the body thinks its own natural antibodies are foreign, it produces antibodies called rheumatoid factors (RF) that fight against its own natural antibodies. The disease starts with a simple synovitis and can progress through several stages, the last being joint immobility. Because of the role of RF antibodies, an RF test confirms RA.
	    The inflammation is initiated by RF antibodies producing an inflammatory exudate called **pannus.** Movement is difficult and painful because the thick pannus adheres to the joint surfaces, producing **ankylosis.**
	    Diagnostic tests may include **analysis of synovial fluid, antinuclear antibody, latex fixation tests,** and **rheumatoid factors.** (For a detailed description of these and other tests, see laboratory tests below.)

osteoarthritis (OA)	**Osteoarthritis** is a degenerative disease of the joint and is a normal part of aging. Although the exact cause is unknown, the articular cartilage wears away, often because of overuse, exposing underlying bone. Pain is caused by the friction between the two bones as they glide across each other without the protection of the articular cartilage. The most effective treatment for both RA and OA is **acetylsalicylic acids,** such as aspirin, and **nonsteroidal anti-inflammatory drugs (NSAID).** Diagnosis is made by skeletal x-ray of arthritic joint.
Dislocations	A dislocation is the displacement of a bone from its socket, usually caused by trauma. The types of dislocations include **compound** or open, which is the complete displacement of the bone from its socket along with a break in the skin so that the joint communicates with the air; **complete,** which is the complete displacement of the bone from its socket with no break in the skin; and **incomplete, subluxation,** or **partial,** which is the slight displacement of the bone from its socket and does not involve communication with the air.
Gout	This is a metabolic disease characterized by increased production of uric acid with deposits of uric acid crystals in the joint, usually the big toe. Chronic gout is characterized by **tophi,** which are nodules around the joint that are filled with sodium urate crystals.

CONDITION	DESCRIPTION
internal derangement of the knee joint	disruption in the arrangement of the structure and therefore affecting the function of the knee
bucket handle tear	A **bucket handle tear** includes abnormalities of the internal structures of the knee joint such as c-shaped meniscus tears on the medial or lateral edge with the opposite side still attached. The torn edge resembles a bucket handle.
joint mice	**Joint mice,** so called because of loose particles within the joint, are caused by repeated trauma to the knee. Joint mice often create a constant irritation within the joint cavity, which produces an excess of synovial fluid. When a particle becomes lodged between articulating surfaces, pain or a locking of the joint may occur.

Diseases of the Vertebrae

CONDITION	DESCRIPTION
ankylosing spondylitis (AS)	non-rheumatoid arthritis of the sacroiliac joint with eventual involvement of the entire spine, ultimately leading to spinal fusion or ankylosis
herniated disc; herniated nucleus pulposis	displacement of the nucleus pulposus through a weakened annulus fibrosus **Note:** The nucleus puts pressure on a nerve, which produces lower back pain. The sciatic nerve, a large nerve running the length of the leg, is commonly involved. In many cases, the lower back pain will go away spontaneously following bed rest and localized heat. If the patient fails to respond to conservative treatment, surgery may be necessary to remove the displaced disc.

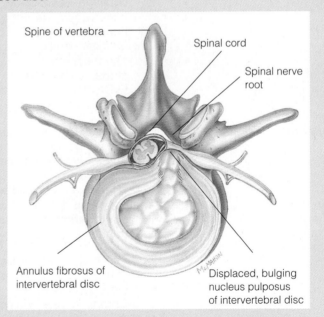

Spine of vertebra

Spinal cord

Spinal nerve root

Annulus fibrosus of intervertebral disc

Displaced, bulging nucleus pulposus of intervertebral disc

sciatica	pain anywhere along the sciatic nerve is called **sciatica** **Note:** The cause is often the rupture or displacement of an intervertebral disc, or osteoarthrosis of lumbosacral vertebrae.

CONDITION	DESCRIPTION
bunion	a bony protuberance on the medial aspect of the first metatarsal The condition is associated with **hallux valgus** deformity. A bony prominence projecting from a bone is called an **exostosis**.

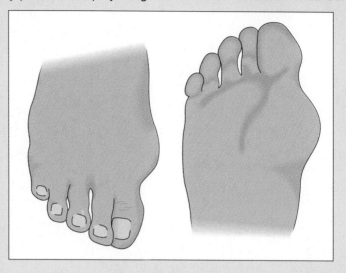

ganglion of tendon sheath	a cystic growth commonly occurring on the dorsum of the wrist

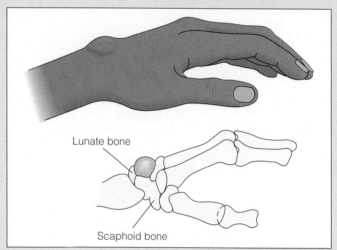

Lunate bone

Scaphoid bone

Osteopathies and Chondropathies

CONDITION	DESCRIPTION
osteomalacia	a softening of bone caused by abnormal calcium deposits **Note:** It can be caused by a lack of vitamin D or by malabsorption of calcium and is called rickets in children.
osteomyelitis	inflammation of the bone and sometimes of the bone marrow **Note: Osteomyelitis** is caused by the presence of pyogenic bacteria, usually *staphylococcus*. The infection can spread to the bone through the blood from a previously injured site, or the microorganism can infiltrate the bone directly following open fractures, surgical reductions, or other exposures to the air.

CONDITION	DESCRIPTION
osteoporosis	condition of decreased bone density due to a loss of bony substance and diminished osteogenesis—the bone becomes porous and fragile, and fractures are common

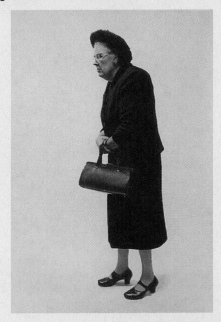

CONDITION	DESCRIPTION
primary osteoporosis	**Primary osteoporosis** is idiopathic; however, contributing factors include reduction in calcium intake and hormonal imbalance. It is most commonly seen in postmenopausal women.
secondary osteoporosis	**Secondary osteoporosis** is caused by extended drug use, particularly steroids, or by extended periods of inactivity. In general, osteoporosis is usually seen in elderly women who first come to a health care facility complaining of back pain, as the vertebral column is most commonly affected. Diagnosis is mainly through x-rays of the thoracic and lumbar vertebrae. Treatment is preventive by increasing bone mass through proper dietary consumption of calcium and vitamin D and through exercise.

Acquired Deformities of the Toe

CONDITION	DESCRIPTION
Hallux valgus	the outward turning of the great toe away from the midline
Hallux varus	the inward turning of the great toe toward the midline
hammer toe, claw toe, mallet toe	acquired or congenital deformities of the toes as a result of abnormal positioning of the interphalangeal joints

Acquired Deformities of the Hip

CONDITION	DESCRIPTION
coxa valga	outward turning of the hip joint
coxa vara	inward turning of the hip joint
genu valgum	knock-kneed; the knees are in close position and the space between the ankles is increased

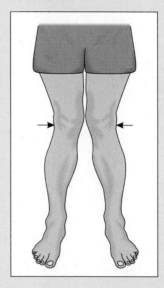

genu varum	bow-legged; the space between the knees is abnormally increased and the lower leg bows inwardly

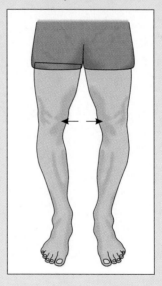

Acquired Curvatures of the Spine

CONDITION	DESCRIPTION
kyphosis	exaggerated posterior curvature of the thoracic spine, also known as humpback or hunchback

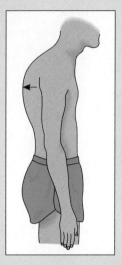

lordosis — exaggerated anterior curvature of the lumbar and cervical spines, also known as swayback

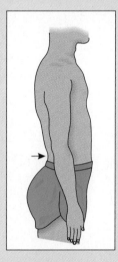

scoliosis — abnormal lateral curvature of the thoracic spine

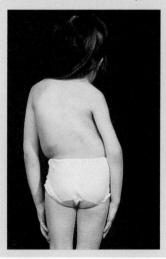

CONDITION	DESCRIPTION
spondylolisthesis	forward displacement of one of the vertebrae, usually the 5th lumbar vertebra over the 1st sacral vertebra

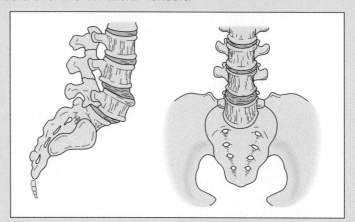

Congenital Anomalies

Note: Congenital anomalies are abnormalities that are present at birth. Included are the following:

CONDITION	DESCRIPTION
congenital dislocation of the hip (CDH)	displacement of the head of the femur from the acetabulum
spina bifida	incomplete neural arch **Note:** In this condition, segments of the vertebra(e) do not fuse posteriorly, leaving a gap in the neural arch. This skeletal problem may lead to a neural defect that involves the displacement of the spinal cord and its membranes and sometimes the spinal cord outside its bony encasement.
talipes equinovarus	plantar flexion of the foot with the heel turned inward, toward the midline, commonly called clubfoot 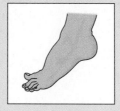
talipes equinus	because of shortened tendons posteriorly, the heel does not touch the ground, which forces the patient to walk on the toes with the foot plantar flexed 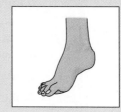

CONDITION	DESCRIPTION
talipes valgus	turning outward of the foot away from the midline 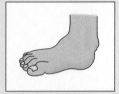
talipes varus	turning inward of the foot toward the midline 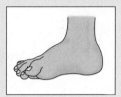

Note: all varieties of talipes can be acquired.

Injuries

CONDITION	DESCRIPTION
fractures	discontinuity of the normal alignment of bone **Note:** Most fractures are caused by accidents, although some are **pathological** (fractures caused by diseased bones).
Classification of fractures	Fractures can be grouped according to the following list: a. whether or not the bone pierces the skin If the bone pierces the skin, it is called a **compound** or **open fracture.** If the fracture does not pierce the skin, it is called a **simple** or **closed fracture.** b. fracture line through the bone If the fracture line is continuous through the bone, it is called **complete.** If the fracture line is not continuous through the bone, it is called **incomplete** or **partial.** A type of partial fracture is a **greenstick** fracture, which like a green stick or twig from a tree, will bend on one side and break on the other. c. direction of the fracture line **linear fracture** where the line of the fracture runs parallel to the axis of the bone **spiral fracture** where the fracture line curves around the bone **transverse fracture** where the fracture line is across the bone **intra-articular fracture** where the fracture line is on the joint surfaces of bone d. miscellaneous fractures **Pott's fracture,** a break of the lower fibula, is an outdated term. **Colles' fracture** is a break of the distal radius.

Injuries (continued)

CONDITION	DESCRIPTION

Classification of fractures (*continued*)

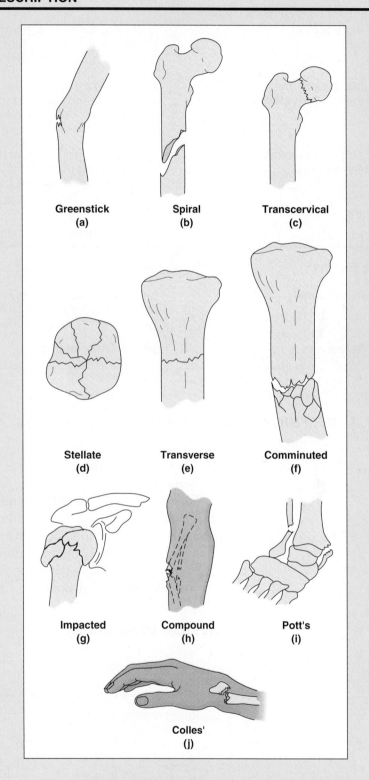

Greenstick
(a)

Spiral
(b)

Transcervical
(c)

Stellate
(d)

Transverse
(e)

Comminuted
(f)

Impacted
(g)

Compound
(h)

Pott's
(i)

Colles'
(j)

sprains — injury to the joint characterized by the rupture of some or all fibers of the supporting ligament

II–7

Malignant Neoplasms

CONDITION	DESCRIPTION
Ewing's tumor	malignant tumor of bone affecting mostly boys between 5 and 15 years of age; the cure rate is currently greater than 60% with proper treatment such as chemotherapy, radiation therapy, and surgery
multiple myeloma; plasma cell myeloma	malignant neoplasm of the marrow plasma cells resulting in bone destruction and overproduction of immunoglobulins and Bence Jones protein (see laboratory procedures) **Note:** Treatment is chemotherapy.
osteogenic sarcoma; osteosarcoma	malignant tumor of the long bones, particularly the femur, commonly metastasizing to the lungs **Note:** Treatment is chemotherapy and surgery.

Benign Neoplasms

CONDITION	DESCRIPTION
chondroma	benign tumor of cartilage.
giant cell tumor	tumor of the epiphysis of long bones, particularly the distal femur at the knee, commonly seen in the 20 to 40 age group. **Note:** Treatment is removal of the tumor followed by bone grafting.
Osteoma	benign tumor of bone.

7.6 PHYSICAL EXAMINATION, DIAGNOSIS, AND TREATMENT

An examination of the skeletal structures includes inspection and palpation for bone abnormalities, along with observation of ligament stability and ranges of joint motion.

Diagnosis of skeletal abnormalities may require a wide range of laboratory tests. For example, a laboratory examination of synovial fluid may help in the diagnosis of various kinds of arthritis, and bacterial cultures sometimes help the physician to identify microorganisms that cause bone disease.

Treatments include everything from simple analgesics to bone grafts and other complex surgical procedures.

Physical Examination

TERM	DESCRIPTION
range of motion (ROM)	degree to which a joint can be moved in any range, including abduction, flexion, extension, dorsiflexion. **Note:** Range is measured in degrees. For example, limited joint movement may be 55 degrees, or full range movement, 360 degrees.
Lachman and Drawer	tests ligament stability of the knee
sulcus test	tests ligament stability of the shoulder

Laboratory Tests

TEST	DESCRIPTION
analysis of synovial fluid	Synovial fluid is aspirated (withdrawn) and then examined. This test is used to distinguish between osteoarthritis, rheumatoid arthritis, traumatic arthritis, infectious arthritis, and gout. In rheumatoid arthritis, rheumatoid factors are present in the synovial fluid.
antinuclear antibody (ANA)	**ANAs** are antibodies the body produces against its own nuclear material; their presence indicates autoimmune diseases such as systemic lupus erythematosus.
Bence Jones protein	Bence Jones protein is produced by malignant plasma cells and secreted by the bone marrow in multiple myeloma. Initially, this protein is catabolized by the kidneys; however, as the disease progresses, the protein is produced in such large amounts that the kidneys are unable to cope. The excess spills over into the urine where it can be detected by laboratory examination.
cultures	Cultures are used to isolate and identify microorganisms causing disease. These tests are used in diagnosing infectious diseases such as osteomyelitis and septic arthritis.
erythrocyte sedimentation rate (ESR)	This test measures the rate at which red blood cells fall or settle to the bottom of a tube. Red blood cells fall faster during inflammations, elevating the **ESR** above its normal value. This test, in conjunction with other tests, helps diagnose inflammatory conditions such as ankylosing spondylitis and rheumatoid arthritis.
human leukocyte antigen B-27(HLA)	HLAs are proteins found on white blood cells. The occurrence of HLA-B27 is seen in ankylosing spondylitis.
latex fixation tests (agglutination tests)	This test is used to diagnose rheumatoid arthritis because it detects rheumatoid factors.
serum and urinary calcium and phosphorus	Calcium and phosphorus are important constituents of bone. Abnormal values are present in osteoporosis and osteomalacia.
rheumatoid factors (RF)	This test measures the quantity of **RF** in the blood. Rheumatoid factors are proteins present in the blood and synovial fluid of patients with rheumatoid arthritis.

TEST	DESCRIPTION
serum alkaline phosphatase (SAP)	Alkaline phosphatase is important in the building of new bone. However, increased levels indicate bone disease such as multiple myeloma, osteomalacia, osteogenic sarcoma, and rheumatoid disease.
serum urate	Elevated amounts of serum urate are present in gout.
urinary uric acid	Elevated amounts of urinary uric acid are found in patients with gout.

Radiology and Diagnostic Imaging

TEST	DESCRIPTION
arthrography	X-ray of a joint after injection of a contrast medium.
bone scans	A visual image of bone is displayed following injection of technetium (^{99m}Tc), a radioactive substance. This substance is picked up by bone undergoing abnormal metabolic activity and shows up as dark areas on the image. Bone scans are useful in detecting tumors and are used to distinguish between osteomyelitis and cellulitis. (See figure 18–4.)
computed tomography (CT)	A CT scan is an x-ray of an organ or body detailing that structure at various depths. Multiple radiographs are taken at multiple angles, and the computer reconstructs these images to represent a cross-section or "slice" of the structure.
magnetic resonance imaging (MRI); nuclear magnetic resonance (NMR)	This is a noninvasive imaging technique that relies on the body's responses to a strong magnetic field
skeletal x-rays	This simple x-ray of bone is often used to initially evaluate patient's complaints. No contrast media or radioactive substances are used.

Clinical Procedures

PROCEDURE	DESCRIPTION
arthrocentesis (aspiration of synovial fluid)	removal of synovial fluid for analysis in such conditions as gout, rheumatoid arthritis, hematoma, and infection
arthroscopy	diagnostic and therapeutic procedure used to inspect certain joint cavities. The instrument used is an arthroscope. The scope houses a video camera, and the image is projected onto a television monitor. Arthroscopy is most commonly used on the knee joint. The advantages of this procedure include the use of local anesthetic, a quick recovery time, and a reduced hospital stay.

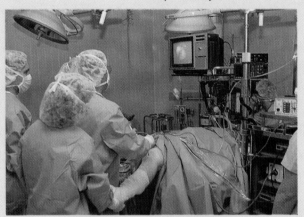

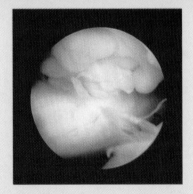

aspiration of bone marrow	withdrawal of bone marrow for the evaluation of bone marrow disease, such as blood dyscrasias (abnormalities) and multiple myeloma
biopsy	removal of a piece of bone that is to be examined by a pathologist for diagnostic purposes **Note:** This test is used to diagnose tumors and chronic infections such as osteomyelitis.

Treatment

Medical Treatment

TREATMENT	DESCRIPTION
analgesics	given to relieve pain on movement in such conditions as osteoarthritis; example: aspirin
antibiotics	drugs used against bacterial diseases such as osteomyelitis
colchicine	a drug given to treat gout by reducing the urate crystal deposits
corticosteroids	injected into a joint to relieve tenderness
nonsteroidal anti-inflammatory drugs (NSAIDs)	helps facilitate exercise and other supportive measures by suppressing articular inflammation, pain, and spasm **Note:** Used to relieve pain due to inflammation such as in bursitis, tenosynovitis, and tendinitis.
physiotherapy; physical therapy	clinically controlled exercise to help maintain joint motion and promote muscle strength
immobilization	prevents movement of a skeletal structure by means of splints, plaster casts, traction, braces, or bed rest

Surgical Treatment

TREATMENT	DESCRIPTION
arthrodesis	surgical fixation of a joint to accomplish fusion of the joint surfaces by promoting the proliferation of bone cells; used in certain cases of osteoarthritis
arthroplasty	surgical reconstruction of a joint using prosthetic devices

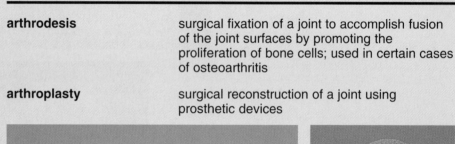
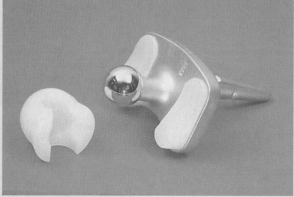
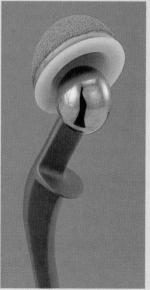

Prosthetic devices. Left: artificial knee joint; right: artificial hip joint.

TREATMENT	DESCRIPTION
bone grafting	transplantation of bone from one site to another; used occasionally to replace malignant bone tissue that has been excised but most commonly for fractures that will not heal
reduction of fractures and immobilization	the placement of the bone into its normal alignment Bone can be reduced in several ways: **Traction** is a considerable pull, aligning the distal fragment with the proximal fragment **Closed reduction** is a surgical procedure involving the manual manipulation of the ends of the fractured bone so that normal alignment is maintained. The procedure is performed under local anaesthetic. There is no incision through the skin, subcutaneous tissue, or muscle. **Open reduction** involves manipulating the ends of the fractured bone under direct vision. This procedure is performed under general anesthetic, and an incision is made into the skin and underlying tissues. Following reduction, the bone is **immobilized** by plaster casts to prevent further damage by prohibiting movement.
internal fixation	At times, **internal fixation** is needed to immobilize the bone pieces by means of screws, plates, pins, wires, nails, or rods. Examples of internal fixations are screws, wires such as Kirschner (kersh'ner), plates such as Austin-Moore, and nails and pins such as Steinman.
resection	the partial or total excision of tissue In the case of malignant tumors of bone, total resection is necessary for the prevention of recurrence.

II–7

▶ 7.7 ABBREVIATIONS

ABBREVIATION	MEANING
AC joint	acromioclavicular joint
AIIS	anterior inferior iliac spine
ANA	antinuclear antibody
AS	ankylosing spondylitis
ASIS	anterior superior iliac spine
C	cervical
C1, C2 . . . C7	1st cervical vertebra, 2nd cervical vertebra . . . 7th cervical vertebra
C1–C2 . . . C6–C7	intervertebral disc space between the 1st and 2nd cervical vertebrae . . . intervertebral disc space between 6th and 7th cervical vertebrae
Ca	calcium
CDH	congenital dislocation of hip
DDH	developmental dysplasia of hip
DIP joint	distal interphalangeal joint
Fx	fracture
HLA	human leukocyte antigen
IP joint	interphalangeal joint
L	lumbar
L1, L2 . . . L5	1st lumbar vertebra, 2nd lumbar vertebra . . . 5th lumbar vertebra
L1–L2 . . . L4–L5	intervertebral disc space between the 1st and 2nd lumbar vertebrae . . . intervertebral disc space between 4th and 5th lumbar vertebrae

ABBREVIATION	MEANING
MCP joint	metacarpophalangeal joint
MSS	musculoskeletal system
OA	osteoarthritis
ortho	orthopedics
P	phosphorus
PIP joint	proximal interphalangeal joint
RA	rheumatoid arthritis
RF	rheumatoid factor
ROM	range of motion
S1, S2 . . . S5	1st sacral vertebra, 2nd sacral vertebra . . . 5th sacral vertebra
S1–S2 . . . S4–S5	intervertebral disc space between the 1st and 2nd sacral vertebrae . . . intervertebral disc space between 4th and 5th sacral vertebrae
SAP	serum alkaline phosphatase
T	thoracic
T1, T2 . . . T12	1st thoracic vertebra, 2nd thoracic vertebra . . . 12th thoracic vertebra
T1–T2 . . . T11–T12	intervertebral disc space between the 1st and 2nd thoracic vertebrae . . . intervertebral disc space between 11th and 12th thoracic vertebrae

Definitions

Give the common term for the following bones

Answers to the exercise questions appear in Appendix A.

1. acetabulum _____

2. calcaneus _____

3. coccyx _____

4. clavicle _____

5. femur _____

6. humerus _____

7. mandible _____

8. maxilla _____

9. olecranon _____

10. patella _____

11. sternum _____

12. scapula _____

13. thorax _____

14. fibula _____

Write the terms that correspond with the following abbreviations.

15. AC joint _____

16. ANA _____

17. AS _____

18. C _____

19. C1, C2, etc. _____

20. Ca _____

21. CDH _____

22. DDH _____

23. DIP joint _____

24. Fx _____

25. IP _____

26. L _____

27. L1, L2, etc. _____

28. MCP joint _____

29. MSS _____

30. OA _____

31. ortho _____

32. P _____

33. PIP joint _____

34. RA _____

35. RF _____

36. ROM _____

37. SAP _____

38. T _____

39. T1, T2, etc. _____

▶EXERCISE 7–2

Word Building

_____

Word Building

Build medical terms for the following phrases.

1. joint pain _____

2. surgical fusion of a joint _____

▶EXERCISE 7–3

Practice Quiz

Short Answer

Answer the following questions briefly.

1. List the five functions of the skeletal system. _____

_____

_____

_____

2. Name the four bone shapes. _____

_____

3. To what do the terms diaphysis and endosteum refer? _____

_____

4. What is hematopoiesis? _____

_____

5. What bone may be described as resembling the wings of a bat? _____

_____

6. The cranial bones come together to form immovable joints called

_____ .

7. The inferior nasal conchae are also known as _____ .

8. The mandible and the temporal bone unite at a joint called the _____

_____ .

9. What bone supports the tongue? _____

10. How many vertebrae make up the spinal column? _____

11. How many cervical vertebrae are there? _____

12. Which vertebra is called atlas? _____

Matching Terms with Meanings

Matching

Match the term in Column A with its definition in Column B.

Column A	Column B
1. rheumatoid arthritis _____	A. inflammation of the synovial membrane
2. synovitis _____	B. pain along the sciatic nerve
3. greenstick _____	C. collar bone
4. osteomalacia _____	D. a small rounded process
5. humerus _____	E. softening of bone
6. tibia _____	F. a type of fracture
7. tubercle _____	G. a long bone in the upper arm
8. clavicle _____	H. a chronic systemic disease that can strike people of any age
9. sciatica _____	I. the shinbone

Match each item in Column A with a corresponding item in Column B.

Column A	Column B
10. occipital bone _____	A. cranial bone
11. palatine _____	B. cranial suture
12. a body, two pedicles, and two laminae _____	C. facial bone
13. sagittal _____	D. vertebral column
14. ulna _____	E. lower extremities
15. fibula _____	F. pectoral girdle
16. talus _____	G. pelvic girdle
17. scapula _____	H. upper extremities
18. ilium _____	
19. obturator foramen _____	

Match the bone marking in Column A with the definition in Column B. Definitions in Column B will be used more than once.

Column A

20. crest _____
21. head _____
22. fossa _____
23. foramen _____
24. tuberosity _____
25. condyle _____
26. trochanter _____
27. facet _____
28. tubercle _____
29. meatus _____
30. spinous process _____
31. sinus _____

Column B

A. a projection that fits into a joint

B. a projection that acts as an attachment for tendons and ligaments

C. a depression

Match the term in Column A with its meaning in Column B.

Column A

32. flexion _____
33. extension _____
34. hyperextension _____
35. abduction _____
36. adduction _____
37. circumduction _____
38. supination _____
39. pronation _____
40. inversion _____
41. eversion _____
42. elevation _____
43. depression _____
44. protraction _____
45. retraction _____
46. plantar flexion _____
47. dorsiflexion _____

Column B

A. movement, usually of the palm of the hand forward, as in the anatomical position; or movement of the body lying on a table so that the ventral cavity is facing up

B. movement that raises a part; moving the shoulders up

C. decreasing the angle between two bones at a joint

D. movement, usually of the palm of the hand backward; or movement of the body lying on a table so that the ventral cavity is facing down

E. increasing the angle between two bones at a joint; return from flexion

F. flexing the foot toward the sole

G. flexing the foot dorsally

H. overextending the joint or extending it beyond the anatomical position

I. movement of a joint in a circular manner

Column A	Column B
	J. movement away from the medial line of the body, usually involving the upper or lower extremities
	K. movement toward the medial line of the body, usually involving the upper or lower extremities
	L. moving of a part backward; moving the lower jaw back
	M. movement of the tarsals so that the sole of the foot is facing away from the midline
	N. movement that lowers a part; moving the shoulders down
	O. movement of a part forward; moving the lower jaw forward
	P. movement of the tarsals so that the sole of the foot is facing toward the midline

▶EXERCISE 7–5

Spelling Practice

Spelling

Place a check mark beside all misspelled words in the following list. Correctly spell those that you checked off.

1. ostioblast ☐ _____
2. osteocyte ☐ _____
3. humorus ☐ _____
4. stermun ☐ _____
5. endosteum ☐ _____
6. cartalige ☐ _____
7. hematapoeisis ☐ _____
8. tubercal ☐ _____
9. trochanter ☐ _____
10. fosca ☐ _____
11. condile ☐ _____
12. sella turcika ☐ _____
13. foramen ☐ _____
14. ethmoid ☐ _____
15. hyoid ☐ _____
16. coccyx ☐ _____

17. phalanxes ☐ _____

18. olecranen ☐ _____

19. supanation ☐ _____

20. osteomylitis ☐ _____

Use of Medical Terms in Context

Medical Terms in Context

Define the underlined terms as they are used in context.

UNIVERSITY HOSPITAL ✚   **RADIOLOGY REPORT**

SHOULDER, RIGHT

Severe arthropathy in the shoulder predominantly involves the glenohumeral joint where articular cartilage has been obliterated and extensive subchondral sclerosis has developed. The superior aspect of the humeral head and inferior surface of the acromion are somewhat irregular in contour. The AC joint is widely separated, but no definite erosion is identified.

OPINION:

Clearly there are severe degenerative changes in the right glenohumeral joint, although it is not clear whether this is secondary to an underlying inflammatory arthropathy.

SIGNATURE OF DOCTOR IN CHARGE _____

---

1. arthropathy _____

2. glenohumeral joint _____

3. articular cartilage _____

4. subchondral sclerosis _____

5. superior _____

6. humeral head _____

7. inferior _____

8. acromion _____

9. AC joint _____

10. inflammatory _____

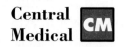

Central Medical CM

RADIOLOGY REPORT

ANKLE, RIGHT

Open reduction and internal fixation have been performed on a previously noted fracture of the lateral malleolus. The internal fixation has been performed with a metallic plate and six metal screws. Lateral examination of the ankle demonstrates a posterior malleolar fracture that is displaced approximately 1 mm dorsally and 1 to 2 mm inferiorly, resulting in a small deformity at the posterior mid-surface of the right ankle. The fibular fracture is in near-anatomic position. A small joint effusion is noted on the lateral film. Examination of the remainder of the foot demonstrates no evidence of fractures or dislocations.

SIGNATURE OF DOCTOR IN CHARGE _____

11. open reduction _____

12. internal fixation _____

13. fracture _____

14. lateral malleolus _____

15. dorsally _____

16. inferiorly _____

17. fibular _____

18. joint effusion _____

19. dislocations _____

**Crossword
Puzzle**

Joint Movement

Across

1. Movement toward the medial line of the body
4. Decreasing the angle between two bones at a joint
7. Extending the joint beyond the anatomical position
8. Movement forward, usually of the palm of the hand
9. Movement of the tarsals so that the sole of the foot is facing away from the midline
10. Movement that lowers a part of the body
11. Movement of a part in a backwards direction
12. Movement of a part in a forward direction

Down

1. Movement away from the medial line of the body
2. Circular movement of a joint
3. Movement of the tarsals so that the sole of the foot faces the midline
5. Return from flexion
6. Backwards movement of the palm of the hand
9. Movement away from the medial line of the body

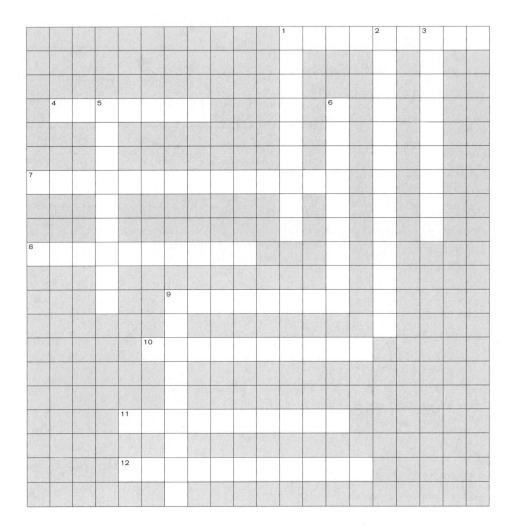

II—7

_____

_____

_____

_____

_____

_____

_____

_____

_____

_____

_____

_____

_____

_____

_____

_____

_____

_____

_____

_____

_____

_____

_____

8 THE MUSCULAR SYSTEM

CHAPTER OBJECTIVES

Upon successful completion of this chapter, the student will be able to do the following:

1. List and differentiate between the three types of muscle tissue.
2. Define terms relating to skeletal muscle organization.
3. State the functions of skeletal muscles.
4. List and define muscular actions.
5. Define insertion, origin, tendon, ligament, and aponeurosis.
6. Describe how muscles are named and give examples.
7. Name and locate major skeletal muscles.
8. Pronounce, analyze, define, and spell terms relating to the muscular system.
9. List and define terms describing the physical examination, abnormal conditions, and diagnostic and therapeutic procedures common to the muscular system.
10. Define abbreviations related to the muscular system.

WORD ELEMENT	TYPE	MEANING	WORD ELEMENT	TYPE	MEANING
-asthenia	suffix	without strength	ligament/o	root	ligament
duct/o	root	to lead; to carry	my/o; muscul/o; myos/o	root	muscle
fasci/o	root	fascia	ten/o; tendin/o	root	tendon
-kinesia; -kinesis	suffix	movement	tenosynov/i/o	root	tendon sheath
kinesi/o	root	movement			

▶ 8.1 MUSCLE TISSUE

The body's muscles make movement possible, not just the movement necessary for walking, running, swimming, lifting, and so on, but also the movement needed for us to breathe, digest food, and carry out all the other functions of the body.

Muscle Types

There are three different types of muscular tissue: **cardiac, visceral,** and **skeletal. Cardiac muscle,** located in the heart, is also known as **striated, involuntary muscle.** See Figure 8–1.

FIGURE 8–1

Cardiac Muscle Tissue

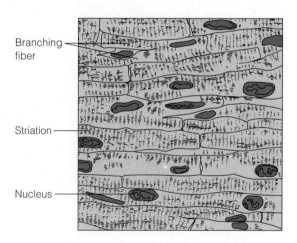

Branching fiber

Striation

Nucleus

Striated refers to the striped appearance of the tissue, and involuntary means that the action occurs spontaneously. **Visceral muscles,** located within organs, are known as nonstriated, or as **smooth, involuntary muscle.** See Figure 8–2.

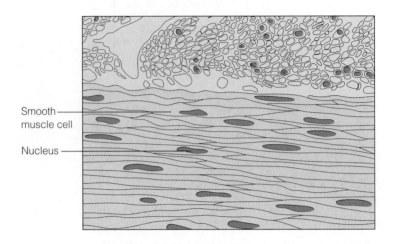

Smooth refers to the nonstriped appearance. **Skeletal muscle,** located on top of bone, is called **striated, voluntary.** Voluntary is the act of intentionally moving a muscle. See Figure 8–3.

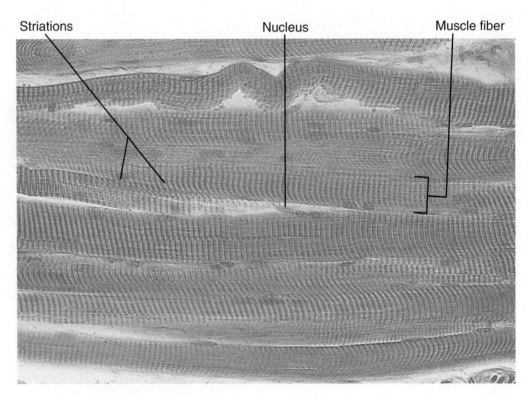

Cardiac and visceral muscles are discussed in their respective systems. This chapter deals only with the skeletal muscles.

Muscle Organization

The cells of a skeletal muscle are long and slender rather than the usual spherical shape. Because of this shape, muscle cells are often known as **muscle fibers.** Like all cells, muscle fibers contain a plasma membrane called **sarcolemma** and a cytoplasm called **sarcoplasm.** Smaller units of muscle tissue are packaged together to form larger units. The units fit together like the sections of a folding telescope, each smaller unit sliding into another larger unit. Each unit is held together by a band of connective tissue. For example, each muscle fiber is surrounded by **endomysium.** A group of muscle fibers are packaged into larger units called **fasciculi.** Each fasciculus is surrounded by **perimysium.** The fasciculi are grouped together to form a larger unit, the muscle, that is surrounded by **epimysium,** also known as **deep fascia.**

The muscle itself resembles parallel strands of spaghetti (see Figure 8–4) that contract (shorten) and pull on bone, resulting in movement, one of the functions of the muscular system. Such movements include flexion, extension, abduction, adduction, elevation, depression, **rotation, supination, pronation,** and **reduction in the size of an opening.** This latter movement involves a **sphincter muscle,** a ringlike muscle that closes an opening or passageway.

Other muscular system functions include **production of heat,** made possible by muscle contraction. **Shivering** is a form of muscle contraction that increases the core body temperature.

Exercise also produces body heat. The final function of muscles is the **maintenance of posture,** the positioning and alignment of body parts.

FIGURE 8–4 **Skeletal Muscle Anatomy** a. The muscle belly is attached to skeletal structures on both ends. b. Muscle fibers are grouped together to form fasciculi; fasciculi are grouped together to form the muscle. Each unit is held together by connective tissue, the endomysium, perimysium, or epimysium.

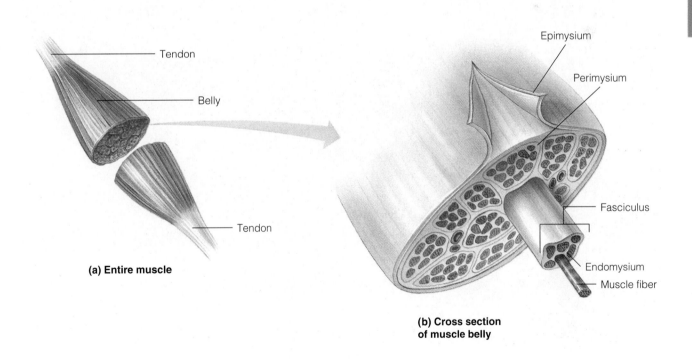

(a) Entire muscle

(b) Cross section of muscle belly

Skeletal muscles are held in place at points of attachment on two bones. The **origin** is an attachment of the muscle to the bone that does not move when a muscle contracts. The **insertion** is the attachment of the muscle to the bone that moves when the muscle contracts. For example, the **biceps muscle,** a muscle lying over the humerus, has its origin on the scapula, the bone that remains stable when the muscle contracts; its insertion is on the radius, the bone the muscle pulls, thereby flexing the forearm. See Figure 8–5.

Tendons function in the attachment of muscles to bone. They are composed of dense connective tissue and contain a large amount of **collagen.** It is the collagen bundles in the tendons that give them their strength and shiny, white appearance. An example of a tendon is the **Achilles tendon,** which attaches the distal end of the gastrocnemius (a calf muscle) to the heel.

Usually, tendons are long and slender; however, if they appear to be broad and flat, they are called **aponeuroses** (ăp″-ō-nū-rō′-sēz). An example of an aponeurosis is the **galea aponeurotica** (gā′-lĭ-ă ăp″-ō-nū-rŏt′-ĭk-ă) of the scalp—a wide, broad tendon sitting on the top of the scalp like a helmet.

Ligaments are fibrous bands of connective tissue connecting bone to bone. See Figure 8–6.

FIGURE 8–5 Origin and Insertion of the Biceps Muscle

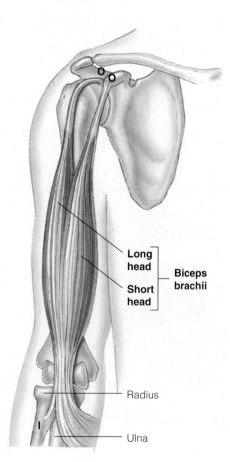

Long head
Short head
Biceps brachii
Radius
Ulna

FIGURE 8–6 Ligaments

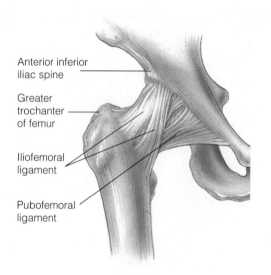

Anterior inferior iliac spine
Greater trochanter of femur
Iliofemoral ligament
Pubofemoral ligament

Naming of Skeletal Muscles

Muscles are named as follows:

Action   Muscles are often named for the movement they cause. For example, the **adductor brevis** (ăd-dŭk′-tor brē′-vĭs) muscle of the medial thigh pulls the leg toward the body (toward the midline). Flexor muscles decrease the angle of a joint. The **flexor digitorum superficialis** (flĕks′-or dĭ-gĭ-tor′-ŭm soo″-pĕr-fĭsh-ē-ăl′-ĭs) flexes the digits, or fingers.

Point of Attachment   Some muscles are named after the bones to which they are attached. The **sternocleidomastoid** (stĕr″-nō-klī″-dō-măs′-toyd) **muscle,** for example, attaches to the sternum, the clavicle, and the mastoid process.

Location   Muscles are sometimes named for their locations. For example, the **rectus femoris** (rĕk′-tŭs fĕm′-ō-rĭs) muscle is located on the femur, and the **tibialis anterior** (tĭb-ĭ-ā′-lĭs) muscle is located on the anterior aspect of the tibia.

Direction of Muscle Fibers   Muscle fibers can follow any number of lines. If the muscle fibers run straight up and down, they are called **rectus,** as in the rectus femoris muscle. The name **transversus abdominis** (trăns-vĕr′-sŭs ăb-dŏm′-ĭn-ŭs) indicates that the muscle fibers run across the abdomen.

Shape   The shape of the muscle can be the source of its name. For instance, **cruciate** (kroo′-shē-āt) means crossed. Anterior and posterior cruciate muscles of the knee joint cross each other to form an X.

Size   The size of the muscle is also used for naming. In the name **gluteus maximus** (glū′-tē-ŭs măks′-ĭ-mŭs), maximus refers to the large size of the buttocks.

Muscular Divisions   The **biceps** (bī′-sĕps) muscle on its proximal end divides into two tendons, attaching the biceps to the scapula in two places. It is said that the biceps has two heads. The **triceps** (trī′-sĕps) muscle on its proximal end divides into three tendinous attachments. It is said that the triceps has three heads.

8–II

FIGURE 8–7   Muscles of the Head and Neck (Anterior)

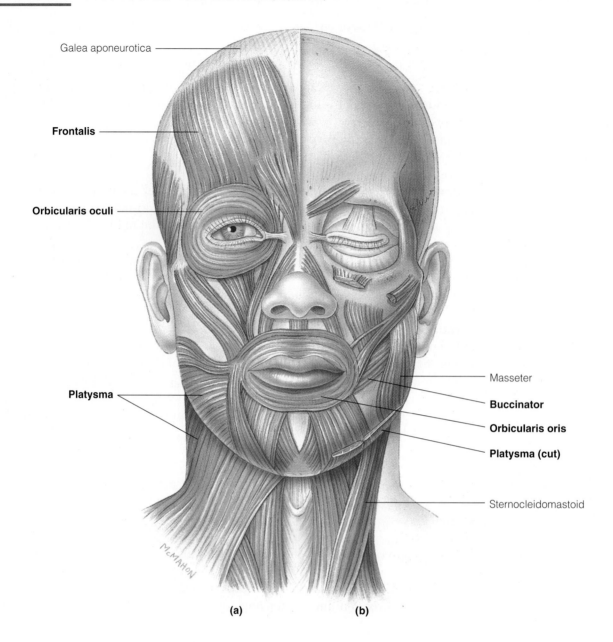

Galea aponeurotica

Frontalis

Orbicularis oculi

Platysma

Masseter

Buccinator

Orbicularis oris

Platysma (cut)

Sternocleidomastoid

(a)   (b)

Major Skeletal Muscles

Head and Neck Muscles   Using Figures 8–7 and 8–8 as references, locate the following muscles of the head and neck:

buccinator (bŭk′-sĭn-ā-tŏr)
epicranials (ĕp″-ĭ-krā′-nĭ-ăls)
  frontalis (frŏn′-tă-lĭs)
  occipitalis (ŏk-sĭp″-ĭ-tā′-lĭs)
  temporalis (tĕm″-pō-rā′-lĭs)
  galea aponeurotica
  (galea, Latin for helmet, is a broad tendinous attachment over the upper part of the cranium connecting the temporalis with the parietalis muscles and the temporalis with the occipitalis muscles)

FIGURE 8–8 Muscles of the Head and Neck (Lateral)

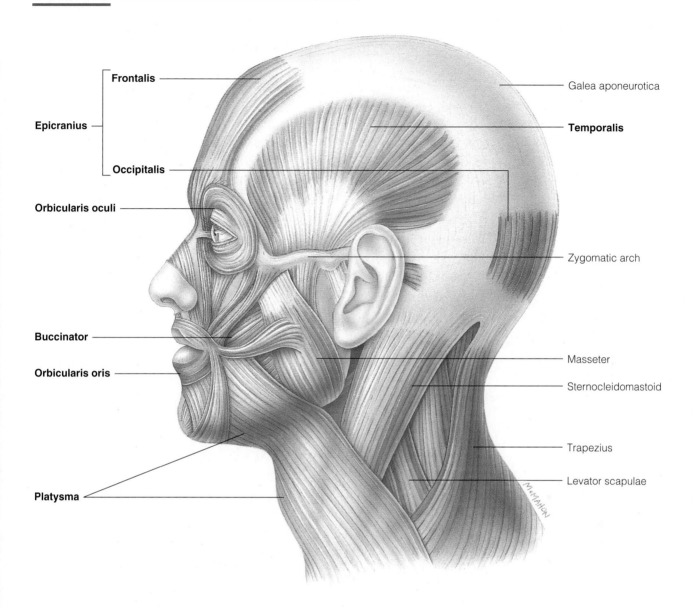

Frontalis — Galea aponeurotica

Epicranius

Temporalis

Occipitalis

Orbicularis oculi

Zygomatic arch

Buccinator

Masseter

Orbicularis oris

Sternocleidomastoid

Trapezius

Levator scapulae

Platysma

levator scapula (lĕ-vā′-tōr skăp′-ū-lă)
masseter (măs-sē′-tĕr)
orbicularis oculi (ŏr″-bĭk′-ū-lă′-rĭs ŏk′-ū-lī)
orbicularis oris (ŏr″-bĭk-ū-lă′-rĭs ōr′-ĭs)
platysma (plă-tĭz′-mă)
pterygoid (tĕr′-ĭ-goyd) (not shown; deep muscle of the cheek)
sternocleidomastoid (stĕr″-nō-klī″-dō-măs′-toyd)

Using Figures 8–9 and 8–10 as references, locate the following muscles:

Thoracic Muscles
intercostal muscles (not shown; located between the ribs)
pectoralis major (pĕk″-tō-rā′-lĭš)
pectoralis minor (not shown; deep to the pectoralis major)
serratus anterior (sĕr-ră′-tŭs)

Anterior Abdominal Muscles   Muscles are listed from most superficial to deepest.
rectus abdominis (rĕk′-tŭs ăb-dŏm′-ĭn-ŭs)
external oblique
internal oblique (not shown)
transversus abdominis (not shown)
linea alba (lĭn′-ē-ă ăl′-bă) (white line) not a muscle belly but formed by fibers of the right abdominal muscles, interlacing with fibers from the left abdominal muscles, anchoring the layers of muscles; extends from the xiphoid process to the symphysis pubis

Posterior Abdominal Muscles
iliopsoas (ĭl″-ĭ-ŏp-sō′-ăs) muscle (not shown, lies deep in the abdomen)

Back Muscles
infraspinatus (ĭn″-fră-spĭn-ă′-tŭs)
latissimus dorsi (lă-tĭ′-sĭ-mŭs dōr′-sī)
rhomboideus major (rŏm-bō-ĭd′-ĭ-ŭs)
teres major (tē′-rēz)
teres minor
trapezius (tră-pē′-zĭ-ŭs)

Shoulder Muscles
deltoid (dĕl′-toyd) (covers the shoulder anteriorly, posteriorly, and laterally)
serratus anterior

Upper Arm Muscles
biceps brachii (bī′-sĕps brā′-kĭ)
brachialis (brā-kĭ-ăl′-ĭs)
triceps brachii (trī′-sĕps brā-kĭ)

Forearm Muscles   Although there are many muscles of the forearm, each individually named, they can be placed into two groups:

flexors of the hand, located anteriorly
extensors of the hand, located posteriorly

FIGURE 8–9   Major Superficial Muscles of the Body (Anterior)

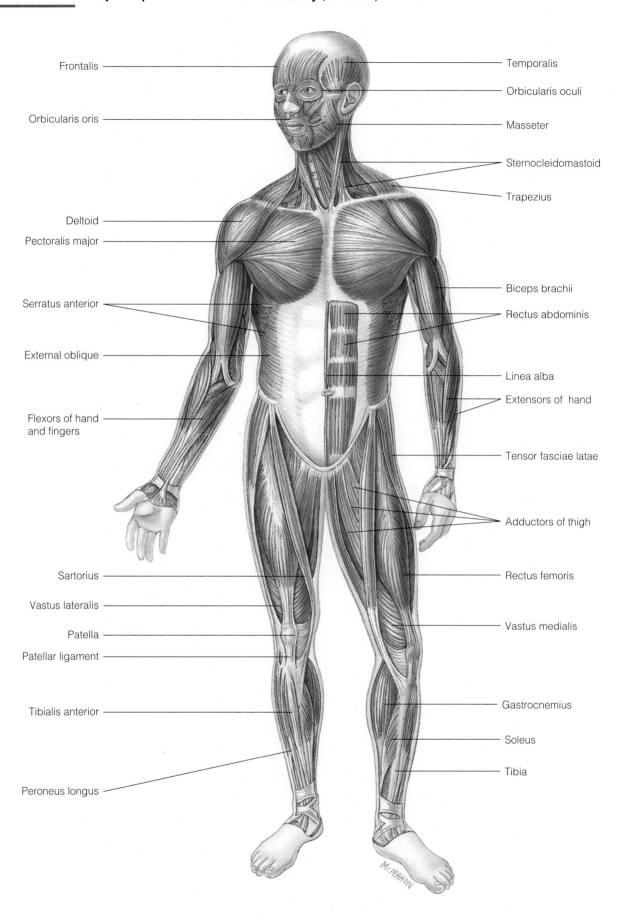

Frontalis

Orbicularis oris

Deltoid

Pectoralis major

Serratus anterior

External oblique

Flexors of hand
and fingers

Sartorius

Vastus lateralis

Patella

Patellar ligament

Tibialis anterior

Peroneus longus

Temporalis

Orbicularis oculi

Masseter

Sternocleidomastoid

Trapezius

Biceps brachii

Rectus abdominis

Linea alba

Extensors of hand

Tensor fasciae latae

Adductors of thigh

Rectus femoris

Vastus medialis

Gastrocnemius

Soleus

Tibia

8—II

FIGURE 8–10 Major Superficial Muscles of the Body (Posterior)

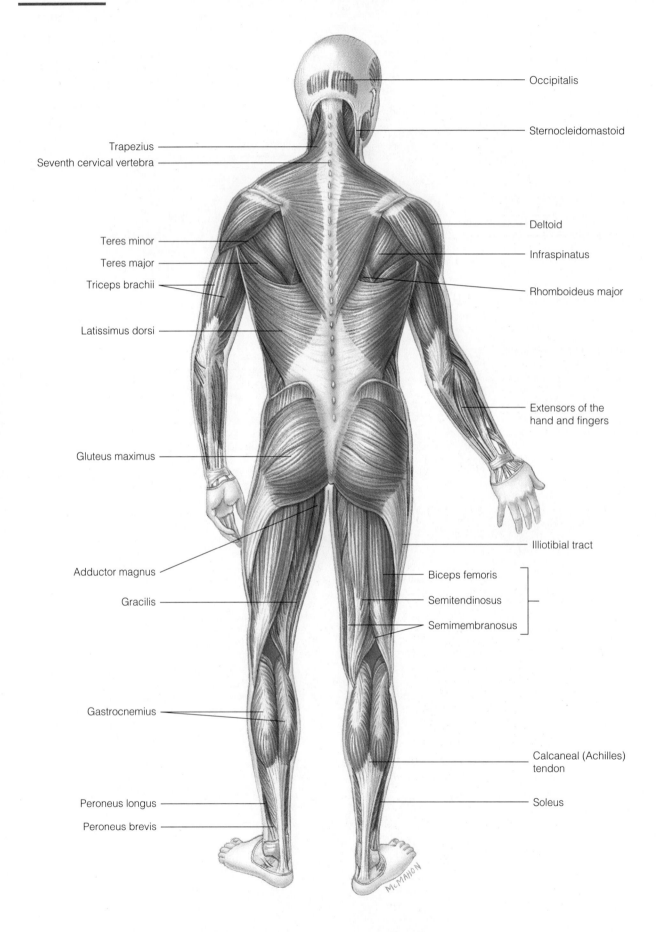

Occipitalis

Sternocleidomastoid

Trapezius

Seventh cervical vertebra

Deltoid

Teres minor

Teres major

Infraspinatus

Triceps brachii

Rhomboideus major

Latissimus dorsi

Extensors of the
hand and fingers

Gluteus maximus

Illiotibial tract

Biceps femoris

Adductor magnus

Semitendinosus

Gracilis

Semimembranosus

Gastrocnemius

Calcaneal (Achilles)
tendon

Peroneus longus

Soleus

Peroneus brevis

Thigh Muscles

ANTERIOR:

quadriceps (kwăd′-rĭ-sĕps)

  rectus femoris

  vastus intermedius (văs′-tŭs ĭn-tĕr-mē′-dĭ-ŭs) (not shown; deep to rectus femoris)

  vastus medialis (văs′-tŭs mē-dĭ-ā′-lĭs)

  vastus lateralis (văs′-tŭs lăt-ēr-ā′-lĭs)

sartorius (săr-tō′-rĭ-ŭs)

POSTERIOR

gracilis (grăs′-ĭ-lĭs)

hamstrings

  biceps femoris (bī′-sĕps fĕm′-ō-rĭs)

  semimembranosus (sĕm-″ĭ-mĕm-bră-nō′-sŭs)

  semitendinosus (sĕm″-ĭ-tĕn-dĭ-nō′-sŭs)

MEDIAL

adductors

  adductor magnus (ăd-dŭk′-tŏr măg′-nŭs)

  adductor brevis (not shown) (brevis-short)

  adductor longus (ăd-dŭk′-tŏr lŏng′-gŭs) (not shown)

LATERAL

tensor fasciae latae (tĕn′-sōr făs′-ĭ-ē lā′-tē) (the tendinous attachment of the tensor fascia lata is called the iliotibial tract)

Buttocks Muscles

gluteus maximus

gluteus minimus (glū′-tē-ŭs mĭn′-ĭ-mŭs) (not shown; deep to the gluteus maximus)

Lower Leg Muscles

ANTERIOR

tibialis anterior

POSTERIOR

gastrocnemius (găs-trŏk-nē′-mĭ-ŭs) (tendinous attachment is the Achilles tendon)

soleus (sō′-lē-ŭs)

LATERAL

peroneus brevis (pĕr-ō-nē′-ŭs brē′-vĭs)

peroneus longus (pĕr-ō-nē′-ŭs lŏng′-gŭs)

8—II

Pelvic Floor Muscles   See Figure 8–11.

      levator ani (lē-vā′-tōr ā′-nī)
      coccygeus (kŏk-sĭj′ ē-ūs)
      sphincter ani (sfĭnk-tĕr ā-nī) (the sphincter ani opens and closes the anus)

FIGURE 8–11   Muscles of the Pelvic Floor and Perineum

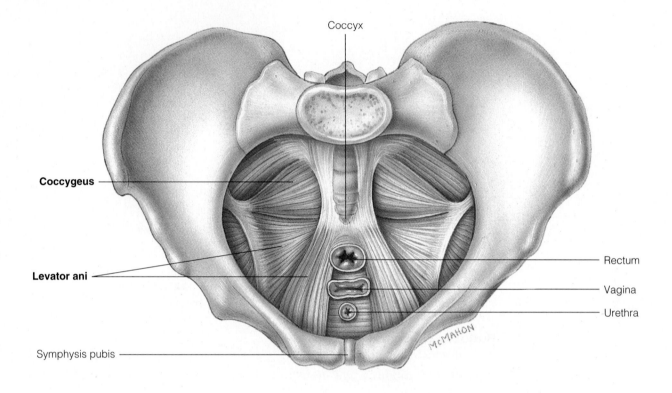

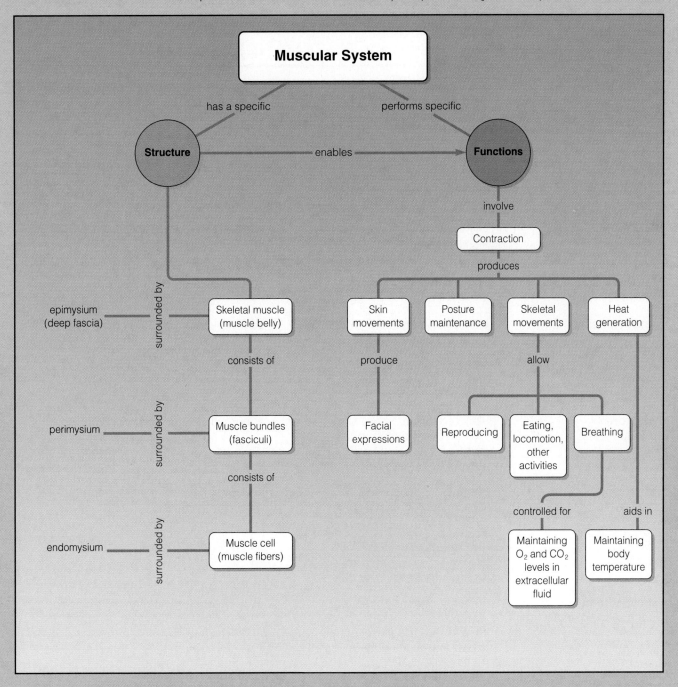

II—8

TERM WITH PRONUNCIATION	ANALYSIS	DEFINITION
abductor ăb-dŭk-tor	-or = person or thing that does something ab- = away from duct/o = to draw	refers to muscles that move a part away from the midline
adductor ă-dŭk′-tor	-or = person or thing that does something ad- = toward duct/o = to draw	refers to muscles that move a part toward the midline
atonic ă-tŏn′-ĭk	-ic = pertaining to a- = no; not ton/o = tone; tension	a muscle that has no tone or tension; atony
atrophy ăt′-rō-fē	-trophy = nourishment a- = no; not	wasting away of the muscle
bradykinesia brăd″-ē-kĭ-nē′-sē-ă	-kinesia = movement; motion brady- = slow	slow movement
dyskinesia dĭs″-kĭ-nē′-sē-ă	-kinesia = movement dys- = bad; difficult; painful; poor	impairment of muscle movement
dystonia dĭs-tō′-nē-ă	-ia = condition dys- = bad; painful; difficult; poor ton/o = tone; tension	abnormal tone or tension of muscle
dystrophy dĭs′-trō-fē	-trophy = nourishment dys- = poor; bad; difficult; painful	abnormal development, especially muscular dystrophy
fascial făsh′-ē-ăl	-al = pertaining to fasci/o = fascia (band of tissue surrounding the muscle)	pertaining to the fascia
fasciectomy făsh″-ē-ĕk′-tō-mē	-ectomy = excision; surgical removal fasci/o = fascia (band of tissue surrounding the muscle)	excision or surgical removal of fascia
fasciitis; fascitis făsh-ē-ī′-tĭs fă-sī′-tĭs	-itis = inflammation fasci/o = fascia (band of tissue surrounding the muscle)	inflammation of fascia
fasciorrhaphy făsh-ē-or′-ă-fē	-rrhaphy = suturing fasci/o = fascia (band of tissue surrounding the muscle)	suturing the fascia
hyperkinesia hī″-pĕr-kĭ-nē′-zē-ă	-kinesia = movement hyper- = excessive; above	excessive movement
hypertrophy hī-pĕr′-trō-fē	-trophy = nourishment hyper- = excessive; above	enlargement of an organ (due to an increase in the size of its cells)
kinesiology kĭ-nē″-sē-ŏl′-ō-jē	-logy = study of kinesi/o = movement	study of movement

TERM WITH PRONUNCIATION	ANALYSIS	DEFINITION
kinesimeter kĭn″-ĕ-sĭm′-ĕ-tĕr	-meter = instrument used to measure kinesi/o = movement	instrument used to measure movement
leiomyoma lī″-ō-mī-ō′-mă	-oma = tumor or mass lei/o = smooth my/o = muscle	tumor of smooth muscle; fibromyoma
leiomyosarcoma lī″-ō-mī″-ō-săr-kō′-mă	-sarcoma = malignant tumor of connective tissue lei/o = smooth my/o = muscle	malignant tumor of smooth muscle
ligamentous lĭg″-ă-mĕn′-tŭs	-ous = pertaining to ligament/o = ligament (tissue connecting bone to bone)	pertaining to ligaments
muscular mŭs′-kū-lăr	-ar = pertaining to muscul/o = muscle	pertaining to muscle
myalgia mī-ăl′-jē-ă	-algia = pain my/o = muscle	muscle pain
myasthenia mī-ăs-thē-nē-ă	-asthenia = condition of no strength my/o = muscle	no muscle strength
myoclonus mī-ŏk′-lō-nŭs	-clonus = turmoil my/o = muscle	alternate muscular relaxation and contraction in rapid succession
myofibrosis mī″-ō-fī-brō′-sĭs	-osis = abnormal condition my/o = muscle fibr/o = fibers	replacement of muscle tissue with fibrous tissue
myopathy mī-ŏp′-ă-thē	-pathy = disease my/o = muscle	disease of the muscles
myositis mī-ō-sī′-tĭs	-itis = inflammation myos/o = muscle	inflammation of muscle
myotonia mī″-ō-tō′-nē-ă	-ia = condition my/o = muscle ton/o = tone; tension	inability of the muscle to relax after increased muscular contraction; tonic spasm of a muscle
polymyositis pŏl″-ē-mī″-ō-sī′-tĭs	-itis = inflammation poly- = many myos/o = muscle	inflammation of many muscles
rhabdomyolysis răb″-dō-mī-ŏl′-ĭ-sĭs	-lysis = destruction; breakdown rhabd/o = rod-shaped; striped my/o = muscle	destruction of striated muscle tissue
rhabdomyoma răb″-dō-mī-ō′-mă	-oma = tumor or mass rhabd/o = rod/shaped; striped my/o = muscle	tumor of striated muscle
rhabdomyosarcoma răb″-dō-mī″-ō-săr-kō′-mă	-sarcoma = malignant tumor of connective tissue rhabd/o = rod-shaped; striped my/o = muscle	malignant tumor of striated muscle

8–II

TERM WITH PRONUNCIATION	ANALYSIS	DEFINITION
tendinitis tĕn″-dĭn-ī′-tĭs	-itis = inflammation tendin/o = tendon	inflammation of a tendon
tendinous tĕn′-dĭ-nŭs	-ous = pertaining to tendin/o = tendon	pertaining to a tendon
tenosynovitis tĕn″-ō-sĭn″-ō-vī′-tĭs	-itis = inflammation tenosynov/i/o = tendon sheath	inflammation of the tendon sheath
tenotomy tĕ-nŏt′-ō-mē	-tomy = to cut; incise ten/o = tendon	cutting of a tendon
tonic tŏn′-ĭk	-ic = pertaining to ton/o = tone; tension	pertaining to tone or tension

▷ 8.5 ABNORMAL CONDITIONS

PATHOLOGY	DESCRIPTION
contracture	shortening of muscle fibers, preventing stretching of the muscle
Dupuytren's contracture	shortening of the palmer fascia (fibrous tissue surrounding the muscle in the palm of the hand) resulting in flexion of the fingers, making normal use impossible
Volkmann's contracture	flexion deformity of the fingers due to a lack of blood supply to the muscle
muscular dystrophy	Muscular dystrophy is a broad term used to describe several types of congenital conditions, all of which are characterized by wasting of the muscles. **Note:** This condition is a genetic disorder most often seen in boys. The skeletal muscles are first affected, followed by the involuntary muscles. The muscles appear bulky and strong, which belies the loss of muscle tissue that is taking place. This false appearance is due to the infiltration of fat and fibrous tissue into the muscle. In the late stages of the disease, the involuntary muscles of the heart are affected, resulting in cardiac and pulmonary complications and eventual heart failure. Diagnosis is confirmed by three tests: muscle biopsy, which shows replacement of muscle tissue with fat and fibrous tissue; EMG, which shows weak muscle activity; and laboratory tests, which show increased amounts of creatinine phosphokinase (CPK) in the serum indicating muscular wasting. There is no cure, and patients succumb to the disease usually in their twenties.
strain	overstretching of a muscle usually due to overexercise or overuse **Note:** Compare with another common injury, the **sprain,** which is injury to a joint (see skeletal system, Chapter 7).
torticollis	a congenital or acquired contracture of the sternocleidomastoid muscles resulting in flexion of the head toward the injured side; wryneck

During the muscular system examination, which most often accompanies a skeletal system examination, the physician pays close attention to the range of motion, ligament stability, and muscle power. (Range of motion and ligament stability are discussed in Chapter 7.)

Muscle power varies from individual to individual, depending on size, sex, age, and muscular development. It is usually tested by asking the patient to move a body part while the physician applies resistance. The muscle power is graded from 0–5 where:

0 = no power or muscle contraction exhibited

1 = flicker of muscle contraction

2 = movement of a body part but not against gravity

3 = movement of a body part against gravity

4 = movement against gravity with minimal resistance applied

5 = movement of a body part against strong resistance with no evidence of muscular fatigue, indicating normal muscle strength

Laboratory Tests Used in Diagnosing Muscular Pathology

TEST	DESCRIPTION
serum creatine phosphokinase (CPK); also known as creatine kinase (CK)	CPK is an enzyme found in cardiac and skeletal muscle tissue as well as brain tissue. **Note:** Following skeletal muscle trauma or myocardial damage, the muscle cells release CPK. Increased levels of this enzyme in the blood is a good indicator of muscle disease.
urine creatine	Creatine is found in muscle and is usually excreted in the urine as **creatinine.** In certain muscular disease, such as muscular dystrophy, creatine is released from the muscle in such large amounts that it spills over into the urine, where it is detected by laboratory test.

Radiology and Diagnostic Imaging Used in Diagnosing Muscular Pathology

computerized axial tomography	a technique that uses x-ray technology and a computer to obtain cross-sectional images detailing the structure at various depths
magnetic resonance imaging	a technique that relies on a strong magnetic field into which the patient is placed; a three-dimensional record is made of the area imaged through computer calculation of the body's response to the strong magnetic field

8–II

Clinical Procedures	
electromyography (EMG)	recording of the electrical characteristics of muscle Note: Electrical activity is produced in a muscle when it is stimulated by a nerve.
biopsy	removal of a piece of muscle, which is then examined by a pathologist for diagnostic purposes

Treatment Methods for Muscular Disorders

MEDICAL TREATMENT	DESCRIPTION
diathermy	heat applied to deep tissues
muscle relaxants	drugs used to relieve pain and stiffness of skeletal muscles; used extensively for various orthopedic disorders, injuries, and back pain

8.7 ABBREVIATIONS

ABBREVIATION	DEFINITION	ABBREVIATION	DEFINITION
CPK; CK	creatine phosphokinase; creatine kinase	IM	intramuscular
EMG	electromyography	RICE	rest, ice, compression, elevation

▶EXERCISE 8–1

Short Answer

Briefly answer the following questions.
Answers to all exercise questions appear in Appendix A.

Practice Quiz

1. List and differentiate between the three types of muscle tissue. _____

    _____

    _____

    _____

    _____

2. What is the major function of the skeletal muscles? _____

    _____

3. What shape are the cells that make up skeletal muscles? _____

_____

4. What is another name for muscle cells? _____

5. Muscle fibers form larger units known as _____.

6. What is another term for epimysium? _____

7. Briefly discuss the difference between origin and insertion as these terms relate to muscle/skeletal attachment. _____

_____

_____

8. A broad, flat tendon is called _____.

9. What is the term that describes a fibrous band of connective tissue that connects bone to bone? _____

10. What term refers to muscles that move a part away from the midline? ___

_____

▶EXERCISE 8–2

Matching Terms with Meanings

Matching

Match the term in Column A with its meaning in Column B.

Column A		Column B
1. aponeurosis	_____	A. suturing of the fascia
2. ligaments	_____	B. enlargement of an organ owing to increased cell size
3. fasciorrhaphy	_____	
4. myasthenia	_____	C. abnormal tone of a muscle
5. myopathy	_____	D. a broad, flat tendon
6. hypertrophy	_____	E. refers to a muscle that moves a part toward the midline
7. bradykinesia	_____	F. muscular disease
8. dystonia	_____	G. fibrous bands of connective tissue connecting bone to bone
9. abductor	_____	H. refers to a muscle that moves a part away from the midline
10. adductor	_____	I. slow movement
		J. absence of muscle strength

Match the term in Column A with its location in Column B. Use more than one letter if required.

Column A		Column B
11. levator ani	_____	A. head and neck
12. buccinator	_____	B. thorax
13. coccygeus	_____	C. abdomen
14. platysma	_____	D. back
15. pectoralis major	_____	E. upper arm
16. levator scapula	_____	F. forearm
17. external oblique	_____	G. thigh
18. serratus anterior	_____	H. pelvic floor
19. brachialis	_____	
20. gracilis	_____	

▶ **EXERCISE 8–3**

Spelling

Place a check mark beside all misspelled words in the list that follows. Correctly spell those that you checked off.

Spelling Practice

1. bucinator ☐ _____

2. platisma ☐ _____

3. pectorialis major ☐ _____

4. transversus abdominus ☐ _____

5. byceps femorus ☐ _____

6. fasciorrhaphy ☐ _____

7. distrophy ☐ _____

8. ligamentus ☐ _____

9. muscular ☐ _____

10. myopathy ☐ _____

11. myositus ☐ _____

12. tonic ☐ _____

13. pterygoid ☐ _____

14. visceral muscles ☐ _____

15. striated ☐ _____

16. tendin ☐ _____

17. ligament ☐ _____

18. muscle fibres ☐ _____

19. fasciculus ☐ _____

20. perimysium ☐ _____

Vocabulary Study

Using the phonetic pronunciations appearing throughout the text and using the list of word elements at the beginning of the chapter, pronounce each term aloud and write its definition.

1. atonic _____

2. atrophy _____

3. dyskinesia _____

4. dystrophy _____

5. fascial _____

6. fasciectomy _____

7. fasciitis _____

8. hyperkinesia _____

9. kinesiology _____

10. kinesiometer _____

11. leiomyoma _____

12. leiomyosarcoma _____

13. ligamentous _____

14. muscular _____

15. myalgia _____

16. myoclonus _____

17. myofibrosis _____

18. myositis _____

19. myotonia _____

20. polymyositis _____

21. rhabdomyolysis _____

22. rhabdomyoma _____

23. rhabdomyosarcoma _____

24. tonic _____

25. tendinitis _____

26. tendinous _____

27. tenosynovitis _____

28. tenotomy _____

Medical Terms in Context

Define the underlined terms as they are used in context.

UNIVERSITY HOSPITAL ✚

SUMMARY RECORD

ADMISSION DATE: FEBRUARY 24, 1995

DISCHARGE DATE: FEBRUARY 26, 1995

DISCHARGE DIAGNOSIS: LEFT HAND, *DUPUYTREN'S CONTRACTURE*

This is a 65-year-old male patient who is known to have Dupuytren's disease in both hands, with the left hand more extensively involved than the opposite one. The patient had a previous fasciectomy approximately five years ago, but the disease recurred on the palmar surface of the fifth digit, and with tendinous contracture, it pulled the MCP and the PIP joint into a flexion deformity. The patient was admitted for fasciectomy.

SIGNATURE OF DOCTOR IN CHARGE _____

---

1. Dupuytren's contracture _____

2. fasciectomy _____

3. digit _____

4. tendinous contracture _____

5. MCP _____

6. PIP _____

7. flexion deformity _____

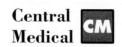

SUMMARY RECORD

ADMISSION DATE: AUGUST 10, 1995

DISCHARGE DATE: AUGUST 12, 1995

HISTORY OF PRESENT ILLNESS:

The patient is a seven-year-old boy who was first noticed to have
signs of weakness at age 2-3 years. The diagnosis of muscular
dystrophy was confirmed by an elevated CK and muscular degeneration
on the biopsy. He is still ambulatory and was started on drug
therapy three months ago.

PHYSICAL EXAMINATION:

On examination, the patient is a pleasant young fellow. He has
proximal muscle weakness. He has calf hypertrophy and some
contractures of the heel tendons. General physical examination is
within normal limits.

COURSE IN HOSPITAL:

While in the hospital, an intravenous line was started, and blood
samples were taken for CK during a 24-hour period. He also underwent
a 24-hour urine collection. All of these samples were sent to a
central laboratory for analysis, and results are unavailable at the
time of this dictation.

The course in hospital was uneventful.

MOST RESPONSIBLE DIAGNOSIS: MUSCULAR DYSTROPHY

SIGNATURE OF DOCTOR IN CHARGE _____

8. muscular dystrophy   _____

9. CK   _____

10. biopsy   _____

11. ambulatory   _____

12. hypertrophy   _____

13. contractures   _____

14. tendons   _____

Crossword Puzzle

Terms of the Muscular System

Across

3. Inflammation of the tendon sheath
4. Muscle that moves a part away from the midline
6. Fast movement
7. Pertaining to muscle tone
8. Abnormal development
10. Slow movement
13. Bending
14. Muscle pain

Down

1. Wasting away
2. Without tone
4. A muscle that moves a part toward the midline
5. Muscular disability
8. Difficult movement
9. Destruction of striated muscle tissue
11. Abnormal muscle tone
12. Study of movement

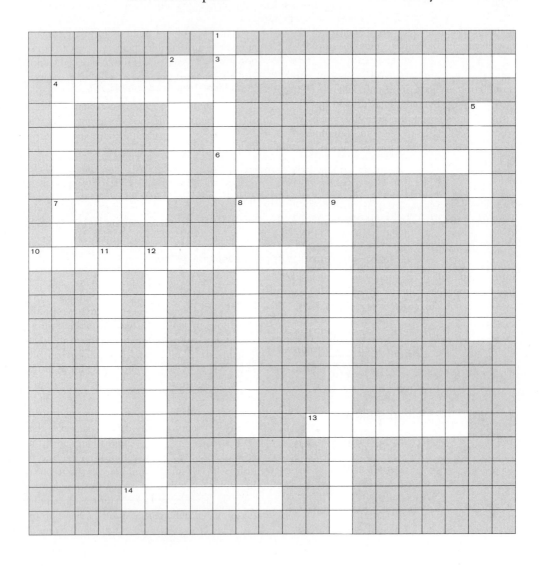

8—11

9

THE NERVOUS SYSTEM

CHAPTER OBJECTIVES

Upon successful completion of this chapter, the student will be able to do the following:

1. Name and describe the major divisions and subdivisions of the nervous system.
2. State the major functions of the nervous system.
3. Name and describe the cells of the nervous system.
4. Differentiate between a neuron, nerve fiber, nerve, nerve tract, and ganglion.
5. Describe a synapse.
6. List and describe the major divisions of the brain.
7. Discuss the anatomical structures of the spinal cord.
8. Name and describe the protective coverings of the brain and spinal cord.
9. Describe cerebrospinal fluid and its functions.
10. Name three divisions of the peripheral nervous system.
11. Name and number the cranial nerves in the correct sequence as they emerge from the anterior to posterior aspect of the brain.
12. List the functions of the cranial nerves.
13. Define plexus and name four plexuses arising from the spinal cord.
14. Name the major nerves arising from each plexus.
15. Define reflex.
16. Differentiate between superficial and deep tendon reflexes.
17. Name five common reflexes and the associated normal response.
18. Define Babinski's reflex.
19. Name two subdivisions of the autonomic nervous system.
20. Describe the function of the autonomic nervous system.
21. Pronounce, analyze, define, and spell common terms of the nervous system.
22. Define terms relating to the physical examination, abnormal conditions, signs and symptoms, diagnostic, and therapeutic procedures common to the nervous system.
23. Define common abbreviations of the nervous system.

WORD ELEMENT	TYPE	MEANING	WORD ELEMENT	TYPE	MEANING
cerebell/o	root	cerebellum	mening/o	root	membrane; meninges
cerebr/o	root	brain; cerebrum	myelin/o	root	myelin sheath
cortic/o	root	cortex; outer layer	myel/o	root	spinal cord; bone marrow
dur/o	root	dura mater			
encephal/o	root	brain	neur/o	root	nerve
gangli/o	root	ganglion	pont/o	root	pons; bridge
ganglion/o	root	ganglion	somn/o	root	sleep
lept/o	root	thin; slender; delicate	radicul/o; rhiz/o	root	nerve root
			thalam/o	root	thalamus
medull/o	root	medulla oblongata	ventricul/o	root	ventricle

⧫ 9.1 OVERVIEW OF THE NERVOUS SYSTEM

Computer networking "highways" have now developed to the point that millions of messages are exchanged daily by personal computers throughout the world. People marvel at the complexity of this technology, perhaps never stopping to consider that their own nervous systems are much more intricate and vastly more efficient information networks. This chapter will give you a basic understanding of the structure of the nervous system and how it functions and will introduce you to the most common terms associated with this magnificent system.

Divisions of the Nervous System

The nervous system consists of the **central nervous system (CNS)** and the **peripheral nervous system (PNS)** (see Figure 9–1). The CNS consists of the brain and spinal cord. The brain receives information about the changing environment, associates the data, and initiates a response. The spinal cord carries information back and forth between the brain and the PNS.

The PNS consists of **nerves** and **ganglia.** The **nerves** are grouped into the **sensory (afferent) system** and the **motor (efferent) system.** The neurons of the sensory system receive messages about changes in the environment to which the body should respond. These messages are transferred into electrical impulses and carried toward the brain. The neurons of the motor system carry information away from the brain to stimulate (innervate) the skeletal muscles, glands, or internal organs, enacting an appropriate response. **Ganglia** are groups of nerve cell bodies located outside the brain and spinal cord.

9–1

FIGURE 9–1 Divisions of the Nervous System

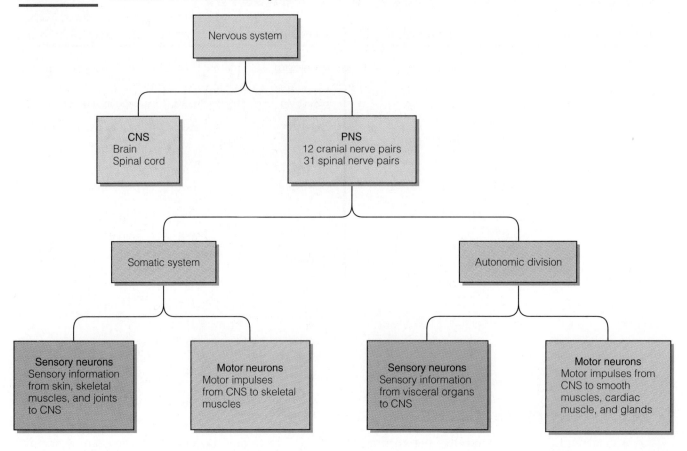

Both sensory and motor neurons are present in the **somatic** and **autonomic** **systems.** The **somatic system** is voluntary and innervates the skeletal muscles in controlling activities such as running. The autonomic system is involuntary; it innervates smooth muscle, cardiac muscle, and glands to control unconscious functions such as the beating of the heart.

Functions of the Nervous System

The nervous system has three functions: sensory, motor, and integrative. **Sensory** functions involve the detection of ongoing changes in the body and the environment. Information about these changes is transmitted to the spinal cord and brain.

Motor functions are those that relate to the movement of muscles and the actions of glands. In this context, muscles and glands are referred to as **effectors,** because they **effect change** in the body.

The **integrative** function is performed by the brain and the spinal cord. They receive incoming information from the sensory system, process it, and initiate the appropriate response through the motor system.

Nerve Cells

Nervous tissue is made up of two types of cells: **neuroglia** (nū-rō-glē'-ă) and **neurons.** The neuroglia are found between the neurons, connecting them and providing support and protection, (see Figure 9–2).

Neuroglial cells do not carry electrical impulses. Their function is to protect the neurons through **phagocytosis** (engulfing of unwanted substances by phagocytes) and to provide nutrients by attaching blood vessels to the neurons. They look like fluffy clouds that seem to be floating between the neurons. See Table 9-1.

FIGURE 9–2 Types of Neuroglia Found in the Central Nervous System

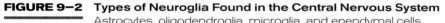

Astrocytes, oligodendroglia, microglia, and ependymal cells

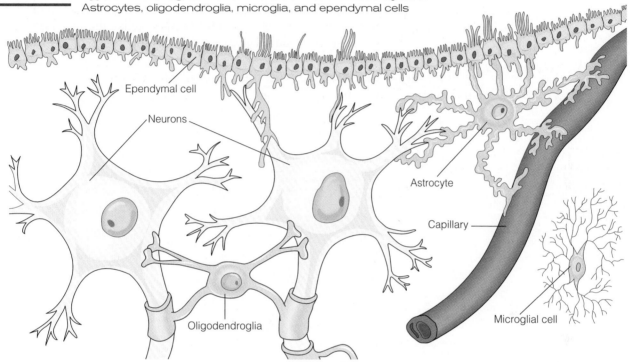

- Ependymal cell
- Neurons
- Astrocyte
- Capillary
- Oligodendroglia
- Microglial cell

TABLE 9–1

Types of Neuroglia

TYPE	DESCRIPTION
astrocytes ăs'-trō-sīts	star-shaped cells that function in the blood-brain barrier to prevent toxic substances from entering the brain
oligodendroglia ŏl"-ĭ-gō-děn-drŏg'-lē-ă	provide support and connection
microglia mī-krŏg'-lē-ă	involved in the phagocytosis of unwanted substances
ependyma ĕp-ĕn'-dĭ-mă	form the lining of the cavities in the brain and spinal cord
Schwann cells shvŏn	located only in the peripheral nervous system and make up the **neurilemma** and **myelin sheath** (see below)

Neurons perform the work of the nervous system, which is to transmit electrical impulses. There are several types: **sensory (afferent)** neurons transmit impulses to the brain and spinal cord, making the body aware of changes in the environment; **motor (efferent)** neurons transmit impulses away from the brain and spinal cord to **effectors,** either muscles or glands, that respond to the changes in the environment; and **interneurons** transmit impulses between sensory and motor neurons.

Unlike conventional cells, which are spherical, neurons are long and narrow. Each neuron contains one **cell body,** many **dendrites** (děn′-drīts), and one **axon** (ăx′-ŏn). Dendrites and axons are also known as **nerve cell fibers.** For an example of a neuron, see Figure 9–3.

The **cell body** is the main part of the neuron. It contains the organelles important to any cell type, including the nucleus, mitochondria, Golgi apparatus, and endoplasmic reticulum. But unlike other cells, the cell body of a neuron contains a substance called **nissl** (nĭs′-l) **bodies,** important to protein synthesis.

Dendrites are short branches that receive information from the internal and external environments. A single neuron has many dendrites that resemble

FIGURE 9–3

Neurons

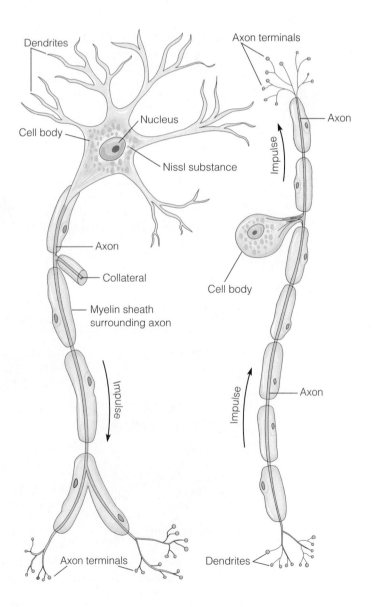

branches of a tree, reaching out to receive the various stimuli from the changing environment. The distal dendrites of sensory neurons contain receptors that receive initial stimuli, such as sound, and change it into electrical impulses that act as messages to other neurons.

Axons conduct impulses away from the cell body and **synapses** (sĭn′-ăps) (connect) with dendrites from other neurons, other cell bodies, or organs such as muscles or glands. Although an axon is a single extension from the cell body, it has branches called **collateral axons,** which transmit the impulses.

All neurons, whether they are in the central or peripheral nervous system, contain cell bodies, dendrites, and axons. However, only the neurons of the peripheral nervous system have the **myelin sheath** (mī′-ĕ-lĭn shēth), which is a fatty substance made of **Schwann cells.** Axons that are surrounded by myelin are referred to as **myelinated** (mī″-ĕl-in-āt′-ĕd); those that are not are **unmyelinated** (ŭn-mī′-ĕ-lĭ-nāt″-ĕd). See Figure 9–4.

FIGURE 9–4

Axon and Its Covering

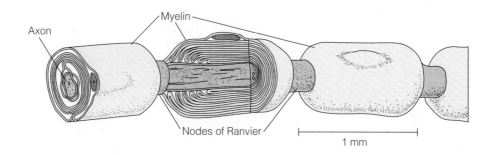

The myelin sheath wraps itself around the axon in a jelly-roll fashion. It acts as an insulator, keeping the electrical impulse travelling towards its destination without any loss of momentum. The entire axon is not covered, however. Small gaps appear at regular intervals. These gaps are called **nodes of Ranvier** (rŏn′-vē-ā). Electrical impulses jump from node to node, which greatly increases the speed of the impulse.

The outermost layer of the myelin sheath is called the **neurilemma** (nū-rĭ-lē′-mă). It is found only in the PNS and plays a central role in regenerating injured nerve tissue.

You will frequently encounter the terms nerve fibers, nerves, tracts, and ganglions when dealing with the nervous system. It is important to understand the difference. A **nerve fiber** is a process or projection extending from the cell body. Axons or dendrites are examples. A **nerve** is a group of nerve fibers outside the CNS. Nerves of similar function are arranged in **tracts. Ascending tracts** carry impulses to the brain; **descending tracts** carry impulses away from the brain.

Synapses

A light switch works by moving a tiny piece of metal back and forth. When the switch is turned on, the metal contacts another piece of metal and completes the electrical circuit. Flick the switch the other way, and the metal pieces are separated, breaking the circuit.

A **synapse** functions very much like a light switch. It is the junction between two neurons or between a neuron and a muscle. When the right stimulus comes along, the synapse is triggered and completes a circuit between two neurons, or between a neuron and a muscle (see Figure 9–5).

FIGURE 9–5

Synapse at the Myoneural Junction

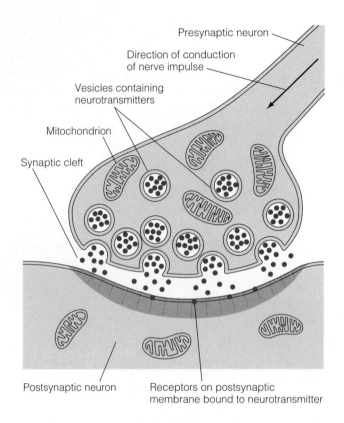

Presynaptic neuron

Direction of conduction of nerve impulse

Vesicles containing neurotransmitters

Mitochondrion

Synaptic cleft

Postsynaptic neuron

Receptors on postsynaptic membrane bound to neurotransmitter

As an electrical impulse travels down the neuron and reaches the synapse, the neurotransmitter **acetylcholine** (ACh) is released from a little sac or vesicle. This neurotransmitter migrates across the synaptic cleft and acts on the muscle, causing it to generate its own electrical impulse that produces a muscle contraction. Also present at the neuromuscular junction is **acetylcholinesterase,** an enzyme needed to eliminate ACh once it has done its work, returning the muscle to its original state.

There are many neurotransmitters. Acetylcholine and **norepinephrine** are just two examples.

◢ 9.2 CENTRAL NERVOUS SYSTEM

Brain

As mentioned previously, the **central nervous system** (CNS) consists of the brain and the spinal cord. The structures of the brain are as follows: the **cerebrum** (sĕr′-ĕ-brŭm), including the **cerebral cortex;** the **diencephalon** (dī″-ĕn-sĕf′-ă-lŏn), which includes the **thalamus** (thăl′-ă-mŭs) and the **hypothalamus** (hī″-pō-thăl′-ă-mŭs); the **brain stem,** which includes the **midbrain,** the **pons** (ponz), and the **medulla oblongata** (mĕ-dūl′-lă ŏb″-lŏng-gă′-tă); and the **cerebellum** (sĕr-ĕ-bĕl′-ŭm). See Figure 9–6.

FIGURE 9–6

Brain–Lateral View

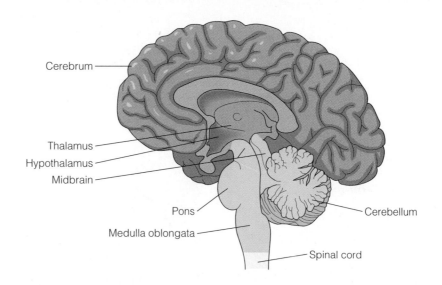

The **cerebrum** is the largest part of the brain. It receives sensory impulses from the peripheral nerves and initiates motor impulses to the viscera, especially muscles. It is the site of higher intellectual function. The cerebrum is divided into right and left hemispheres by the **longitudinal fissure.** The **hemispheres** are joined by the **corpus callosum** (kōr′-pŭs kă-lō′-sŭm), which consists of bundles of nerve fibers that allow the two hemispheres to share information.

The entire cerebrum is covered by a thin gray layer called the **cerebral cortex,** which is involved in sensory and motor functions as well as thought, judgment, and perception. The surface of the cerebrum has the appearance of little gray bulges that look somewhat like sausages. These bulges are also known as **convolutions** or **gyri** (jī′-rĭ). Each gyri is separated by shallow grooves called **sulci** (sŭl′-kĭ) or deeper grooves called **fissures.** See Figure 9–7.

FIGURE 9–7 Photograph of an Adult Human Brain, Lateral View

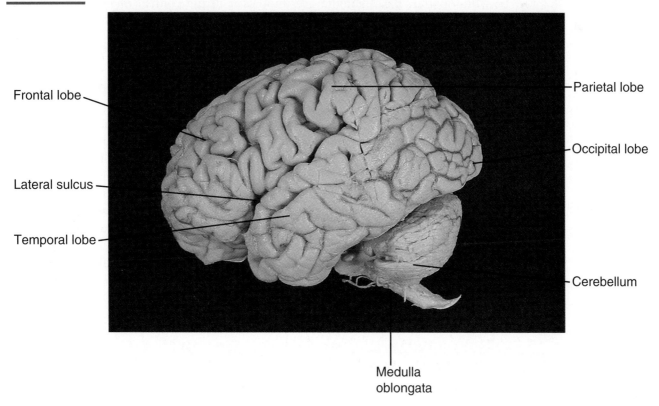

Fissures divide the cerebrum into lobes named after the bones of the skull under which they lie: **frontal lobe, parietal lobe, temporal lobe,** and **occipital lobe.** A fifth lobe, the **insula,** is embedded deep in the **lateral sulcus.** The **central sulcus** separates the frontal and parietal lobes, and the **lateral fissure** separates the cerebrum into frontal, parietal, and temporal lobes. See Figure 9–8.

FIGURE 9–8

Right and Left Cerebral Hemispheres
Frontal section showing the cerebrum in the anterior view. Notice the cerebral cortex, basal ganglia, fissures, sulci, thalamus, and ventricles.

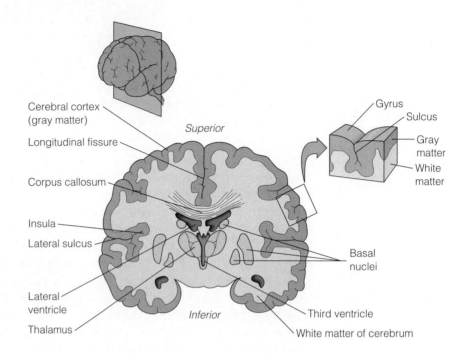

The interior of the cerebrum is made up of white and gray matter. Islands of gray matter, known as the **basal ganglia** or **basal nuclei,** are embedded in the white matter. Basal ganglia are important in the control of motor functions. Injury results in tremors and rigidity, as seen in Parkinson's disease, if the cells that produce and secrete **dopamine,** a neurotransmitter of the central nervous system, are destroyed. Also within the interior of the cerebrum are four hollow spaces called **ventricles.** The ventricles are referred to as first, second, third, and fourth. The first and second are also referred to as **lateral ventricles.** (CSF collects in the first and second ventricles and flows to the third through a passageway called the **interventricular foramen,** or **foramen of Monro.** From there, it flows to the fourth ventricle through the cerebral aqueduct and into the spinal canal. Ultimately, it is reabsorbed into the bloodstream and filtered out again into the ventricles. (See Protective coverings—Cerebrospinal fluid.)

The **diencephalon** is made up of the **thalamus** and the **hypothalamus.** The **thalamus,** located deep in the cerebrum, acts as a relay station in which sensory neurons synapse with other sensory neurons. When impulses travel to the brain, they stop at the thalamus, where the stimulus is recognized as pain, temperature, touch, etc. The thalamus then sends the impulse to the cerebral cortex for interpretation.

The **hypothalamus** is located below the thalamus. It helps regulate the autonomic nervous system by maintaining homeostasis of appetite, thirst, temperature, and water. It is also associated with the endocrine system and is extensively involved with emotional and basic behavioral patterns.

The **brain stem** consists of the **midbrain,** the **pons,** and the **medulla oblongata.** Each structure is continuous with the other. The midbrain is the superior part of the brain stem, and the pons is located between the midbrain and the medulla. The medulla, the most inferior part of the brain stem, is continuous with the spinal cord.

The **midbrain** is involved with visual and auditory reflexes, such as moving the head and eyes to view objects or turning of the head so that sound can be heard directly. The **pons** serves as a relay station for sensory stimuli passing through on the way to the brain. The **medulla oblongata** contains descending and ascending tracts and is the vital link for eyes, ears, respiratory, and circulatory functions. The mixed gray and white matter of the medulla integrates information from the sensory systems with cortical activity. Various specialized structures within the medulla control arousal, heart rate, blood pressure, and respiration. Two large bundles of nerve fibers on the ventral surface of the medulla, the **pyramids,** carry the impulses that control the skeletal muscles. The majority of these fibers cross from one side to the other, and thus the right hemisphere of the brain controls the left side of the body, and vice versa.

The **cerebellum** is tucked under the occipital lobe of the cerebrum and protrudes dorsally. It is important in maintaining balance, muscle coordination, and equilibrium. Any cerebellar disease is marked with **ataxia** (lack of muscular coordination) and loss of balance.

Spinal Cord

The **spinal cord** is made up of nerves that are protected by a bony encasement, the vertebrae (see Figure 9–9).

The spinal cord extends from the medulla oblongata to approximately the second lumbar vertebra. It ends in a cone-shaped structure called the **conus medullaris** (kō′-nŭs měd′ū-lăr-ĭs), from which the nerves extend downward, resembling a horse's tail, and is referred to as the **cauda equina** (kŏ′ dă ē-kwĭn′-ă).

FIGURE 9–9

Spinal Cord Posterior View

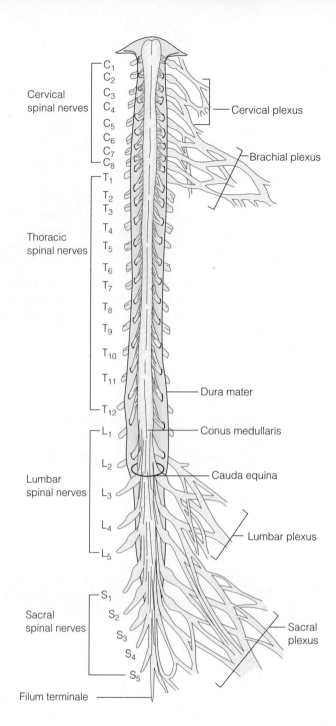

The spinal cord branches into 31 pairs of spinal nerves. Each pair extends from the spinal cord bilaterally throughout its entire length. Each spinal nerve is attached to the spinal cord via the **dorsal** and **ventral nerve roots.** See Figure 9–10.

FIGURE 9—10 Cross-sectional View of the Spinal Cord

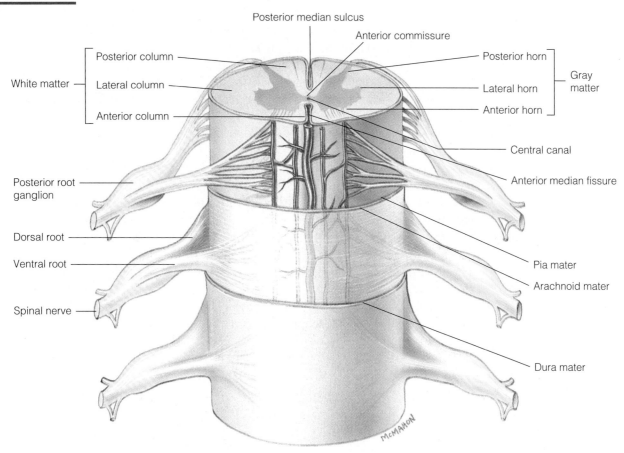

The dorsal and ventral roots emerge from each segment of the spinal cord and converge to form a spinal nerve. Of the 31 pairs of spinal nerves, eight pairs are **cervical,** twelve pairs are **thoracic,** five pairs are **lumbar,** five pairs are **sacral,** and one is **coccygeal.**

Like the brain, the spinal cord is made up of white and gray matter, with the white surrounding the gray. The white matter is separated into **posterior, lateral,** and **anterior columns.** These columns contain the axons and dendrites arranged into ascending and descending tracts. The ascending tracts carry impulses to the brain, and the descending tracts carry impulses away from the brain.

The gray matter is shaped like an H. The four extensions of the H are called **horns.** The two anterior extensions of the H are called **anterior horns,** and the two posterior ones are called **posterior horns.** The horns are connected by the **anterior commissure** (kŏm′-ĭ-shŭr). The gray matter contains cell bodies, dendrites, and axons.

Running throughout the length of the spinal cord is a canal called the **spinal (central) canal.** It is lined with ependymal cells and is filled with cerebrospinal fluid.

9–11

Protective Coverings

Because of its relative fragility and critical importance to life, the CNS is provided with considerable protection. The brain is surrounded by thick bones, which form the cranium. The spinal cord is encased in a long chain of thorny bones, called vertebrae. Both the brain and the spinal cord are also protected by membranes called **meninges** (měn-ĭn′-jēz) and **cerebrospinal fluid (CSF)**. The brain also has a protective covering referred to as the **blood-brain barrier.**

Meninges   Three meninges, or membranes, protect the brain and spinal cord (see Figure 9–11).

The outermost membrane is the **dura mater** (dū′-ră mă′-těr), also called **pachymeninges** (păk-ĭ-měn-ĭn′-jēz). It is tough and thick. The middle layer is called the **arachnoid** (ă-răk′-noyd) **membrane.** This layer has a spider web appearance because of tiny projections extending into the **pia mater** (pĭ′-ă mă-těr), the innermost layer that contains many blood vessels. The pia mater runs down the spinal cord to the end, called the **filum terminale** (fī′-lŭm těr-mĭ-năl′). The arachnoid and pia mater together may be called the **leptomeninges** (lěp″-tō-měn-ĭn′-jēz), referring to the thinness of both layers. The space below the dura mater is called the **subdural space.** The space below the arachnoid membrane is called the **subarachnoid space.**

FIGURE 9–11   Meninges

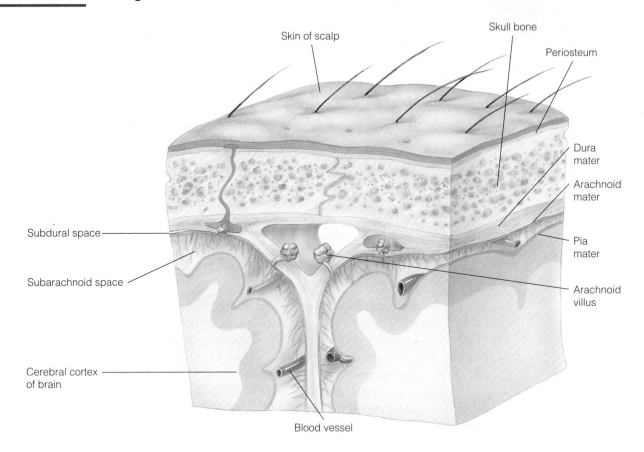

Cerebrospinal Fluid The **cerebrospinal fluid** is a clear fluid containing protein, chloride, and white blood cells. It is located in the subarachnoid space around the brain and spinal cord, within the central canal of the spinal cord, and in the ventricles of the brain. See Figure 9–12.

FIGURE 9–12

Ventricles of the Brain

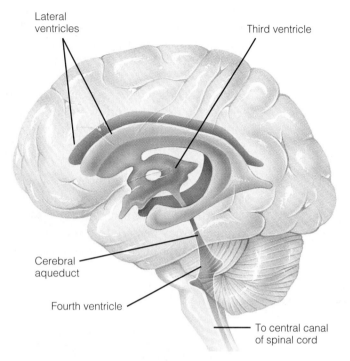

Ventricle of the brain

CSF is continually produced through a filtration process. The filter is a network of blood vessels that covers the ventricles, known as the **choroid plexus.** The filtrate is the CSF formed as the blood passes over the ventricles. This fluid is continually circulated through the ventricles and the spinal canal and is finally reabsorbed into the bloodstream via fingerlike projections called **arachnoid villi.**

Blood-Brain Barrier The **blood-brain barrier (BBB)** is a protective mechanism that prevents toxic substances from entering the brain, while at the same time allowing needed substances, such as glucose and oxygen, to enter.

▶ 9.3 PERIPHERAL NERVOUS SYSTEM

The **peripheral nervous system (PNS)** consists of the nerves and ganglia. The **nerves** originate in the brain or spinal cord and extend to the periphery. They include the **cranial nerves,** the **spinal nerves,** and the **autonomic nervous system (ANS). Ganglia** are nerve cell bodies located outside the brain and spinal cord.

Cranial Nerves

Twelve pairs of **cranial nerves** emerge from the brain bilaterally to innervate the muscles of the head, neck, and trunk (see Figure 9–13).

Each pair of cranial nerves is given a name and number. The name often relates to the organ it innervates, and the number indicates the part of the brain it originates in. The lower the number, the more anterior the origin. Cranial nerves can also be described by their function. Some of the nerves have sensory functions, some motor functions, and some a combination of both sensory and motor functions.

Table 9–2 lists the name, number, and functions of the cranial nerves in sequence as they emerge from the brain from anterior to posterior. Many students have used the following mnemonic devices (memorization by means of a nonsense sentence) to help them remember the cranial nerves.

The following phrase may help you learn the names of the cranial nerves as they emerge from the brain: On One Occasion, Tina Took Alice For Very Good Veggies and Hashbrowns. The first letter of the word in the phrase is the same as the first letter of the cranial nerve.

The phrase Sally Said Meet Me By My Boat So Bob Brought Mackerel Munchies may be used to remember the functions of the cranial nerves. S means sensory, M means motor, B means both sensory and motor functions.

FIGURE 9–13 Cranial Nerves

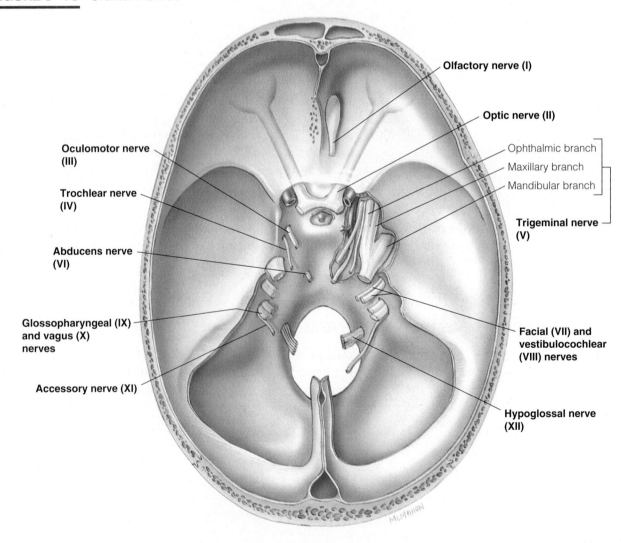

TABLE 9–2

Cranial Nerves

NUMBER	NAME AND PRONUNCIATION	FUNCTION
I	Olfactory ŏl-făk′-tō-rē	**sensory:** smell
II	Optic op′-tik	**sensory:** vision
III	Oculomotor ŏk″-ū-lō-mō-tor	**motor:** movement of the eyeball, regulation of the size of the pupil
IV	Trochlear trŏk′-lē-ăr	**motor:** eye movements
V	Trigeminal tri-jĕm′-ĭn-ăl	**sensory:** sensations of head and face; muscle sense **motor:** mastication **Note:** Divided into three branches: the ophthalmic branch, the maxillary branch, and the mandibular branch.
VI	Abducens ab-dū′-senz	**motor:** movement of the eyeball, particularly abduction
VII	Facial	**sensory:** taste **motor:** facial expressions; secretions of saliva
VIII	Vestibulocochlear vĕs-tĭb′-ū-lō-kŏk′-lē-ăr	**sensory:** balance; hearing **Note:** Divided into two branches: the vestibular branch responsible for balance and the cochlear branch responsible for hearing.
IX	Glossopharyngeal glŏs″-ō-fă-rĭn′-jē-ăl	**sensory:** taste **motor:** swallowing; secretion of saliva
X	Vagus va′-gŭs	**sensory:** sensation of organs supplied **motor:** movement of organs supplied **Note:** Supplies the head, pharynx, bronchus, esophagus, liver, and stomach.
XI	Accessory	**motor:** shoulder movement; turning of head; voice production
XII	Hypoglossal hī″-pō-glŏs′-ăl	**motor:** tongue movements

Spinal Nerves

As mentioned previously, a **spinal nerve** is the union between the dorsal and ventral nerve roots. The **dorsal root,** recognized because of the **spinal ganglion,** contains nerve fibers from sensory neurons that transmit sensory information from the periphery to the brain and spinal cord. The **ventral root** does not have a spinal ganglion and is involved with motor neurons carrying information away from the CNS to the periphery, resulting in a response to a stimulus. Since a spinal nerve is a combination of the dorsal and ventral nerve fibers, a single nerve is a collection of sensory and motor neurons traveling toward and away from the brain and spinal cord.

In some areas of the body, spinal nerves form a network called a **plexus** (pl. = **plexuses**). These plexuses are named **cervical, brachial, lumbar,** and **sacral.** From them, specific peripheral nerves emerge (see Table 9–3 and Figure 9–14).

TABLE 9–3

Major Spinal Nerves Emerging from a Plexus

PLEXUS	MAJOR SPINAL NERVES EMERGING FROM A PLEXUS
cervical	phrenic (frĕn′-ĭk) spinal
brachial	musculocutaneous radial median ulnar axillary
lumbar	lateral femoral cutaneous femoral ilioinguinal (ĭl″-ĭ-ō-ĭn′-gwĭ-năl) iliohypogastric (ĭl″-ĭ-ō-hī-pō-găs′-trĭk)
sacral	sciatic (sī-ăt′-ĭk) pudendal (pū-dĕn′-dăl) common peroneal (pĕr″-ō-nē′-ăl) tibial

FIGURE 9—14

Peripheral Nerves and some Cranial Nerves

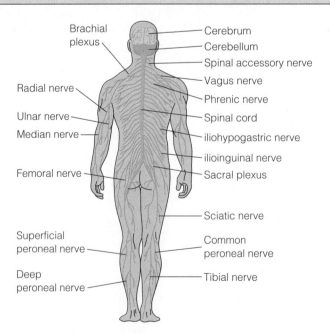

Brachial plexus — Cerebrum — Cerebellum — Spinal accessory nerve — Vagus nerve — Radial nerve — Phrenic nerve — Ulnar nerve — Spinal cord — Median nerve — iliohypogastric nerve — ilioinguinal nerve — Femoral nerve — Sacral plexus — Sciatic nerve — Superficial peroneal nerve — Common peroneal nerve — Deep peroneal nerve — Tibial nerve

Reflex

A **reflex** is an involuntary response to a stimulus. Reflexes allow our bodies to react to situations before we are consciously aware of them. The simplest type of reflex is the knee jerk. More complex reflexes allow us to pull a body part, such as the hand, away from a source of pain, such as a hot stove, before the brain is aware of the situation. If we were to wait until the brain became consciously aware of the hot stove, a more severe burn would occur.

Some reflexes are initiated by stimulation of the skin, and thus are referred to as **superficial** reflexes. Tickle someone lightly on the abdomen, and their abdominal muscles reflexively tighten (the **abdominal reflex**). Other reflexes are initiated by the stimulation of a tendon and are thus called **deep tendon reflexes.** The Achilles reflex is an example. Tap the Achilles tendon and the resulting muscle contraction causes the foot to plantar flex.

Reflex response to a stimulus, whether hyperactive or diminished, can indicate any number of diseases of the nervous system. The more common reflexes and the normal response are listed in the Table 9–4.

TABLE 9–4

Common Reflexes and Their Normal Response

REFLEX	RESPONSE
plantar reflex	Stroking the sole of the foot results in flexion of the toes. **Note:** An abnormal response to the plantar reflex is the **Babinski's reflex,** which is dorsiflexion of the great toe when the sole of the foot is stimulated. This reflex is normal in newborns, but disappears after two years of age.

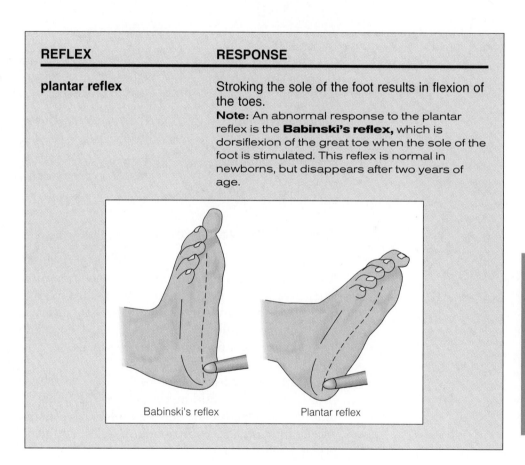

Babinski's reflex   Plantar reflex

9–11

TABLE 9–4

**Common Reflexes and
Their Normal Response**
(concluded)

REFLEX	RESPONSE
knee jerk; patellar reflex	tapping the patellar ligament results in the lower leg extending

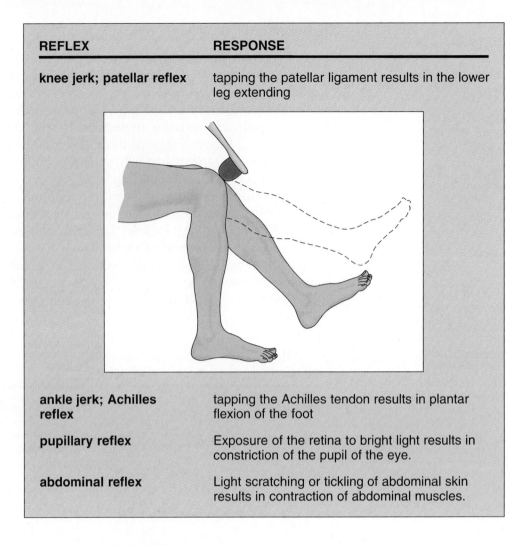

ankle jerk; Achilles reflex	tapping the Achilles tendon results in plantar flexion of the foot
pupillary reflex	Exposure of the retina to bright light results in constriction of the pupil of the eye.
abdominal reflex	Light scratching or tickling of abdominal skin results in contraction of abdominal muscles.

Autonomic Nervous System

The **autonomic nervous system (ANS)** is part of the peripheral nervous system. It functions mainly in homeostasis. The neurons involved are primarily efferent. They extend from the brain and spinal cord to govern (without conscious control) glands and involuntary muscles of the heart, digestive, circulatory, respiratory, urinary, and endocrine systems. Two subdivisions of the ANS are the **sympathethic** and **parasympathetic systems.**

Sympathetic System The nerve fibers of the **sympathetic system** originate from the thoracic and lumbar area of the spinal cord and end in involuntary muscles and glands. The nerve impulses have an excitatory effect on the body, accelerating organs, constricting muscles, and generally increasing the rate of organ activity.

Parasympathetic System The nerve fibers of the **parasympathetic system** originate in the cranial and sacral areas and end in muscles and glands. The nerve impulses have an inhibitory effect on the body, preparing it for rest and repose.

Effect on Body Organs The sympathetic system is predominant in times of stress, and the parasympathetic system is predominant in times of relaxation. Each system has the opposite effect on a body part, but both work continuously and well together to maintain homeostasis.

TERM WITH PRONUNCIATION	ANALYSIS	DEFINITION
anencephaly ăn″-ĕn-sĕf′-ă-lē	-y = condition a- = no; not encephal/o = brain	congenital absence of the brain
cerebellitis sĕr″-ĕ-bĕl-ī′-tĭs	-itis = inflammation cerebell/o = cerebellum	inflammation of the cerebellum
cerebral sĕr′-ĕ-brăl	-al = pertaining to cerebr/o = brain	pertaining to the brain
cerebrospinal sĕr″-ĕ-brō-spī′-năl	-al = pertaining to cerebr/o = brain spin/o = spine; vertebral column	pertaining to the brain and spine
cerebrovascular sĕr″-ĕ-brō-văs′-kū-lăr	-ar = pertaining to cerebr/o = brain vascul/o = vessel	pertaining to the blood vessels of the brain
cortical kŏr′-tĭ-kăl	-al = pertaining to cortic/o = cortex; outer layer	pertaining to the outer layer of the brain
demyelination dē-mī″-ĕ-lī-nā′-shŭn	-ion = process de- = lack of; removal myelin/o = myelin sheath	lack of the myelin sheath
encephalitis ĕn-sĕf″-ă-lī′-tĭs	-itis = inflammation encephal/o = brain	inflammation of the brain
encephalomalacia ĕn-sĕf″-ă-lō-mă-lā′-sē-a	-malacia = softening encephal/o = brain	softening of the brain
encephalomyelitis ĕn-sĕf″-ă-lō-mī-ĕl-ī′-tĭs	-itis = inflammation encephal/o = brain myel/o = spinal cord	inflammation of the brain and spinal cord
epidural ĕp″-ĭ-dŭ′-răl	-al = pertaining to epi- = on; upon; above dur/o = dura mater	pertaining to above the dura mater
ganglioneuroma găng″-lē-ō-nū-rō′-mă	-oma = tumor or mass ganglin/o = ganglion	tumor made up of ganglions and nerves
ganglionectomy găng″-lē-ō-nĕk′-tō-mē	-ectomy = excision; removal ganglion/o = ganglion	removal of a ganglion
glioma glī-ō′-mă	-oma = tumor or mass gli/o = glue	tumor of the neuroglial cells
intramedullary ĭn″-tră-mĕd′-ū-lăr″-ē	-ary = pertaining to intra- = within medull/o = medulla oblongata	pertaining to within the medulla oblongata
laminectomy lăm″-ĭ-nĕk-tō-mē	-ectomy = excision; removal lamin/o = lamina (portion of the vertebra)	excision of the lamina

9–11

TERM WITH PRONUNCIATION	ANALYSIS	DEFINITION
leptomeningeal lĕp″-tō-mĕn-ĭn′-jē-ăl	-eal = pertaining to lept/o = slender; thin; delicate mening/o = membranes; meninges	pertaining to the leptomeninges (the arachnoid membrane and the pia mater together)
meningioma mĕn-ĭn″-jē-ō′-mă	-oma = tumor or mass mening/o = membranes; meninges	tumor of the meninges
meningitis mĕn-ĭn-jī′-tĭs	-itis = inflammation mening/o = membranes; meninges	inflammation of the meninges
meningoencephalitis mĕn-ĭn″-gō-ĕn-sĕf″-ă-lī′-tĭs	-itis = inflammation mening/o = membranes; meninges encephal/o = brain	inflammation of the meninges and brain
meningoencephalocele mĕn-ĭn″-gō-ĕn-sĕf′-ăl-ō-sēl	-cele = hernia mening/o = membranes; meninges encephal/o = brain	hernia or protrusion of the meninges and brain through a defect in the skull
meningomyelocele mĕn-ĭn″-gō-mī-ĕl′-ō-sēl	-cele = hernia mening/o = membranes; meninges myel/o = spinal cord	hernia or protrusion of the meninges and spinal cord through a defect in the vertebrae
myelitis mī-ĕ-lī′-tĭs	-itis = inflammation myel/o = spinal cord	inflammation of the spinal cord
myelogram mī′-ĕ-lō-grăm	-gram = record; x-ray myel/o = spinal cord	record or x-ray of the spinal cord
narcolepsy năr′-kō-lĕp″-sē	-lepsy = seizure narc/o = sleep	a condition characterized by an uncontrollable desire to sleep
neuritis nū-rī′-tĭs	-itis = inflammation neur/o = nerve	inflammation of a nerve
neurolysis nū-rōl′-ĭs-ĭs	-lysis = to loosen; breakdown; destruction; separate neur/o = nerve	to loosen a nerve sheath; destruction of a nerve
neuromuscular nū″-rō-mŭs′-kū-lăr	-ar = pertaining to neur/o = nerve muscul/o = muscle	pertaining to the nerves and muscles
neurotripsy nū″-rō-trĭp′-sē	-tripsy = crushing neur/o = nerve	crushing of a nerve
pachymeningitis pak-ē-mĕn″-ĭn-jī′-tĭs	-itis = inflammation pachy- = thick mening/o = membrane; meninges	inflammation of the pachymeninges (dura mater)
poliomyelitis pōl-ē-ō mī″-ĕl-ī′-tĭs	-itis = inflammation poli/o = gray myel/o = spinal cord	inflammation of the gray matter of the spinal cord

TERM WITH PRONUNCIATION	ANALYSIS	DEFINITION
polyneuropathy pŏl″-ē-nū-rŏp′-ă-thē	-pathy = disease poly- = many neur/o = nerve	disease of many nerves
pontocerebellar pŏn″-tō-sĕr″-ĕ-bĕl′-ăr	-ar = pertaining to pont/o = pons (bridge between the medulla oblongata and midbrain) cerebell/o = cerebellum	pertaining to the pons and cerebellum
radiculitis ră-dĭk″-ū-lī′-tĭs	-itis = inflammation radicul/o = nerve root	inflammation of nerve roots
radiculopathy ră-dĭk″-ū-lŏp′-ă-thē	-pathy = disease radicul/o = nerve roots	disease of the nerve root
thalamic thăl-ăm′-ĭk	-ic = pertaining to thalam/o = thalamus	pertaining to the thalamus
thalamocortical thăl″-ăm-ō-kōr′-tĭ-kăl	-al = pertaining to thalam/o = thalamus cortic/o = cortex	pertaining to the thalamus and cerebral cortex
ventriculoperitoneal vĕn-trĭk″-ū-lō-pĕr″-ĭ-tō-nē′-ăl	-al = pertaining to ventricul/o = ventricles peritone/o = peritoneum	pertaining to the ventricle and peritoneum

▸ 9.5 ABNORMAL CONDITIONS

Central Nervous System Disorders

DISORDER	DESCRIPTION
Alzheimer's disease 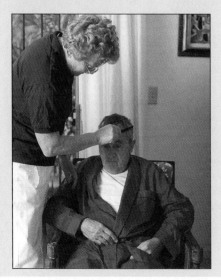	dementia or mental disorder due to the degeneration of brain tissue, resulting in impairment of intellectual abilities such as memory, judgment, and abstract thinking, as well as changes in personality and behavior Loss of memory is the most notable early symptom. As the disease continues, subtle mental lapses and slight personality changes progress to more obvious disturbances in brain function to the point that the patient is unable to care for him or herself. Onset is usually between the ages of 50 and 70. Death is inevitable.

DISORDER	DESCRIPTION
amyotrophic lateral sclerosis (ALS); Lou Gehrig's disease	progressive motor neuron disease causing death of nerve cells in the brain and spinal cord and resulting in muscular degeneration; typically fatal within 3 to 5 years
cerebral palsy (CP)	a congenital anomaly due to injury of the CNS resulting from trauma in the prenatal, perinatal, or postnatal periods **Note:** CP is difficult to diagnose immediately after birth, as the characteristic motor disturbances do not appear until the motor system is more fully developed.
spastic CP	**Spastic,** the most common type of CP, is characterized by toe-walking, scissors gait, and paralysis such as hemiplegia, quadriplegia, or paraplegia.
athetoid CP	**Athetoid,** the next most common type of CP, involves purposeless, slow, writhing, and jerky movements.
ataxic CP	**Ataxic CP** is characterized by weakness, loss of equilibrium, and a wide and unsteady gait. There are also mixed forms of the above CP classifications, with spastic-athetoid being the most common.
seizure disorders; epilepsy 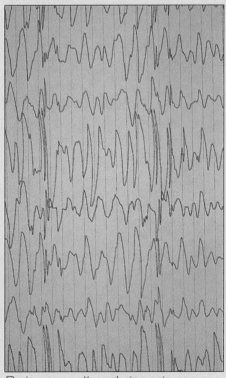 Brain wave pattern during seizure	paroxysmal (sudden starting and stopping) attacks of altered cerebral functions due to uncoordinated and disorganized electrical impulses in the brain **Note:** The seizure is characterized by abnormalities in consciousness, sensory disturbances, and impaired motor functions. In the majority of cases the cause is unknown. In other cases, the possible causes may include high fevers, brain tumors, CNS infections, anoxia, toxic agents, and cerebral injury. The characteristic sign is a seizure that can be described as **partial** or **generalized.** Partial seizures originate in a focal (localized) point in the brain. Generalized seizures involve widespread areas of the brain. An example of a partial seizure is **jacksonian seizure,** which begins in one finger or toe and travels upward, eventually involving the entire extremity. The jacksonian seizure can also involve the corner of the mouth, moving to include the face. **Absence** (ăb′-sĕnz) and **tonic-clonic** are examples of generalized seizures. **Absence (petit mal)** are brief attacks lasting 1 to 30 seconds, usually in children. The seizure is manifested by blank stares, eye disturbances, and changes in the levels of consciousness. **Tonic-clonic (grand-mal)** is characterized by alternating tonic contractions (prolonged contractions with no periodic relaxation of the muscle) and clonic contractions (alternating muscular contractions and relaxations).

DISORDER	DESCRIPTION
seizure disorders; epilepsy (continued)	An **aura** is an abnormal sensation that may precede a seizure, whether partial or generalized. These are warning signs to the patient that a seizure is starting. Auras can include abnormal smells, tastes, and visual and gastrointestinal disturbances. They represent the localized area of the brain where the seizure occurs.
	Status epilepticus is the occurrence of one seizure after another; can occur in both partial and general seizures. This condition can be fatal.
	Diagnosis is made by the succession of seizures. A common diagnostic test is the electroencephalogram.
	Seizures are effectively controlled but not cured by drugs. Some common drugs include Dilantin (dī-lăn′-tĭn), phenoybarbital (fē-nō-băr′-bĭ-tŏl), and valproic (văl-prō′-ĭc) acid.
Huntington's chorea; Huntington's disease (HD)	inherited disease resulting in degeneration of the basal ganglia and cerebral cortex; characterized by rapid, jerky movements, called chorea, and mental deterioration with eventual dementia (mental disorder).
	Genetically transmitted by either parent; the offspring of the affected parent has a 50% chance of being affected. The disease does not favor one sex over the other.
migraine	paroxysmal attacks of headaches of unknown cause that are associated with cerebrovascular constriction and dilation, usually on one side of the head
	Visual and gastrointestinal disturbances may also occur. No cure, treatment is palliative. Resting in a darkened room gives some relief.
multiple sclerosis (MS)	inflammation of the myelin sheath leading to demyelination around the axon. Demyelination and the ensuing sclerotic patches are scattered throughout the brain and spinal cord, resulting in a variety of neurological disorders such as visual disturbances, urinary dysfunctions, emotional instability, muscle weakness, paresthesia, and paralysis. Most often females are affected, the average age of onset being 30.

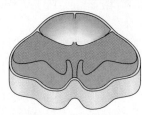 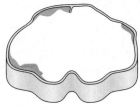

(a) Partial demyelination of posterior column.

(b) Almost complete demyelination

The cause of MS is unknown; however, there seem to be environmental factors at play, as MS is more common in temperate climates than in the tropics. Other common theories include an allergic reaction to an infectious substance, a viral infection, or an autoimmune reaction.

9–11

DISORDER	DESCRIPTION
multiple sclerosis (MS) (continued)	MS is difficult to diagnose, and diagnosis is often made based on the exacerbations and remissions characteristic of MS, and the presence of sclerotic patches.
	Diagnostic tests include **lumbar puncture (LP),** showing elevated gamma globulin in the CSF; **electroencephalogram (EEG),** showing abnormalities; **magnetic resonance imaging (MRI);** and **evoked potentials,** which record responses to electrical stimulation of a sensory neuron (see diagnostic procedures).
	There is no cure for MS. Treatment is aimed at alleviating the symptoms. The progress of MS is varied. A patient may live a productive life with few exacerbations, or the disease may progress rapidly, incapacitating the patient, resulting in death soon after onset of the disease.
Parkinson's disease (PD); paralysis agitans; shaking palsy 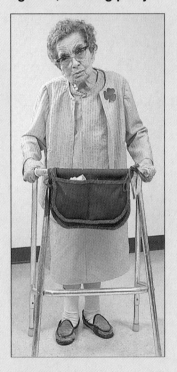	chronic, progressive disorder characterized by bradykinesia, muscular rigidity, resting tremors, and slow gait. Onset is in middle age, beginning with tremors followed by bradykinesia and rigidity.
	Although parkinsonism is idiopathic, it is characterized by a decrease in dopamine (a neurotransmitter) and loss of cells in the basal ganglia.
	Characteristic tremor is the resting tremor called **pill-rolling tremor.** It involves the thumb and fingers and is present at rest but disappears when the part moves. Also characteristic is muscle rigidity: the muscle resists passive muscle stretching. When this resistance is uniform and unyielding, it is termed **lead pipe rigidity.** When the rigidity is jerky, it is called **cogwheel rigidity.**
	There are no specific diagnostic tests and no cure. Treatment is palliative, consisting of drugs such as **levodopa,** which increases levels of dopamine, and physical therapy to keep the patient as active as possible.
Reye's syndrome; acute encephalopathy and fatty degeneration of the viscera (AEFDV)	pathology of the brain with the accumulation of fat in the viscera such as the pancreas, heart, kidney, lymph nodes, and spleen
	Etiology is unknown, but a viral infection tends to precede the onset of Reye's syndrome. Affects children under 18 years, usually following a bout of influenza. There is evidence that the use of salicylates during an attack of influenza increases the chances of Reye's syndrome.

DISORDER	DESCRIPTION
Bell's palsy	paralysis of one side of the face involving the facial nerve (7th cranial nerve). The cause is unknown, although nerve damage may be due to a viral disease. 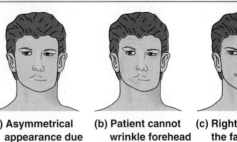 **(a) Asymmetrical appearance due to left side facial paralysis.**　**(b) Patient cannot wrinkle forehead on paralyzed left side.**　**(c) Right side of the face is smiling, left side distorted.**
carpal tunnel syndrome (CTS)	compression or entrapment of the median nerve at the carpal tunnel, which is a passageway for the median nerve and the flexor tendons of the forearm. Compression may occur spontaneously or may be due to overuse, particularly where a keyboard is used on a daily basis. Compression results in pain and paresthesia of the radial-palmar aspect of the hand. Although many cases do not require treatment, surgery may be required to relieve the pressure off the median nerve (decompression).
Guillain-Barré syndrome (gĕ-yā′ bă-rā′)	acute, progressive polyneuritis, resulting in muscle weakness and moderate sensory loss. Often may follow a mild infection with spontaneous recovery in the majority of cases. However, in some cases, the disease is fatal. The cause is unknown, although a viral infection is implicated. Symptoms are caused by demyelination of the peripheral nerves. Since the PNS is affected, regeneration and complete recovery are possible.
myasthenia gravis	progressive weakening and fatigue of the skeletal muscles due to abnormalities at the neuromuscular junction Many of the cases are not life threatening, as the disease is well controlled by drugs. However, there is no cure, and as the disease advances, it may prove life-threatening when involuntary muscles of the respiratory system are affected. Although the exact cause is not known, there are several reasons for the underperformance of skeletal muscles. Included are an autoimmune response, insufficient amounts of acetylcholine (ACh), and an inability of the muscle fibers to respond in a normal fashion. Muscle fatigue and weakness are the major symptoms, but the diagnosis is confirmed by giving the patient an **anticholinesterase drug** such as **neostigmine,** which increases the amount of ACh available at the neuromuscular junction, thereby improving muscle strength immediately.

9—II

DISORDER	DESCRIPTION
trigeminal neuralgia; tic douloureux (tĭk-doo-loo-roo′)	intense pain along one or more branches of the trigeminal nerve (5th cranial nerve), often set off by stimulation of a trigger point. Trigger point is a specific area of the body that when stimulated will result in an abnormal sensation. Drug treatment includes anticonvulsants such as phenytoin (fĕn′-ĭ-tō-ĭn). Surgical treatment involves rhizolysis to reduce pain.

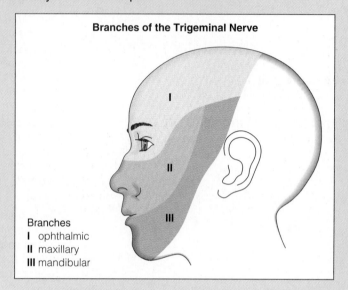

Branches of the Trigeminal Nerve

Branches
I ophthalmic
II maxillary
III mandibular

Infectious Diseases of the Nervous System

DISORDER	DESCRIPTION
herpes zoster; shingles	an infection of the CNS that inflames the dorsal root ganglia, resulting in pus-filled vesicles of the skin and neuralgia in areas stimulated by the nerves. A disease of adults usually past 50 years of age, herpes zoster is caused by the varicella-zoster virus, which also causes chicken pox in children. The skin lesions are the same in both diseases, causing pain and pruritus that are difficult to control even with analgesics.

Inflammatory Diseases

DISORDER	DESCRIPTION
meningitis	inflammation of the meninges, the membranes that cover the brain and spinal cord, caused by a bacterial infection such as *Neisseria meningitidis* or *Streptococcus pneumoniae* and transmitted by the respiratory tract; it is highly contagious Signs and symptoms may include extreme headaches, vomiting, increased intracranial pressure, neck rigidity, and positive Brudzinski's and Kernig's signs (see signs and symptoms). Lumbar puncture confirms the diagnosis. Treatment is antibiotics.

Inflammatory Diseases (continued)

DISORDER	DESCRIPTION
intracranial abscess	an abscess is the accumulation of bacterial exudate within a walled-off area that prevents the spread of the infection to other sites; this abscess is within the skull

Follows a purulent infection from such bacteria as *Staphylococcus aureus* and *Streptococcus virdidans,* although any pyogenic bacteria can cause the abscess. |

Congenital Diseases

DISORDER	DESCRIPTION
hydrocephalus 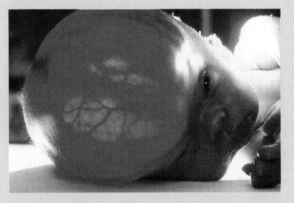	increased intracranial pressure with accumulation of cerebrospinal fluid (CSF) in the brain due to blockage of the natural flow of CSF through the ventricles

Newborns are mostly affected by hydrocephalus, although adults can develop intracranial tumors that can block the outflow of CSF.

Diagnosis is made by CT scans and MRI which show the obstructed area and ventricular size.

Surgery using a ventriculoperitoneal shunt (device used to bypass fluid around a blockage) to divert the CSF from the ventricles to the peritoneum is the treatment of choice. |
| **spina bifida** | a developmental abnormality occurring in the first three months of gestation, resulting in incomplete closure of the vertebrae around the spinal cord.

The severity of the incomplete closure can vary greatly, as described below: |
| **spina bifida occulta** | incomplete closure of the neural arch. It is difficult to diagnose (occult = hidden), as the vertebral opening is slight, and there may be no neurological defects. There is no protrusion of the spinal cord or membranes. It is sometimes accompanied by a depression in the skin, with a patch of hair and port-wine nevi over the defect. |

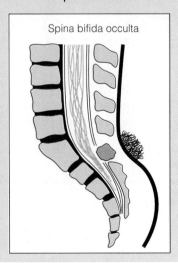

Spina bifida occulta

DISORDER	DESCRIPTION
spina bifida cystica	through a fissure in the vertebrae **(rachischisis),** there is a protrusion of the spinal cord and/or meninges resulting in a saclike structure **(cystica).** If the sac contains meninges, it is called **meningocele;** if it contains the spinal cord, it is called **myelocele;** if it contains both the meninges and the spinal cord, it is called **myelomeningocele.**
	The degree of neurological dysfunction depends upon the amount of spinal cord that is affected. There may be no impairment, as with meningocele and spina bifida occulta, or there may be loss of bladder and bowel control and paralysis of the legs, as often seen in spina bifida cystica.
	Associated with spina bifida cystica is **kyphosis** and **hydrocephalus.**
	Diagnosis can be made by ultrasound, which shows any bony abnormalities, and by **amniocentesis** (surgical puncture of the sac in which the fetus lies), which shows an abnormal increase in the amount of **alpha-fetoprotein (AFP),** a protein secreted by the fetus.
	Treatment varies depending on severity. Spina bifida occulta requires no treatment; spina bifida cystica requires reduction of the protrusion and closure of the defect. If there is spinal cord involvement with resulting neurological deficits, support measures must be taken.

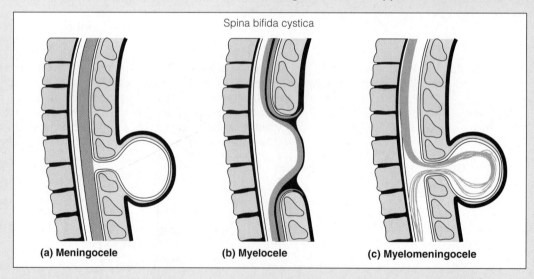

Spina bifida cystica

(a) Meningocele   (b) Myelocele   (c) Myelomeningocele

Brain Hemorrhage

DISORDER	DESCRIPTION
hemorrhage; hematoma	**hemorrhage** is the escape of blood from a blood vessel into the surrounding tissue, and a **hematoma** is the accumulation of escaped blood into the surrounding tissue
	Damage to the brain is proportional to the loss of blood and to the pressure on the brain substance by the hematoma.

DISORDER	DESCRIPTION
hemorrhage; hematoma (continued)	Hemorrhages or hematomas are named according to the site of bleeding. For example: a **subarachnoid hemorrhage** is bleeding in the subarachnoid space; **extradural hemorrhage** is bleeding outside the dura mater; and **subdural hemorrhage** is bleeding under the dura mater.

Tumors

DISORDER	DESCRIPTION
intracranial tumors	Tumors of the nervous system include intracranial tumors, tumors of the peripheral nervous system (**neurofibromas**), and spinal tumors. Intracranial tumors are the most common. There are two types of intracranial tumors: those within the brain substance and those outside it. A type of primary brain tumor located within the brain substance is a **glioma.** They invade the supporting structures within the brain. Gliomas are usually derived from astrocytes and can be well differentiated, slow-growing **astrocytomas,** or poorly differentiated, fast-growing, quickly fatal, **glioblastoma multiformes.** Intracranial tumors do not metastasize, as they cannot pass through the cranial vault, but tumors from elsewhere in the body (*i.e.* lung, breast, kidney, melanoma) may metastasize to the brain. A type of intracranial tumor located outside the brain substance is a benign, slow-growing, encapsulated tumor of the meninges called **meningoma.** Although benign, these tumors should be removed to alleviate any symptoms.

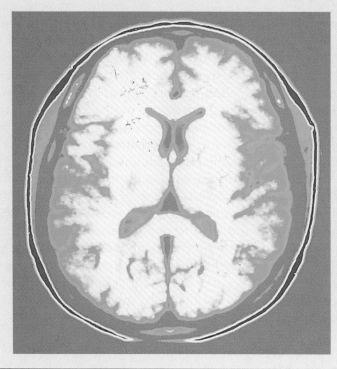
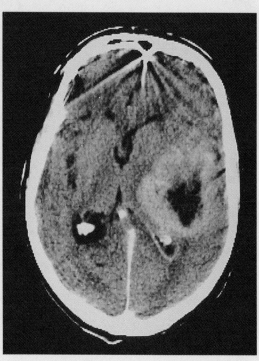

Physical Examination

Neurological examination involves assessment of the cranial nerves, sensory and motor systems, and any abnormalities of speech, as well as a **psychological examination,** which gives clues to any cortical dysfunction through observation of the patient's behaviors, attitudes, dress, memory, and language.

Each **cranial nerve** is tested systematically for proper functioning. Functions tested include smell, vision, eye movements, facial sensations, and weakness, hearing, balance, movement of neck and upper back muscles, and movements of the tongue.

Examination of the **sensory system** includes assessment of the response to such stimuli as pain, temperature, touch, vibration, position sense, and discriminative sensations. Discriminative sensations means that the skin is stimulated to see if the patient can differentiate between dull and sharp pain and between hot and cold temperatures. Variations in sensitivity to normal stimulation, particularly touch, can be described as follows: **hypoesthesia** is an abnormal decrease in one's sensitivity to normal stimulation; **hyperesthesia** is an abnormal increase in one's sensitivity to normal stimulation; **anesthesia** is loss of sensation; **dysesthesia** is an irritative sensation in response to normal stimuli; and **paresthesias** are abnormal sensations such as numbness and tingling.

Postural sense is determined by how well the patient perceives changes in body position and movement. A positive **Romberg's sign** is when the patient is unable to stand with the feet together and eyes closed. In some pathology, **discriminative sense** is impaired. A **2-point discrimination test** may identify such pathology by touching two points on a structure, e.g., the arm or finger. As the two points are moved closer together, the patient is observed for difficulty in differentiating two points from one.

On initial examination of the **motor system,** the patient's general appearance is assessed for evidence of contractures or abnormal **gait** (walk). Unsteady or uncoordinated walking is called **ataxic gait.** The patient is also assessed for signs of **muscular atrophy, impaired coordination, abnormal movements, muscle spasms,** or **paralyses.**

Impaired coordination includes **apraxia,** the inability to perform skilled movements such as brushing teeth or tying shoes; and **ataxia,** the lack of coordination. Abnormal movements include **tremors,** which are involuntary trembling or quivering muscular actions. **Resting tremors** are tremors that occur at rest but disappear with action. **Intention tremors** appear when an action is intended. **Fasciculations** are fine twitching movements of small segments of resting skeletal muscles. **Muscle spasms** are sudden, cramping, involuntary contractions of a muscle. Types include **clonic,** an alternating contraction and relaxation of the muscle in rapid succession; **tonic,** continuous contraction either brief or prolonged; **clonic-tonic,** alternating tonic and clonic spasms; and **tic,** rapidly repetitive nervous twitches. **Paralysis** is the loss of motor function, either temporary or permanent. Paralysis can be described as **spastic,** in which there is loss of motor function but with muscle tone and increased tendon reflexes, or **flaccid,** in which there is loss of motor function with loss of muscle tone and tendon reflexes. Other paralyses include **hemiplegia,** paralysis of either the right or left side of the body; **quadriplegia,** paralysis of all four extremities; **paraplegia,** paralysis of the legs and lower part of the body; **monoplegia,** paralysis of one limb: and **diplegia,** paralysis of like parts on both sides of the body.

Signs and Symptoms

Symptoms are numerous and varied and are based on the part of the nervous system affected by disease. For example, a tumor in the left temporal lobe of the brain may affect speech, while a tumor in the occipital lobe of the brain will affect vision.

Signs and Symptoms

SIGN OR SYMPTOM	DESCRIPTION
aphasia	inability or impairment to speak or write due to a brain defect
motor aphasia	a loss of the power of expression in speech or in writing
sensory aphasia	the inability to understand spoken or written language
amnesia	inability to remember; loss of memory
analgesia	lack of sensitivity to pain
apraxis	inability to perform skilled movements
bradykinesia	slow movement
comatose	pertaining to a coma, an unconscious state from which the patient cannot be aroused
dysarthria	difficulty in articulating speech due to muscular incoordination resulting from damage to the nerves
dysphasia	difficulty in speaking
myasthenia	muscle weakness
neurasthenia	nerve weakness
syncope	fainting
Kernig's sign	an indication of meningitis

There is a positive Kernig's sign when the patient shows pain or resistance to flexion of the knee and hip.

Signs and Symptoms (continued)

SIGN OR SYMPTOM	DESCRIPTION
Brudzinski's sign (brū-jĭn′-skēz)	an indication of meningitis

There is a positive Brudzinski's sign when the patient shows pain or resistance to forward flexion of the neck, with simultaneous flexion of hips and knees.

Romberg's sign	an indication of loss of position sense
Babinski's sign	an indication of a central nervous system disorder

Diagnostic Procedures

Radiology

PROCEDURE	DESCRIPTION
computerized tomography (CT) scan	x-ray of an organ or the body detailing a structure at various depths Multiple radiographs are taken at multiple angles, and the computer reconstructs these images to represent a cross-section or "slice" of the structure.
myelography	following injection of contrast medium into subarachnoid space, the spinal cord is x-rayed
magnetic resonance imaging (MRI)	a 3-dimensional record is made of the area imaged through computer calculation of the responses of the specific body area to a strong magnetic field
brain scan	following intravenous injection of a radioactive substance, an image is produced by the uptake of a radioactive substance into the brain
positron emission tomography (PET)	used to study metabolic processes in the brain, particularly glucose metabolism

Ultrasound

PROCEDURE	DESCRIPTION
echoencephalography	use of high frequency sound waves in diagnosing pathology of the brain

Clinical Procedures

PROCEDURE	DESCRIPTION
electroencephalography (EEG)	process of recording the electrical impulses of the brain
electromyelography	combination of electromyography that records the electrical currents in a muscle and nerve conduction procedure that records the speed at which nerve impulses travel through a nerve when stimulated Used to evaluate neuromuscular pathology
evoked responses	auditory, visual, or tactile stimuli that activate their corresponding neural pathways and result in a response that tests the functional ability of the path traveled by the nerve impulse to the brain
lumbar puncture (LP); spinal tap	insertion of a needle into the subarachnoid space between L3-L4 or L4-L5 to withdraw cerebrospinal fluid for diagnostic purposes such as in confirming infectious diseases (e.g., meningitis), or for therapeutic purposes (e.g., reducing intracranial pressure) Correct placement of the needle between the lumbar vertebrae is important so as not to damage nerve roots.

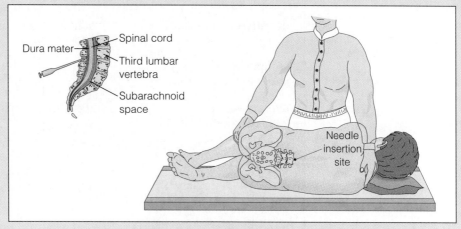

9–11

Treatment

For many neurological abnormalities, treatment is for relief of symptoms so that the patient is able to carry on as normally as possible. In many cases, drugs are used to this end.

Treatment Using Pharmacological Agents

TREATMENT	DESCRIPTION
analgesics	for relief of pain Most common type of analgesia is acetylsalicylic acid. Other analgesics include codeine, morphine, and Demerol.
antibiotics	antibacterial agents used to treat infections such as meningitis
anticonvulsants	used to inhibit seizure activity by reducing the excessive neural excitability in the brain (examples are phenobarbital and valproic acid)
levodopa (lĕv″-ō-dō′-pă)	a dopamine replacement used to treat Parkinson's disease
parasympatholytic drugs (păr″-ă-sĭm″-pă-thō-lĭt′-ĭk)	used to block the effects of the parasympathetic system An example is **atropine,** for reducing smooth muscle spasms.
parasympathomimetic drugs (păr″-ă-sĭm″-pă-thō-mĭm-ĕt′-ĭk)	drugs that mimic the parasympathetic system. An example is the **anticholinesterase** drug **neostigmine,** used to treat myasthenia gravis by prolonging the action of acetylcholine.
sedative and hypnotics	reduce anxiety, calm nervousness, and produce sleep
sympatholytic drugs (sĭm-pă″-thō-lit′-ĭk)	used to block the effects of the sympathetic nervous system
sympathomimetic drugs (sĭm-pă″-thō-mĭm-ĕt′ik)	drugs used to mimic the sympathetic nervous system Examples include **epinephrine** (ĕp-ĭ-nĕf′-rĭn), used as an emergency treatment of asthma and for bronchospasm, and **norepinephrine** used to increase blood pressure
tranquilizers	used as a mild sedative, and for anxiety reduction Examples are Valium and Librium.

Surgical Treatment

TREATMENT	DESCRIPTION
chordotomy	incision of the spinal cord to interrupt pain impulses to the brain
ganglionectomy	excision of a ganglion

Surgical Treatment (continued)

TREATMENT	DESCRIPTION
neurolysis	destruction of a nerve
rhizotomy	incision into the spinal nerve roots for relief of pain
stereotaxic neurosurgery	method of precisely locating areas in the brain using a 3-dimensional measurement; essential for certain neurological procedures
sympathectomy	partial excision of a part of the sympathetic nervous pathways
ventriculostomy	surgical creation of a new opening in the ventricles

Other Therapies

TREATMENT	DESCRIPTION
radiation therapy	use of radioactive substances to treat benign and malignant tumors
chemotherapy	a broad term, meaning treatment with drugs **Note:** Chemotherapy can be applied to a regime of antibiotics used to treat bacterial infections, but most commonly refers to the use of drugs in treating benign and malignant tumors.
physiotherapy	use of physical exercise in such conditions as multiple sclerosis, amyotrophic lateral sclerosis, and muscular dystrophy

◀▷ 9.7 ABBREVIATIONS

ACh	acetylcholine	CTS	carpal tunnel syndrome
AEFDV	acute encephalopathy and fatty degeneration of viscera	EEG	electroencephalography
AFP	alpha-fetoprotein	EMG	electromyogram
ALS	amyotrophic lateral sclerosis	GABA	gamma-aminobutyric acid
ANS	autonomic nervous system	HD	Huntington's disease
BBB	blood-brain barrier	LP	lumbar puncture
CNS	central nervous system	MS	multiple sclerosis
CP	cerebral palsy	PD	Parkinson's disease
CSF	cerebrospinal fluid	PNS	peripheral nervous system

► EXERCISE 9–1

Definitions

Define the following suffixes
and roots.

*Answers to all exercise
questions appear in
Appendix A.*

Definitions

1. encephal/o _____
2. rhiz/o _____
3. myelin/o _____
4. cortic/o _____
5. gli/o _____
6. polio- _____
7. pont/o _____
8. mening/o _____
9. neur/o _____
10. pachy- _____
11. radicul/o _____
12. narc/o _____
13. -lepsy _____
14. -tripsy _____
15. myel/o _____

Write definitions for the
following terms.

16. amyotrophic lateral sclerosis _____
_____
_____

17. cerebral palsy _____
_____
_____

18. jacksonian seizure _____
_____
_____

19. Reye's syndrome _____
_____
_____

20. Guillian-Barré syndrome _____
_____
_____

21. myasthenia gravis _____
_____
_____

22. spina bifida occulta _____

_____

23. glioblastoma multiforme _____

_____

24. Parkinson's disease _____

_____

25. multiple sclerosis _____

_____

26. Huntington's chorea _____

_____

27. seizure disorder _____

_____

Give the number and function for the following cranial nerves.

28. trochlear _____ _____

29. hypoglossal _____ _____

30. facial _____ _____

31. spinal accessory _____ _____

32. abducens _____ _____

33. trigeminal _____ _____

Write the meaning of the abbreviation in the space provided

34. CTS _____

35. CP _____

36. CNS _____

37. EMG _____

38. HD _____

39. EEG _____

40. ANS _____

41. ACh _____

42. AEFDV _____

43. BBB _____

9—11

Word Building

Give the correct prefix, suffix, or root for the following.

1. ventricles _____

2. cortex; outer layer _____

3. ganglion _____

4. thin _____

5. myelin sheath _____

6. spinal cord; bone marrow _____

7. glue _____

8. seizure _____

9. thick _____

10. nerve _____

11. brain _____

12. medulla oblongata _____

13. bridge _____

14. nerve root _____

15. crushing _____

Write the correct medical term for the following.

16. inflammation of the cerebellum _____

17. pertaining to the outer layer _____

18. lack of myelin sheath _____

19. inflammation of the brain and spinal cord _____

20. pertaining to above the dura mater _____

21. removal of a ganglion _____

22. pertaining to within the medulla oblongata _____

23. hernia or protrusion of the meninges and brain through a defect in the skull _____

24. record or x-ray of the spinal cord _____

25. pertaining to the muscle and nerve _____

26. destruction of a nerve _____

27. crushing of a nerve _____

28. inflammation of the gray matter of the spinal cord _____

29. disease of the nerve root _____

30. pertaining to the thalamus _____

Matching

Match the term from Column A with its definition in Column B.

Column A

1. Alzheimer's disease _____
2. Parkinson's disease _____
3. myasthenia gravis _____
4. shingles _____
5. seizure disorder _____
6. carpal tunnel syndrome _____
7. hydrocephalus _____
8. multiple sclerosis _____
9. meningioma _____
10. glioblastoma multiforme _____

Column B

A. paroxysmal attacks of altered cerebral function due to disorganized nerve impulses in the brain

B. characterized by muscular rigidity and resting tremors

C. presenile dementia

D. compression of the median nerve in the wrist area

E. scattered patches of demyelination in the brain and spinal cord

F. malignant tumor of the brain

G. progressive weakening and fatigue of the skeletal muscles due to abnormalities at the neuromuscular junction

H. a disease occurring in adulthood, caused by the varicella zoster virus

I. tumor located outside the brain substance

J. accumulation of cerebrospinal fluid resulting in increased intracranial pressure

9–II

Match the term in Column A
with its definition in
Column B.

Column A

11. cerebral cortex _____

12. brain stem _____

13. hypothalamus _____

14. ventricles _____

15. dura mater _____

16. leptomeninges _____

17. spinal nerve _____

18. reflex _____

19. plexus _____

20. demyelination _____

Column B

A. the arachnoid membrane and pia mater, taken together

B. maintains homeostasis of appetite, thirst, temperature, and water

C. the outermost meninges

D. a thin, gray layer covering the entire cerebrum

E. an involuntary response to a stimulus

F. midbrain, pons, and medulla oblongata

G. network of nerves

H. removal of the myelin sheath

I. hollow, fluid-filled spaces in the brain

J. union between the dorsal and ventral nerve roots

Match the term in Column A with its definition in Column B. Some definitions may be used more than once.

Column A

21. motor aphasia _____
22. apraxis _____
23. dysphasia _____
24. Kernig's sign _____
25. sensory aphasia _____
26. bradykinesia _____
27. myasthenia _____
28. Brudzinski's sign _____
29. amnesia _____
30. comatose _____
31. neurasthenia _____
32. Romberg's sign _____
33. analgesia _____
34. dysarthria _____
35. syncope _____
36. paresthesia _____

Column B

A. Lack of sensitivity to pain

B. slow movement

C. loss of power of expression in speech or in writing

D. abnormal sensations

E. an indication of meningitis

F. fainting

G. lack of understanding the spoken or written language

H. difficulty in speaking

I. difficulty in speaking caused by lack of muscle coordination

J. inability to perform skilled movements

K. an indication of loss of position sense

L. muscle weakness

M. nerve weakness

N. loss of memory

O. pertaining to a state of unconsciousness

▶**EXERCISE 9–4**

Short Answer

Practice Quiz

1. Name the two primary divisions of the nervous system. _____

_____

2. What are three functions of the neuroglia? _____

_____

3. Name the neuron types. _____

_____

4. What is a synapse? _____

_____

5. What is the largest sub-part of the brain? _____

_____

9–II

6. After what other anatomical parts are the lobes of the brain named?

_____

_____

7. How many pairs of cranial nerves are there? _____

8. What phrase helps us to remember the functions of the cranial nerves?

_____

_____

9. What is a reflex? _____

_____

10. Name the two subdivisions of the autonomic nervous system. _____

_____

▶EXERCISE 9–5   **Fill in the Blank**

Fill in the Blank

1. The star-shaped neuroglia that prevent toxic substances from entering the brain are called _____ .

2. The nerve cell fiber that carries nerve impulses away from the cell body is the _____ .

3. The basal ganglia are located in the _____ .

_____

4. The brain stem includes the _____ ,

_____ , _____ .

5. The _____ joins the right and left sides of the brain.

6. The inferior portion of the spinal cord, resembling a horse's tail is called the _____ _____ .

7. Cerebrospinal fluid is produced by a network of capillaries called the

_____ .

8. The interventricular foramen through which cerebrospinal fluid passes is also known as the _____ .

9. An abnormal response to the plantar reflex is the _____ .

10. Jessie is afraid of a dog that is chasing her. Which division of the autonomic nervous system is predominant in this situation? _____ .

11. The femoral nerve is a branch of the _____ plexus.

Spelling Practice

Spelling

Place a check mark beside all misspelled words in the list that follows. Correctly spell those that you checked off.

1. neuraglial ☐ _____
2. sinapse ☐ _____
3. myelin sheath ☐ _____
4. norypinophrene ☐ _____
5. corpus callosum ☐ _____
6. pariatil lobe ☐ _____
7. dyencephalon ☐ _____
8. hypothalmus ☐ _____
9. medulla oblongata ☐ _____
10. cerrebelum ☐ _____
11. fileum terminal ☐ _____
12. subdurral space ☐ _____
13. aqueduct of Sylvia ☐ _____
14. lateral ventricals ☐ _____
15. olfactory ☐ _____
16. trigeminal ☐ _____
17. glossapharingeal ☐ _____
18. plexus ☐ _____
19. skiatic nerve ☐ _____
20. parasympathetic ☐ _____

Medical Terms in Context

Define the underlined terms as they are used in context.

UNIVERSITY HOSPITAL ✚   **SUMMARY RECORD**

ADMISSION DATE: JUNE 22, 1995

DISCHARGE DATE: JUNE 27, 1995

ADMISSION DIAGNOSIS: POSSIBLE NORMAL PRESSURE <u>HYDROCEPHALUS</u>

HISTORY OF PRESENT ILLNESS:

This 66-year-old black gentleman, right handed, was admitted because of at least a several month history of increasing cognitive deterioration, memory deficits, and early <u>ataxia</u>. Previous <u>CT scan</u> had demonstrated moderate hydrocephalus.

On this admission he underwent <u>magnetic resonance imaging</u> that confirmed the CT findings and did not reveal anything else significant. His history was once again reviewed. The patient was a former professional football player and in this activity had undergone numerous minor head injuries, but had never suffered major head injury. There was no history of <u>subarachnoid hemorrhage</u> or <u>meningitis</u>.

He was seen in consultation by <u>Neurology</u>, who felt that his diagnosis might be consistent with normal pressure hydrocephalus.

He underwent a <u>ventriculoperitoneal shunt</u> on the 25th of June, inserting a medium pressure valve. This went without complication.

His postoperative course was good, without any complications or untoward effects with shunting. He was discharged home on the second postoperative day, and a scheduled follow-up and CT scan have been planned.

DISCHARGE DIAGNOSIS: POSSIBLE NORMAL PRESSURE HYDROCEPHALUS

SIGNATURE OF DOCTOR IN CHARGE _____

---

1. hydrocephalus   _____

2. ataxia   _____

3. CT scan   _____

4. magnetic resonance imaging _____

5. subarachnoid hemorrhage _____

6. meningitis   _____

7. neurology   _____

8. ventriculoperitoneal shunt _____

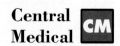

Central Medical **CM**

Operative Report

PROCEDURE: VENTRICULOPERITONEAL SHUNT

OPERATIVE REPORT

PREPOPERATIVE DIAGNOSIS: NORMAL PRESSURE HYDROCEPHALAUS

OPERATION PROPOSED: RIGHT <u>VENTRICULOPERITONEAL SHUNT</u>

PROCEDURE:

The region above and behind his right ear was shaved, prepped, and draped in the usual fashion as well as the anterior neck and chest and upper abdomen. A <u>midline incision</u> in the <u>subxiphoid</u> region and the peritoneum was identified and picked up through <u>linea alba</u>. A crescent-shaped incision was made above and behind the right ear and a hole created using a <u>trephine.</u> We first passed into the right <u>lateral ventricle</u>, and clear <u>CSF</u> was obtained and sent for sampling. Pressure moderately increased but not measured. A <u>ventriculoperitoneal</u> tubing had been passed between the two incisions previously, and a medium pressure valve had been attached to the upper end. The whole system was connected and internalized and the incisions closed in layers. No complications. Sponge and instrument count correct.

POSTOPERATIVE DIAGNOSIS: NORMAL PRESSURE HYDROCEPHALUS

Authorized Health Care Practitioner _____

9. midline incision   _____

10. subxiphoid   _____

11. linea alba   _____

12. trephine   _____

13. lateral ventricle   _____

14. CSF   _____

15. ventriculoperitoneal   _____

9–11

10

THE EYES AND EARS

CHAPTER OBJECTIVES

Upon successful completion of this chapter, the student will be able to do the following:

1. List and describe the external and internal structures of the eye.
2. Differentiate between anterior and posterior cavities and anterior and posterior chambers of the eye.
3. Identify the terms relating to the outer, middle, and inner ear.
4. Describe the physiology of vision and hearing.
5. Analyze, pronounce, define, and spell medical terms related to the eye and ear.
6. List and define abnormal conditions of the eyes and ears.
7. Define terms related to the examination, diagnosis, and treatment of the eyes and ears.
8. Give meanings for abbreviations related to the eyes and ears.

THE EYE WORD ELEMENT	MEANING
chori/o; choriod/o	choroid
cochle/o	cochlea
conjunctiv/o	conjunctiva
core/o	pupil
corne/o; kerat/o	cornea
cycl/o	ciliary body
dacry/o	tears
dacryoaden/o	tear gland
dacryocyst/o	tear sac; lacrimal sac
irid/o; ir/o	iris
lacrim/o	tears
mi/o	lessening; contraction
mydr/o	wide
ocul/o	eye
ophthalm/o	eye
opt/o	vision
palpebr/o	eyelid
phak/o; phac/o	lens
phot/o	light
pupill/o	pupil
retin/o	retina
scler/o	sclera
uve/o	uvea; middle layer (choroid, ciliary body, and iris)

THE EAR WORD ELEMENT	MEANING
acoust/o	sound
audi/o	hearing
aur/o	ear
auricul/o	ear
labyrinth/o	labyrinth
mastoid/o	mastoid process
myring/o	tympanic membrane
ot/o	ear
salping/o	eustachian tube
staped/o	stapes
tympan/o	tympanic membrane

▷ 10.1 ANATOMY AND PHYSIOLOGY OF THE EYE

The eye is very similar to a video camera. It can move from object to object, just as a camera pans across the visual field. The pupil of the eye constricts in bright light, like the aperture of a camera, so that less light is allowed in. The lens of the eye adjusts, so that both near and far objects can be brought into focus. Light entering the eye is transformed into electrical signals, to be processed in the occipital lobe of the brain.

Inner Eye

The eye is a sphere with an outer layer, a middle layer, and an inner layer (see Figure 10–1).

FIGURE 10–1 **Structures of the Eye** (a) Sagittal view. (b) Anterior view.

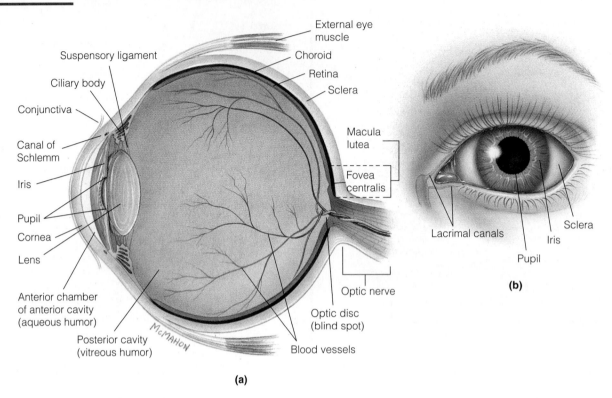

(a)

(b)

Outer Layer The outer layer of the eyeball is called the **fibrous tunic.** Its transparent anterior portion, the **cornea** (kor′-nē-ă), allows light into the eyeball while keeping dust and foreign matter out. Its smooth, firm, white posterior portion, the **sclera** (sklĕr′-ă), maintains the eye's spherical shape. The sclera is sometimes referred to as the "white" of the eye.

Middle Layer The middle layer, known as the **vascular tunic,** or **uvea** (ū′-vē-ă), includes the **choroid** (kor′-oyd), the **ciliary body,** and the **iris.** The **choroid** is the dark colored inner lining of the sclera. It contains the blood vessels that supply nutrition to the eye. At the anterior edge of the choroid is the **ciliary body,** consisting of the ciliary muscles and the ciliary processes (see Figure 10–2).

The **ciliary muscles** adjust the shape of the lens, allowing the eye to focus on objects at various distances. The **ciliary processes,** projections from the ciliary muscle, produce a watery fluid called aqueous humor, which bathes the anterior region. Attached to the ciliary body and forming the anterior portion of the vascular tunic is the **iris,** a flat, circular structure with a round opening at its center. The pigment in the iris gives the eye its brown, blue, or green color. The central opening, called the **pupil,** regulates the amount of light that passes into the eye. The iris has two types of muscles that function to open and close the pupil. In dim light, the **radial** muscle fibers of the iris contract, **dilating** (enlarging) the pupil. In bright light, the **circular** muscle fibers of the iris contract, constricting the pupil.

FIGURE 10–2 Uvea, Lens, and Other Structures of the Eye

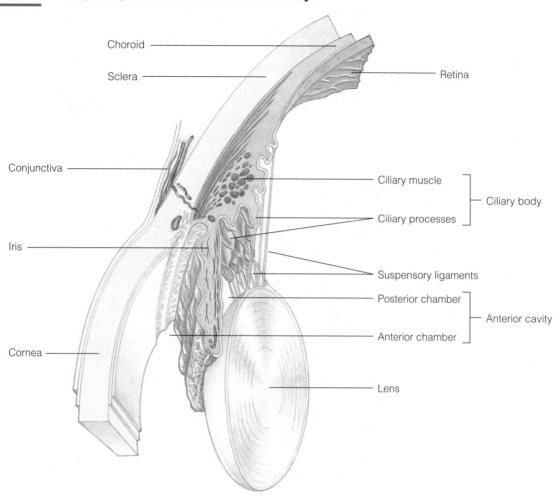

Choroid

Sclera

Retina

Conjunctiva

Ciliary muscle

Ciliary processes

Ciliary body

Iris

Suspensory ligaments

Posterior chamber

Anterior cavity

Anterior chamber

Cornea

Lens

Inner Layer The inner layer of the eyeball, the **retina**, consists of several layers of nervous tissue (see Figure 10–3). This nervous tissue contains photoreceptor cells called **rods** and **cones**, which change light energy into nerve impulses. Close to the center of the retina is a small, yellowish area called the **macula lutea**, and

FIGURE 10–3

Retina Seen on Ophthalmoscopy The back wall of the eye is shown focusing on the macula lutea and optic disc.

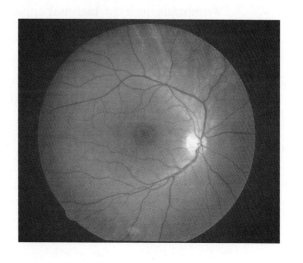

set within the macula lutea is a small depression called the **fovea centralis,** where a high number of cones are located. These cones are responsible for central vision and for the contrast and color differentiation that is possible in daylight vision. The rods, which are located in the periphery of the retina, away from the macula lutea, are responsible for peripheral vision and dim-light vision. In dim-light conditions, the body manufactures a pigment called **rhodopsin,** which increases the rods' responsiveness to light. Vitamin A is needed to manufacture rhodopsin; hence, Vitamin A deficiency can lead to night blindness.

One small area of the retina, medial to the fovea centralis, has no rods or cones and thus produces no visual image. This area, called the **optic disc** or **blind spot,** is the point at which the optic nerve begins. It is also the entry point for the major blood vessels of the eye.

Lens and Suspensory Ligaments Two additional internal structures that are not part of any of the layers so far mentioned are the **lens** and the **suspensory ligaments** (see Figure 10-2). The lens, located posterior to the iris and held in place by the suspensory ligaments, refracts (bends) light rays reflected from an object and focuses these light rays onto the retina.

Cavities and Humors The internal eye has two separate cavities: the **posterior cavity** is behind the lens, and the **anterior cavity** is in front of it (see Figure 10-1). The anterior cavity is separated by the iris into two chambers: the **posterior chamber,** between the iris and the lens, and the **anterior chamber,** between the iris and the cornea. The anterior cavity is filled with a watery fluid called **aqueous humor,** which flows freely between the two chambers by passing through the pupil. As this substance is produced and secreted by the ciliary processes, an equal amount is constantly drained through a lattice-type or meshwork structure called the **trabecula** (tră-běk′-ū-lă) into the canal of Schlemm (shlěm) and into the venous system. If the aqueous humor is unable to drain through the canal, a condition called **glaucoma** results. This equality between production and drainage helps maintain the equilibrium of the intraocular pressure.

The posterior cavity of the eye is filled with **vitreous** (vĭt′-rē-ŭs) **humor,** a clear, jellylike, material that maintains the spherical shape of the eyeball, holds the retina firmly against the choroid, and transmits light.

Outer Eye

The **orbital cavity,** the **extrinsic ocular muscles,** the **eyelids,** the **conjunctival membrane,** and the **lacrimal apparatus** all contribute to the proper functioning of the eye (see Figure 10-4).

Orbital Cavity The **orbital cavity,** or **orbit,** is the bony depression of the skull, below the frontal bone, into which the eyeball fits. The eyeball is protected from injury by the bony orbital rim and by the fatty tissue that lines the orbital cavity.

Extrinsic Ocular Muscles Six extrinsic ocular muscles are attached to the sclera of each eye. Stimulated by the third, fourth, and sixth cranial nerves, these muscles can move the eye in any direction. They are named according to their location and orientation, **rectus** meaning straight and **oblique** meaning slanted. The **superior rectus, inferior rectus, medial rectus,** and **lateral rectus**

FIGURE 10—4

External Anatomy of the Eye (a) Eyebrow, conjunctiva, orbit, ocular muscles, optic nerve. (b) Lacrimal apparatus.

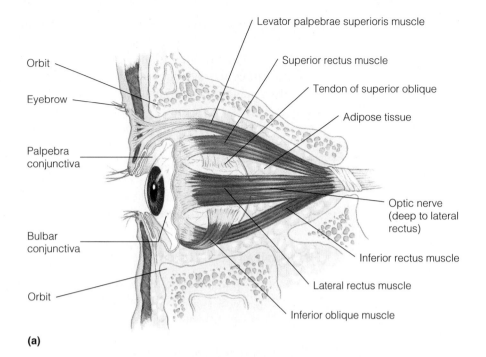

(a)

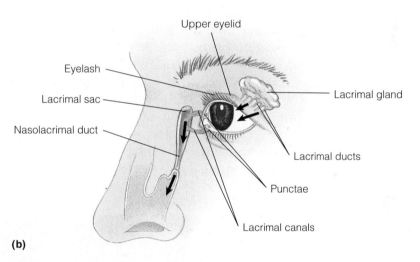

(b)

respectively turn the eyeball upward, downward, medially, and laterally. The **superior oblique** turns the eye downward laterally; the **inferior oblique** turns it upward laterally.

Eyelids   The eyelids, or **palpebrae** (păl′-pĕ-brī), are movable and are located in front of the eyeball. They shield the eye from dust, extreme light, and trauma. The **superior palpebra** and the **inferior palpebra** (upper and lower eyelids) meet laterally at a point called the **external canthus** and medially at a point called the **internal canthus.**

Conjunctival Membrane   A thin layer of mucous membrane called the **conjunctival membrane** lines the anterior part of the eye exposed to air. The part of this membrane lining the inside of the eyelids is called the **palpebral conjunctiva;** the part covering the surface of the eyeball is called the **bulbar conjunctiva.**

II—10

Lacrimal Apparatus   The lacrimal apparatus of each eye includes the lacrimal gland, the lacrimal duct, the lacrimal canal, the lacrimal sac, and the nasolacrimal duct. The **lacrimal glands,** located in the superior, lateral region of each orbit, produce tears, which cleanse and lubricate the conjunctiva. Since tears contain **lysozyme** (lī'-sō-zīm), an antibacterial enzyme, they also kill microorganisms. Tears run steadily from the glands, through the **lacrimal ducts,** across the eye, and into two small openings called **punctae** at the medial corner of each eyelid. The punctae connect to the lacrimal canals, which carry the tears into the lacrimal sac, which is the bulbous, proximal portion of the nasolacrimal duct. The nasolacrimal duct extends from the lacrimal sac into the distal segment of the nose. If any of these ducts become plugged, from a cold for example, the tears flow from the eyes instead of draining into the nose.

Physiology of Vision

The process of vision begins when an image is formed on the retina. The photoreceptors are stimulated, causing nerve impulses to travel to the cerebral cortex of the occipital lobe, where they are interpreted.

Retinal Image   Refraction, lens accommodation, convergence, and **pupillary accommodation** are essential for formation of a clear image on the retina.

Refraction, the bending of light, occurs when light passes through tissue of a certain density at an oblique angle (see Figure 10–5). As light travels through the cornea, aqueous humor, lens, and vitreous humor, it is refracted and comes together at the same time and at the same point on the retinas of both eyes. This phenomenon is known as **binocular vision** (seeing one object instead of two). The importance of refraction is better understood if one thinks of the light rays reflected from an object as being scattered and disorganized. The eye structures take these disorganized light rays and refract them so that they come together at a single point on the retina. See Figure 10–6.

FIGURE 10–5

Refraction Light bends as it travels from a denser medium, like the water in the glass, to a less dense medium, like air. Therefore, the position of the portion of the pencil immersed in water appears to be different than the position of the portion not immersed. The pencil appears bent, because the light waves travelling from the water to the air bend.

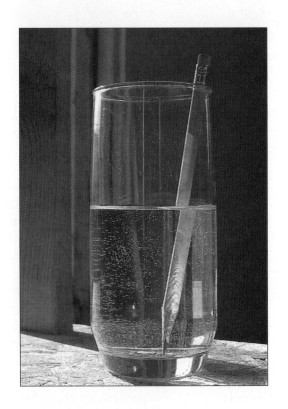

FIGURE 10-6

**Focusing of Light Rays
onto the Retina**

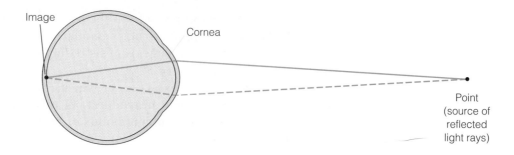

Lens accommodation is the ability of the lens to adjust to make far and near vision possible. The elastic quality of the lens allows it to adapt to objects of varying distances. When an object is near, the light rays have to be refracted sharply, and so the lens becomes rounded, bending the light to a greater degree. However, with distant objects, the lens retains a flattened shape, refracting the light rays less as they pass through the various refracting media (see Figure 10–7). Therefore, the degree to which the lens refracts light rays depends on

FIGURE 10–7 **Lens Accommodation** (a) The suspensory ligaments are attached to the lens and ciliary body. (b) For near vision, the suspensory ligaments relax, lens becomes rounded, bending the light rays to a greater degree. (c) For far vision, the suspensory ligaments tighten, flattening the lens.

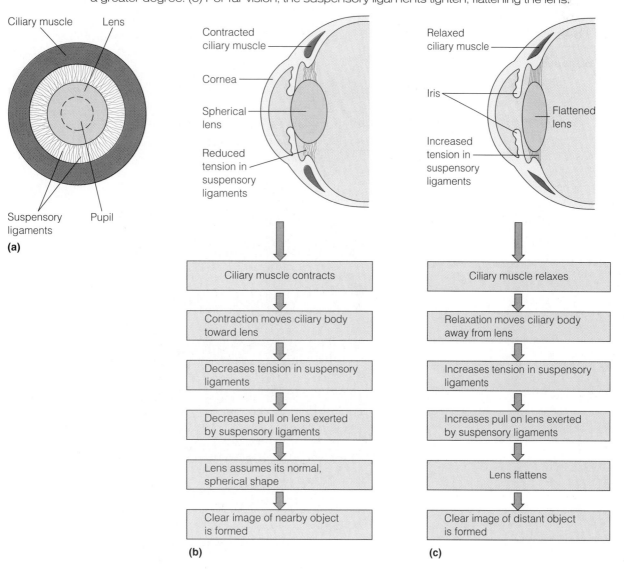

the distance of the object away from the lens. With age, the lens loses its elasticity and therefore its ability to accommodate. Vision is impaired and we start to need reading glasses or bifocals. This reduction of vision due to old age is known as **presbyopia.**

Convergence is a reflex action in which the two eyeballs move medially when they are focusing on a near object. In this manner, light rays from the object will focus on corresponding points of both retinae simultaneously, producing binocular vision.

Pupillary accommodation describes the ability of the pupil to adapt by dilating for distant objects and constricting for near ones.

Neural Pathways At the retina, light is transformed into nerve impulses that travel along the optic nerve from each eye. They meet at the **optic chiasm** (kī'-ăzm), where an interesting thing happens: nerve fibers from the medial portion of each eye cross each other and link up with nerve fibers from the lateral portion of the opposite eye. Thus, the fibers from the inner portion of the right eye join fibers from the outer portion of the left eye.

On leaving the optic chiasm, the light impulse travels the optic tract to the thalamus. From the thalamus, the impulse travels to the cerebral cortex of the occipital lobe of the brain, where it is interpreted (see Figure 10–8).

FIGURE 10–8

Neural Pathways

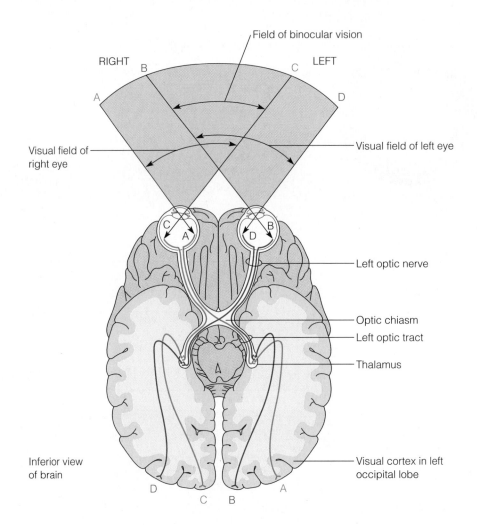

In summary, the following flow chart simplifies the visual pathway.

FIGURE 10–9

Flow Chart of Visual Pathway

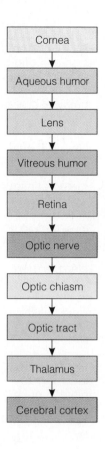

Cornea → Aqueous humor → Lens → Vitreous humor → Retina → Optic nerve → Optic chiasm → Optic tract → Thalamus → Cerebral cortex

◗ 10.2 TERM ANALYSIS FOR THE EYE

TERM WITH PRONUNCIATION	ANALYSIS	DEFINITION
anisocoria ăn-ĭ″-sō-kō′-rē-ă	-ia = condition an- = no; not is/o = equal core/o = pupil	inequality in the size of the pupil
aphakia ă-fā′-kē-ă	-ia = condition a- = no; not phak/o = lens	absence of lens
aqueous ā′-kwē-ŭs	-ous = pertaining to aque/o = water	pertaining to water
blepharochalasis blĕf″-ăr-ō-kăl′-ă-sĭs	-chalasis = relaxation blephar/o = eyelid	relaxation of the eyelid
blepharoptosis blĕf″-ă-rō-tō′-sĭs	-ptosis-drooping; sagging; prolapse blephar/o = eyelid	drooping of the eyelid
blepharospasm blĕf′-ă-rō-spăsm	-spasm = sudden violent contraction blephar/o = eyelid	sudden, involuntary contraction of the eyelid

II–10

TERM WITH PRONUNCIATION	ANALYSIS	DEFINITION
chorioretinitis kō″-rē-ō-rĕt″-ĭn-ī′-tĭs	-itis = inflammation chori/o = choroid retin/o = retina	inflammation of the choroid and retina
choroidopathy kō-roy-dŏp′-ă-thē	-pathy = disease choroid/o = choroid	disease of the choroid
conjunctivitis kŏn-juňk″-tĭ-vī′-tĭs	-itis = inflammation conjunctiv/o = conjunctiva	inflammation of the conjunctiva
coreometer kō″-rē-ŏm′-ĕ-tĕr	-meter = instrument to measure core/o = pupil	instrument to measure the diameter of the pupil
corneal kor′-nē-ăl	-al = pertaining to corne/o = cornea	pertaining to the cornea
cycloplegic sī″-klō-plē′-jĭk	-plegic = pertaining to paralysis cycl/o = ciliary body	pertaining to paralysis of the ciliary body
dacryoadenitis dăk-rē-ō-ăd″-ĕn-ī′-tĭs	-itis = inflammation dacryoaden/o = tear glands; lacrimal glands	inflammation of the tear glands (lacrimal glands)
dacryocystorhinostomy dăk″-rē-ō-sĭs″-tō-rī-nŏs′-tō-mē	-stomy = new opening dacryocyst/o = tear sac; lacrimal sac rhin/o = nose	surgical creation of a new opening between the lacrimal sac and the nose
dacryorrhea dăk″-rē-ō-rē′-ă	-rrhea = discharge; flow dacry/o = tears	excessive flow of tears
ectropion ĕk-trō′-pē-ŏn	-tropion = turn ec- = outward	outward turning of the eyelid
emmetropia ĕm′-mĕ-trō-pē-ă	-opia = vision emmetr/o = in normal measure	normal vision
entropion ĕn-trō′-pē-ŏn	-tropion = turn en- = inward	inward turning of the eyelid
episcleritis ĕp″-ĭ-sklĕ-rī′-tĭs	-itis = inflammation epi- = upon; on; above scler/o = sclera	inflammation (of the tissues) upon the sclera
esotropia ĕs-ō-trō′-pē-ă	-tropia = turning eso- = inward	turning inward of the eye
exotropia ĕks″-ō-trō′-pē-ă	-tropia = turning exo- = outward	turning outward of the eye
extraocular ĕks″-tră-ŏk′-ū-lăr	-ar = pertaining to extra- = outside ocul/o = eye	pertaining to outside the eye
hemianopia; hemianopsia hĕm″-ē-ă-nŏ′-pē-ă hĕm″-ē-ă-nŏp′-sē-ă	-opia = visual condition hemi- = half an- = no; not	lack of vision in half the visual field

TERM WITH PRONUNCIATION	ANALYSIS	DEFINITION
iridocyclitis ĭr″-ĭd-ō-sī-klī′-tĭs	-itis = inflammation irid/o = iris cycl/o = ciliary body	inflammation of the iris and ciliary body
iritis ĭ-rī′-tĭs	-itis = inflammation ir/o = iris	inflammation of the iris
keratoconjunctivitis kĕr″-ă-tō-kŏn-jŭnk″-tĭ-vī′-tĭs	-itis = inflammation kerat/o = cornea conjunctiv/o = conjunctiva	inflammation of the cornea and conjunctiva
keratoconus kĕr-ă-tō-kō′-nŭs	-conus = cone-shaped kerat/o = cornea	abnormal, outward, cone-shaped protrusion of the cornea
keratomycosis kĕr″-ă-tō-mī-kō′-sĭs	-osis = abnormal condition kerat/o = cornea myc/o = fungus	fungal infection of the cornea
lacrimal lăk′-rĭm-ăl	-al = pertaining to lacrim/o = tears	pertaining to tears
miosis mī-ō′-sĭs	-sis = state of; condition; process mi/o = contraction; less	contraction of the pupil
mydriasis mĭd-rī′-ă-sĭs	-iasis = condition; process mydr/o = wide; dilation	dilation of the pupil
nasolacrimal nā″-zō-lăk′-rĭm-ăl	-al = pertaining to nas/o = nose lacrim/o = tears	pertaining to the nose and lacrimal apparatus
ophthalmologist ŏf-thăl-mŏl′-ō-jĭst	-logist = specialist in the study of ophthalm/o = eye	a physician who specializes in the diagnosis and medical and surgical treatment of eye disorders
ophthalmopathy ŏf″-thăl-mŏp′-ă-thē	-pathy = disease ophthalm/o = eye	disease of the eye
optic ŏp′-tĭk	-ic = pertaining to opt/o = vision; sight	pertaining to vision or sight
optician ŏp-tĭsh′-ăn	-ician = specialist; one who specializes; expert opt/o = vision; sight	expert who fills prescriptions for eyeglasses and contact lens **Note:** Opticians are not physicians and do not carry out medical and surgical treatment of eye conditions.
optometrist ŏp-tŏm′-ĕ-trĭst	-metrist = specialist in the measurement of opt/o = vision; sight	specialist in the testing of visual function and in the diagnosis and nonsurgical treatment of eye conditions **Note:** Optometrists prescribe eyeglasses and contact lens and are licensed in some areas to prescribe medication. They do not have a degree in medicine.

TERM WITH PRONUNCIATION	ANALYSIS	DEFINITION
palpebral păl′-pĕ-brăl	-al = pertaining to palpebr/o = eyelid	pertaining to the eyelid
phacomalacia făk″-ō-mă-lā′-shē-ă	-malacia = soft phac/o = lens	softening of the lens
pseudophakia sū-dō-fā′-kē-ă	-ia = condition pseudo- = false phak/o = lens	condition characterized by replacement of the lens with connective tissue
pupillary pū′-pĭ-lĕr-ē	-ary = pertaining to pupill/o = pupil	pertaining to the pupil
retinopathy rĕt″-ĭn-ŏp′-ă-thē	-pathy = disease retin/o = retina	disease of the retina
retinopexy rĕt″-ĭn-ō′-pĕk-sē	-pexy = surgical fixation retin/o = retina	surgical fixation of the retina
retinoschisis rĕt″-ĭ-nŏs′-kĭ-sĭs	-schisis = splitting; division retin/o = retina	splitting of the retina
sclerectomy sklĕ-rĕk′-tō-mē	-ectomy = excision; removal scler/o = sclera	excision of the sclera
uveitis ū′-vē-ī′-tĭs	-itis = inflammation uve/o = uvea, including the choroid, ciliary body, and iris	inflammation of the uvea
vitreous vĭt′-rē′-ŭs	-ous = pertaining to vitre/o = glasslike; gel-like	pertaining to the vitreous humor, a gel-like, glassy substance in the posterior cavity

◊ 10.3 ABNORMAL CONDITIONS OF THE EYE

The most common abnormal eye conditions are focusing disorders. They are referred to as errors of refraction and include myopia (mī-ō′-pē-ă), hyperopia (hī-pĕr-ō′-pē-ă) [also known as hypermetropia (hī-pĕr-mē-trō′-pē-ă)], and astigmatism (ă-stĭg′-mă-tĭzm). Myopia and hyperopia are commonly called nearsightedness and farsightedness, respectively. In myopia, the image is focused before it reaches the retina. Myopia is corrected by placement of a concave lens in front of the eye to spread the image so that it is in focus when it reaches the retina. In hyperopia, the image is focused behind the retina. Placing a convex lens in front of the eye narrows the image slightly so that it is in focus when it reaches the retina. In astigmatism, light is not focused properly on the retina because the asymmetrical curvature of the cornea or lens results in blurred vision. Placing a lens with the proper curvature corrects this problem. See Figure 10–10.

FIGURE 10-10 **Errors of Refraction** (a) Myopia (nearsightedness), in which light rays focus in front of retina is corrected by concave lens. (b) Hyperopia (farsightedness), in which light rays focus behind the retina, is corrected by convex lens. (c) Astigmatism as a result of an asymmetrical cornea. (d) Astigmatism as a result of an asymmetrical lens.

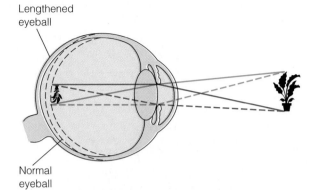

Lengthened eyeball

Normal eyeball

(a) Myopia (nearsightedness) uncorrected

Concave lens

Myopia (nearsightedness) corrected

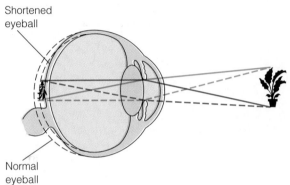

Shortened eyeball

Normal eyeball

(b) Hyperopia (farsightedness) uncorrected

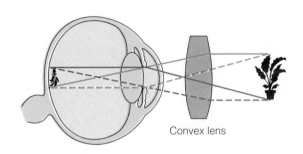

Convex lens

Hyperopia (farsightedness) corrected

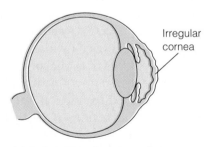

Irregular cornea

(c) Astigmatism from irregular cornea

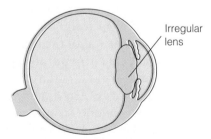

Irregular lens

(d) Astigmatism from irregular lens

Color blindness affects approximately 1 in 13 males, but it is relatively rare in females. It is a genetically transmitted disorder, more often involving the absence of red or green cones in the retina (see Figure 10–11). Severity can range from the total inability to detect color to the much more common problem of inability to distinguish red from green.

FIGURE 10–11

Test for Color Blindness
A figure like this is used to detect red-green color blindness. Diagnosis is positive when the number cannot be seen.

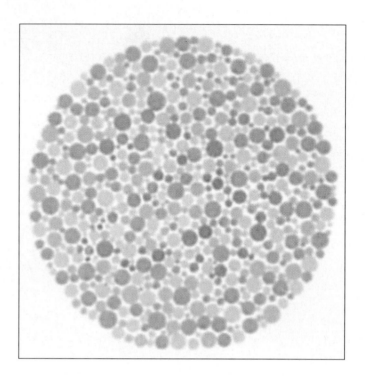

Cataracts (kăt′-ă-răkts) are opaque areas in the lens of the eye (see Figure 10–12). Cataracts sometimes accompany the aging process and were once a leading cause of serious vision loss, but are now routinely removed surgically. One surgical technique is **extracapsular cataract extraction (ECCE),** which is partial removal of the lens and lens capsule followed by insertion of a prosthetic implant called an **intraocular lens.** A type of ECCE is **phacoemulsification** (făk″-ō-ē-mŭl′-sĭ-fĭ-kā″-shŭn),which destroys the cataract by means of ultrasonic sound waves. Any fragments left are removed by suction and aspiration. Another technique is **intracapsular cataract extraction (ICCE),** which is the removal of the entire lens and lens capsule (see Figure 10–13).

FIGURE 10–12

Cataracts

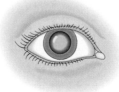

FIGURE 10–13

Types of Cataract Extraction (a) Intracapsular cataract extraction removes the entire lens within its capsule. (b) Extracapsular cataract extraction removes the lens within its anterior capsule, leaving the posterior capsule intact.

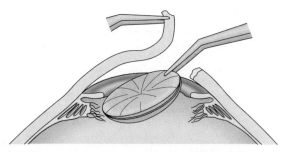

(a) Intracapsular cataract extraction: Removal of the entire lens and lens capsule.

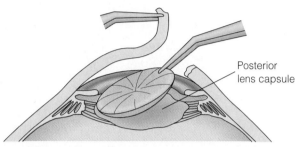

Posterior lens capsule

(b) Extracapsular cataract extraction: Lens is removed with its anterior capsule, leaving posterior capsule intact.

Glaucoma (glaw-kō′-mă) is characterized by increased **intraocular pressure (IOP),** resulting in deterioration of the retina and optic nerve (see Figure 10–14). Normally aqueous humor is continuously being produced and drained from the eye through the canal of Schlemm. In glaucoma, the aqueous humor fails to drain away and accumulates in the eye, increasing IOP. If early treatment is not prescribed, glaucoma damages the optic disc and results in blindness. Approximately half of all cases of adult blindness are caused by glaucoma.

FIGURE 10–14

Glaucoma

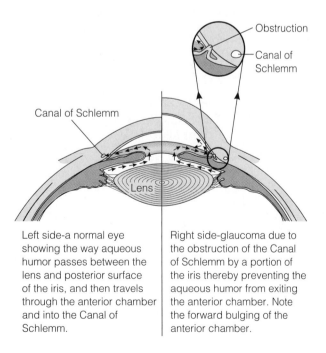

Obstruction

Canal of Schlemm

Canal of Schlemm

Lens

Left side-a normal eye showing the way aqueous humor passes between the lens and posterior surface of the iris, and then travels through the anterior chamber and into the Canal of Schlemm.

Right side-glaucoma due to the obstruction of the Canal of Schlemm by a portion of the iris thereby preventing the aqueous humor from exiting the anterior chamber. Note the forward bulging of the anterior chamber.

CONDITION	DESCRIPTION
acute conjunctivitis kŏn-jŭnk″-tĭ-vī-tĭs	contagious bacterial infection causing inflammation of the conjunctiva; may also be known as **pink-eye**
chalazion kă-lā′-zē-ŏn	a cyst of the eyelid, also known as a meibomian (mī-bō′-mĭ-ăn) cyst

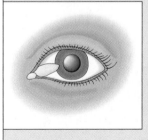

CONDITION	DESCRIPTION
exophthalmia ĕks″-ŏf-thăl′-mē-ă	outward protrusion of the eyeball
hordeolum hor-dē′-ō-lŭm	inflammation of one or more sebaceous glands of the eyelid characterized by pustular lesions; commonly know as a sty (stye) **Note:** Compare chalazion and hordeolum. The chalazion is **cystic;** the hordeolum is **pustular.**
hyphema; hyphemia hī-fē′-mă; hī-fē′-mē-ă	bleeding into the anterior chamber of the eye
ophthalmia neonatorum ŏf-thăl′-mē-ă nē-ō-nă-tōr′-um	gonococcal infection of the newborn, transmitted from mother to baby during pregnancy
ptosis tō′-sĭs	drooping of the eyelid
pterygium tĕr-ĭj′-ē-ŭm	thick, triangular-shaped growth extending from the canthus, to the conjunctiva, to the cornea thereby reducing vision and necessitating removal (usually by laser)
punctal stenosis pŭnk′-tăl stĕ-nō′-sĭs	narrowing of the punctae, which means that tears cannot flow into the nose through the lacrimal ducts (a common condition in infants)

CONDITION	DESCRIPTION
retinal tears	weak spots on the retina that develop as a result of shrinkage of the vitreous body with age (As the vitreous shrinks, it pulls on and tears the retina. If left untreated, the vitreous humor can seep behind the retina and slowly peel it from the choroid [**retinal detachment**].) **Note: Laser photocoagulation** can repair retinal tears and prevent retinal detachment. However, it is ineffective in fixing retinal detachments.

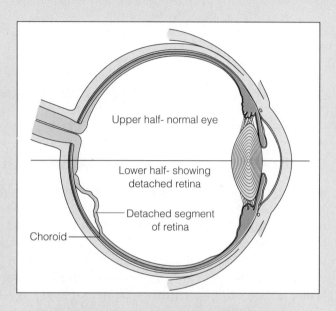

Upper half- normal eye

Lower half- showing detached retina

Detached segment of retina

Choroid

strabismus strǎ-bĭz'-mǔs	the absence of coordinated directional control of both eyes; example: crossed-eyes. There are four types of strabismus: **esotropia**— an inward turning of the eye **exotropia**— an outward turning of the eye **hypertropia**— an upward turning of the eye **hypotropia**— a downward turning of the eye

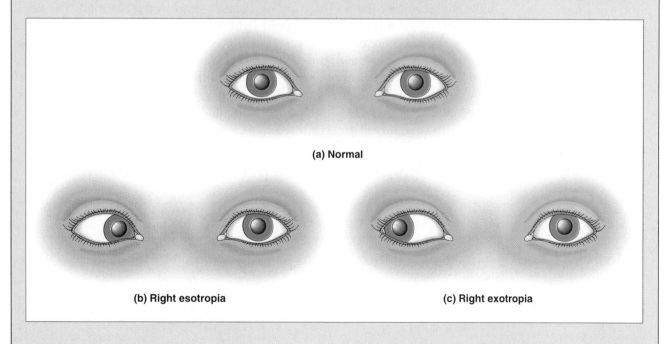

(a) Normal

(b) Right esotropia

(c) Right exotropia

CONDITION	DESCRIPTION
symblepharon sim-blĕf′-ă-rŏn	adhesion of the eyeball and the eyelid
synechiae sĭn-ĕk′-ē-ă	adhesions of surfaces **Note:** Adhesion of the iris to the cornea is called **anterior synechiae;** adhesion of the iris to the lens is called **posterior synechiae.**
trachoma trā-kō′-mă	bacterial infection causing chronic conjunctivits

◈ 10.4 PHYSICAL EXAMINATION, DIAGNOSIS, AND TREATMENT FOR CONDITIONS OF THE EYE

Diagnosis of Abnormal Eye Conditions

The **Snellen Eye Chart,** composed of letters of the alphabet, is used to examine **visual acuity** (sharpness of vision), which is expressed as a fraction. The two numbers, both the numerator (the top number) and the denominator (the bottom number), stand for distance in feet. The numerator represents the examinee's distance from the chart, and the denominator represents the distance at which a normal eye can read a given line on the chart. Thus, 20/20 is normal visual acuity, 20/30 is below normal, and 20/15 is above normal.

The examining health care practitioner will also examine the visual field of each eye by bringing an object such as a pen into the field of vision from the periphery. The object is brought into the visual field from several directions, and any abnormalities are noted. Extraocular movements, such as **nystagmus,** are also noted.

The health care practitioner will also examine for pupillary reaction to light and accommodation (reaction to distance of objects). Normally the pupil constricts when it is exposed to bright light or objects that are near and dilates when exposed to dim light or distant objects. The instrument used to assess pupillary reaction is the ophthalmoscope, or **funduscope** (fŭn′-dŭ-skōp). With it, the health care practitioner observes the fundus, which is the posterior portion of the eye. The fundus includes the retina, retinal arteries and veins, optic nerve, and optic discs. The tables below include terms relating to the signs and symptoms, diagnostic procedures, and treatment of abnormal eye conditions.

Signs and Symptoms of Abnormal Eye Conditions

SIGN OR SYMPTOM	DEFINITION
amblyopia ăm″-blē-ō′-pē-ă	dimness of vision not caused by organic defect or refractive error
Argyll-Robertson pupil	pupil reacts to accommodation but not to light
diplopia dĭp-lō′-pē-ă	double vision

SIGN OR SYMPTOM	DEFINITION
flashes	quick one- or two-second flashes of light coming from the pulling on the retina by the vitreous. A symptom of retinal detachment.
floaters	spots seen by the patient in front of one or both eyes **Note:** These spots represent small bits of protein or cells floating in the vitreous humor and are symptomatic of harmless ocular deterioration. In some patients, floaters may be symptomatic of retinal tears where blood from the torn retina seeps into the vitreous humor, with the patient seeing the blood as floating spots.
lacrimation lăk″-rĭ-mā′-shŭn	production of tears
nystagmus nĭs-tăg′-mŭs	rapid, involuntary movement of the eyeball
papilledema; choked disc păp″-ĭl-ĕ-dē′-mă	accumulation of fluid at the optic disc
photophobia fō″-tō-fō′-bē-ă	intolerance or sensitivity to light
scotoma skō-tō′-mă	an area of depressed vision within the visual field

Diagnostic Procedures for Abnormal Eye Conditions

PROCEDURE	DEFINITION
electronystagmography (ENG) (ĕ-lĕk″-trō-nĭs″-tăg-mŏg′-ră-fē)	the process of recording the electrical activity of the extraocular muscles during nystagmic activity
electroretinography ē-lĕk″-trō-rĕt″-ĭn-ŏg′-ră-fē	process of recording the electrical impulses of the retina following stimulation by light
fluorescein staining floo″-ō-rĕs′-ē-ĭn	detection of foreign bodies, corneal abrasion, and ulcers by the use of a powdered dye called fluorescein
funduscopy; fundoscopy; ophthalmoscopy (fŭn-dŭs′-kō-pē, fŭn-dŏs′-kō-pē; ŏf-thăl-mŏs′-kō-pē)	visual examination of the inside of the eye with a funduscope
gonioscopy gō′-nē-ŏs′-kō-pē	examination of the angle of the anterior chamber of the eye, a common diagnostic procedure for detection of glaucoma
tonometry tōn-ŏm′-ĕ-trē	measurement of intraocular pressure, another common diagnostic procedure for the detection of glaucoma

Treatment of Abnormal Eye Conditions

MEDICAL TREATMENT	DEFINITION
antiallergy	for symptomatic relief of allergic conditions such as hay fever and rhinitis

antinfectives
    antibiotics
    antifungals
    antivirals
	for diseases of the eye caused by bacterial, fungal, or viral infection

corticosteroids	for inflammatory and chronic allergic conditions involving the eye, such as iritis, uveitis, and allergic conjunctivitis
cycloplegics	for relaxation of the iris and ciliary muscles and for inflammation of the iris, choroid, and cornea
idoxuridine (IDU) (ī-dŏks-ūr′-ĭ-dēn)	for viral conditions
miotics	drugs used to constrict the pupil
mydriatics	drugs used to widen the pupil

SURGICAL TREATMENT	DEFINITION
corneal transplant; keratoplasty	restoration of vision by taking the cornea from one individual and grafting it to the eye of another **Note:** Corneal transplants are of two types: **whole thickness graft (penetrating graft),** in which the entire depth of the cornea is replaced; and **partial thickness graft (lamellar),** in which the transplanted corneal tissue is of partial depth
evisceration (ē-vĭs″-ĕr-ā′-shŭn)	removal of the contents of the eyeball except for the sclera
intraocular lens implant	fixation of an artificial lens in place of a cataract lens following extracapsular cataract extraction
retinopexy	reattachment of the retina to the choroid for repair of retinal detachment **Note:** Several methods of reattachment are used such as the application of cold **(cryotherapy)**, the application of heat **(diathermy),** and **scleral buckling,** in which the sclera is indented toward the retina at the area of detachment.
trabeculectomy	partial removal of trabecular tissue to increase the outflow of aqueous humor
trabeculotomy	incision into the trabecular meshwork to improve drainage of aqueous humor

EYE SURGERY USING LASERS	DEFINITION
cyclophotocoagulation (sī″-klō-fō″-tō-kō-ăg-ū-lā′-shŭn)	destruction of a portion of the ciliary body using laser to reduce the production of aqueous humor **Note:** used to treat glaucoma
iridectomy	The beam from the laser creates a tiny hole in the iris through which aqueous humor can drain, detouring past the blockage. **Note:** used to treat narrow angle glaucoma

EYE SURGERY USING LASERS	DEFINITION
photorefractive keratectomy (PRK)	A laser is used to reshape the layers of the cornea to improve its refractive powers. **Note:** Used in the treatment of myopia, hypermetropia, and astigmatism. Following this procedure, the patient has improved vision without glasses or contact lenses.
retinal photocoagulation	A beam from a laser is aimed at the site of injury to condense the retinal tissue, thus sealing the tear.
trabeculoplasty	The open spaces of the trabecular meshwork are enlarged by the laser, which allows the aqueous humor to flow out of the eye, reducing intraocular pressure. **Note:** used to treat open angle glaucoma

▶ 10.5 ABBREVIATIONS FOR THE EYE

DCR	dacryocystorhinostomy	OD (oculus dextra)	right eye
ECCE	extracapsular cataract extraction	OS (oculus sinistra)	left eye
ENG	electronystagmography	OU (oculus unitas)	both eyes
EOM	extraocular movement	PERLA	pupils equal; react to light and accommodation
ERG	electroretinography		
ICCE	intracapsular cataract extraction	PERRLA	pupils equal; round, regular, react to light and accommodation
IDU	idoxuridine	PRK	photorefractive keratectomy
IOP	intraocular pressure		

▶ 10.6 ANATOMY AND PHYSIOLOGY OF THE EAR

Our ears perform two important jobs for us: they allow us to hear and they assist us in keeping our balance. The hearing process consists of detection and **transduction.** Detection involves receiving the sound stimulus. Transduction involves converting the detected sound into an electrical signal that is sent on to the brain for processing. Body balance is maintained through the interaction of visual signals and the balance mechanisms of the inner ear.

The ear is made up of three distinct sections: the external ear, the middle ear, and the inner ear (see Figure 10–15).

II–10

FIGURE 10–15 External, Middle, and Inner Ear

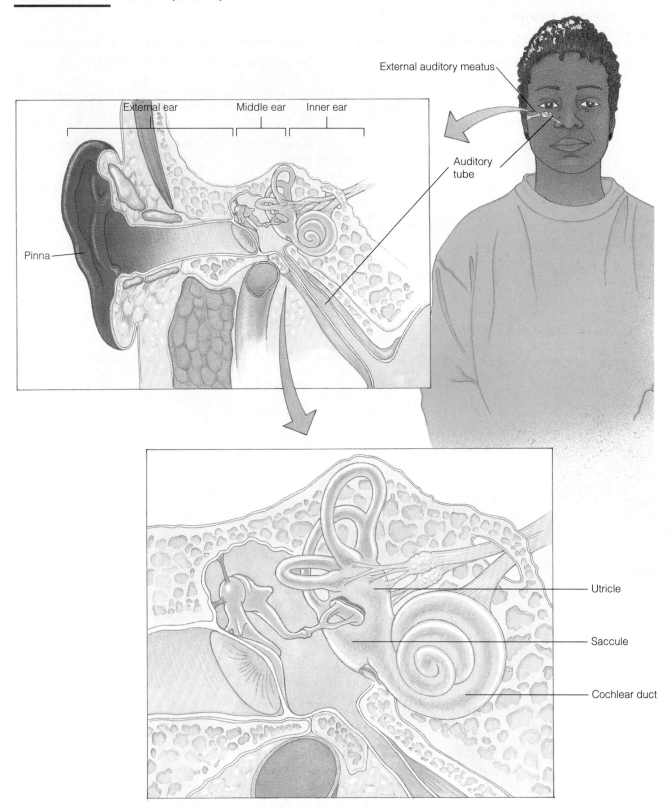

External Ear

The external ear is composed of three parts: the **auricle** (aw′-rĭ-kl), or **pinna** (pĭn′-ă); the **external acoustic (auditory) meatus** (mē′-ā′-tŭs); and the eardrum or **tympanic** (tĭm-păn′-ĭk) **membrane.** The auricle is the part of the ear that we call the "ear" in nontechnical conversation. The external acoustic meatus is the canal that leads to the eardrum. It transmits sound to the tympanic membrane and produces a protective waxy substance called **cerumen.** The transmitted sound causes the tympanic membrane to vibrate, sending the sound waves into the middle ear.

Middle Ear

The middle ear includes the three bones called the **malleus** (măl′-ē-ŭs), the **incus** (ĭng′-kŭs), and the **stapes** (stā-pēz), known collectively as the **auditory ossicles** (ŏs′-ĭ-klz). They are also called the hammer, the anvil, and the stirrup. Sound is transmitted from the malleus to the incus and to the stapes. The stapes vibrates against the **oval window,** which transmits the amplified sound to the inner ear, where it is changed to electrical impulses that the brain can detect and interpret. Also included in the middle ear are two muscles that help prevent loud sounds from damaging the ear. When loud noises occur, the **tensor tympani** (těn′-sor tĭm-păn′-ē) tightens the eardrum to reduce the amount of sound that enters the middle ear, and the **stapedius** (stā-pē′-dē-ŭs) dampens the movement of the auditory ossicles.

The **eustachian** (ū-stā′-shěn) **tube** (auditory tube) connects the middle ear to the throat. It opens when we yawn or swallow so that the air pressure on the inside of the eardrum is equalized with the air pressure on the outside. If the air pressure is not equal, the eardrum is not able to vibrate freely, resulting in temporary hearing impairment. Usually, a popping sound is heard when the pressure is equalized, resulting in restored hearing and elimination of the feeling of pressure in the ear.

Inner Ear

The inner ear is a series of sacs and canals encased in bone, much like the passageways of a cave. The passageways of the inner ear are called the **bony labyrinth** (lăb′-ĭ-rĭnth) and are filled with fluid called **perilymph** (pěr′-ĭ-lĭmf). Tubes called the **membranous labyrinth** are encased in the bony labyrinth. These tubes are filled with another fluid called **endolymph** (ěn′-dō-lĭmf). Portions of the bony labyrinth are the vestibule, semicircular canals and the cochlea. The vestibule, located next to the stapes, contains the utricle (ū′-trĭk′l) and saccule (săk′-ŭl), which are membranous sacs that aid in maintaining balance; the semicircular canals, behind the vestibule, house the membranous semicircular ducts, also involved in balance; and the cochlea contains the cochlear duct, a membranous structure responsible for hearing (see Figure 10–16).

As was stated in the previous sections, sound is transmitted to the inner ear by the action of the stapes vibrating against the oval window. Although the process of transforming the vibrations of the stapes into electrical impulses in the inner ear is very complex, it can be simply described as follows. The receptor

10–II

FIGURE 10–16

Inner Ear

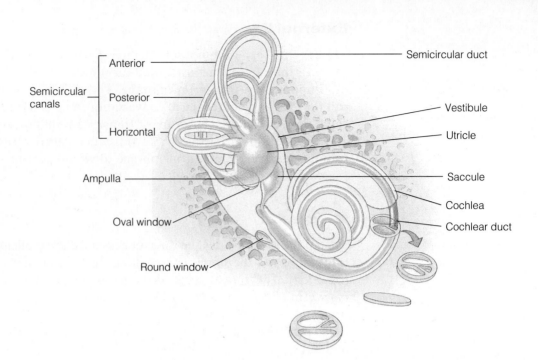

organ for hearing in the inner ear is the **organ of Corti** (kor′-tē), lying within the cochlear (kŏk′-lē-ăr) duct. It contains sensitive hair cells, which react to the vibrations of the stapes by moving, much as tall grass sways in the wind. The movement of the hair cells stimulates underlying nerve cell fibers that create the nerve impulses which travel to the brain. (See Figure 10–17.)

FIGURE 10–17   **Terminology of the Middle and Inner Ear**

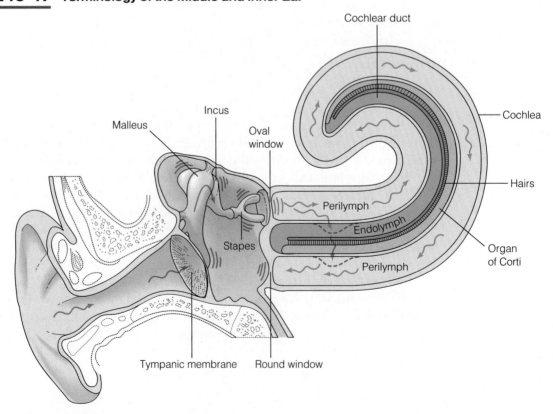

In summary, the following flow chart shows the auditory pathway.

FIGURE 10–18

Flow Chart of the Auditory Process

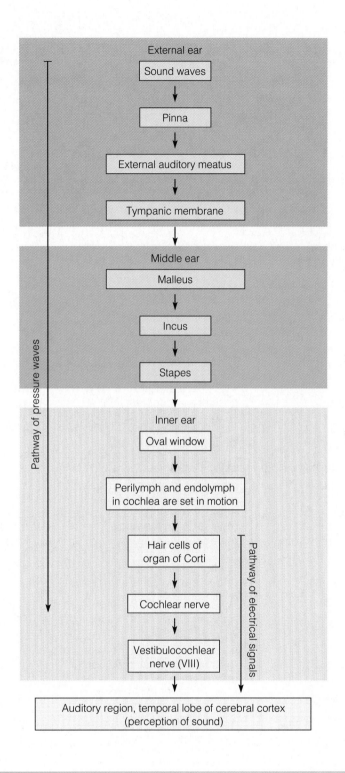

TERM WITH PRONUNCIATION	ANALYSIS	DEFINITION
acoustic ă-koos′-tĭk	-ic = pertaining to acoust/o = sound	pertaining to sound
audiogram ăw′-dē-ō-grăm″	-gram = record audi/o = hearing	record of a patient's hearing ability
auditory ăw′-dĭ-tō″-rē	-ory = pertaining to audit/o = hearing	pertaining to hearing
aural aw′-răl	-al = pertaining to aur/o = ear	pertaining to the ear
auriculotemporal aw-rĭk″-ū-lō-tĕm′-pŏ-răl	-al = pertaining to auricul/o = ear tempor/o = temporal region; temporal bone	pertaining to the ear and temporal region
barotitis media băr″-ō-tī′-tĭs mē′-dē-ă	-itis = inflammation bar/o = pressure ot/o = ear media = middle	inflammation of the middle ear caused by changes in atmospheric pressure as can occur in a descending airplane or in deep-sea diving
cochlear kŏk′-lē-ăr	-ar = pertaining to cochle/o = cochlea	pertaining to the cochlea
labyrinthitis lăb″-ĭ-rĭn-thī′-tĭs	-itis = inflammation labyrinth/o = inner ear	inflammation of the inner ear
mastoiditis măs-toyd-ī-′-tĭs	-itis = inflammation mastoid/o = mastoid process	inflammation of the mastoid process
myringotomy mĭr-ĭn-gŏt′-ō-mē	-tomy = incision myring/o = tympanic membrane; eardrum	incision into the tympanic membrane to remove fluid from the middle ear; also known as tympanocentesis
otalgia ō-tăl′-jē-ă	-algia = pain ot/o = ear	earache
otitis media ō-tī′-tĭs mē′-dē-ă	-itis = inflammation ot/o = ear media = middle	inflammation of the middle ear
otomycosis ō″-tō-mī-kō′-sĭs	-osis = abnormal condition ot/o = ear myc/o = fungus	fungal infection of the ear
otorrhea ŏ″-tō-rē′-ă	-rrhea = flow; discharge ot/o = ear	discharge from the ear
presbycusis prĕz-bĭ-kū′-sĭs	-cusis = hearing presby- = old age	diminished hearing due to old age
salpingoscope săl-pĭng′-gō-skōp	-scope = instrument used to view salping/o = eustachian tube	instrument used to view the eustachian tube
stapedectomy stā″-pē-dĕk′-tō-mē	-ectomy = excision; removal staped/o = stapes	excision of the stapes

TERM WITH PRONUNCIATION	ANALYSIS	DEFINITION
tympanoplasty tĭm″-păn-ō-plăs′-tē	-plasty = surgical reconstruction tympan/o = eardrum; tympanic membrane	surgical reconstruction of the eardrum
vestibulocochlear vĕs-tĭb″-ū-lō-kŏk′-lē-ăr	-ar = pertaining to vestibul/o = cavity or space near the entrance to a canal cochle/o = cochlea	pertaining to the vestibule and cochlea

▶ 10.8 ABNORMAL CONDITIONS OF THE EAR

CONDITION	DESCRIPTION
cholesteatoma (kō″-lĕ-stē-ă-tō′-mă)	a chronic condition, associated with severe otitis media, that has caused the rupture of the tympanic membrane **Note:** Through this perforation, epithelial cells move from the outer ear into the middle ear and become trapped. These cells grow and form a cystic mass filled with debris, including cholesterol. Treatment involves the surgical removal of the growth before it destroys the adjacent tissues.
deafness	diminished or total loss of hearing
conductive	**conductive deafness** is caused by obstruction of the path traveled by sound waves from the external ear to the inner ear **Note:** Examples of obstruction are a buildup of cerumen or a foreign body lodged in the external auditory meatus.
sensorineural	**sensorineural deafness** results from damage to the auditory nerve by loud noises **Note:** Hearing aids are used to amplify the sound.
Meniere's disease (mān″-ē-ārz′)	a condition of the inner ear that includes the following symptoms: **vertigo** (dizziness), hearing loss, **tinnitus** (ringing in the ears), and a sensation of pressure in the ear **Note:** This condition is difficult to treat, as the cause is unknown.
otitis media	inflammation of the middle ear **Note:** This condition is common in young children because a child's eustachian tube is more horizontal than vertical. Because of this position, the eustachian tube may not drain the middle ear properly, and it may fill with fluid. Infection can result if bacteria invades the middle ear from the nose and throat. Types of otitis media include: **serous otitis media** and **purulent otitis media.** The terms serous and purulent describe the consistency of the inflammatory exudate. Serous fluid is watery; purulent fluid is pus-filled. Signs and symptoms may include otorrhea, otalgia, hearing loss, nausea, and vomiting. If antibiotic treatment fails to clear the middle ear of infection, a **myringotomy** may be performed. Myringotomy is the insertion of draining tubes (T-tubes) into the tympanic membrane; these tubes fall out months after the operation.

CONDITION	DESCRIPTION
otosclerosis	a condition affecting the bony middle ear, particularly the stapes **Note:** New immature bone forms onto the footplate of the stapes, adhering the stapes to the oval window. This adherence, called **ankylosis,** prevents sound from reaching the inner ear. Treatment involves stapedectomy and replacement with a prosthetic stapes.
perforation of typanic membrane	tear of the eardrum caused by physical injury

10.9 PHYSICAL EXAMINATION, DIAGNOSIS, AND TREATMENT FOR CONDITIONS OF THE EAR

Physical Examination

A complete history and physical examination of the ears and adjacent structures are necessary for patients presenting with common symptoms such as tinnitus, vertigo, otorrhea, and otalgia. Initial examination should be on the ears, nose, throat, and paranasal sinuses, with further evaluation of the tongue, teeth, tonsils, larynx, and temporomandibular joint.

Diagnostic Procedures for Abnormal Ear Conditions

PROCEDURES	DEFINITION
audiometry	examination of hearing acuity by measuring the patient's ability to hear sound at different frequencies and different intensities **Note:** The extent and type of hearing loss are plotted on a graph called an audiogram.
electrocochleography (ĕ-lĕk″-trō-kŏk-lē-ŏg′-ră-fē)	process of recording the electrical activity of the cochlea
otoscopy	the process of viewing the outer, middle, and inner ear by using an otoscope or aural speculum
tuning fork tests	examination of hearing acuity through use of a tuning fork
Weber's test	The **Weber's test** determines whether or not sound can be heard equally in both ears. The base of the tuning fork is placed on top and in the middle of the head. Normally, a patient can hear the sound equally in both ears.
Rinne test	The **Rinne test** compares air conduction (AC) with bone conduction (BC). The vibrating tuning fork is placed over the mastoid process until the patient can no longer hear the sound. Then it is placed over the external ear. In the normal ear, the patient can hear the sound vibrating through air longer than through bone (AC>BC).

Surgical Treatment of Abnormal Ear Conditions

TREATMENT	DEFINITION
otoplasty	surgical reconstruction of the ear following trauma or for cosmetic reasons
stapedectomy	removal of the stapes and replacement with a prosthetic stapes that will restore hearing **Note:** Stapedectomies can also be performed using lasers.
hearing aids	devices that amplify sound

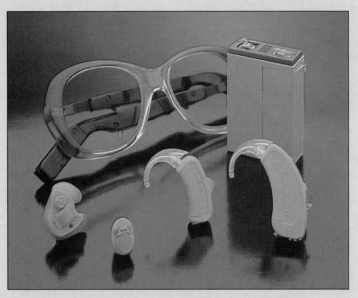

Note: There are bone conduction and air conduction hearing aids, which help persons with both sensorineural and conductive deafness.

10.10 ABBREVIATIONS FOR THE EAR

ABR	auditory brainstem response	**BC**	bone conduction
AC	air conduction	**dB**	decibel
AD (auris dextra)	right ear	**EENT**	eyes, ears, nose, throat
AS (auris sinistra)	left ear	**ENT**	ear, nose, and throat
AU (auris unitas)	both ears	**TM**	tympanic membrane

Practice Quiz

Briefly answer the following questions.
Answers to exercises in this chapter appear in Appendix A.

1. What is the outer layer of the eye called? _____

2. What are the three parts of the vascular tunic? _____
   _____

3. Name the muscles that shape the lens of the eye. _____
   _____
   _____

4. What regulates the amount of light that enters the eye? _____
   _____

5. What three bones are known as the auditory ossicles? _____
   _____

6. The ciliary processes produce a watery fluid called _____ .

7. Into what body cavity does the eyeball fit? _____
   _____

8. What is the abbreviation for auditory brainstem response? _____

9. What is another name for the auricle? _____

10. The stapes transmits sound to the inner ear through what? _____
    _____

11. Name the two fluids contained in the inner ear.
    _____

▶**EXERCISE 10–2** **Multiple Choice**

Multiple Choice

Circle the letter next to the correct answer.

1. core/o means
   a. cornea
   b. lens
   c. pupil
   d. sclera

2. blephar/o means
   a. eyelid
   b. eye
   c. lens
   d. pupil

3. cycl/o means
   a. ciliary body
   b. iris
   c. tears
   d. retina

4. -chalasis means
   a. constriction
   b. dilation
   c. involuntary contraction
   d. relaxation

5. -tropia means
   a. bend
   b. flex
   c. stretch
   d. turn

6. mydr/o means
   a. contraction
   b. narrowing
   c. turning
   d. wide

7. -schisis means
   a. fixation
   b. fusion
   c. paralysis
   d. splitting

8. aur/o means
   a. ear
   b. eye
   c. hearing
   d. vision

9. salping/o means
   a. acoustic meatus
   b. conjunctival membrane
   c. eustachian tube
   d. tympanic membrane

10. myring/o means
    a. acoustic meatus
    b. conjunctival membrane
    c. eustachian tube
    d. tympanic membrane

▶EXERCISE 10–3

Definitions

Give the prefix, suffix, or root for the following.

Definitions

1. lens _____

2. water _____

3. drooping _____

4. lacrimal sac _____

5. visual condition _____

6. contraction, less _____

7. eye _____

8. glasslike _____

9. pressure _____

10. stapes _____

Write the terms that correspond with the following abbreviations.

11. ABR _____

12. AC _____

13. AD _____

14. AS _____

15. BC _____

16. dB _____

17. ENG _____

18. ENT _____

19. DCR _____

20. ICCE _____

21. PERLA _____

22. EOM _____

23. IDU _____

24. EENT _____

II–10

Using the pronunciations
appearing throughout the
text and using the list of
word elements at the
beginning of the chapter,
pronounce each term and
write its definition.

25. amblyopia _____

26. aqueous humor _____

27. astigmatism _____

_____

28. audiometry _____

29. auditory ossicles _____

30. auricle _____

31. binocular vision _____

32. bulbar conjunctiva _____

33. cataracts _____

34. chalazion _____

35. cholesteatoma _____

_____

_____

36. choroid _____

37. ciliary body _____

38. ciliary muscles _____

39. cochlea _____

40. conjunctivitis _____

41. conjunctival membrane _____

42. convergence _____

_____

_____

43. cornea _____

44. diplopia _____

45. electrocochleography _____

_____

_____

46. electroretinography _____

_____

_____

47. endolymph _____

_____

48. eustachian tube   _____

49. evisceration   _____

50. exophthalmia   _____

51. external acoustic meatus   _____

52. extrinsic ocular muscles   _____

_____

53. fibrous tunic   _____

_____

54. fovea centralis   _____

_____

55. glaucoma   _____

56. gonioscopy   _____

57. hordeolum   _____

58. hyperopia   _____

59. hyphema   _____

60. incus   _____

61. iris   _____

62. lacrimal glands   _____

63. macula lutea   _____

64. malleus   _____

65. Ménière's disease   _____

_____

_____

66. myopia   _____

67. myringotomy   _____

68. nystagmus   _____

69. ophthalmia neonatorum   _____

_____

70. ophthalmopathy   _____

71. optic disc   _____

72. organ of Corti   _____

_____

73. otitis media   _____

74. otoscope _____

75. otoplasty _____

76. oval window _____

77. palpebrae _____

78. papilledema _____

79. perilymph _____

80. photophobia _____

81. pupil _____

82. retina _____

83. retinitis _____

84. retinopathy _____

85. rhodopsin _____

86. Rinne test _____

87. rods and cones _____

88. sclera _____

89. scotoma _____

90. stapedectomy _____

91. stapedius _____

92. stapes _____

93. ptosis _____

94. strabismus _____

95. symblepharon _____

96. synechiae _____

97. tensor tympani _____

98. tonometry _____

99. trachoma _____

100. transduction _____

101. uveitis _____

102. vascular tunic (uvea) _____

103. vitreous humor _____

104. Weber's test _____

Word Building

1. surgical reconstruction of the tympanic membrane   _____

2. fungal infection of the ear   _____

3. diminished hearing due to old age   _____

4. inflammation of the middle ear   _____

5. earache   _____

6. discharge from the ear   _____

7. inflammation of the middle ear caused by changes in atmospheric pressure   _____

8. a physician who specializes in the diagnosis and medical and surgical treatment of eye disorders   _____

9. expert who fills prescriptions for eyeglasses and contact lens   _____

10. a practitioner who does not have a medical degree but is a specialist in the testing of visual function and in the diagnosis and nonsurgical treatment of eye conditions   _____

Matching Terms with Meanings

Column A		Column B
1. amblyopia	_____	A. meibomian cyst
2. photophobia	_____	B. dimness of vision not caused by organic defect or refractive error
3. uveitis	_____	
4. chalazion	_____	C. an area of depressed vision within the visual field
5. scotoma	_____	D. intolerance to light
6. ICCE	_____	E. change of form of energy
7. otoplasty	_____	F. the outer layer of the eye
8. fibrous tunic	_____	G. inflammation of the uvea
9. retina	_____	H. surgical reconstruction of the ear
10. transduction	_____	I. intracapsular cataract extraction
		J. inner layer of the eyeball

Match the term in Column A
with its location in Column B.
Some letters may be used
more than once.

Column A		Column B
11. cornea	_____	A. inner eye
12. ciliary processes	_____	B. outer eye
13. auricle	_____	C. external ear
14. incus	_____	D. middle ear
15. saccule	_____	E. inner ear
16. sclera	_____	
17. conjunctival membrane	_____	
18. superior rectus	_____	
19. perilymph	_____	
20. choroid	_____	

▶EXERCISE 10–6

Spelling

Place a check mark beside
all misspelled words in the
list that follows. Correctly
spell those that you checked
off.

Spelling Practice

1. eustacian ☐ _____

2. oteitis ☐ _____

3. amblyopia ☐ _____

4. audeometry ☐ _____

5. endosteum ☐ _____

6. electroretinography ☐ _____

7. opthamalogist ☐ _____

8. option ☐ _____

9. optomotrist ☐ _____

10. coroid ☐ _____

11. aurical ☐ _____

12. stapes ☐ _____

13. audatory ☐ _____

14. accoustic ☐ _____

15. conjunctavits ☐ _____

16. cochlea ☐ _____

17. organ of Corte ☐ _____

18. endolimph ☐ _____

19. miopia ☐ _____

Medical Terms in Context

Describe and define the underlined terms as they are used in context.

UNIVERSITY HOSPITAL ✚   SUMMARY RECORD

ADMISSION DIAGNOSIS: <u>BILATERAL SEROUS OTITIS MEDIA</u>
HISTORY:

This three-year-old child had problems with recurrent ear infections. He was on <u>prophylactic antibiotics.</u>

PHYSICAL EXAMINATION:

He was noted to have bilateral serous otitis media more severe on the left where he had a previous <u>perforation.</u> The remainder of his physical exam was unremarkable.

OPERATION PERFORMED:

On the day of admission, the patient underwent <u>bilateral myringotomies</u> and <u>insertion of T-tubes.</u>

Postoperative course was uneventful, and he was well enough to be discharged later that day.

DISCHARGE DIAGNOSIS: BILATERAL SEROUS OTITIS MEDIA

SIGNATURE OF DOCTOR IN CHARGE _____

---

1. bilateral serous otitis media _____

2. prophylactic antibiotics _____

3. perforation _____

4. bilateral myringotomies _____

5. insertion of T-tubes _____

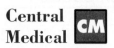

Central Medical CM

OPERATIVE REPORT

PRE-OPERATIVE DIAGNOSIS: BILATERAL SEROUS OTITIS MEDIA

OPERATION PROPOSED: BILATERAL MYRINGOTOMY AND T-TUBE INSERTION

OPERATIVE NOTE:

The patient was brought to the operating room, placed in the <u>supine position,</u> and given a general anesthetic. Using the operative <u>microscope,</u> the right ear canal was cleaned of a small amount of <u>cerumen</u> revealing a <u>retracted tympanic membrane</u> with yellow <u>effusion.</u> An <u>anterosuperior myringotomy</u> was performed and the effusion was suctioned. A drainage T-tube was inserted. The procedure was then performed on the left side with a similar technique and a finding of serous effusion. The patient was then allowed to recover from anesthetic and taken to the recovery room in good condition.

POST-OPERATIVE DIAGNOSIS: RECURRENT OTITIS MEDIA

OPERATION PERFORMED: BILATERAL MYRINGOTOMY AND T-TUBE INSERTION

Authorized Health Care Practitioner _____

6. supine position   _____

7. microscope   _____

8. cerumen   _____

9. retracted tympanic
   membrane   _____

10. effusion   _____

11. anterosuperior
    myringotomy   _____

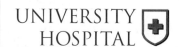

UNIVERSITY HOSPITAL

SUMMARY RECORD

ADMISSION DIAGNOSIS: LEFT <u>CATARACT</u> FOR <u>EXTRACTION</u>

HISTORY:

Mrs. B. had noted progressive deteriorating vision in the left eye over a number of years. Remainder of medical history is unremarkable.

PHYSICAL EXAMINATION:

Best corrected <u>visual acuity</u> was <u>20/70</u> in the left eye.

COURSE IN HOSPITAL:

On June 21, Mrs B. underwent an uneventful left <u>phacoemulsification</u> cataract extraction with insertion of <u>posterior chamber intraocular lens.</u> On the first postoperative day, she was discharged home.

DISCHARGE DIAGNOSIS: LEFT CATARACT

OPERATION PERFORMED: LEFT PHACOEMULSIFICATION CATARACT

EXTRACTION WITH INSERTION OF POSTERIOR CHAMBER INTRAOCULAR LENS.

SIGNATURE OF DOCTOR IN CHARGE _____

12. cataract   _____

13. extraction   _____

14. visual acuity   _____

15. 20/70   _____

16. phacoemulsification   _____

17. posterior chamber
    intraocular lens   _____

II—10

Crossword Puzzle

The Eyes and Ears

Across

2 Expert who fills prescriptions for eyeglasses
4 Inequality in pupil size
10 Drooping of the eyelid
12 Turning outward of the eye
13 Dilation of the pupil

Down

1 Turning inward of the eye
3 An adjective describing paralysis of the ciliary body
4 Absence of lens
5 Inflammation of the choroid and retina
6 Waterlike
7 Tear like
8 Instrument for measuring the pupil's diameter
9 Pertaining to the vitreous humor
10 Involuntary contraction of the eyelid muscle
11 Pertaining to the eyelid

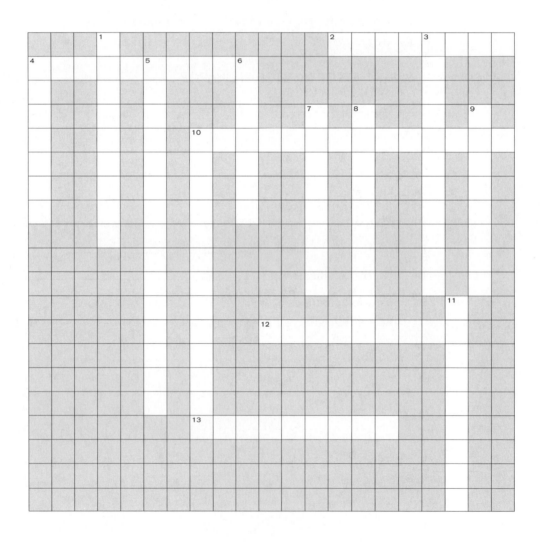

CHAPTER

11

THE DIGESTIVE SYSTEM

CHAPTER ORGANIZATION

This chapter has been designed to help the student learn terms and abbreviations related to the digestive system.

CHAPTER OBJECTIVES

Upon successful completion of this chapter, the student will be able to do the following:

1. Name the six major organs of the digestive tract and describe their functions.
2. Name the accessory organs of the digestive system and describe their functions.
3. Describe the peritoneum.
4. Define digestion and describe the process.
5. Define absorption and describe the process.
6. Describe the function of the digestive system.
7. List the roles of the digestive tract wall.
8. Name the tunics of the wall of the digestive tract.
9. Name the major exocrine and endocrine secretions of the digestive tract.
10. Name the three regions of the small intestine.
11. Name the four sections of the large intestine.
12. Pronounce, analyze, define, and spell terms relating to the digestive system.
13. List and define the terms describing common digestive disorders, the physical examination, signs and symptoms, and diagnostic and therapeutic procedures.
14. Define abbreviations common to the digestive system.

WORD ELEMENT	MEANING	WORD ELEMENT	MEANING
aliment/o	nutrition	gingiv/o	gums
an/o	anus	gloss/o; lingu/o	tongue
append/o; appendic/o	appendix	gluco/o; glyc/o	sugar
		glycogen/o	glycogen
bil/i	bile	hepat/o	liver
bilirubin/o	bilirubin	ile/o	ileum
bucc/o	cheek	jejun/o	jejunum
cec/o	cecum	labi/o	lips
celi/o	abdomen	lapar/o	flank; abdomen
cheil/o	lips	or/o; stomat/o	mouth
chlorhydr/o	hydrochloric acid	pancreat/o	pancreas
cholang/o	bile duct	peritone/o	peritoneum
cholecyst/o	gallbladder	pharyng/o	pharynx
col/o	colon	ptyal/o	saliva
colon/o	colon	proct/o	rectum and anus
dent/o odont/o	tooth	pylor/o	pylorus
duoden/o	duodenum	rect/o	rectum
enter/o	small intestine	sialaden/o	salivary glands
esophag/o	esophagus	sigmoid/o	sigmoid colon
gastr/o	stomach		

▷ 11.1 GENERAL ANATOMY AND PHYSIOLOGY OF THE DIGESTIVE SYSTEM

The digestive system consists of the digestive tract, which is an approximately 16-foot-long tube (5m) that extends from the mouth to the anus, and four accessory organs connected to the tract by ducts: the salivary glands, the pancreas, the liver, and the gallbladder. Along the length of the digestive tract, also called the **gastrointestinal tract,** or **alimentary** (al″-ĭ-mĕn′-tăr-ē) canal, are six specialized regions that have specific names: the oral cavity (mouth); the throat or **pharynx** (făr′-ĭnks); the **esophagus** (ē-sŏf′-ă-gŭs); the stomach; the small intestine; and the large intestine or colon (see Figure 11–1).

FIGURE 11-1

The Digestive System

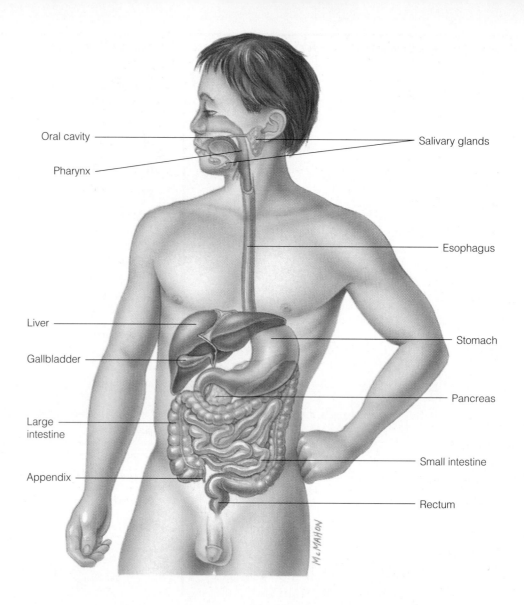

The function of the digestive system is to convert food into the nutrients that are required for the growth, repair, and energy of the body. The process of breaking down large, complex food molecules into simpler molecules is called **digestion**. The process of moving these simpler molecules across the wall of the digestive tract into blood and lymph for transport throughout the body is called **absorption**.

The four accessory organs of the digestive system secrete substances into the digestive tract to assist the processes of digestion and absorption.

Wall of Digestive Tract

During digestion, the mixture of food molecules and the enzymes which break them down is confined to the hollow center of the digestive tract, called the **lumen**. Undigested residue remains in the lumen and is moved out of the body. The wall of the digestive tract functions to fulfill these roles of mixing, absorbing, and moving nutrients through the body.

The wall of the tract is formed of four layers of tissue surrounding the lumen, as illustrated in Figure 11–2.

1) The innermost layer adjacent to the lumen is the **mucosa** (mū-kō-să), which digests, absorbs, protects, and secretes.

2) The **submucosa**, the second layer, contains lymph and blood vessels, as well as a network of neurons called the **Meissner's plexus.**

3) The third layer, the **muscularis externa**, is composed of muscle tissue that contracts to move food through the tract by the process of **peristaltic** (pĕr′-ĭ-stăl′-tĭk) **waves.** These waves are generated by neurons in the **Auerbach's** (ŏw′-ĕr-băks) **plexus** within the muscularis externa.

4) The fourth, outermost layer is called the **adventitia** (ăd″-vĕn-tĭsh′-ē-ă) in the esophagus. Below the esophagus, in the stomach and the two intestines, the outer layer is called the **serosa** (sē-rō′-să).

FIGURE 11–2 **Walls of the Digestive Tract**

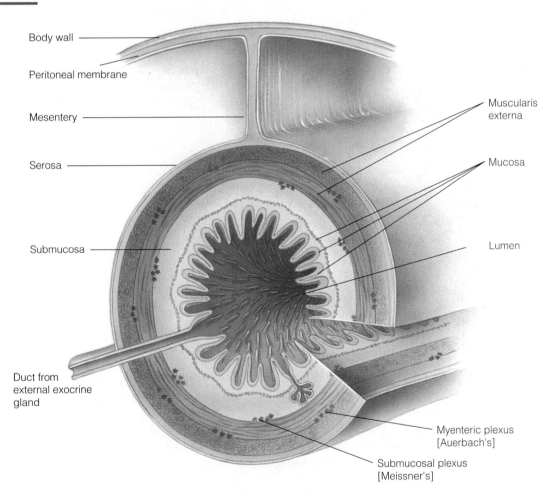

Oral Cavity

The opening to the digestive tract, the mouth, is called the **oral** or **buccal** (bŭk′-kal) **cavity**. The lips are muscular folds connected to the gums by mucous membranes, a part of which is called the **labial frenulum** (lā′-bē-ăl frĕn′-ū-lŭm). The **palate** (the roof of the mouth) separates the nasal cavity from the oral cavity. By placing your tongue on the anterior portion of the palate, you will feel the hard palate, made of bone. Dragging your tongue over the posterior palate, you will feel the soft palate, made up of muscle and connective tissue. At the back of the palate is the **uvula** (ū′-vū-lă), which hangs into the throat and closes off the nasal passage during swallowing. See Figure 11–3.

FIGURE 11–3

Oral Cavity

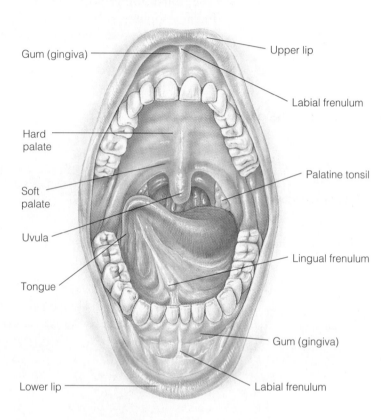

Gum (gingiva) · Upper lip · Labial frenulum · Hard palate · Soft palate · Uvula · Tongue · Palatine tonsil · Lingual frenulum · Gum (gingiva) · Lower lip · Labial frenulum

Tongue The tongue is a muscle used in chewing and swallowing food. It is connected to the bottom of the mouth by mucous membranes, the central portion of which is the **lingual frenulum** (lǐng′-gwăl frĕn′-ū-lŭm). The rough surface of the tongue is caused by projections called **papillae** (pă-pǐl-ī). The **filiform papillae** at the front of the tongue add roughness to aid licking. The **fungiform** (fŭn′-jǐ-form) and **circumvallate** (sĕr″-kŭm-văl′-lāt) **papillae** at the back of the tongue contain taste buds; there are four primary tastes: sweet, sour, salt, and bitter (see Figure 11–4).

FIGURE 11–4

The Papillae of the Tongue

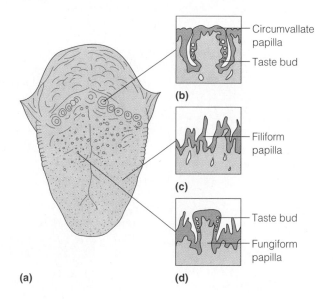

(b) Circumvallate papilla — Taste bud

(c) Filiform papilla

(d) Taste bud — Fungiform papilla

(a)

Teeth   The digestive process begins when food is ground up by the teeth and softened by saliva. The process of chewing is called **mastication**. Twenty temporary, or **deciduous** (dē-sĭd-ū-ŭs), teeth appear in infants between the age of six months and two years. Thirty-two permanent teeth replace the deciduous ones by age 13. The tooth is anchored in its socket by the **periodontal** (pĕr″-ē-ō-dŏn′-tăl) **ligament**.

Incisors, canines, and molars are the terms given to the various teeth according to their respective shapes and functions (see Figure 11–5).

The **molars** have three projections or cusps and are also known as **tricuspids** (trī-kŭs-pĭds). The **premolars**, with two cusps, are called **bicuspids**. Both types of molars grind food. The **canine** teeth, with one cusp, are called **cuspids** (kŭs′-pĭds) and tear food. The four front teeth, the **incisors** (ĭn-sī′-zors), are used for cutting.

The tooth fits into a bony socket called the **alveolus** (ăl-vē′-ō-lŭs), with only a small part of the tooth visible above the gum or **gingiva** (jĭn-jĭ′-vă). The visible part is called the **crown** and is covered with enamel. Beneath the gum line lies the neck of the tooth and the root, surrounded by **cementum** (sē-mĕn′-tŭm). The entire tooth is surrounded by a layer of **dentin**, and beneath the dentin is the pulp cavity containing **pulp** made up of blood vessels and nerves that extend into the root through the **root canal**. These blood vessels and nerves enter the tooth at the tip of the root through an opening called the **apical foramen** (ăp′-ĭ-kăl fōr-ā′-mĕn).

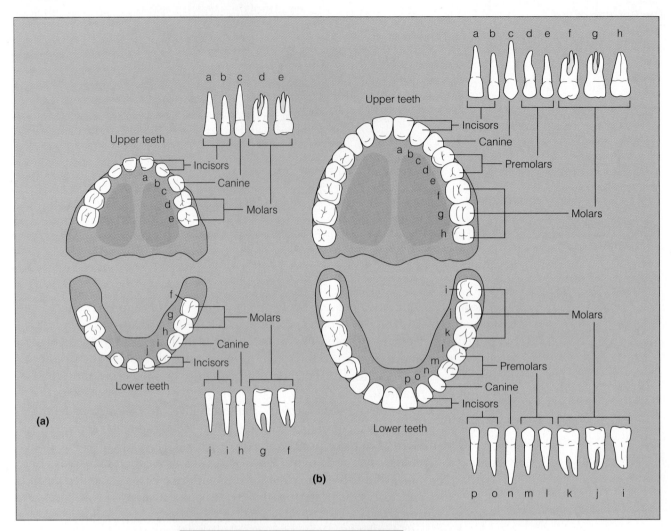

(a)

(b)

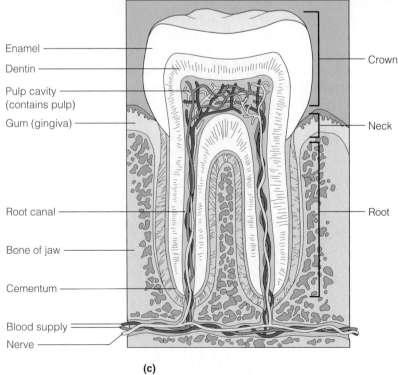

Enamel

Dentin

Pulp cavity
(contains pulp)

Gum (gingiva)

Root canal

Bone of jaw

Cementum

Blood supply

Nerve

Crown

Neck

Root

(c)

Pharynx

Both food and air pass through the **pharynx**. The section of the pharynx behind the nasal cavity is the **nasopharynx** (nā″-zō-făr′-ĭnks), which is a passageway for air. Food passes through the other two sections, the **oropharynx** and the **laryngopharynx** (lăr-ĭn″-gō-făr-ĭnks).

Swallowing, or **deglutition** (dē″-gloo-tĭsh′-ŭn), is initiated when the tongue pushes a ball of softened food, called a **bolus** (bō′-lŭs), into the pharnyx, as shown in Figure 11–6. The bolus moves from the pharynx through the esophagus to the stomach by involuntary peristalsis. Involuntary reflexes also coordinate the movement of the uvula and the upper esophageal sphincter, which opens to admit the bolus to the esophagus.

FIGURE 11–6 **Swallowing** (a) Bolus is pushed through the esophagus by peristaltic waves; lower esophageal sphincter is closed. (b) Lower esophageal sphincter is open, and the bolus enters the stomach.

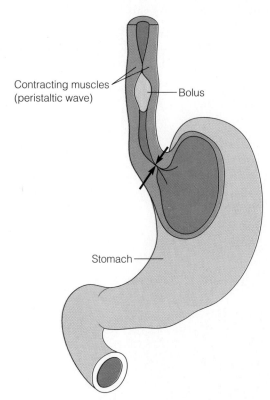

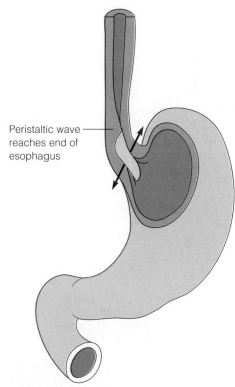

(a) Bolus is swept along esophagus by peristaltic contractions; lower esophageal sphincter (arrows) is closed

(b) Lower esophageal sphincter (arrows) opens; bolus moves into stomach

Esophagus

The esophagus is a 10-inch (25 cm) muscular tube between the pharynx and the stomach, with a **sphincter** (sfĭngk′-tĕr) at each end. A sphincter is a circular muscle that allows passage of material when relaxed and restricts the passage of material when contracted. The upper esophageal sphincter, the **pharnygo-esophageal** (fă-rĭng″-gō-ē-sŏf′-ă-jē″-ăl) **sphincter**, opens at the approach of food and closes at other times to prevent air from entering the stomach. The lower esophageal sphincter, the **cardiac sphincter**, opens to allow passage of food into the stomach and closes to prevent stomach contents from re-entering the esophagus.

The esophagus enters the abdominal cavity through the esophageal **hiatus** (hī-ā′-tŭs), an opening in the diaphragm, then attaches to the stomach.

Stomach

The stomach is a J-shaped sac divided into four regions: the **cardia** (kăr′-dē-ă), the **fundus** (fŭn′-dŭs), the **body**, and the **antrum**. As shown in Figure 11–7, this latter section ends at the **pyloric sphincter**, which permits passage of food from the stomach to the small intestine. The medial curve of the stomach is called the **lesser curvature**, and the lateral curve is called the **greater curvature**.

FIGURE 11–7 Stomach

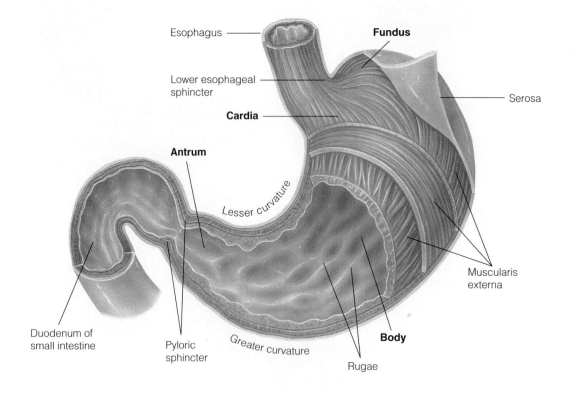

The inner surface of the stomach is formed of folds called rugae (roo´-gī). These folds permit the stomach wall to stretch as food enters. The taste and smell of food initiate gastric secretions in the stomach, which are regulated by both hormonal and neural control. Four exocrine secretions are produced by the gastric glands: mucus; hydrochloric acid; a molecule called **intrinsic factor**, and **pepsinogen** (pĕp-sĭn´-ō-jĕn), an inactive digestive enzyme. The combination of these exocrine secretions is called **gastric juice**. Pepsinogen and intrinsic factor are imperative for the absorption of vitamin B_{12}, which in turn is required for production of red blood cells. Endocrine secretions of the hormone **gastrin** are also produced in the stomach. Muscle action in the stomach causes churning, which mixes food with the secretions. This mixture of food and secretions is called **chyme** (kīm).

Small Intestine

The small intestine, so named because of its 1-inch (2.54 cm) diameter, is the longest part of the digestive tract and is coiled within the abdominopelvic cavity (see Figure 11–1). It is divided into three regions: the **duodenum** (dū″-ō-dē´-nŭm), the **jejunum** (jē-jū´-nŭm), and the **ileum** (ĭl-ē-ŭm) (see Figure 11–8). The **ileocecal** (ĭ´-lē-ō-sē´-kăl) valve between the ileum and large intestine prevents contents of the large intestine from entering the small intestine. Bile and pancreatic secretions from the liver, gallbladder, and pancreas enter the small intestine at the duodenum.

FIGURE 11–8

The Small Intestine

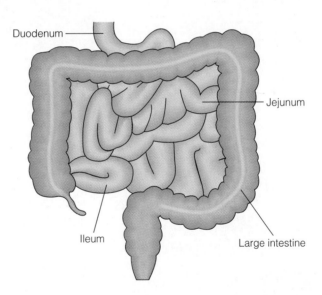

Absorption of nutrients takes place in the small intestine. Absorption is accomplished through physical contact of digested nutrients with the surface area of the intestine.

This surface area is increased hundreds of times by the presence of folds called **plicae circulares** (plī´-kā sĭr´-cū-lăr-ēz). Projecting from these folds are

villi, which are fingerlike projections, and projecting from these villi are **micro-villi,** which are hairlike projections. Digested nutrients are thus absorbed into the blood through the villi and microvilli (see Figure 11–9).

Most of the secretions from the small intestine such as water, ions, and mucus are produced by intestinal glands called **crypts of Lieberkuhn** (lē-běr-kēn). Additional mucus is secreted by **goblet cells** and by **Brunner's** (brŭn′-ĕrz) **glands.**

FIGURE 11–9 **Absorption Features of the Small Intestine** (a) Plicae circulares. (b) Vili. (c) Goblet cells. (d) Microvili.

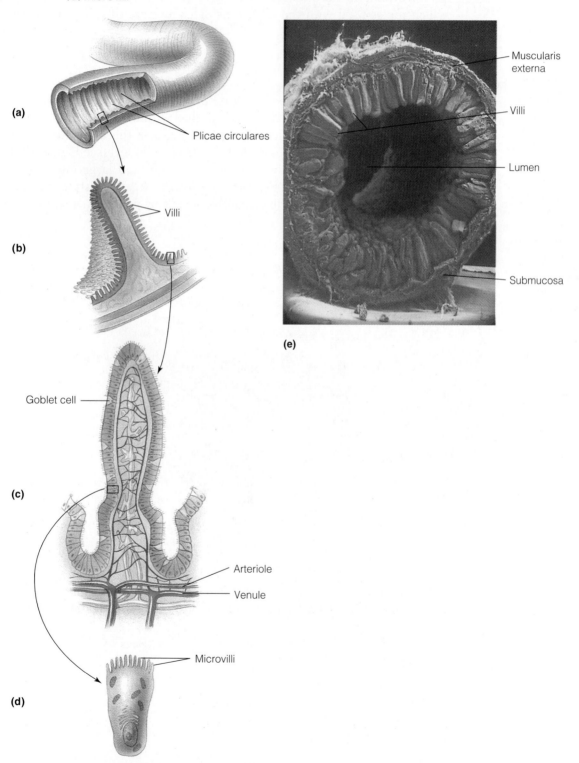

Large Intestine

The large intestine, named for its large diameter of approximately 2.4 inches (6 cm), is made up of three sections: a pouch called the **cecum** (sē′-kŭm), the **colon**, and the **rectum**, which includes the **anal** (ā′-nŭl) **canal** and the **anus** (ā′-nŭs).

The colon is divided into four sections: the **ascending colon**, the **transverse colon**, the **descending colon**, and the **sigmoid colon**. The arrangement of these sections within the abdominopelvic cavity resembles a square arch. The ascending colon proceeds vertically, then turns to the horizontal at the **hepatic flexure** below the liver, where it becomes the transverse colon. The transverse colon turns downward and becomes the descending colon at the **splenic flexure** below the spleen (see Figure 11–10).

FIGURE 11–10 **The Large Intestine**

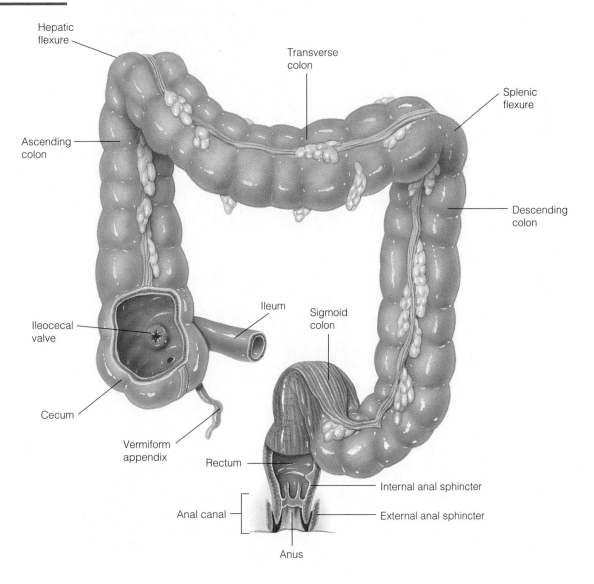

The **vermiform appendix**, which has no known function, projects from the cecum. The area of the abdomen in the right lower quadrant above the appendix is known as **McBurney's point**.

As mentioned in the discussion of the digestive tract wall, one of its roles is to keep digestive tract contents separate from the body. This function is especially important with respect to the large intestine and the appendix. The large intestine contains millions of bacteria that play a beneficial role within the intestinal lumen but which may be toxic outside the intestine. Likewise, an infected appendix contains material that is toxic to the body. Therefore, a large intestine that becomes punctured or an infected appendix that ruptures can cause a life-threatening condition called **peritonitis** (pĕr-ĭ-tō-nī′-tĭs).

The large intestine plays no part in absorption of nutrients except for the absorption of water, vitamin K, and some B vitamins that are produced by bacterial action in the intestine. Therefore, no villi are present in the large intestine. These are, however, numerous goblet cells that produce mucus to aid in lubricating undigested residue during its passage. The **rectum** is the last segment of the large intestine and is approximately 8 inches long. It is lined with mucous folds, each supplied with arteries and veins. The final segment of the rectum is the **anal canal**, which is surrounded by an **internal sphincter** and an **external sphincter**. Evacuation of feces, or **defecation** through the anus, is regulated by the external sphincter.

▶ 11.2 ACCESSORY ORGANS

Salivary Glands

There are three pairs of **salivary** (săl′-ĭ-vĕr-ē) **glands**: the **parotid** (pă-rŏt′-ĭd), **submandibular** (sŭb″-măn-dĭb-ū-lăr), and **sublingual** glands. These glands are located outside of the mouth and drain saliva into the oral cavity via salivary ducts, as illustrated in Figure 11–11.

FIGURE 11–11

Salivary Glands

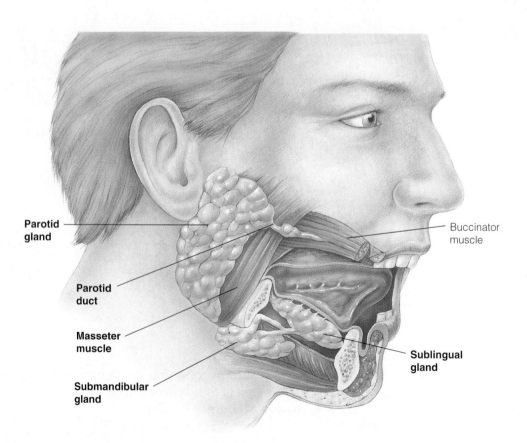

Parotid gland

Parotid duct

Masseter muscle

Submandibular gland

Buccinator muscle

Sublingual gland

Secretions of enzymes and mucus are carried to the mouth from the salivary glands through numerous ducts. The major enzyme in saliva is called **salivary amylase** (ăm′-ĭ-lās), which begins the digestion of carbohydrates. The combination of mucus and enzymes in the saliva softens the bolus in preparation for swallowing.

Pancreas

The pancreas is shaped like a fish and is located behind the stomach (see Figure 11–12). It produces both endocrine and exocrine secretions. The exocrine secretions of enzymes by the acinar cells and sodium bicarbonate by the duct cells are collectively known as **pancreatic juice**. The sodium bicarbonate in pancreatic juice neutralizes the acid in chyme, thereby producing a proper environment for the action of the enzymes.

FIGURE 11–12 Pancreas

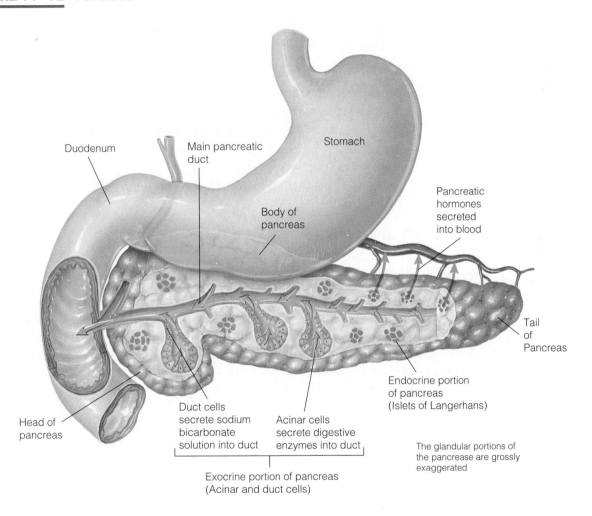

Duodenum

Main pancreatic duct

Stomach

Body of pancreas

Pancreatic hormones secreted into blood

Tail of Pancreas

Endocrine portion of pancreas (Islets of Langerhans)

Head of pancreas

Duct cells secrete sodium bicarbonate solution into duct

Acinar cells secrete digestive enzymes into duct

The glandular portions of the pancrease are grossly exaggerated

Exocrine portion of pancreas (Acinar and duct cells)

Pancreatic juice is carried to the duodenum by the main pancreatic duct, which fuses with the common bile duct from the liver. The resulting fused duct empties into the duodenum at the **ampulla** (ăm-pŭl′-lă) **of Vater** (fā′-tĕr). The **sphincter of Oddi** in the ampulla of Vater regulates the flow of pancreatic juice into the duodenum.

The endocrine cells of the pancreas are clusters called **islets of Langerhans** (lŏng'-ĕr-hănz). Within these islets are **alpha cells**, which secrete the hormone glucagon (gloo'-kă-gŏn), and **beta cells**, which secrete the hormone insulin. Insulin and glucagon work together to regulate the amount of sugar in the bloodstream. When there is an excess of glucose in the blood, it is converted by insulin to **glycogen** (glī'-kō-jĕn) for storage in the liver. This process is known as **glycogenesis** (glī″-kō-jĕn'-ĭ-sĭs). When there is a decrease of glucose in the blood, glycogen is converted back to glucose by glucagon. This process is called **glycogenolysis** (glī″-kō-jĕn-ŏl'-ĭ-sĭs).

In cases where there is a shortage of carbohydrates to provide glucose for body energy, the body synthesizes glucose and glycogen from fats and proteins stimulated by the action of **cortisol**. This process is called **gluconeogenesis** (gloo″-kō-nē-ō-jĕn'-ĕ-sĭs).

Liver and Gallbladder

The liver, which secretes bile for emulsifying fat, is located under the diaphragm in the right upper quadrant of the abdomen. It is divided anteriorly into right and left lobes and inferiorly into **caudate** (kaw'-dāt) and **quadrate** (kwŏd-rāt) lobes. The liver performs the following functions:

1. produces bile, which consists of water, cholesterol, and bile pigments
2. breaks down carbohydrates, fats, and proteins so that they can be absorbed or stored for later use
3. stores sugar (as glycogen); vitamins A, D, E, and K; iron; and copper
4. detoxifies harmful substances by the action of phagocytic cells called **Kupffer's** (koop'-fĕrz) **cells**
5. synthesizes **prothrombin** and **fibrinogen**, which are necessary for blood clotting

The gallbladder, in which the bile is stored, is located in a small depression under the surface of the liver.

The liver and gallbladder, together with their ducts, are called the **biliary** (bĭl'-ē-ār-ē) **system**. The **hepatic duct** carries bile from the liver. The **cystic duct** carries bile to and from the gallbladder. The cystic and hepatic ducts unite to form the **common bile duct**, which drains into the duodenum (Figure 11–13). Liver cells called **hepatocytes** (hĕp-ă'-tō-sītz) produce the bile. Hepatocytes also process absorbed nutrients that have been carried to the liver through the blood. Endocrine glands in the liver produce **somatomedin** (sō″-mă-tō-mĕ'-dĭn), which acts on cartilage to stimulate skeletal growth.

FIGURE 11–13

Liver and Gallbladder

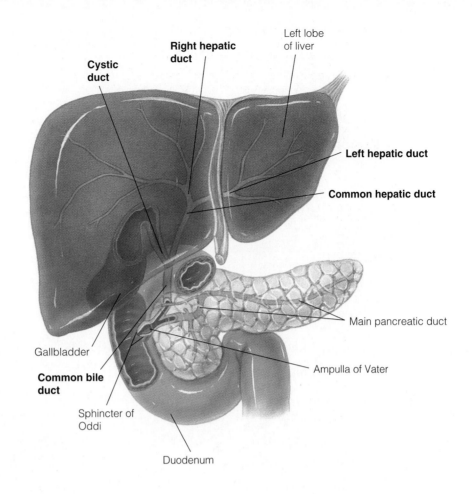

Cystic duct
Right hepatic duct
Left lobe of liver
Left hepatic duct
Common hepatic duct
Main pancreatic duct
Ampulla of Vater
Gallbladder
Common bile duct
Sphincter of Oddi
Duodenum

▷▷ 11.3 PERITONEUM

The abdominal cavity is the space between the diaphragm and pelvis. It is lined with **parietal peritoneum** and contains the stomach and large and small intestines, which are covered with **visceral peritoneum** or **serosa** (see Figure 11–14). The space between the parietal and visceral peritoneum is called the **peritoneal** (pĕr″-ĭ-tō-nē′-ăl) **cavity** and is filled with a small quantity of serous fluid that prevents friction between the parietal and visceral layers. There are some organs, near the posterior abdominal wall, that lie outside the peritoneal cavity, such as the kidneys. This position is called **retroperitoneal** (rĕt″-rō-pĕr-ĭ-tō-nē′-ăl).

FIGURE 11–14 **The Peritoneum** (a) Peritoneum shown in midsagittal view. (b) Anterior view of abdominopelvic cavity. Notice the lifting of the greater omentum to show the mesentery proper and mesocolon. (c) Anterior view of abdominal cavity showing the lesser omentum.

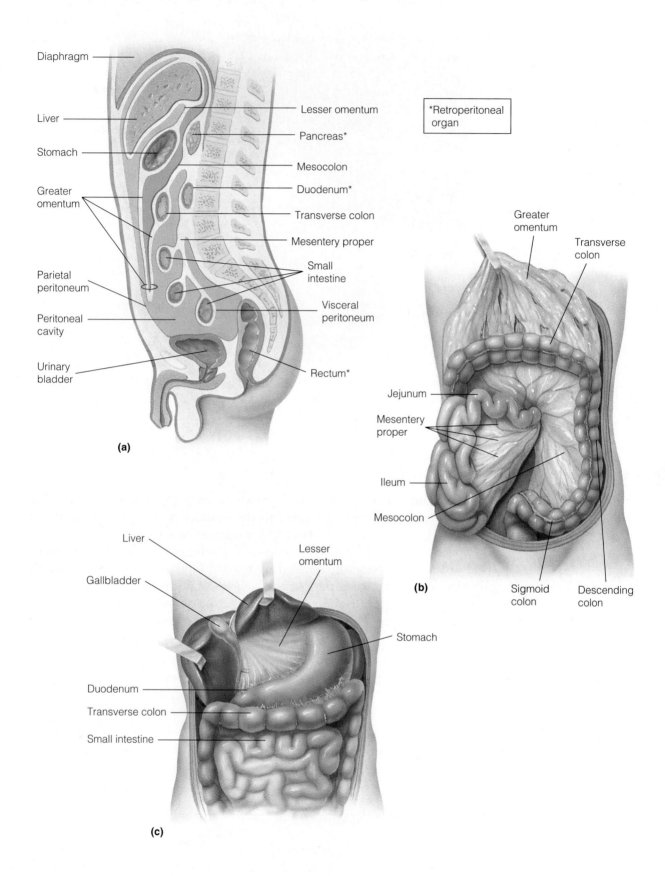

The peritoneum is given various names, depending upon its location. **Mesentery** (měs′-ĕn-tĕr′-ē) attaches the small intestine to the posterior abdominal wall. **Mesocolon** (měs″-ō-kō′-lŏn) attaches the colon to the abdominal wall. **Transverse mesocolon** attaches the transverse colon to the posterior abdominal wall. The **greater omentum** (ō-mĕn′-tŭm), a double fold of peritoneum, extends from the greater curvature of the stomach like an apron, folding upon itself, returning superiorly, and attaching to the transverse colon. The **lesser omentum** passes from the lesser curvature to the stomach to the liver (see Figure 11–15).

FIGURE 11–15

The Abdominal Cavity and Peritoneal Membranes

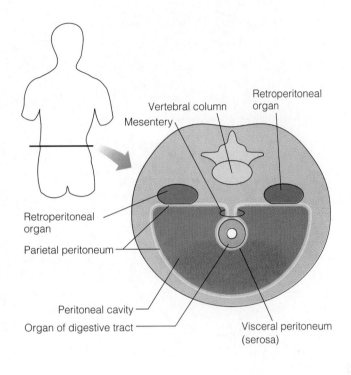

Vertebral column

Retroperitoneal organ

Mesentery

Retroperitoneal organ

Parietal peritoneum

Peritoneal cavity

Organ of digestive tract

Visceral peritoneum (serosa)

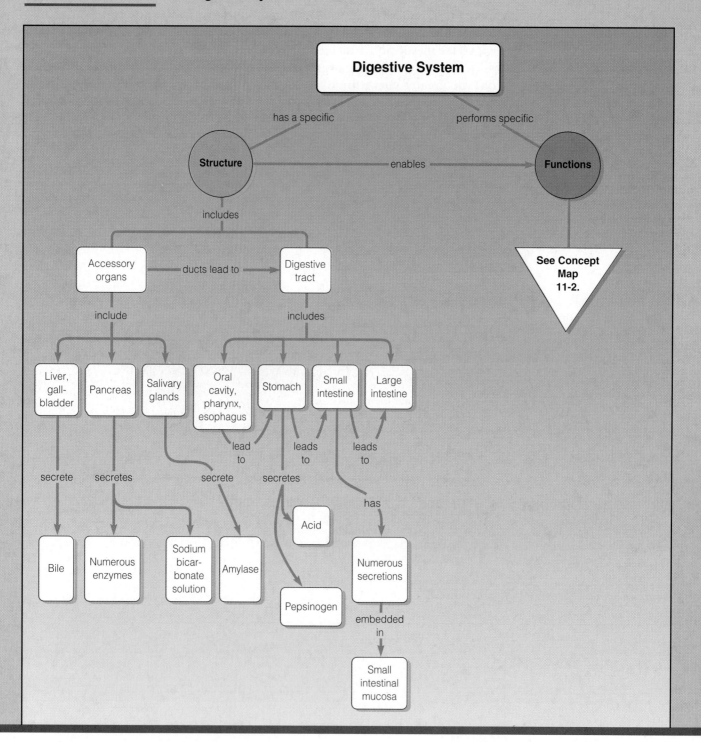

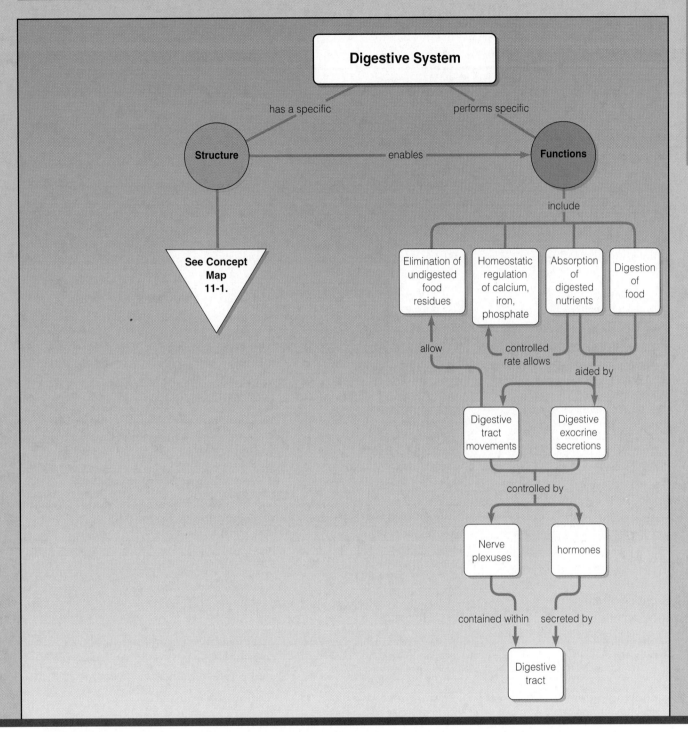

TERM WITH PRONUNCIATION	ANALYSIS	DEFINITION
achalasia ăk″-ă-lā′-zē-ă	-ia—state of; condition a- = no; not chalas/o = relaxation	inability of the muscles of the digestive tract to relax
alimentary ăl″-ĭ-měn′-tăr-ē	-ary = pertaining to aliment/o = food; nutrition	pertaining to food or nutrition
ankyloglossia ăng″-kĭ-lō-glŏs′-sē-ă	-ia = condition; state of ankyl/o = fusion of parts; stiff gloss/o = tongue	restrained tongue movements due to a shortened frenulum; tongue-tied
anodontia ăn″-ō-dŏn′-shē-ă	-ia = state of; condition an- = no; not odont/o = tooth	condition of no teeth (a developmental condition)
anorectal ān-ō-rĕk′-tăl	-al = pertaining to an/o = anus rect/o = rectum	pertaining to the anus and rectum
appendectomy ăp″-ĕn-dĕk′-tō-mē	-ectomy = excision; removal appendo/o = appendix	excision of the appendix
appendicitis ă-pĕn″-dĭ-sī′-tĭs	-itis = inflammation append/o = appendix	inflammation of the appendix
buccal mucosa bŭk′-ăl mū-kō′-să	-al = pertaining to bucc/o = cheek	pertaining to the mucous membrane of the cheek **Note:** Mucosa refers to mucous membrane.
cecopexy sē′-kō-pĕk″-sē	-pexy = surgical fixation cec/o = cecum	surgical fixation of the cecum
celiac sē′-lē-ăk	-ac = pertaining to celi/o = abdomen	pertaining to the abdomen
cheilorrhaphy kī-lōr′-ă-fē	-rrhaphy = suture cheil/o = lips	suturing of lips
cheilosis kī-lō′-sĭs	-osis = abnormal condition cheil/o = lips	abnormal condition of the lips characterized by deep, cracklike sores known as fissures
cholangiogram kō-lăn′-jē-ō-grăm	-gram = record; x-ray cholangi/o = bile vessel	x-ray of a bile vessel
cholecystectomy kō″-lē-sĭs-tĕk′-tō-mē	-ectomy = excision; removal cholecyst/o = gallbladder	excision of the gallbladder
cholecystitis kō″-lē-sĭs-tī′-tĭs	-itis = inflammation cholecyst/o = gallbladder	inflammation of the gallbladder
cholecystolithiasis kō″-lē-sĭs″-tō-lĭ-thī′-ă-sĭs	-iasis = abnormal condition cholecyst/o = gallbladder lith/o = stone	condition of stones in the gallbladder

TERM WITH PRONUNCIATION	ANALYSIS	DEFINITION
choledochectomy kō-lĕd″-ō-kĕk′-tō-mē	-ectomy = excision; removal choledoch/o = common bile duct	excision of the common bile duct
cholelithiasis kō″-lē-lĭ-thī′-ă-sĭs	-iasis = condition chol/e = bile; gall lith/o = stone	gallstones
cholestasis kō-lē-stā′-sĭs	-stasis = stoppage chol/e = bile; gall	stoppage of the flow of bile through the biliary system
colitis kō-lī′-tĭs	-itis = inflammation col/o = colon	inflammation of the colon
colonoscopy kō″-lŏn-ŏs′-kō-pē	-scopy = process of visually examining colon/o = colon	process of visually examining the colon
duodenojejunostomy dū″-ō-dē″-nō-jĕ-joo- nŏs′-tō-mē	-stomy = new opening duoden/o = duodenum jejun/o = jejunum	surgical creation of a new opening between the duodenum and the jejunum; in other words, an **anastomosis** between the duodenum and the jejunum **Note:** The surgical joining of two structures that are normally separate is called **anastomosis**. Duodenojejunostomy is an anastomosis between the duodenum and jejunum. When a new opening is made between two or more **organs**, both word roots of the organs involved are used in the medical term (compare with ileostomy).
endodontist ĕn″-dō-dŏn′-tĭst	-ist = specialist endo- = within odont/o = tooth	dentist who specializes in the diagnosis and treatment of diseases within the tooth including the dental pulp and related structures
enteritis ĕn″-tĕr-ī-tĭs	-itis = inflammation enter/o = small intestine	inflammation of the small intestine
esophageal atresia ē-sŏf″-ă-jē′ -ăl ă′-trē-zhă	-tresia = opening a- = no; not	closure of the esophageal lumen (space within the esophagus)
gastrospasm găs′-trō-spăzm	-spasm = sudden, involuntary, violent contractions gastr/o = stomach	sudden, involuntary contractions of the stomach
gingivobuccal jĭn″-jĭ-vō-bŭk′-ăl	-al = pertaining to gingiv/o = gums bucc/o = cheek	pertaining to the gums and cheek
gluconeogenesis gloo″-kō-nē″-ō-jĕn′-ĕ-sĭs	-genesis = production; formation gluc/o = sugar ne/o = new	formation of sugar from proteins and carbohydrates

TERM WITH PRONUNCIATION	ANALYSIS	DEFINITION
glycogenolysis glī″-kō-jĕn-ŏl′-ĭ-sĭs	-lysis = breakdown; separate; destruction glycogen/o = glycogen	the breakdown of glycogen to form glucose
hepatocyte hĕp′-ă-tō-sīt	-cyte = cell hepat/o = liver	liver cell
hyperbilirubinemia hī″-pĕr-bĭl″-ĭ-roo-bĭn-ē′-mē-ă	-emia = blood condition hyper- = excessive; above; more than the normal number bilirubin/o = bilirubin	excessive amounts of bilirubin in the blood
hypoglycemia hī″-pō-glī-sē′-mē-ă	-emia = blood condition hypo- = deficient; below normal; under glyc/o = sugar	deficient amounts of sugar in the blood
ileostomy ĭl″-ē-ŏs′-tŏ-mē	-stomy = new opening ile/o = ileum	surgical creation of a new opening in the ileum by bringing the ileum through the abdominal wall **Note:** When a new opening is made between an organ and the abdominal wall, only one root word is used in the medical term.
labioglossopharyngeal lā″-bē-ō-glŏs″-ō-făr-ĭn′-jē-ăl	-eal = pertaining to labi/o = lips gloss/o = tongue pharyng/o = pharynx; throat	pertaining to the lips, tongue, and throat
laparoscope lăp′-ă-rō-skōp″	-scope = instrument used to visually examine lapar/o = flank; abdomen	instrument used to visually examine the abdominal and pelvic contents
leukoplakia loo″-kō-plā′-kē-ă	-plakia = patch; plate leuk/o = white	condition of white patches on the mucous membrane
odontalgia ō″-dŏn-tăl′-jē-ă	-algia = pain odont/o = tooth	toothache
orthodontist or″-thō-dŏn′-tĭst	-ist = specialist ortho- = straight odont/o = tooth	a dentist who specializes in the correction of deformed or maloccluded teeth
pancreatogenic păn″-krē-ă-tō-jĕn′-ĭk	-genic = produced by; formed in pancreat/o = pancreas	produced by or formed in the pancreas
parenteral păr-ĕn′-tĕr-ăl	-al = pertaining to para- = beside enter/o = small intestine	refers to methods of placing pharmacological agents into the body via routes other than the digestive tract, for example, intramuscular or intravenous injection
perianal pĕr-ē-ā′-năl	-al = pertaining to peri- = surrounding an/o = anus	pertaining to around the anus

TERM WITH PRONUNCIATION	ANALYSIS	DEFINITION
periodontitis pĕr″-ē-ō-dŏn-tī′-tĭs	-itis = inflammation peri- = surrounding odont/o = tooth	inflammation involving the structures surrounding the tooth, including gums, cementum, periodontal ligament, and bony socket
peritonitis pĕr″-ĭ-tō-nī′-tĭs	-itis = inflammation peritone/o = peritoneum	inflammation of the peritoneum
proctoclysis prŏk-tŏk-lĭ-sĭs	-clysis = irrigation; washing proct/o = rectum	irrigation of the rectum
ptyalism tī′-ă-lĭzm	-ism = state of; condition ptyal/o = saliva	excessive secretion of saliva
pyloromyotomy pī-lōr″-ō-mī-ŏt′-ō-mē	-tomy = incision; to cut; incise pylor/o = pylorus; pyloric sphincter my/o = muscle	incision into the pyloric sphincter
pylorospasm pī-lōr′-ō-spăzm	-spasm = sudden, involuntary, contraction pylor/o = pylorus; pyloric sphincter	sudden, involuntary contraction of the pyloric sphincter
retroperitoneal rēt″-rō-pĕr″-ĭ-tō-nē″-ăl	-eal = pertaining to retro- = behind peritone/o = peritoneum	pertaining to behind the peritoneum
sialadenitis sī″-ăl-ăd″-ĕ-nī′-tĭs	-itis = inflammation sialaden/o = salivary glands	inflammation of the salivary glands
sialolith sī-ăl′-ō-lĭth	-lith = stone sial/o = saliva	stone in the saliva
sigmoidoscopy sĭg″-mŏy-dŏs′-kō-pē	-scopy = process of visually examining sigmoid/o = sigmoid colon	process of visually examining the sigmoid colon
stomatitis stō″-mă-tī′-tĭs	-itis = inflammation stomat/o = mouth	inflammation of the mouth
sublingual sŭb-lĭng′-gwăl	-al = pertaining to sub- = under; below lingu/o = tongue	pertaining to under the tongue

Oral Cavity, Teeth, and Salivary Glands

CONDITION	DESCRIPTION
aphthous (ăf′-thŭs) stomatitis; canker sores; oral aphthae (ăf′-thē)	recurring ulcers of the oral mucosa that are caused by the herpes simplex virus or are idiopathic
cleft palate; cleft lip	incomplete closure of the hard and/or soft palate, which results in fissuring of the lips (cleft lip) or palate (cleft palate)
dental caries	dental cavities
	Note: Dental caries are caused by the action of bacteria on the teeth. The accumulation of bacteria and detritus is called dental plaque. If plaque is not removed with normal brushing of the teeth, tooth decay results and the tooth can be lost.
thrush	fungal infection of the mucous membrane of the oral cavity, caused by the microorganism **Candida albicans**

The Esophagus and Stomach

CONDITION	DESCRIPTION
esophageal varices	dilated, tortuous veins of the esophagus
peptic ulcers	a wearing away and necrosis of the mucous membrane lining the digestive tract (peptic means pertaining to digestion)
	Note: Following necrosis, the dead tissue is sloughed off, leaving an open sore (the ulcer) that extends to the muscularis mucosa.
	Ulcers may involve the distal esophagus, stomach, pyloric antrum, duodenum, and jejunum, although most ulcers are duodenal.
	Heliobacter pylori, a bacterium, is now known to be a cause of many peptic ulcers.

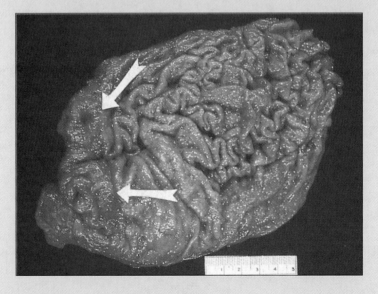

The Small and Large Intestines

CONDITION	DESCRIPTION
anal fissure; fissure in ano	a cracklike sore in the anal canal

CONDITION	DESCRIPTION
anal fistula; fistula in ano	abnormal passage in the anal area
	Note: A fistula is an abnormal canal leading from an abscess to another organ or cavity. This canal acts as a passage for purulent material as it drains from the abscess.
celiac disease; celiac sprue (sē′-lē-ăk)	hereditary condition characterized by malabsorption of food caused by an intolerance to gluten, a protein found in wheat products (celiac means related to the abdomen and sprue means intestinal malabsorption)
	Note: Prognosis is good if gluten is eliminated from the patient's diet.
Crohn's disease	form of inflammatory bowel disease which may involve any part of the digestive tract but usually the distal ileum
	Note: In Crohn's disease all layers of the intestinal wall may be affected. Often called **regional enteritis,** as the diseased portions of the intestine are well demarcated (marked) from normal areas. If the large intestine is involved, it is called **colitis**; if the small and large intestine are involved, it is called **ileocolitis**. The etiology is unknown. While it may be placed into remission, there is no cure.
diverticulum	pockets (**diverticulum**) in the mucous membrane occurring at any point along the digestive tract but usually in the sigmoid colon, duodenum, and jejunum
	Note: Diverticulosis describes a condition characterized by many **diverticula**. These pockets easily trap bacteria and bits of food, which inflame the diverticula, a condition called **diverticulitis**.
	Severity varies from asymptomatic or mild diverticulitis to clinically significant, chronic diverticulitis that does not respond to medical treatment.

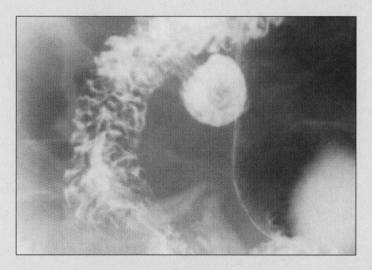

Meckel's diverticulum	**Meckel's diverticulum** is a congenital condition caused by failure of a fetal duct to be obliterated, as it normally is in early fetal life. Remnants of this duct can form an intestinal pocket, which can cause ulceration, bleeding, abdominal pain, and vomiting.
hemorrhoids; piles	dilatation of the veins of the anal canal often referred to as internal or external hemorrhoids depending on the location of the affected veins
Hirschsprung's disease; congenital megacolon	obstruction of colonic contents caused by congenital absence of nerves innervating the large intestine
	Note: can result in constipation and large, dilated colon (megacolon)

CONDITION	DESCRIPTION
intestinal obstruction	intestinal obstruction occurs when the contents of the digestive tract fail to move toward the rectum

Note: Causes include **intussuception, volvulus, paralytic ileus**, adhesions, and hernias.

Intussuception (ĭn-tŭ-sŭ-sĕp′-shŭn) is the telescoping of one segment of bowel into another.

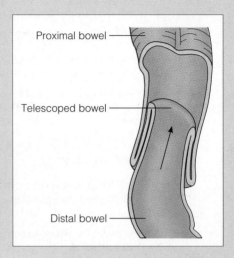

Volvulus (vŏl′-vū-lŭs) is the twisting of one segment of bowel around another.

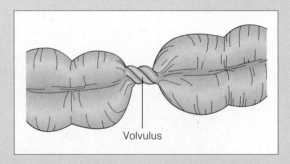

Paralytic ileus, or **ileus,** is the temporary loss of peristaltic waves along the small intestine. This can be caused by inflammation, trauma, or following bowel surgery.

CONDITION	DESCRIPTION
irritable bowel syndrome (IBS); spastic colon	common condition characterized by abdominal pain, diarrhea, and constipation

Note: can be the result of stress, the ingestion of toxins and irritating substances such as laxatives, or more commonly, has no known etiology

CONDITION	DESCRIPTION
polyps	benign growth of tissue originating from the mucous membrane and extending into the lumen of the gastrointestinal tract (see Chapter 6, The Integumentary System)

CONDITION	DESCRIPTION
cirrhosis of the liver	hepatocelluar degeneration caused by the effects of hepatitis or most commonly alcoholism (Laënnec's cirrhosis) **Note:** Effects on the liver include necrosis, fatty infiltration, fibrosis, scarring, and nodule formation.
cholelithiasis	accumulation of stones or calculi in the gallbladder **Note:** Stones, which develop from an accumulation of cholesterol and a variety of bile components, block the passage of bile from the gallbladder. If the stone emerges from the gallbladder but gets stuck in the biliary ducts, the condition is called **choledocholithiasis**.

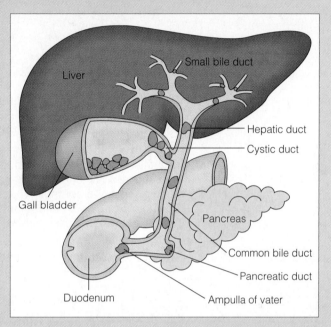

Conventional treatment involves any one of the following surgeries: cholelithotomy, cholecystectomy, choledocholithotomy. However, recent advances in nonsurgical treatments to remove calculi are becoming the preference. Included is the **dissolution of the stones** following the oral administration of a drug or by direct administration of the drug into the gallbladder via catheter; **lithotripsy**, which uses ultrasonic shock waves to shatter the gallstones allowing the fragments to pass freely through the biliary system into the duodenum; and **endoscopic retrograde sphincterotomy (ERS)**, which utilizes heat to widen the ducts to allow the release of the stones into the duodenum. **Laparoscopic cholecystectomy** is a modern technique that removes the gallbladder via a laparoscope that has been inserted through a small incision in the abdominal wall.

CONDITION	DESCRIPTION
hepatitis	inflammation of the liver

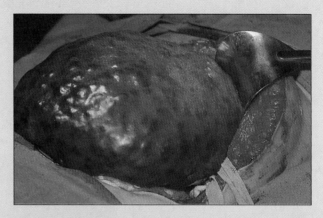

viral hepatitis	Viral hepatitis includes **hepatitis A (HAV)** (formerly called infectious hepatitis); **hepatitis B (HBV)** (formerly called serum hepatits); **hepatitis C (HCV)** (formerly called non-A, non-B hepatitis); **hepatitis D (HDV)**, and **hepatitis E (HEV)**.
	Hepatitis A is transmitted through contaminated feces and water and food such as raw shellfish. Hepatitis B is transmitted by contaminated blood and sexual contact. Hepatitis C is transmitted by blood, hepatitis D is transmitted by sexual contact and contaminated blood, and hepatitis E, the newest form, is transmitted through contaminated feces, water, and food.
nonviral hepatitis	**Nonviral hepatitis** is caused by toxins such as alcohol or drugs.

The Abdominal Wall

CONDITION	DESCRIPTION
hernia	protrusion or displacement of an organ through the membrane that normally contains it

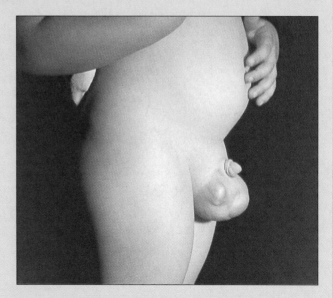

Note: The most common type of hernia is the inguinal hernia. Other hernias include: femoral, umbilical, ventral (incisional) and diaphragmatic hernia.

CONDITION	DESCRIPTION
inguinal hernia	The **inguinal hernia** is the displacement of abdominal contents into the inguinal canal. (The inguinal canal is a 1-inch long channel in either side of the lower abdominal wall. In the male it serves for the passage of nerves and some reproductive organs. In the female, it serves for the passage of ligaments and nerves. Terms often associated with the inguinal canal are internal and external inguinal rings, which are the entrance and exit of the inguinal canal respectively.) The inguinal hernia can be described as **direct** or **indirect,** depending upon the route the abdominal contents take through the canal. The indirect is the most common and most often occurs in males. 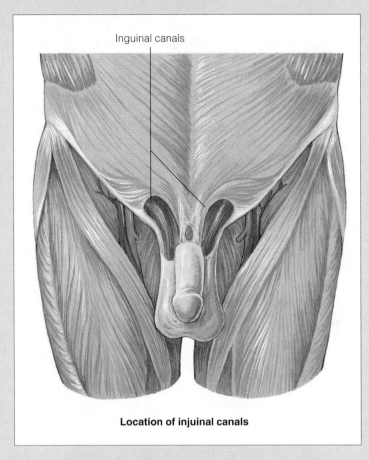 Inguinal canals **Location of injuinal canals**
femoral hernia	The **femoral hernia** is the displacement of abdominal contents into the femoral canal. (The femoral canal is a small tubular channel for the passage of blood vessels and nerves to the thigh.) Most often occurs in women.
ventral or incisional hernia	The **ventral hernia,** or **incisional hernia,** develops at the site of a previous surgery, as the site of an incision is a weak spot in the abdominal wall.
diaphragmatic hernia	**Diaphragmatic (hiatal) hernia** involves the protrusion of abdominal contents through the hiatal opening in the esophagus.
umbilical hernia	An **umbilical hernia** results from weak muscular structure around the umbilicus. Most often occurs in newborns.

The structures that can be manually examined by the physician include the mouth, lips, pharynx, abdomen, rectum, and anus.

When examining the mouth, the health care practitioner looks at the teeth for any signs of dental caries, odontorrhagia, or any abnormalities in tooth development. The buccal mucosa is examined for canker sores, gingivitis, or gingivorrhagia. Color is observed. White patches may indicate leukoplakia; red patches, inflammation. **Halitosis** (hăl-ĭ-tō′-sĭs) (bad breath) may indicate dietary deficiencies or infection. Also noted is whether the tonsils are enlarged. Lips are examined for fissures, ulcers, and abnormal color.

The pharynx is examined for any changes in color and for any sign of ulcers or inflammation.

The health care practitioner systematically applies pressure (palpation) to all four quadrants of the abdomen and observes any **guarding** or **rigidity** of abdominal muscles, which may indicate abdominal pain or tenderness. Pain on release of the pressure is called **rebound tenderness**. Rebound tenderness over McBurney's point may indicate appendicitis. Enlargement of the abdominal organs such as the spleen, liver, or kidney is noted at this time.

Percussion helps the health care practitioner observe any abnormal masses or organic abnormalities such as edema or enlargement. The health care practitioner taps the abdomen and listens to the sounds resonating from the abdominal cavity. Different sounds occur depending upon the density of the underlying structures. **Tympany**, a bell-like sound of high resonance, is normal and predominates when there are gas bubbles in the digestive tract. **Dullness** (low resonance) is normal for solid organs such as the liver and spleen. **Flatness** means no resonance at all.

Auscultation helps in evaluating peristalsis, bowel functions, and possible vascular obstructions. Often heard are normal gurgling sounds called **borborygmi** (bōr″-bō-rig′-mē) from the digestive tract.

The health care practitioner inspects and palpates the anus and rectum. Inspection identifies any inflammation, lesions, or excoriations. (Remember from the integumentary system in Chapter 6 that excoriation means abrasions or scratches). Palpation with a gloved finger helps diagnose abnormalities of the reproductive system: specifically, the prostate in the male and the cervix in the female. Any abnormalities of the anal canal and anal sphincters are also noted.

Signs and Symptoms

SYMPTOM	DEFINITION
achlorhydria ă-klor-hī′-drē-ă	absence of hydrochloric acid (HCL) in the stomach
anorexia ăn-ō-rĕks′-ē-ă	loss of appetite caused by disorder of the digestive system **Note:** not to be confused with **anorexia nervosa**, a psychiatric problem
aphagia ā-fā′-jē-ă	not eating

SYMPTOM	DEFINITION
ascites ă-sī′-tĕz	accumulation of fluid in the abdominal cavity
constipation	difficulty in producing bowel movement
diarrhea	watery discharge from the bowel caused by irritants such as toxins and microorganisms
dyspepsia	indigestion
dysphagia	difficulty in swallowing
emaciation	extreme thinness

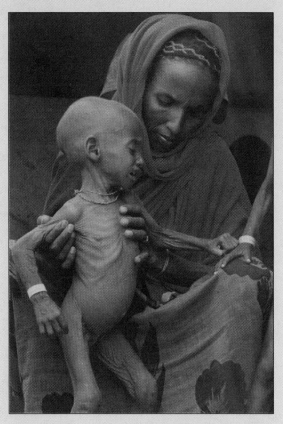

Note: seen in cancer patients, the malnourished, and those with gastrointestinal disorders

emesis	vomiting
	Note: The expulsion of gastric contents through the mouth. Excessive vomiting is called **hyperemesis** (hī″-pĕr-ĕm′-ĕ-sĭs). The vomiting of blood is **hematemesis** (hĕm″-ă-tĕm′-ĕ-sĭs).
eructation	expulsion of gastric gas or air through the mouth
gastroesopha-geal reflux	backward flow of gastric contents into the esophagus
flatulence	distention of the abdomen caused by increased amounts of air or gas in the intestine or stomach
	Note: The expulsion of gas through the anus is known as **flatus**.

SYMPTOM	DEFINITION
jaundice	yellow pigmentation of the skin caused by liver disease or obstruction of the passage of bile to the duodenum
melena	black tarry stools caused by the mixture of intestinal juices with blood
melanemesis	black vomit caused by blood from bleeding ulcers mixing with food
nausea	feeling of discomfort associated with vomiting
pruritus ani	severe itching of the anus
steatorrhea	discharge of fat in the feces in celiac disease

The following table lists various procedures used in the diagnosis of digestive system abnormalities.

Diagnostic Procedures

RADIOLOGY AND DIAGNOSTIC IMAGING	DEFINITION
flat plate of abdomen	x-ray of abdominal organs without use of a contrast medium (see Chapter 19, Medical Imaging) **Note:** This is sometimes called **KUB** for kidney, ureters, and bladder (see Chapter 13, Urinary System), as these organs are clearly evident on the x-ray.
barium enema (BE)	x-ray and fluoroscopic (see below) examination of the large bowel following injection of barium sulfate as a contrast medium into the rectum **Note:** Barium sulfate is a chalky tasting thick liquid that is used as a contrast medium in gastrointestinal studies.
barium swallow	x-ray and fluoroscopic examination of the pharynx and esophagus, following oral intake of barium sulfate
fluoroscopy	x-ray examination of a moving image, such as the movement of substances through the digestive tract **Note:** Fluoroscopy has the advantage of revealing subtle changes in anatomic structures that may obstruct the normal passage of intestinal contents.
small bowel series	x-ray and fluoroscopic examination of the duodenum, ileum, and jejunum, following oral intake of barium sulfate

RADIOLOGY TESTS	DEFINITION
upper gastrointestinal series (UGI)	barium swallow (fluoroscopic x-ray of the pharynx and esophagus) plus fluoroscopic x-ray of the distal esophagus, stomach, and proximal dudodenum following oral intake of barium sulfate
cholaniography	process of recording (x-raying) the biliary ducts (hepatic, cystic, and common bile ducts) following the insertion of a contrast medium into the body
Intravenous cholangiogram	**Intravenous cholangiogram** (IVC) is named for the injection of contrast medium into a vein.
T-tube cholangiogram	**T-tube cholangiogram** is named for the injection of contrast medium through a T-tube catheter.
operative cholangiogram	**operative cholangiogram** involves the injection of the contrast medium into the biliary ducts at the time of surgery
cholecystography	x-ray of the gallbladder following oral injection of the contrast medium Telepaque **Note:** Also known as **oral cholecystogram (OCG)**. This test is being replaced by radionuclide scanning, MRI, CT scans, and ultrasound.
percutaneous transhepatic cholangiography (PTC)	fluoroscopic examination of the biliary system following injection of contrast medium through the skin into the liver's duct system
endoscopic retrograde cholangiopancreatography (ERCP) (kō-lăn″-jē-ō-păn-krē-ă-tŏg′-ră-fē)	x-rays of biliary and pancreatic system, including the ampulla of Vater, using an endoscope and following insertion of a contrast medium
computerized tomography (CT) scans	provides a 3-dimensional view of an organ rather than the 2-dimensional view of conventional x-rays; used to identify tumors, cysts, lesions, and other abnormal masses **Note:** contrast medium may or may not be used
ultrasound	high frequency sounds waves used to produce an image or picture of an organ or tissue onto a screen **Note:** Using ultrasonography, health care practitioners can identify disease processes such as lesions, neoplasms, and hematomas of many gastrointestinal structures including the pancreas, liver, spleen, and gallbladder.

RADIOLOGY TESTS	DEFINITION
Magnetic Resonance Imaging (MRI)	The use of a magnetic field and radiowaves, not x-rays, to take images is based on the relative water content of body tissues. The image has the major advantage of being clearer and more precise than conventional x-rays, and is used to identify diseased tissue such as tumors, and infections.

LABORATORY TESTS	DEFINITION
amylase	increased levels of amylase in the blood indicate pancreatic or salivary gland disease
gastric analysis	study of gastric contents for levels of hydrochloric acid and pepsinogen; aids in the diagnosis of stomach cancer and duodenal ulcers
hepatitis B surface antigen	presence of hepatitis B antigen in the blood indicates hepatitis B infection

liver function tests (LFT):
  liver enzymes
    alkaline phosphatase
    gamma-glytamyl
    transpeptidase (GGT)
    asparate transaminase
    (AST, previously SGOT)
    alanine transaminase
    (ALT, previously
    SGPT)
  lactic dehydrogenase (LDH)
	a damaged liver liberates enzymes into the bloodstream; high levels of serum liver enzymes may indicate liver dysfunction
	
	Note: High levels of these enzymes do not signify liver dysfunction exclusively. AST, ALT, and LDH, for example, are elevated in certain cardiac conditions. GGT levels are high in alcoholism and some urinary dysfunctions.

stool analysis	examination of stool for microorganisms and blood **Note:** Microorganisms are detected through stool cultures and blood by the **occult blood test**. This test is aided by **guaiac** (gwī′-ăk), a substance which is added to the stool to reveal hidden blood.
total serum bilirubin	tests for the level of bilirubin **Note:** Increased levels of bilirubin indicate liver or biliary disease.
urinary bilirubin	presence usually indicates disease of liver and biliary system
urobilinogen (ū″-rō-bī-lĭn′-ō-jĕn)	a product of bilirubin metabolism, excreted in the urine **Note:** Increased levels occur in disease of the hepatobiliary system.

CLINICAL PROCEDURES	DEFINITION
abdominal paracentesis	surgical puncture of the peritoneal cavity to remove excess fluid for examination

endoscopy   visual examination of body cavities by inserting a tube equipped with a light and lens system

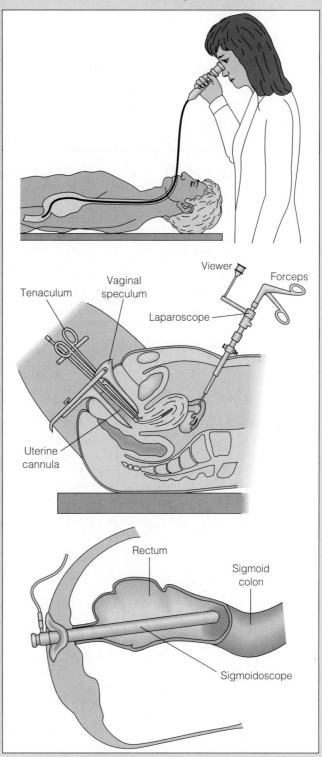

Note: Some examinations of the digestive system using an endoscope include **gastroscopy, colonoscopy, sigmoidoscopy**, and **laparoscopy**.

CLINICAL PROCEDURES	DEFINITION
percutaneous liver biopsy	following insertion of a needle through the skin and into the liver, a piece of hepatic tissue is removed for pathological study

Treatment

MEDICAL TREATMENT	DEFINITION
antibiotics	drugs used to kill bacteria
antiemetics	drugs used to prevent vomiting
emetics	drugs used to stimulate vomiting
gavage (gă-văzh')	instillation of nutritive substances into the stomach via a nasogastric tube
lavage	to irrigate or wash out an organ such as the intestine following ingestion of a toxic substance
litholytic agent	oral drugs used to dissolve gallstones in patients, thereby eliminating the need for surgery
nasogastric intubation	insertion of a soft rubber or plastic tube through the nose into the stomach to relieve gastric pressures, remove toxins, and obtain samples of gastric contents for analysis

SURGICAL PROCEDURES	DEFINITION
cecopexy	surgical fixation of the cecum
cheiloplasty	surgical repair of the lips
cholecystectomy	removal of the gallbladder
colostomy	surgical creation of a new opening between the colon and abdominal wall
colocolostomy	surgical creation of a new opening between two segments of the large intestine
duodenorrhaphy	suturing of the duodenum
endoscopic retrograde sphincterotomy (ERS) (sfĭng″-tĕr-ŏt'-ō-mē)	use of electrocautery to widen the biliary ducts to allow the release of the stones into the duodenum

SURGICAL PROCEDURES	DEFINITION
gastrojejunostomy	surgical creation of a new opening between the stomach and jejunum

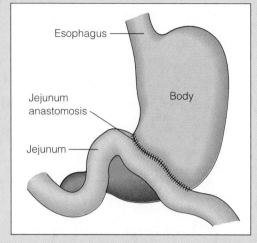

herniorrhaphy	surgical repair of a hernia
ileectomy	removal of the ileum
laparoscopic surgery	use of a laparoscope for removing structures such as the uterus, gallbladder, and kidneys
lithotripsy	use of ultrasonic shock waves to shatter the gallstones, thereby allowing the fragments to pass freely through the biliary system into the duodenum
palatoplasty	surgical repair of cleft palate
pyloromyotomy	incision of the pyloric sphincter

◗ 11.7 ABBREVIATIONS

ALT	alanine transaminase	**GB**	gallbladder
AST	asparate transaminase	**GBS**	gallbladder series
BE	barium enema	**GER**	gastroesophageal reflux
CBD	common bile duct	**GGT**	gamma-glytamyl transpeptidase
ERCP	endoscopic retrograde cholangiopancreatography	**GI**	gastrointestinal
ERS	endoscopic retrograde sphincterotomy	**HAV**	hepatitis A virus

HBV	hepatitis B virus		**N&V**	nausea and vomiting
HCL	hydrochloric acid		**NG**	nasogastric
HCV	hepatitis C virus		**PTC**	percutaneous transhepatic cholangiography
HDV	hepatitis D virus			
IBS	irritable bowel syndrome		**S&D**	stomach and duodenum
IVC	intravenous cholangiogram		**SBS**	small bowel series
LHD	lactic dehydrogenase		**TPN**	total parenteral nutrition
			UGI	upper gastrointestinal

▶ EXERCISE 11–1

Definitions

Definitions

Give the meaning for the following word parts.

Answers to the exercises are found in Appendix A.

Definitions

1. stomat/o _____
2. sialaden/o _____
3. ptyal/o _____
4. col/o _____
5. -chalasia _____
6. ankyl/o _____
7. bucc/o _____
8. proct/o _____
9. -plakia _____
10. lapar/o _____

Give the word part for the following words.

11. vomit _____   17. tongue (2) _____
12. stomach _____   _____
13. sugar _____   18. tooth (2) _____
14. small intestine _____   _____
15. liver _____
16. lips _____

Write the terms that correspond with the following abbreviations.

19. NG _____
20. BE _____
21. N&V _____
22. GER _____
23. IVC _____
24. HAV _____

25. CBD _____

26. S&D _____

27. SBS _____

Write the definition for each of the following terms.

28. gastrointestinal _____

29. lumen _____

30. esophagus _____

31. pharynx _____

32. mucosa _____

33. serosa _____

34. adventitia _____

35. abdominopelvic _____

36. uvula _____

37. palatoglossal _____

38. palatopharyngeal _____

39. circumvallate _____

40. deciduous _____

41. gingiva _____

42. periodontal _____

43. buccal cavity _____

44. labial frenulum _____

45. lingual frenulum _____

46. papillae _____

47. nasopharynx _____

48. oropharynx _____

49. laryngopharynx _____

50. sphincter _____

51. pharyngoesophageal sphincter _____

52. cardia _____

53. fundus _____

54. rugae _____

55. pepsinogen _____

56. anorectal _____

57. chyme _____

58. duodenum _____

59. jejunum _____

60. ileum _____

61. ileocecal valve _____

62. plicae circulares _____

63. villi _____

64. microvilli _____

65. crypts of Lieberkuhn _____

66. colonoscopy _____

67. ileectomy _____

68. sublingual _____

▶EXERCISE 11-2

Word Building

Build the medical word from the following sentences.

1. surgical fixation of the cecum _____

2. suturing of the lips _____

3. x-ray of bile vessels _____

4. conditions of stones in the gallbladder _____

5. surgical creation of a new opening between the ileum and abdominal wall _____

6. inflammation of the colon _____

7. dentist who specializes in the diagnosis and treatment of diseases within the tooth including the dental pulp and related structures _____

8. sudden involuntary spasmodic contractions of the stomach _____

9. formation of sugar from proteins and carbohydrates _____

10. liver cells _____

11. pertaining to the lips, tongue, and throat _____

12. instrument used to visually
examine the abdominal contents _____

13. toothache _____

14. white patches _____

15. inflammation of the peritoneum _____

▶**EXERCISE 11–3**   **Practice Quiz**

Short Answer

Briefly answer the following.

1. Name the papillae that contain taste buds. _____
_____

2. Name the two passages of the pharynx through which food passes. _____
_____

3. What is the term for a circular muscle that regulates passage of material in
the digestive tract? _____

4. What are rugae? _____

5. What are the four exocrine secretions in the stomach? _____
_____

6. What is the composition of pancreatic juice? _____
_____

7. Name the liver cells that produce bile. _____
_____

8. What is a diverticulum? _____

9. What is the sphincter of Oddi? _____
Where is it? _____

10. Where do the majority of peptic ulcers occur? _____

Matching Terms with Meanings

Match the term in Column A with its meaning in Colum B.

Column A

1. adventitia _____
2. plicae circulares _____
3. cardiac _____
4. crypts of Lieberkuhn_____
5. melanemesis _____
6. islets of Langerhans _____
7. filiform _____
8. chyme _____
9. pancreatic duct _____
10. peristaltic waves _____
11. villi and microvilli _____

Column B

A. mixture of food and enzymes in the stomach

B. papillae at the front of the tongue

C. opening through which pancreatic juice passes into the duodenum

D. black vomit

E. lower sphincter of the esophagus

F. the outer tunic of the esophagus

G. intestinal glands that produce most of the secretions in the small intestine

H. folds in the surface of the small intestine

I. endocrine cells of the pancreas

J. projections in the surface of the small intestine

K. muscle contractions that move food through the digestive tract

► EXERCISE 11-5 **Spelling Practice**

Spelling

Place a check mark beside all misspelled words in the list that follows. Correctly spell those that you checked off.

1. labial frenulum ☐ _____
2. saliviary ☐ _____
3. parenteral ☐ _____
4. circumvallate ☐ _____
5. bilary ☐ _____
6. parastalic ☐ _____
7. fundus ☐ _____
8. oxinitic ☐ _____
9. deciduous ☐ _____
10. serosa ☐ _____
11. lacteal ☐ _____
12. duodenal ☐ _____
13. caecum ☐ _____
14. ilectomy ☐ _____
15. parotid ☐ _____

16.	absorbtion	☐	_____
17.	buccal	☐	_____
18.	pyloric	☐	_____
19.	palato	☐	_____
20.	pharyngeal	☐	_____

▶ **EXERCISE 11–6**

Use of Medical Terms in Context

Medical Terms in Context

Describe and define the underlined terms as they are used in context.

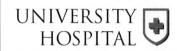
UNIVERSITY HOSPITAL   SUMMARY RECORD

IDENTIFICATION:

Mr. P. is a 48-year-old male who presented to the Emergency Department on June 3, 1995 complaining of <u>nausea</u> and <u>vomiting</u>.

HISTORY OF PRESENT ILLNESS:

Patient has a long history of <u>Crohn's disease</u> and had recently been discharged from hospital. Since discharge he had been doing reasonably well until five days prior to presentation when he developed nausea and vomiting. He also had increasing abdominal cramps. The <u>bowel</u> movements were normal. He had an <u>upper GI series</u> while in the Emergency that showed a normal <u>oropharynx, esophagus, stomach</u> and <u>duodenum</u>. The <u>contrast</u>, however, had a fast run through and therefore the small bowel could not be seen. There was no apparent obstruction.

On his last admission, a <u>colonoscopy</u> showed mainly <u>colon</u> involvement of his Crohn's with subactive disease in the <u>descending colon</u>. He also had a <u>gastroscopy</u> at that time that showed mild <u>gastritis</u> and <u>duodenitis</u> but no <u>ulcer disease</u>.

DISCHARGE DIAGNOSIS: CROHN'S DISEASE

SIGNATURE OF DOCTOR IN CHARGE _____

---

1. nausea   _____

2. vomiting   _____

3. Crohn's disease   _____

                     _____

4. bowel   _____

5. upper GI series   _____

6. oropharynx   _____

7. esophagus   _____

8. stomach   _____

9. duodenum   _____

10. contrast   _____

11. colonoscopy   _____

12. colon   _____

13. descending colon   _____

14. gastroscopy   _____

15. gastritis   _____

16. duodenitis   _____

17. ulcer disease   _____

_____

Central Medical **CM**

OPERATIVE REPORT

PREOPERATIVE DIAGNOSIS: RECURRENT ABDOMINAL PAIN AND DEMONSTRATED
GALLSTONES

OPERATION PROPOSED: LAPAROSCOPIC CHOLECYSTECTOMY

INDICATIONS:

On one of his episodes we thought he had a partial small bowel
obstruction. He subsequently complained of epigastric pain at which
time we demonstrated his gallstones. We therefore decided to proceed
with a laparoscopic cholecystectomy.

PROCEDURE:

A 2.5-inch (1 cm) incision was made immediately below the umbilicus
and the fascia opened under direct vision. Another opening was made
in the subxiphoid region and two openings in the usual positions.
The adhesions from his previous gastrectomy were a bit troublesome
and had to be cleared off the liver and the gallbladder to allow
identification of the gallbladder and performance of the operation.
The cystic duct was revealed. The right upper quadrant was
penetrated and a cholangiogram performed. It revealed no stones in
the proximal and distal ducts. During our dissection we easily
identified the common bile duct. The cystic duct was clipped and
divided. The cystic artery was clipped and the gallbladder was
dissected free. It was extracted through the xiphoid opening.
Several stones in it had to be removed manually before the
gallbladder was removed.

All instruments were removed. The skin was closed at the xiphoid and
umbilicus with intradermal Dexon. Fascia was not closed as the hole
seemed to be quite small. Skin tapes were applied to all wounds.

POST-OPERATIVE DIAGNOSIS: CHRONIC CHOLECYSTITIS; CHOLECYSTOLITHIASIS

OPERATION PERFORMED: LAPAROSCOPIC CHOLECYSTECTOMY

Authorized Health Care Practitioner _____

---

18. laparoscopic cholecystectomy _____

_____

19. bowel obstruction _____

_____

20. epigastric pain _____

21. gallstones _____

_____

22. umbilicus _____

23. fascia _____

24. subxiphoid _____

25. adhesions _____

26. gastrectomy _____

27. cystic duct _____

28. right upper quadrant _____

29. cholangiogram _____

30. proximal and distal ducts _____

_____

31. dissection _____

32. common bile duct _____

33. chronic cholecystitis _____

Crossword Puzzle

The Digestive System

Across

1 Inflammation of the mouth
4 Abnormal lip condition
6 Inability of the digestive tract muscles to relax
9 X-Ray of a bile duct
12 Bleeding from a tooth

Down

2 Under the tongue
3 Excessive saliva secretion
4 Pertaining to the abdomen
5 Inflammation of the gallbladder
6 Restrained tongue movement
7 Without teeth
8 Excision of common bile duct
10 Liver cell
11 Pertaining to the cheek and gums

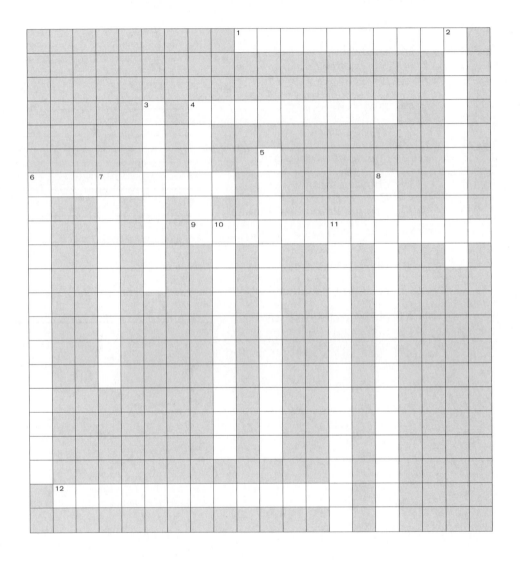

12 THE ENDOCRINE SYSTEM

CHAPTER OBJECTIVES

Upon successful completion of this chapter, the student will be able to complete the following:

1. Differentiate between endocrine and exocrine glands.
2. Differentiate between central and peripheral endocrine glands.
3. Define trophic hormones.
4. Name the secretions of the central endocrine glands.
5. Name the secretions of the thyroid, parathyroid, adrenal, and pineal glands and describe their functions.
6. Identify releasing hormones and describe their actions.
7. Analyze, pronounce, define, and spell terms related to the endocrine system.
8. List and define terms describing common endocrine disorders, diagnosis, and treatment.
9. Define abbreviations common to the endocrine system.

WORD ELEMENTS PROMINENT IN THIS CHAPTER

WORD ELEMENT	ELEMENT TYPE	MEANING
acr/o	root	extremities; top
aden/o	root	gland
adren/o; adrenal/o	root	adrenal gland
andr/o	root	male
cortic/o	root	cortex
-crine	suffix	secrete
estr/o	root	female
gluc/o; glyc/o	root	sugar

WORD ELEMENT	ELEMENT TYPE	MEANING
home/o	root	same
hypophys/o	root	pituitary gland
parathyroid/o	root	parathyroid
pituitar/o	root	pituitary
somat/o	root	body
thyr/o; thyroid/o	root	thyroid
-trophic; -tropic; -trophin; -tropin	suffix	nourishment; stimulation

12.1 GENERAL ANATOMY AND PHYSIOLOGY OF THE ENDOCRINE SYSTEM

The **endocrine** (ĕn′-dō-krĭn) system consists of glands that produce secretions called **hormones**. Hormones are substances that provide a chemical signal to the body as distinguished from a neurological signal of the nervous system, although often one influences the other. Hormones are secreted directly into extracellular fluid. They are then transported via the bloodstream to their target organs and are thus distinguished from **exocrine** (ĕks′-ō-krĭn) secretions, such as saliva, which are transported to their destination by ducts.

The endocrine glands are divided into two categories, the central and the peripheral. Central endocrine glands are the **hypothalamus** (hī″-pō-thăl′-ă-mŭs) and the **pituitary** (pĭ-tū′-ĭ-tār″-ē), both of which are located within the brain. Although the hypothalamus is part of the nervous system, it is also considered part of the endocrine system because it produces and secretes neurohormones, some of which serve as stimulants for the secretions of the peripheral endocrine glands. The pituitary gland is adjacent to the hypothalamus within the brain. The hypothalamus and the pituitary function together to regulate body functions such as growth, metabolism, reproduction, and water and salt balance in the body.

The **peripheral endocrine glands** include the **adrenal** (ăd-rē′-năl), **thyroid**, **parathyroid**, and **pineal** (pĭn′-ē-ăl). These four glands, as well as the pituitary, have as their exclusive function the production and secretion of hormones. There are many additional peripheral endocrine glands located in "mixed function" organs (such as the hypothalamus itself) that have other functions in addition to hormone production. These organs are the thymus, kidneys, digestive tract, pancreas, liver, skin, heart, ovaries, testes, and placenta, as shown in

Figure 12–1. This chapter will cover terminology associated with the two central endocrine glands and the four peripheral glands, whose exclusive function is hormone production. Terminology associated with peripheral endocrine glands located in "mixed function" organs will be discussed in the respective chapters covering those organs.

FIGURE 12–1 Endocrine Glands in "Mixed Function" Organs and in Exclusive Function Glands

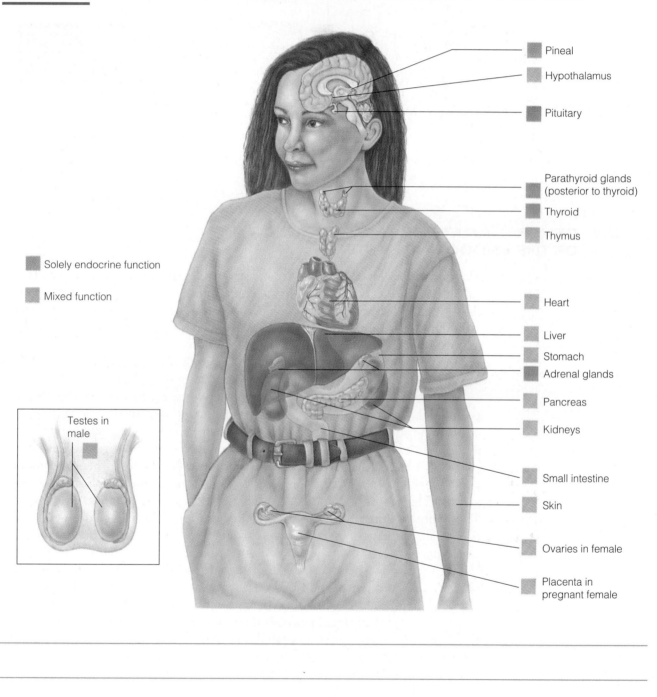

Pineal
Hypothalamus
Pituitary
Parathyroid glands (posterior to thyroid)
Thyroid
Thymus
Heart
Liver
Stomach
Adrenal glands
Pancreas
Kidneys
Small intestine
Skin
Ovaries in female
Placenta in pregnant female
Solely endocrine function
Mixed function
Testes in male

Central Endocrine Glands

Hypothalamus   The hypothalamus is located deep within the central part of the brain (see Figure 12–2). Most of the secretions of the hypothalamus are known as **trophic** (trŏf'-ĭk) hormones. Trophic is a Greek word meaning nourishment or stimulation. The trophic hormones regulate the production and release of hormones from the pituitary gland. The six trophic hormones that *stimulate* the release of pituitary hormones are:

1. growth-hormone-releasing hormone (**GHRH**)
2. thyrotrophin-releasing hormone (**TRH**)
3. corticotrophin-releasing hormone (**CRH**)
4. gonadotrophin-releasing hormone (**GnRH**)
5. prolactin-releasing hormone (**PRH**)
6. melanocyte-releasing hormone (**MRH**)

FIGURE 12–2   Hypothalamus and Pituitary Gland

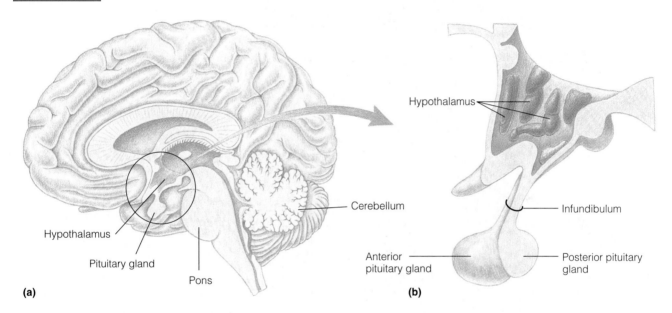

(a)

(b)

The three hypothalamic hormones that *inhibit* the release of pituitary gland hormones are:

1. growth-hormone-inhibiting hormone (**GHIH**)
2. prolactin-inhibiting hormone (**PIH**)
3. melanocyte-inhibiting hormone (**MIH**)

It should be noted that the inhibiting hypothalamic hormones as well as those that stimulate hormone release are referred to as "releasing" hormones.

Two additional hormones are produced by the hypothalamus for storage in the pituitary gland. These latter two hormones are not trophic; that is, they do not stimulate the production of new hormones. These two hormones, **antidiuretic hormone** and **oxytocin**, are stored in and released by the pituitary.

Pituitary Gland

The **pituitary gland**, also known as the **hypophysis** (hī-pŏf′-ĭ-sĭs), is a pea-sized gland hanging from the hypothalamus by a stalk called the **infundibulum** (ĭn″-fŭn-dĭb′-ū-lŭm), as shown in Figure 12–2. The pituitary gland is divided into the **anterior pituitary** or **adenohypophysis** (ăd″-ĕ-nō-hī-pŏf′-ĭ-sĭs), and the **posterior pituitary**, or **neurohypophysis** (nū″-rō-hī-pŏf′-ĭ-sĭs). The anterior pituitary secretes hormones produced by its own cells. This activity is regulated by the trophic hormones secreted by the hypothalamus. The posterior pituitary stores and secretes hormones produced by the hypothalamus (see Figure 12–3).

FIGURE 12–3   Hormonal and Neuronal Influence by the Hypothalamus on the Anterior and Posterior Pituitary

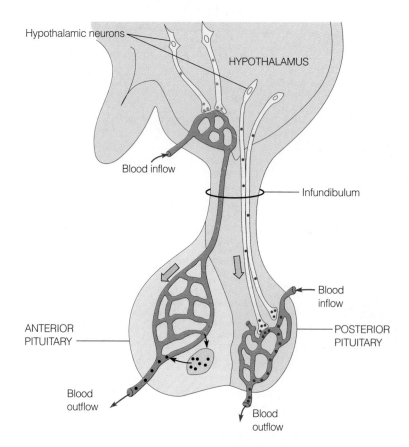

Anterior Pituitary (Adenohypophysis)   The trophic hormones of the hypothalamus trigger the production of seven hormones by the anterior pituitary (see Figure 12–4). Five of these pituitary hormones are themselves trophic hormones, that is, they stimulate hormone release from other glands:

1. **Growth hormone (GH)**, or **somatotrophin**, stimulates growth in all body cells. GH also regulates the release of somatomedin (sō-mă″-tō-mĕd′-ĭn) from the liver, which has an effect on the growth of skeletal structures.

2. **Thyroid-stimulating hormone (TSH)**, or **thyrotrophin**, stimulates the thyroid gland to produce its own hormones **thyroxine** (thī-rŏks′-in) (T_4) and **triiodothyronine** (trī″-ī-ō″-dō-thī′-rō-nēn) (T_3).

3. **Adrenocorticotrophic hormone (ACTH)**, or **corticotrophin**, stimulates the adrenal cortex to release cortisol and aldosterone.
4. **Follicle-stimulating hormone (FSH)** is a **gonadotrophin** involved in the development of the ovaries and testes. In females, this hormone promotes the monthly growth of the ovarian egg and in males it promotes sperm formation.
5. **Luteinizing** (lū'-tē-ĭn-ī-zĭng) **hormone (LH)** is another **gonadotrophin** that triggers ovulation in females. In males it regulates sex hormone secretion and is called **interstitial cell stimulating hormone (ICSH)**.

FIGURE 12–4

Summary of Trophic Hormones

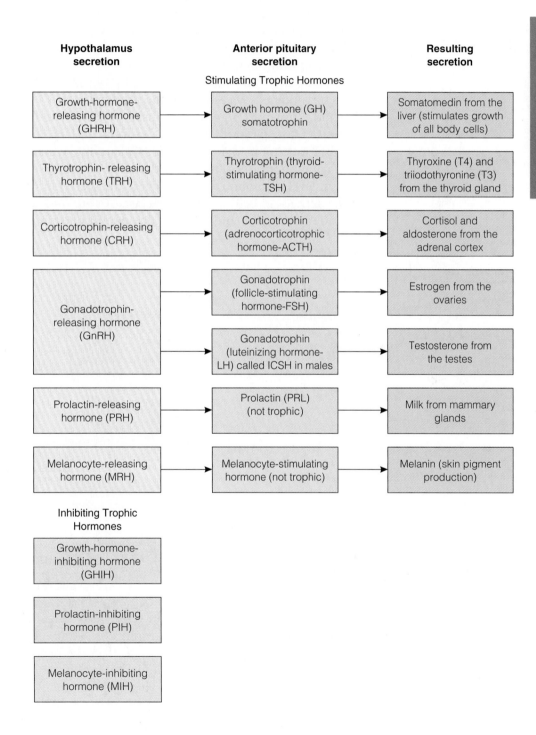

Hypothalamus secretion	Anterior pituitary secretion	Resulting secretion
	Stimulating Trophic Hormones	
Growth-hormone-releasing hormone (GHRH)	Growth hormone (GH) somatotrophin	Somatomedin from the liver (stimulates growth of all body cells)
Thyrotrophin- releasing hormone (TRH)	Thyrotrophin (thyroid-stimulating hormone-TSH)	Thyroxine (T4) and triiodothyronine (T3) from the thyroid gland
Corticotrophin-releasing hormone (CRH)	Corticotrophin (adrenocorticotrophic hormone-ACTH)	Cortisol and aldosterone from the adrenal cortex
Gonadotrophin-releasing hormone (GnRH)	Gonadotrophin (follicle-stimulating hormone-FSH)	Estrogen from the ovaries
	Gonadotrophin (luteinizing hormone-LH) called ICSH in males	Testosterone from the testes
Prolactin-releasing hormone (PRH)	Prolactin (PRL) (not trophic)	Milk from mammary glands
Melanocyte-releasing hormone (MRH)	Melanocyte-stimulating hormone (not trophic)	Melanin (skin pigment production)
Inhibiting Trophic Hormones		
Growth-hormone-inhibiting hormone (GHIH)		
Prolactin-inhibiting hormone (PIH)		
Melanocyte-inhibiting hormone (MIH)		

The sixth and seventh hormones produced by the anterior pituitary are **prolactin (PRL)** and **melanocyte-stimulating hormone (MSH)**. These two are not trophic hormones; that is, they do not stimulate the production of other hormones. Rather, PRL stimulates production of milk in the mammary glands, and MSH enhances the production of melanin, which is required for skin pigmentation.

Thyroid Gland

The thyroid gland is located in the neck below the larynx. It is made up of left and right lobes connected by the **isthmus** (ĭs′-mŭs), as shown in Figure 12–5. Spherical sacs called follicles secrete the two hormones known as the **thyroid hormones**. These are **triiodothyronine (T_3)** and **thyroxine (T_4)**. These hormones are important in growth and metabolism. As the body's needs change, so does the amount of hormones secreted by the gland. It is important to note that dietary iodine is necessary for the production of T_3 and T_4. An enlarged thyroid gland, known as a **goiter**, is caused by lack of iodine in the diet. Between the follicles are **parafollicular** (păr″-ă-fō-lĭk′-ū-lăr) **cells** that secrete a hormone called **calcitonin** (kăl-sĭ-tō′-nĭn). Calcitonin, which is not regulated by hypothalamic hormones, regulates the level of calcium phosphate in the blood. A high level of blood calcium triggers the secretion of calcitonin, which inhibits the activity of cells called **osteoclasts** (ŏs′-tē-ō-klăsts). These are cells that degrade bone tissue and release calcium and phosphates into the blood.

FIGURE 12–5

Thyroid Gland

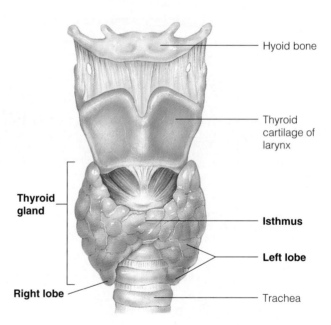

As discussed in the section on central endocrine glands, the production and secretion of the two thyroid hormones are regulated by the central glands. Internal or external conditions that affect the needs of the body, such as cold temperatures, for example, stimulate the hypothalamus to release TRH (thyrotrophin-releasing hormone). This in turn signals the pituitary to release TSH (thyroid-stimulating hormone), which then signals the thyroid to increase the rate of secretion of the thyroid hormones.

Parathyroid Glands

Located posteriorly on each of the two lobes of the thyroid are two small egg-shaped glands called **parathyroid glands** (Figure 12–6). The parathyroids are composed of **chief cells** and **oxyphil** (ŏk′-sē-fĭl) **cells.** The parathyroids secrete one single hormone called **parathyroid hormone** or **parathormone (PTH).** This hormone regulates calcium and phosphate levels in the blood by stimulating the activity of osteoclasts and by increasing the excretion of phosphate in urine.

FIGURE 12–6

Parathyroid Glands

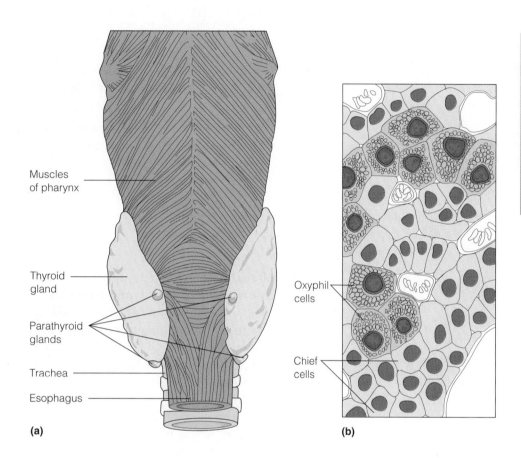

Muscles of pharynx

Thyroid gland

Parathyroid glands

Trachea

Esophagus

(a)

Oxyphil cells

Chief cells

(b)

Adrenal Glands

On top of each kidney is a triangular gland called the **adrenal** (ăd-rē′-năl) **gland.** The outer mass of each adrenal gland, the **adrenal cortex,** surrounds the inner **adrenal medulla,** as shown in Figure 12–7.

FIGURE 12-7

Adrenal Glands

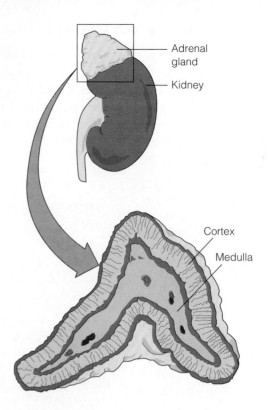

The adrenal cortex is made up of three layers. The outer layer secretes hormones known collectively as **mineralocorticoid** (mĭn″-ĕr-ăl-ō-kōr′-tĭ-koyd) **hormones**. The most important of these is **aldosterone** (ăl-dŏs′-tĕr-ōn), which regulates sodium reabsorption and potassium excretion by the kidneys.

The two inner layers of the cortex secrete **glucocorticoid** (gloo-kō-kōrt′-ĭ-koyd) **hormones** involved in metabolism of carbohydrates, fats, and proteins. The most important of the glucocorticoids is **cortisol (hydrocortisone)**. In addition to its role in metabolism, cortisol is necessary for antibody production and is also involved in response to stress.

The two inner layers of the adrenal cortex also secrete small amounts of the sex hormones estrogen and testosterone. Most of these hormones are produced in the respective reproductive organs of males and females, the testes and ovaries. But small amounts of both hormones are produced by the adrenal cortex in both males and females and contribute to secondary sex characteristics such as beard and breast development.

The adrenal medulla is made up of cells called **chromaffin** (krō-măf′-ĭn). When stimulated, they release two hormones that help the body respond to stress: **epinephrine** (ĕp-ĭ-nĕf′-rĭn) **(adrenaline)** and **norepinephrine** (nŏr-ĕp″-i-nef-rĭn) **(noradrenaline)**. These hormones prepare the body in times of anger, fear, defense, or chase. These two hormones are also released by the brain cells in response to a neural message and act upon specific muscle cells or upon other glands. When adrenaline and noradrenaline are released by the adrenal medulla, they enter the blood and are carried to all body tissues. Epinephrine and norepinephine are known collectively as **catecholamines** (kăt″-ĕ-kōl′-ă-mēnz).

Pineal Gland

The **pineal** (pĭn′-ē-ăl) **gland,** which resembles a pine cone, is located within the brain and is sometimes known as the **epiphysis cerebri** (ĕ-pĭf′-ĭ-sĭs sĕr′-ē-brĭ) (Figure 12–8).

FIGURE 12–8 Pineal Gland

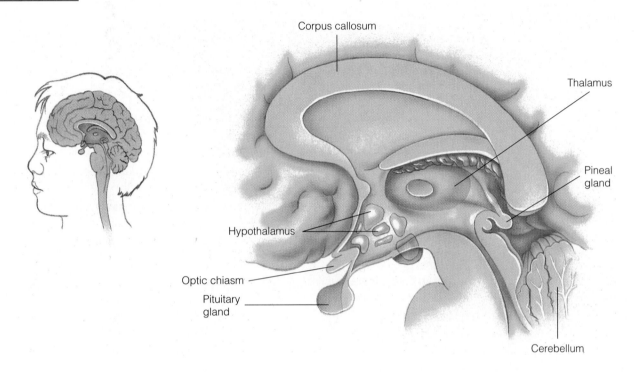

Corpus callosum

Thalamus

Pineal gland

Hypothalamus

Optic chiasm

Pituitary gland

Cerebellum

Because of its location in the brain, the pineal gland is sometimes considered a central rather than a peripheral endocrine gland. However, very little is known about the function of the pineal gland in humans. Some evidence suggests that its secretions are involved with regulating the reproductive system. The hormone secreted by the pineal gland is called **melatonin** (mĕl″-ă-tō′-nĭn). Secretions of melatonin are known to increase in darkness and to decrease when light strikes the eye and travels to the nerves that regulate melatonin production. Recently, the pineal gland has been implicated in the condition known as **seasonally affected disorder (SAD),** a period of mental and physical depression occurring in the winter months.

A summary of the endocrine glands and the hormones they secrete is found in Table 12–1.

TABLE 12–1   Summary of Endocrine Glands and Hormones

GLAND	HORMONE	FUNCTION
hypothalamus	trophic or "releasing" hormones **GHRH,TRH, CRH, GnRH, PRH, MRH, GHIH, PIH,MIH**	hormones that stimulate or inhibit release of pituitary hormones
anterior pituitary (adenohypophysis)	**somatotrophin** growth hormone (GH)	stimulates growth in all body cells
	thyrotrophin thyroid-stimulating hormone (TSH)	stimulates thyroid gland to produce T_3 and T_4
	corticotrophin adrenocorticotrophic hormone (ACTH)	stimulates adrenal cortex to release cortisol and aldosterone
	gonadotrophin follicle-stimulating hormone (FSH)	development of ovaries and testes; promotes monthly growth of ovarian egg in females and sperm production in males
	gonadotrophin luteinizing hormone (LH)	triggers ovulation in females; regulates sex hormone secretion in males
	prolactin (PRL)	stimulates production of milk in mammary gland
	melanocyte-stimulating hormone (MSH)	produces melanin for skin pigmentation
posterior pituitary (neurohypophysis)	**antidiuretic hormone** (ADH) also called vasopressin	regulates water retention in the body
	oxytocin	regulates flow of milk in mammary glands and stimulates uterine contractions during childbirth
thyroid	thyroid hormones **thyroxine (T_4) and triiodothyronine (T_3)**	increase metabolic rate; stimulates growth
	calcitonin	regulates blood calcium
parathyroid	**parathyroid hormone (parathormone) (PTH)**	increases blood calcium; decreases blood phosphate
adrenal cortex	glucocorticoid hormones, including **cortisol**, also called hydrocortisone	antibody production; response to stress; metabolism of carbohydrates, fats, and proteins.
	mineralocorticoid hormones including **aldosterone**	regulates sodium and potassium levels
	sex hormones **estrogen** and **testosterone**	development of secondary female and male characteristics
adrenal medulla	catecholamines: **epinephrine** (adrenaline) and **norepinephrine** (noradrenaline)	help body respond to stress
pineal gland	**melatonin**	function unknown in humans

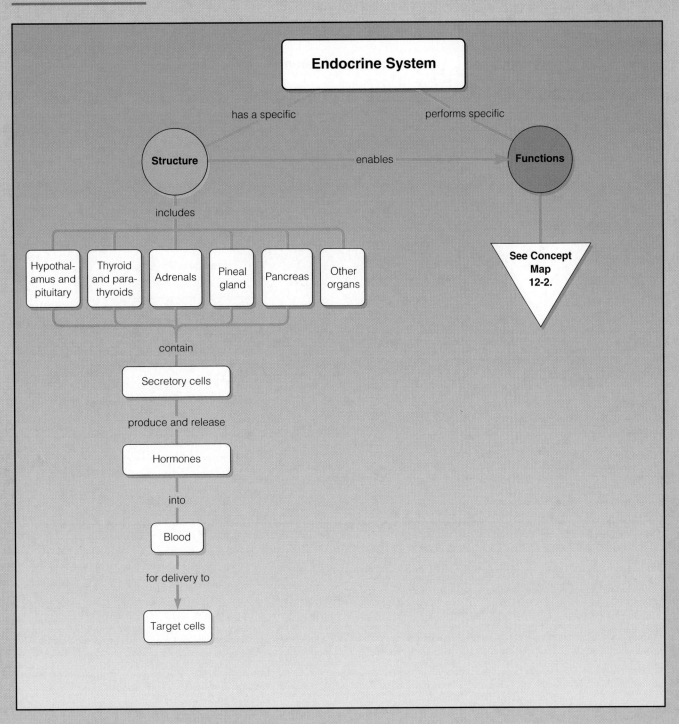

II–12

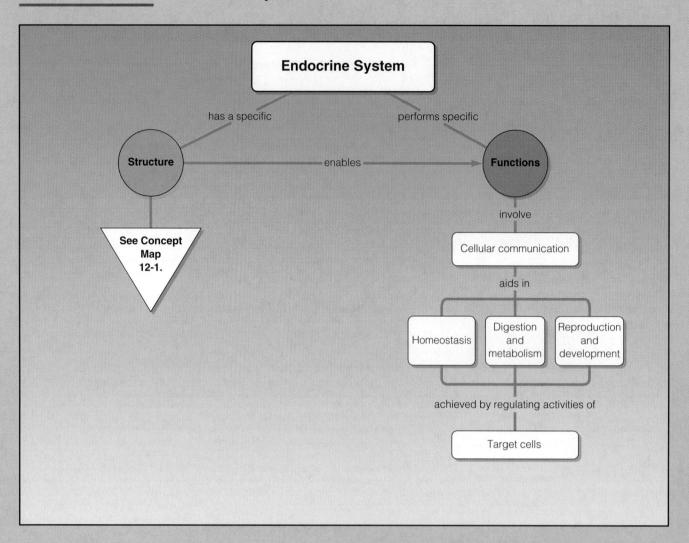

TERM WITH PRONUNCIATION	ANALYSIS	DEFINITION
acromegaly ăk″-rō-mĕg′-ă-lē	-megaly = enlarged acr/o = extremity; top	enlargement of many skeletal structures, particularly the extremities, nose, forehead, and jaw
adenohypophysis ăd″-ĕ-nō-hī-pŏf′-ĭ-sĭs	-physis = to grow aden/o = gland hypo- = under; beneath; deficient; below normal	anterior pituitary gland
adenoma ăd″-ĕ-nō′-mă	-oma = tumor or mass aden/o = gland	tumor of a gland
adrenalectomy ăd-rē″-năl-ĕk′-tō-mē	-ectomy = excision; removal adrenal/o = adrenal gland	excision of the adrenal glands
adrenocortical ăd-rē″-nō-kōr′-tĭ-kăl	-al = pertaining to adren/o = adrenal gland cortic/o = cortex; outer layer	pertaining to the adrenal cortex
androgen ăn′-drō-jĕn	-gen = producing andr/o = male; man	substance producing male characteristics, example: testosterone
antidiuretic ăn″-tĭ-dī-ū-rĕt′-ĭk	-tic = pertaining to anti- = against di(a) = through ure(o) = urea	pertaining to an agent that prevents the loss of excessive amounts of urine **Note:** Urea is the end product of protein metabolism and is found in urine.
endocrine ĕn′-dō-krĭn	-crine = secrete; separate endo- = within	to secrete into the bloodstream
endocrinology ĕn″-dō-krĭn-ŏl′-ō-jē	-logy = study of endo- = within crin/o = secrete	branch of medicine that deals with diagnosis and treatment of endocrine disorders
estrogen ĕs′-trō-jĕn	-gen = producing estr/o = female	female sex hormones
euthyroid ū-thī′-royd	-oid = resembling eu- = good thyr/o = thyroid	normal thyroid gland
exocrine ĕks′-ō-krĭn	-crine = secrete; separate exo- = outside; outward	to secrete outwardly onto the skin or onto the surface of an organ
exophthalmia; exophthalmos ĕks″-ŏf-thăl-mē-ă ĕks″-ŏf-thăl′-mōs	-ia = condition; state of ex- = out of; away from ophthalm/o = eye	abnormal protrusion of the eye
glucogenesis glū-kō-jĕn′-ĕ-sĭs	-genesis = production gluc/o = sugar	production of sugar
gluconeogenesis glū″-kō-nē″-ō-jĕn′-ĕ-sĭs	-genesis = production gluc/o = sugar neo- = new	production of sugar from fats and proteins
glycogenesis glī″-kŏ-jĕn′-ĕ-sĭs	-genesis = production glyc/o = glycogen; sugar	production of glycogen

II–12

TERM WITH PRONUNCIATION	ANALYSIS	DEFINITION
gonadotrophic; **gonadotropic** gŏn″-ă-dō-trŏf′-ĭk gŏn″-ă-dō-trŏ′-pĭk	-trophic; -tropic = pertaining to nourishment gonad/o = gonads; sex glands (ovaries or testes)	pituitary hormone that stimulates the gonads to secrete their own hormones
gynecomastia jī″-nĕ-kō-măs′-tē-ă	-ia = condition gynec/o = woman mast/o = breast	abnormal enlargement of the male breast
hypergonadism hī″-pĕr-gō′-năd-ĭzm	-ism = condition; state of; process hyper- = excessive; above; beyond gonad/o = gonads; sex organs	condition characterized by excessive secretion of gonadal hormones
hyperinsulinism hī″-pĕr-ĭn′-sū-lĭn-ĭzm	-ism = condition; state of; process hyper- = excessive; above; beyond insulin/o = insulin	condition characterized by excessive secretion of insulin
hyperparathyroidism hī″-pĕr-păr″-ă-thī′-rōyd-ĭzm	-ism = condition; state of; process hyper- = excessive; above; beyond parathyroid/o = parathyroid	condition characterized by excessive secretion of the parathyroid hormone
hyperpituitarism hī″-pĕr-pĭ-tū′-ĭ-tăr-ĭsm	-ism = condition; state of; process hyper- = excessive; above; beyond pituitar/o = pituitary	condition characterized by excessive secretion of the pituitary hormones
hyperthyroidism hī″-pĕr-thī′-royd-ĭzm	-ism = condition; state of; process hyper- = excessive; above; beyond thyroid/o = thyroid	condition characterized by excessive secretion of the thyroid hormone
hypocalcemia hī″-pō-kăl-sē′-mē-ă	-emia = presence of a substance in the blood hypo- = deficient; below normal; under; beneath calc/o = calcium	deficient amounts of calcium in the blood
hypokalemia hī″-pō-kă-lē′-mē-ă	-emia = presence of a substance in the blood hypo- = deficient; below normal; under; beneath kal/o = potassium	deficient amounts of potassium in the blood
hyponatremia hī″-pō-nă-trē′-mē-ă	-emia = presence of a substance in the blood hypo- = deficient; below normal; under; beneath natr/o = sodium	deficient amounts of sodium in the blood

TERM WITH PRONUNCIATION	ANALYSIS	DEFINITION
hypophysectomy hī″-pō-fĭ-sĕk′-tō-mē	-ectomy = excision; removal hypophys/o = pituitary gland	excision of the pituitary gland
hypothyroidism hī″-pō-thī′-royd-ĭzm	-ism = condition; state of; process hypo- = deficient; below normal; under; beneath thyroid/o = thyroid gland	condition characterized by a deficient secretion of thyroid hormones
ketoacidosis kē″-tō-ăs-ĭ-dō′-sĭs	-osis = abnormal condition ket/o = ketone bodies acid/o = acid	accumulation of ketones in the body **Note:** When there is an increase in the breakdown of fatty acids for body fuel rather than glucose, ketones, which are acids, build up.
lactogenic lăc″-tō-jĕn′-ĭk	-ic = pertaining to lact/o = milk gen/o = production	pertaining to the production of milk
oxytocin ŏk″-sĭ-tō′-sĭn	-tocin = childbirth; labor oxy- = sharp; quick	pituitary hormone that quickens childbirth
pancreatic păn″-krē-ăt′-ĭk	-ic = pertaining to pancreat/o = pancreas	pertaining to the pancreas
panhypopituitarism păn-hī″-pō-pĭ-tū′-ĭ-tăr-ĭzm	-ism = condition; state of; process pan- = all hypo- = deficient; below normal; under; beneath pituitar/o = pituitary gland	condition characterized by a deficiency of all pituitary hormones
polydipsia pŏl″-ĭ-dĭp′-sē-ă	-dipsia = thirst poly- = many	excessive thirst
somatotrophic hormone; **somatotropic hormone** sō″-mă-tō-trŏf′-ĭk sō″-mă-tō-trō′-pĭc	-trophic; -tropic = pertaining to nourishment somat/o = body	pituitary hormone that stimulates growth of body tissues
thyroiditis thī″-royd-ī′-tĭs	-itis = inflammation thyroid/o = thyroid gland	inflammation of the thyroid gland
thyrotomy thī-rŏt′-ō-mē	-tomy = incision thyr/o = thyroid gland	incision of the thyroid gland
thyrotrophic hormone thī″-rō-trŏf′-ĭk	-trophic; -tropic = nourishment thyr/o = thyroid gland	pituitary hormone that stimulates the thyroid to produce its own hormones

II-12

Pathology of the endocrine system is based on increased or decreased secretions of hormones. Increased amounts of a hormone are indicated by the term **hyper-** followed by the name of the gland involved, for example, hyperpituitarism and hyperthyroidism. Decreased amounts of a hormone are indicated by the term **hypo-** followed by the name of the gland involved, for example, hypopituitarism and hypothyroidism.

Diabetes Mellitus

As shown in the following table, the cause of the diabetes mellitus may be unknown, but many of its symptoms and signs are known extremely well. Because of the lack of insulin to change glucose to glycogen, **hyperglycemia** becomes the main symptom. The sugar remains in the blood and is secreted in the urine (**glycosuria**). Since body tissues have insufficient glucose for energy, proteins and fats are used, a process called **gluconeogenesis**. The result is a breakdown and wasting away of tissue. Other symptoms include **polydipsia** (excessive thirst), **polyuria** (excessive urination), polyphagia (excessive eating), and excessive weight loss.

Types of diabetes mellitus are **type I diabetes mellitus**, formerly known as **insulin dependent diabetes mellitus (IDDM)** and **type II diabetes mellitus**, formerly known as **noninsulin dependent diabetes mellitus (NIDDM)**.

Type I diabetes mellitus is caused by deficiency of insulin as a result of destroyed pancreatic beta cells. It is mostly seen in juveniles but can occur at any age. Because of its juvenile propensity it used to be called juvenile-onset diabetes.

Type II diabetes mellitus is usually seen in adults (previously called adult-onset diabetes).

One of the major complications of diabetes is **ketoacidosis** (a toxic increase in circulating ketones and acids), which is caused by the faulty breakdown of fats. Other complications of diabetes include diabetic retinopathy, nephropathy, neuropathy, and a reduced immunity to infections.

Diagnostic tests include **fasting blood sugar** (FBS), **glucose tolerance test** (GTT), and **postprandial** (PP) test (see diagnostic procedures for definitions).

Treatment for diabetes includes dietary restrictions, hypoglycemic agents, and insulin injections.

Diseases Caused by Hypersecretion of an Endocrine Gland

GLAND	CONDITION	DESCRIPTION
pituitary gland **anterior lobe**	acromegaly	widening of bones, particularly the facial features, hands, and feet caused by increased secretion of the growth hormone **after** the bone has stopped growing

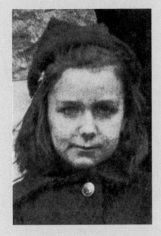 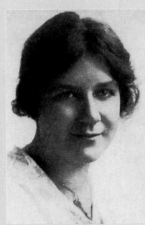 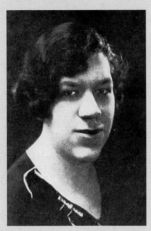 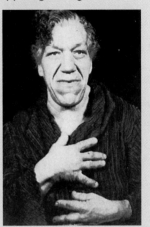

| | giantism | excessive skeletal growth caused by increased secretion of the growth hormone **before** growing has stopped and before the epiphyseal plate closes |

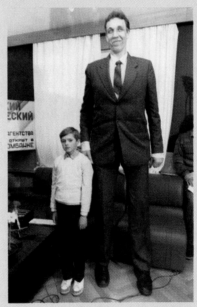

| | galactorrhea | increased prolactin, results in production and secretion of milk in women who are not breast feeding an infant; can also occur in men |
| **posterior lobe** | syndrome of inappropriate secretion of antidiuretic hormone (SIADH) | increased ADH results in fluid retention and hyponatremia |

GLAND	CONDITION	DESCRIPTION
thyroid gland	Graves' disease	characterized by overproduction of thyroid hormone, frequently in association with an enlarged thyroid gland (**goiter**) and protrusion of the eyeball (**exophthalmos**)

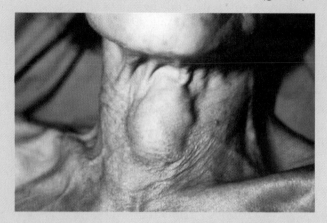 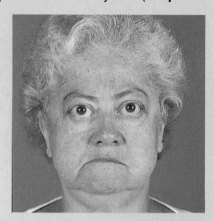

Note: Etiology is unknown but there is evidence of increased amounts of thyroid-stimulating antibodies (**TSAb**), which stimulates the thyroid gland to increase its production of TSH.

adrenal glands		
adrenal cortex	virilism	preponderance of male characteristics caused by an increase in the secretion of **androgens**
		Note: Includes **hirsutism** (hŭr-sūt'-ĭzm) (excessive hair growth), lowering of voice pitch, increased muscle bulk, and baldness. More of a problem in women than in men.
	aldosteronism	increased secretions of aldosterone characterized by water retention, weakness, paresthesias, and tetany (muscle spasms and cramps)
	Cushing's syndrome	caused by an increase of cortisol secretion; the patient exhibits the following characteristics: obesity, moon facies, atrophy of skin, menstrual problems in females

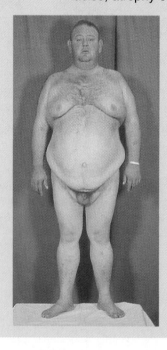

Diseases Caused by Hypersecretion of an Endocrine Gland (continued)

GLAND	CONDITION	DESCRIPTION
adrenal medulla	pheochromocytoma	tumor of the chromaffin cells of adrenal medulla
parathyroid gland	hyperparathyroidism	increased secretion of PTH results in excessive bone loss, which, over time, can lead to pathological fractures or abnormal curvatures of the spine
		Note: With the loss of bone, calcium enters the blood, resulting in hypercalcemia and hypercalciuria.
pancreas	hyperinsulinism	Overproduction of insulin can be organic, due to a disease of the pancreas such as a tumor, or it can be functional, where the cause is unknown.

Diseases Caused by Hyposecretion of an Endocrine Gland

GLAND	CONDITION	DESCRIPTION
pituitary		
anterior lobe	dwarfism	deficiency of growth hormone, resulting in an abnormally small but well-proportioned person

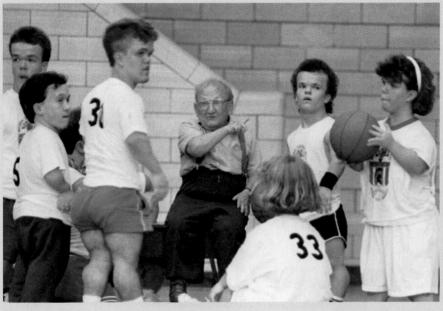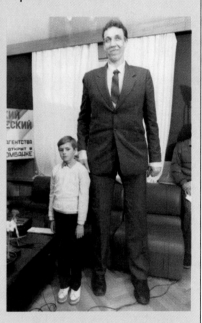

	pituitary neoplasms	pituitary tumors destroy the tissue of the pituitary gland, decreasing the secretion of hormones
	necrosis of the pituitary gland following childbirth	decrease in blood pressure following childbirth results in anoxia followed by necrosis of the pituitary gland
posterior lobe	diabetes insipidus	decrease in antidiuretic hormone resulting in excessive loss of urine accompanied by excessive thirst
	uterine inertia	inability of the uterus to contract during labor

GLAND	CONDITION	DESCRIPTION
thyroid gland	myxedema	an acquired condition in adulthood characterized by a slowing of the metabolic rate caused by low amounts of thyroid hormones
		Note: Symptoms include loss of elasticity of the skin, depression, slowness of activity, puffiness of the skin, dullness of expression.
	cretinism	hypothyroidism in infancy or during fetal development, characterized by the slowing of the metabolic rate manifested as reduced activity and infrequent crying and slow mental and physical growth
		Note: If diagnosed and treated early, these signs of slow mental and physical growth can be reversed.

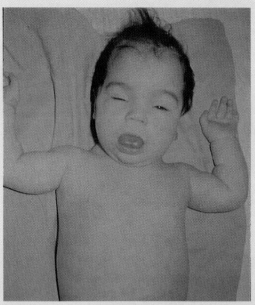

GLAND	CONDITION	DESCRIPTION
adrenal glands		
adrenal cortex	Addison's disease	results in weakness, tiredness, darkened pigmentation of the skin, hypotension
parathyroid gland	hypoparathyroidism	reduced levels of PTH has an effect opposite to hyperparathyroidism; there is decreased bone loss and hypocalcemia and hypocalciuria
	tetany	muscle spasms and cramps
pancreas	diabetes mellitus	a defect in carbohydrate metabolism as insulin is unavailable to change excess glucose to glycogen
		Note: Exact cause is unknown but is characterized by hyposecretion of insulin, which may result from one of the following: beta cell damage, insulin inactivation, increased insulin requirements to meet needs of stress, obesity, or pregnancy.

Abnormal Conditions of the Endocrine System not Caused by Hyper- or Hyposecretion of Hormones

GLAND	CONDITION	DESCRIPTION
thyroid	Hashimoto's thyroiditis	chronic inflammation of the thyroid gland with hypothyroidism; affects mostly women
	euthyroid goiter	enlarged thyroid gland caused by iodine deficiency; no evidence of hypothyroidism

GLAND	CONDITION	DESCRIPTION
pancreas	multiple endocrine neoplasia (MEN)	genetically based disorder characterized by hyperplasia, and benign and/or malignant growth of several endocrine glands
		Note: There are two primary types of MEN: MEN I—the most common type, it involves hyperplasia and benign growth of pancreatic islet cells, pituitary gland, and parathyroid gland.
		MEN II—involves carcinoma of the thyroid, with hyperplasia and benign growth of the adrenal medulla and parathyroids.

▶ 12.4 PHYSICAL EXAMINATION, DIAGNOSIS, AND TREATMENT

Laboratory Tests

Laboratory tests for diagnosis of endocrine disorders are summarized below. In addition to laboratory tests, **thyroid scans, thyroid sonograms,** and **radio-immunoassay tests** are used to diagnose endocrine disorders. These latter tests are described in Chapter 18. Summaries of some of the surgical procedures performed in treatment of endocrine disorders are found below.

GLAND	TESTS
pituitary gland	serum ACTH, serum FSH, blood GH, blood LH, serum calcium, and urine calcium measure the levels of these substances in blood and urine
thyroid gland	**thyroid function tests** include the free thyroxine index, thyroid stimulating hormone, T_3, T_4
	antithyroglobulin antibody: This test looks for the presence of antibodies in the blood that act against thyroglobulin, which is a protein found in inflammatory conditions of the thyroid and hypofunction of the thyroid.
	antimicrosomal antibody: This test checks for antibodies against microsomes (natural substance within the thyroid gland) and are found in the blood during inflammatory conditions of the thyroid and hypofunction of the thyroid.
	thyroid stimulating hormone (TSH): blood test measuring the amount of thyroid stimulating hormone in the blood

GLAND	TESTS
adrenal glands	The **urine** and **serum** are tested for **cortisol, epinephrine, norepinephrine, vanillylmandelic (văn-ĭl″-ĭl-măn-dĕl′-ĭk) acid (VMA), and homovanillic (hō″-mō-văn-ĭl′-ĭk) acid (HVA) levels** to detect hyperfunction and hypofunction of the adrenal glands. **Note:** Both VMA and HVA are end-products of neurotransmitter metabolism. Elevated levels may occur as a result of adrenal tumors.
parathyroid	**Serum calcitonin, serum calcium, urine calcium, blood parathormone, serum phosphorus,** and **urine phosphorus** tests measure the level of calcitonin, calcium, parathormone, and phosphorus in the serum and urine.
pancreas	Blood glucose levels are monitored with the following laboratory tests: **Fasting blood sugar (FBS)** measures blood glucose when the patient is fasting (refrain's from eating for 12–24 hours). **Glucose tolerance test (GTT)** monitors the effect of a measured dose of glucose for 3 to 5 hours. **Postprandial (PP) test** measures blood glucose following a meal.

Treatment Using Pharmacological Agents

TREATMENT	DESCRIPTION
adrenal corticosteroids	suppresses the body's response to inflammation by reducing pain, swelling, and heat; these drugs do not cure but may be used alone or with other drugs to reduce symptoms of allergic reactions, skin conditions and some respiratory disorders Examples include hydrocortisone (Cortef) and prednisone (Prednisone).
antidiabetic agents	
insulin	replacement therapy when the pancreas is unable to supply sufficient amounts of insulin to convert glucose to glycogen; used to treat patients with insulin dependent diabetes mellitus Insulin preparations are injected subcutaneously and can be categorized into rapid-acting, intermediate-acting and long-acting. Examples include Regular Insulin, Humulin R, rapid-acting; Isophane (NPH), Lente, Humulin N, Novolin N, intermediate-acting; and Protaminezine (PZI), Ultralente, and Humulin U, long-acting.

Treatment Using Pharmacological Agents (continued)

TREATMENT	DESCRIPTION
antidiabetic agents (continued)	
oral hypoglycemics	stimulates the secretion of insulin from the pancreas in noninsulin dependent diabetes mellitus; the pancreas is functioning but does not produce sufficient amounts of insulin to meet body demands
	Examples include chlorpropamide (Diabinase) and tolbutamide (Orinase).
antithyroid agents	stops the production of thyroid hormones by interfering with the use of iodine in the manufacture of thyroid hormones; the production of thyroxine or triiodothyronine is not directly affected
	Examples include Tapazole (methimazole) and Propylthiouracil (propylthiouracil).
thyroid agents	replacement therapy for underperforming thyroid glands; used to treat cretinism and myxedema
	Examples include natural thyroid and synthetic Synthyroid.

Surgical Procedures

PROCECURE	DESCRIPTION
adrenalectomy	removal of the adrenal gland
hypophysectomy	removal of the hypophysis (anterior pituitary gland)
lobectomy	excision of a lobe of the thyroid gland
parathyroidectomy	excision of the parathyroid gland
pinealectomy	removal of the pineal gland
thyroidectomy	removal of the thyroid gland

II–12

ACTH	adrenocorticotrophic hormone	**MEN**	multiple endocrine neoplasia
ADH	antidiuretic hormone (vasopressin)	**MRH**	melanocyte-releasing hormone
Ca	calcium	**Na**	sodium
CRH	corticotrophin-releasing hormone	**OT**	oxytocin
DI	diabetes insipidus	**PIH**	prolactin-inhibiting hormone
DKA	diabetic ketoacidosis	**PRH**	prolactin-releasing hormone
FSH	follicle-stimulating hormone	**PRL**	prolactin
GH	growth hormone	**PTH**	parathyroid hormone (parathormone)
GHIH	growth-hormone-inhibiting hormone	**RIA**	radioimmunoassay
GHRH	growth-hormone-releasing hormone	T_3	triiodothyronine
GnRH	gonadotrophin-releasing hormone	T_4	thyroxine
HVA	homovanillic acid	**TRH**	thyrotrophin-releasing hormone
LH	luteinizing hormone	**TSH**	thyroid-stimulating hormone
		VMA	vanillylmandelic acid

▶EXERCISE 12–1

Definitions

Definitions

Give the meaning of the following word parts.

Answers to all exercises in this chapter appear in Appendix A.

1. aden/o _____

2. cortic/o _____

3. diure/o _____

4. -crine _____

5. estr/o _____

6. kal/o _____

7. -dips/o _____

8. lact/o _____

9. oxy- _____

10. somat/o _____

Give the prefix, suffix, or word root for the following.

11. within _____

12. out _____

13. enlargement _____

14. good _____

15. calcium _____

16. extremities, top _____

17. male _____

18. childbirth _____

19. same _____

20. pituitary gland _____

21. sodium _____

22. all _____

23. woman _____

24. nourishment, stimulating _____

Write the terms that correspond with the following abbreviations.

25. GnRH _____

26. CRH _____

27. PIH _____

28. TSH _____

29. LH _____

30. PRL _____

31. ACTH _____

32. T_3 _____

33. DI _____

34. FSH _____

Give the alternate name of the following hormones. Include the abbreviation if applicable.

35. somatotrophin _____

36. triiodothyronine _____

37. cortisol _____

Word Building

Word Building

Build the medical term for the following.

1. excessive thirst _____

2. inflammation of the thyroid _____

3. stimulating the thyroid _____

4. quick birth _____

5. deficiency of all the pituitary hormones _____

6. deficient amounts of calcium in the blood _____

7. deficient amounts of potassium in the blood _____

8. normal thyroid _____

9. abnormal protrusion of the eye _____

10. study of the endocrine system _____

▶**EXERCISE 12–3**   **Practice Quiz**

Short Answer

Briefly answer the following.

1. Which of the central endocrine glands is located in a "mixed function" organ? _____

2. What is the difference between exocrine and endocrine glands? _____

_____

_____

3. What is the definition of a hormone? _____

_____

4. Name four peripheral endocrine glands that have no function other than the production of hormones. _____

_____

5. What is the hormone that stimulates uterine contractions during childbirth? _____Where is it produced?

_____

6. What hormones depend on the presence of dietary iodine for their production? _____

_____

7. Name the hormone produced by the thyroid that is not regulated by a releasing hormone. _____

8. Is aldosterone a mineralocorticoid or a glucocorticoid? _____

9. Describe the action of adrenaline when it is released by the chromaffin cells.

   _____

   How does this action differ from the action of adrenaline that is released by brain cells? _____

   _____

10. Which of the following are releasing hormones: corticotrophin, prolactin, estrogen, somatotrophin, cortisol, GHIH? _____

    _____

11. How is release of hormones from the anterior hypophysis regulated?

    _____

    What are the names of those hormones? _____

    _____

12. Where are hormones of the adenohypophysis produced? _____

    _____

II–12

▶EXERCISE 12–4

Matching Hormones with Glands

Matching

Match hormone in Column A with its gland in Column B. Some answers may be used more than once.

Column A		Column B
1. aldosterone	_____	A. adrenal medulla
2. epinephrine	_____	B. anterior pituitary
3. T$_4$	_____	C. parathyroid
4. calcitonin	_____	D. adenohypophysis
5. parathormone	_____	E. thyroid
6. oxytocin	_____	F. neurohypophysis
7. cortisol	_____	G. adrenal cortex
8. somatotrophin	_____	
9. ACTH	_____	

Spelling Practice

Spelling

Place a check mark beside all misspelled words in the following list. Correctly spell those that you checked off.

1. hypothalmus ☐ _____

2. somatrophin ☐ _____

3. pituitary ☐ _____

4. hypophysis ☐ _____

5. triodothyronine ☐ _____

6. mammary ☐ _____

7. endocrene ☐ _____

8. glucocortocoid ☐ _____

9. oxytocin ☐ _____

10. aldosterone ☐ _____

11. diabetis ☐ _____

12. lutenizing ☐ _____

► EXERCISE 12–6 **Use of Medical Terms in Context**

Medical Terms in Context

Define the underlined terms as they are used in context.

Medical Terminology used in Sentences

1. Two days following admission, the diagnosis of <u>adrenal insufficiency</u> was confirmed. Apparently <u>hypopituitarism</u> was ruled out.

2. Biochemical evaluations ruled out the presence of a <u>pheochromocytoma</u> and, because of the possibility of malignancy, the options were presented to the patient; she has requested to undergo surgery.

3. The patient was evaluated for left upper quadrant pain with an <u>ultrasound</u> followed by a <u>gastroscopy</u>. These investigations suggested the presence of an <u>adenoma</u> pressing on the stomach.

1. adrenal insufficiency _____

2. hypopituitarism _____

3. pheochromocytoma _____

4. ultrasound _____

5. gastroscopy _____

6. adenoma

Crossword Puzzle

The Endocrine System

Across

1 Deficiency of adrenal activity
2 Stimulates milk production in mammary gland
6 Slow mental and physical growth
8 Widening of bones
9 Excessive secretions of aldosterone

Down

1 Decrease in TSH
3 Regulates milk flow in mammary glands
4 Regulates blood calcium
5 Excessive skeletal growth
7 An excessive or spontaneous flow of milk

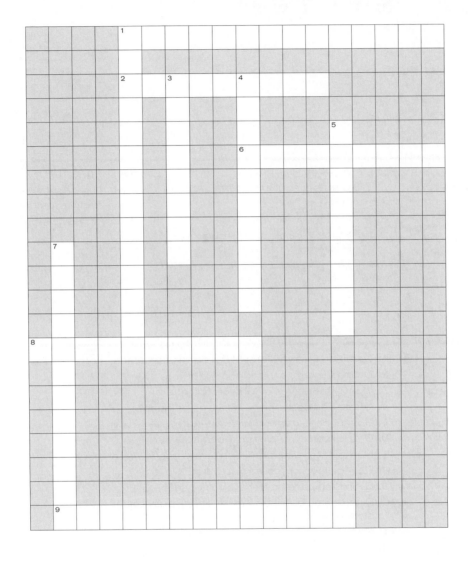

II–12

13 THE CARDIOVASCULAR SYSTEM

CHAPTER ORGANIZATION

This chapter has been designed to help the student learn terms and abbreviations that relate to the cardiovascular system.

CHAPTER OBJECTIVES

Upon successful completion of this chapter, the student will be able to do the following:

1. Describe the functions of the cardiovascular system.
2. Define the terms relating to the heart.
3. Identify the valves of the heart by reference to a diagram.
4. Name and describe the walls of the heart.
5. Describe the conduction system.
6. Define cardiac cycle and heart sounds.
7. Name and define common terms used in an electrocardiogram.
8. Define blood pressure and pulse.
9. Define terms related to blood vessels.
10. Differentiate between the coronary, pulmonary, and systemic circulation systems.
11. Name and locate the major arteries.
12. Name and locate the major veins.
13. Pronounce, analyze, define, and spell the terms relating to the cardiovascular system.
14. List and define terms describing abnormal conditions, the physical examination, diagnosis, and therapeutic procedures common to the cardiovascular system.
15. Define abbreviations common to the cardiovascular system.

ELEMENT	MEANING	ELEMENT	MEANING
angi/o; vas/o; vascul/o	vessel	phleb/o; ven/o	vein
aort/o	aorta	rhythm/o	rhythm
arteri/o	artery	sphygm/o	pulse
ather/o	fatty debris	thromb/o	clot
atri/o	atrium	valvul/o	valve
cardi/o	heart	ventricu/o	ventricle
myel/o	bone marrow		

▷ 13.1 COMPOSITION OF THE CARDIOVASCULAR SYSTEM

The human body contains approximately 75 trillion individual cells, all of which require a continuous supply of oxygen, heat, and nourishment. One might appreciate the complexity of the cardiovascular system by imagining a city with 75 trillion residents (15,000 times the current population of the earth), all of whom expect that food, water, and heat will be dispatched to their homes from a single, central location. Nevertheless, the cardiovascular system miraculously delivers the necessities of life to every cell in the body. The cardiovascular system has two parts: the heart and the circulatory system. The heart provides the mechanical energy to deliver blood, which carries oxygen and nutrients through vessels to all parts of the body.

▷ 13.2 HEART

The heart is a muscular organ located within the thoracic cavity, posterior to the sternum, left of the body's midline. Surrounded by a large, fluid-filled sac called the **pericardium** (pĕr″-ĭ-kăr′-dē-ŭm), the heart is connected to a number of major blood vessels, including the **aorta** (ā-ōr′-tă), the largest artery in the body, the inferior and superior **venae cavae** (vē′-nă kā′-vă), the largest veins of the body, and the **pulmonary veins and arteries**, which lead to and from the lungs (see Figure 13–1).

FIGURE 13–1   Structures of the Heart

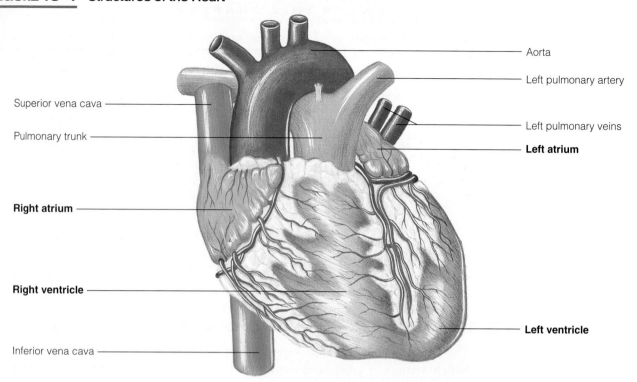

Superior vena cava

Pulmonary trunk

Right atrium

Right ventricle

Inferior vena cava

Aorta

Left pulmonary artery

Left pulmonary veins

Left atrium

Left ventricle

Chambers of the Heart

The heart is composed of four chambers: the right **atrium** (ā′-trē-ŭm), the left atrium, the right **ventricle** (vĕn′-trĭk-l), and the left ventricle. The two sides of the heart are separated by a wall called the **interventricular septum** (ĭn″-tĕr-vĕn-trĭk′-ū-lar sĕp′-tŭm) between the ventricles. The atria are separated by the **interatrial** (ĭn-tĕr-ā′-trē-ăl) **septum**.

   The right side of the heart pumps blood to the lungs, where the blood takes on oxygen. The left side of the heart pumps oxygenated blood to the tissues. Blood flows through the heart in only one direction. (See coronary circulation.)

Valves of the Heart

Two sets of valves in the heart keep the blood flowing in one direction. The **atrioventricular** (AV) **valves** are located between the atrium and the ventricle in each side of the heart. The atrioventricular valve on the right side of the heart is called the **tricuspid** (trī-kŭs′-pĭd) **valve** because it is made up of three triangular bits of tissue called cusps or flaps. The atrioventricular valve on the left side of the heart has only two cusps and is therefore called the **bicuspid** (bī-kŭs′-pĭd) **valve** or, often, the **mitral** (mī′-trăl) **valve** because it resembles a miter (a bishop's hat).

   The cusps of the atrioventricular valves are attached to the myocardium by strong, tough cords called **chordae tendineae**, which ensure that the cusps close tightly, thus preventing any backflow of blood.

The two **semilunar** valves, referred to as such because of the half moon shape of their parts, are located at the entry way to the aorta (the **aortic semilunar valve**) and the pulmonary trunk (the **pulmonary valve**). Figure 13–2 illustrates the interior of the heart, including the four chambers and the valves.

FIGURE 13–2 **The Interior of the Heart** (a) Cross-section of the heart showing the chambers, valves, septum, chordae tendineae, and vessels. (b) Photograph of chordae tendineae. (c) Superior view of valves. (d) Photograph of pulmonary semilunar valve.

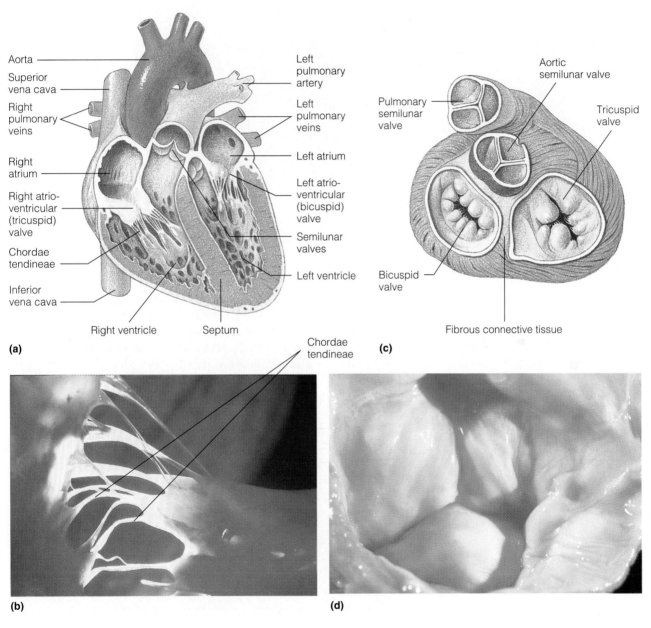

Walls of the Heart

The heart walls are made up of a thick layer of muscle tissue called the **myocardium** (mī″-ō-kar′-dē-ŭm) enclosed by two thin layers of epithelial tissue. The inside layer of epithelial tissue is called the **endocardium** (ĕn-dō-kăr′-dē-ŭm), and the outer layer is called the **epicardium** (ĕp″-ĭ-kăr′-dē-ŭm). See Figure 13–3.

FIGURE 13–3 The Walls of the Heart

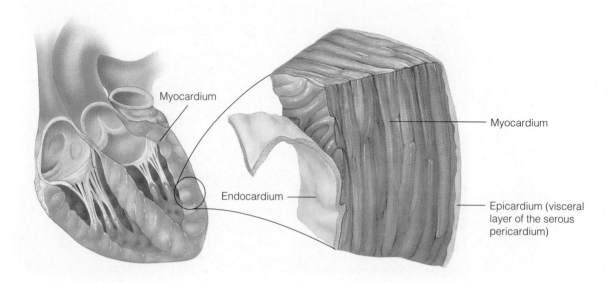

The pericardium surrounds the heart. It has two layers: the **parietal** layer, lining the pericardium; and the **visceral** layer, covering the heart. The visceral layer is the epicardium. Between the parietal and visceral layers is the pericardial cavity, which is filled with a minuscule quantity of pericardial fluid (see Figure 13–4).

FIGURE 13–4

Pericardium Visceral pericardium and parietal pericardium surround but do not enclose the heart. The pericardial cavity is filled with fluid.

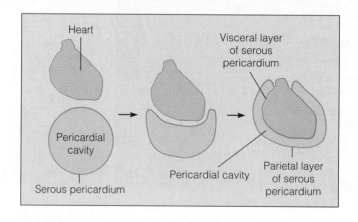

▶ 13.3 CONDUCTION SYSTEM

The heart has its own electrical system which can function independently. A network of muscle cells located within the heart initiates an electrical impulse that begins each heart beat. These electrical impulses spread throughout the heart causing it to contract. This specialized network of muscle cells, called the conduction system, (see Figure 13–5) includes the following structures:

sinoatrial node (SA node)
atrioventricular node (AV node)
atrioventricular bundle (AV bundle, or bundle of His)
right and left bundle branches
Purkinje (pŭr-kĭn′-jē) fibers

FIGURE 13–5

Conduction System of the Heart

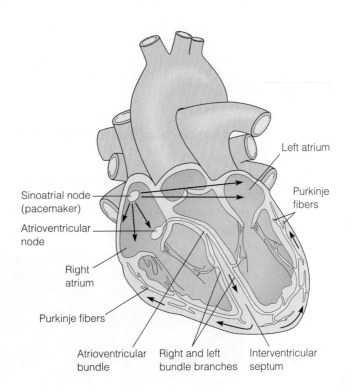

The **sinoatrial node** is located in the right atrial wall. The SA node is called the **pacemaker**, as it sets the heart's basic rhythm (75 to 100 times per minute). It does this by initiating an electrical impulse spontaneously. Once this heart action is initiated, the impulses travel to the **atrioventricular node**. The AV node, also located in the right atrium near the interatrial septum, receives the impulses from the SA node and causes the atria to contract.

The **Bundle of His,** or **AV bundle,** contains fibers that extend from the AV node into the interventricular septum. The bundle branches into smaller branches known as **Purkinje fibers,** which reach deep into the endocardium and produce a simultaneous contraction of the ventricles. The proper conduction of the electrical impulses from the SA node to the Purkinje fibers is called **normal sinus rhythm.**

Cardiac Cycle

The cardiac cycle represents one complete heart beat consisting of a contraction phase, called **systole** (sĭs′-tō-lē), and a relaxation phase called **diastole** (dī-ăs′-tō-lē). The heart beats rhythmically, meaning that the atria contract while the ventricles relax and that the ventricles contract while the atria relax. In this way, both sides of the heart work together to maintain a rhythm.

When the atria contract, blood is pumped into the ventricles through the cuspid valves. When the ventricles contract, the blood from the right ventricle is pumped through the pulmonary artery into the lungs, and the blood from the left ventricle is pumped through the aorta to the body tissues. The amount of blood expelled from the ventricles is the **cardiac output**.

Heart Sounds

Each heart beat consists of two heart sounds created by closure of the valves. The first is recognized by a **"lupp"** sound, the second by a **"dubb"** sound. The "lupp" sound represents the closing of the atrioventricular valves, the first heart sound (S$_1$); the "dubb" sound represents the closing of the semilunar valves, the second heart sound (S$_2$). A complete cardiac cycle consists of a "lupp-dubb" sound. The sound of blood flowing turbulently across the valves is known as a **murmur**.

Electrocardiogram (ECG, EKG)

An ECG (EKG in some countries) is a diagnostic measurement of the electrical activity of the heart. The minute electric currents produced by the heart can be detected by an instrument called an electrocardiograph which records the currents as waves. Different waves, produced by different portions of the cardiac cycle, are named and can be studied in an ECG (see Figure 13–6).

FIGURE 13–6

Electrocardiogram Showing P Waves, QRS Wave, T Wave; P-R interval and S-T interval
Stress test. (a) The heart's function is monitored during exercise. (b) An electrocardiogram.

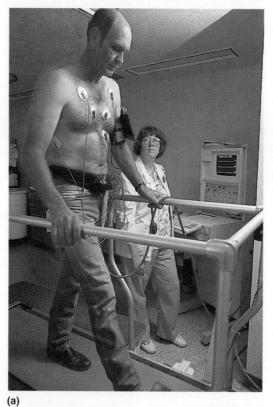

(a)

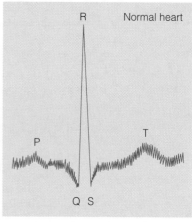

P = strength of atrial contraction.

QRS = strength of ventricular contraction.

T = resting state of ventricles.

P - R interval = time required for impulses to travel from SA node to Purkinje fibres.

(b)

A normal ECG consists of **P waves**, **QRS waves**, **T waves**, a **P-R interval** and an **S-T interval**. The P wave corresponds to the atrial contraction, the QRS corresponds to the ventricular contraction, and the T wave signifies the repolarization of the ventricles. The P-R interval is a measurement of the period of time that impulses take to reach the Purkinje fibers from the SA and AV nodes. The S-T interval is the period of time between ventricular contractions.

13.4 BLOOD VESSELS AND CIRCULATORY ROUTES

Blood vessels are classified as **arteries** (ăr-tĕr′-ĭz), **arterioles** (ar-tē′-rĭ-ōlz), **veins** (vān), **venules** (vĕn′-ūl), and **capillaries** (kăp′-i-lā-rēz). As we have already seen, blood flows from the heart into the arteries and back to the heart through the veins. Arterioles are small arteries that supply capillaries, the connecting vessels between arteries and veins. Venules are small veins. Capillaries serve as the delivery and collection vessels between the bloodstream and the body's cells.

All arteries lead from the heart and, except for the pulmonary artery, contain oxygenated blood. All veins lead to the heart and, except for the pulmonary veins, contain deoxygenated blood.

The walls of arteries and veins comprise three layers: the **tunica intima** (tū-nĭ′-kă ĭn′-tĭ-mă), which is the innermost layer made up of endothelium (a type of epithelium); the **tunica media**, the middle layer made up of muscle; and the **tunica adventitia** (ăd″-vĕn-tĭsh′-ē-ă), the outermost layer made up of connective tissue. Capillary walls are composed only of endothelium. See Figure 13–7.

FIGURE 13–7 The Three Layers of Arteries and Veins

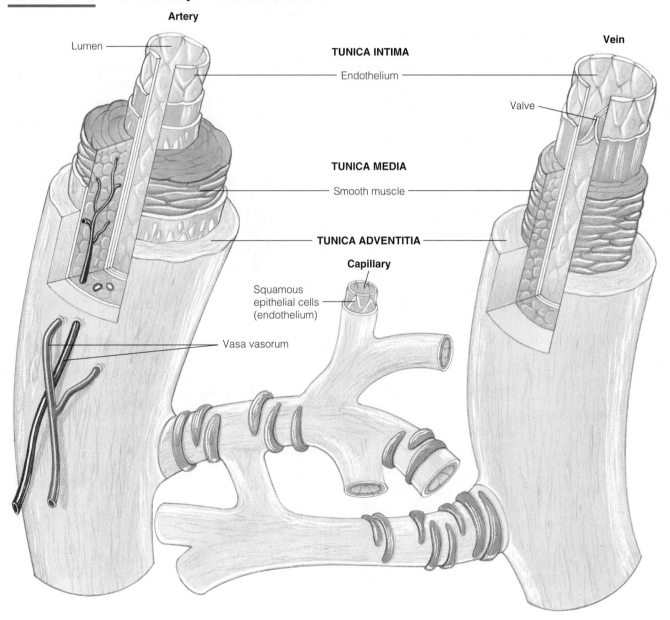

Artery

Lumen

TUNICA INTIMA

Endothelium

Vein

Valve

TUNICA MEDIA

Smooth muscle

TUNICA ADVENTITIA

Capillary

Squamous
epithelial cells
(endothelium)

Vasa vasorum

Arteries have more elastic and muscular tissue than veins or capillaries. Both these tissue types aid in **vasoconstriction**, whereby the lumen, or hollow center, of the artery is made smaller, and in **vasodilation**, whereby the lumen is made larger.

Veins have less elastic and muscular tissue. Because they return blood to the heart, in some cases against gravity, veins have valves within the lumen that help to prevent backflow.

As previously mentioned, capillaries are composed only of the lining of the endothelium. This single-layer allows for easy exchange of nutrients and waste products within the organ.

Blood vessels are sometimes connected in a junction called an **anastomosis** (ă-năs″-tō-mō′-sis), which provides for an alternate path for blood flow around a damaged or blocked area.

Blood Pressure

Blood pressure is a measure of the pressure exerted on the arterial walls during the contraction (systolic) phase and the relaxation (diastolic) phase of the cardiac cycle. It is numerically expressed as a fraction such as 120/80. The first number represents the pressure on the blood vessel wall when the ventricles contract (**systolic pressure**). The second number represents the pressure on the blood vessel wall when the ventricles relax (**diastolic pressure**). Blood pressure is measured by a **sphygmomanometer** (sfĭg″-mō-măn-ŏm′-ĕ-tĕr) (see Figure 13–8). Normal range is approximately 100/60 to 120/80. Blood pressure above the normal range is called **hypertension**. Blood pressure below the normal range is called **hypotension**.

FIGURE 13–8

Sphygmomanometer for Blood Pressure Readings

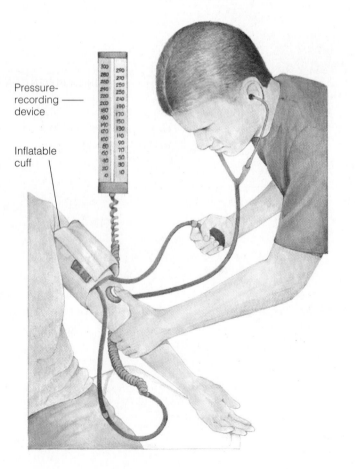

Pressure-recording device

Inflatable cuff

Pulse

The atrial walls dilate and contract in unison with the heartbeat. These movements can be readily detected at certain sites and counted for ascertaining heart rate. Pulses can be felt at the following sites: brachial, temporal, carotid, radial, femoral, popliteal, and dorsalis pedis.

Coronary Circulation

Blood flows through the heart in the following pattern: It goes from the superior and inferior venae cavae to the **right atrium** and then through the **tricuspid valve** into the **right ventricle**. Contraction of the right ventricle pushes the blood into the pulmonary artery to the lungs (see pulmonary circulation, below). From the lungs, the blood returns to the **left atrium** and then through the **mitral valve** into the **left ventricle**. It is then pumped through the **aortic valve** and into the aorta and out to the individual body organs (see Figure 13–9).

FIGURE 13–9 **Coronary and Pulmonary Circulation**

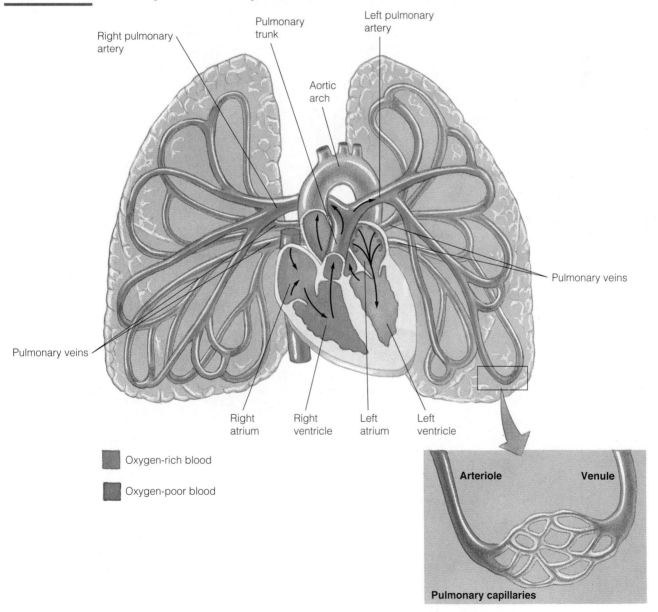

Pulmonary Circulation

The body's cells require oxygen for sustenance. The heart therefore directs **deoxygenated** blood through the lungs so that it can become oxygenated. The path of this circulation begins at the right ventricle of the heart, continues through the pulmonary valve, through the pulmonary trunk, and through the pulmonary arteries to the lungs. In the lungs, carbon dioxide is exchanged for oxygen. The oxygenated blood reenters the heart at the left atrium via the pulmonary veins. See Figure 13–9 and Figure 13–10.

FIGURE 13–10

Schematic Drawing of
Pulmonary and Systemic
Circulations

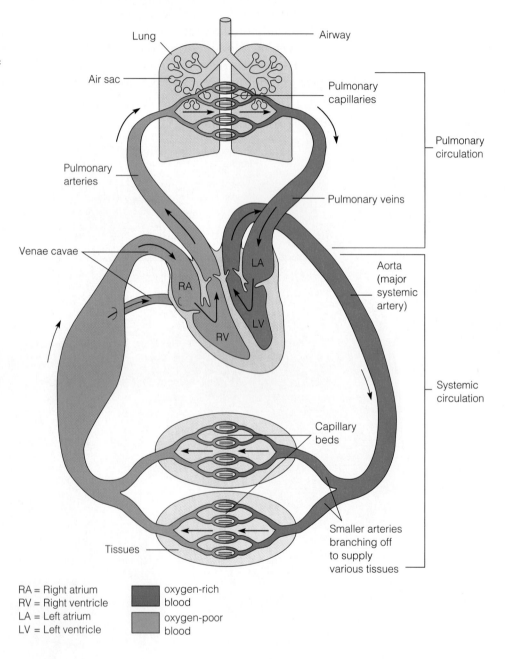

RA = Right atrium
RV = Right ventricle
LA = Left atrium
LV = Left ventricle

oxygen-rich blood

oxygen-poor blood

Systemic Circulation

Systemic Arteries The systemic circulation begins at the aorta, which is connected to the left ventricle of the heart. The aorta conveys blood to all the other arteries, which subsequently branch into arterioles. Figure 13–11 shows the arteries and the areas of the body they serve.

FIGURE 13–11 The Major Arteries of the Systemic Circulation

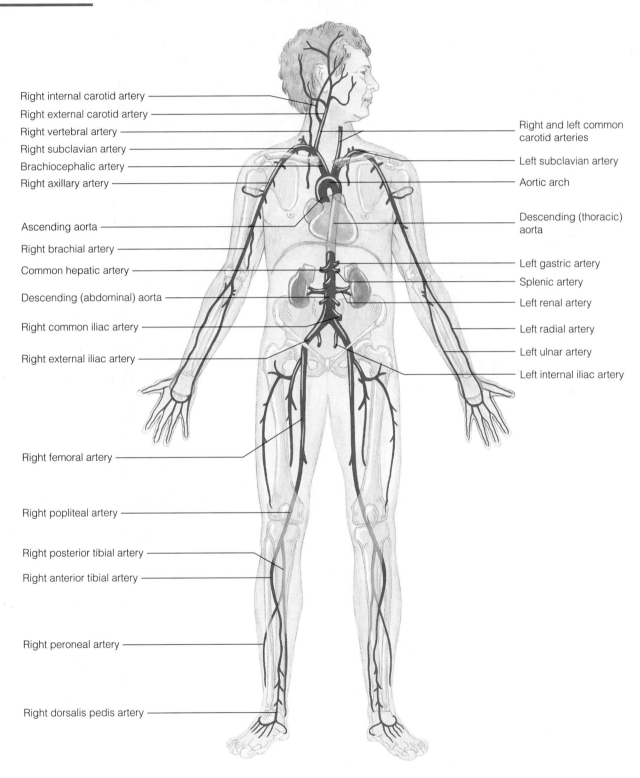

Right internal carotid artery

Right external carotid artery

Right vertebral artery

Right subclavian artery

Brachiocephalic artery

Right axillary artery

Ascending aorta

Right brachial artery

Common hepatic artery

Descending (abdominal) aorta

Right common iliac artery

Right external iliac artery

Right femoral artery

Right popliteal artery

Right posterior tibial artery

Right anterior tibial artery

Right peroneal artery

Right dorsalis pedis artery

Right and left common carotid arteries

Left subclavian artery

Aortic arch

Descending (thoracic) aorta

Left gastric artery

Splenic artery

Left renal artery

Left radial artery

Left ulnar artery

Left internal iliac artery

Systemic Veins Blood flows from the capillaries into venules and from venules into veins, eventually flowing through either the superior or inferior vena cava into the right atrium of the heart. Figure 13–12 shows the major veins.

FIGURE 13–12 Major Veins of the Body

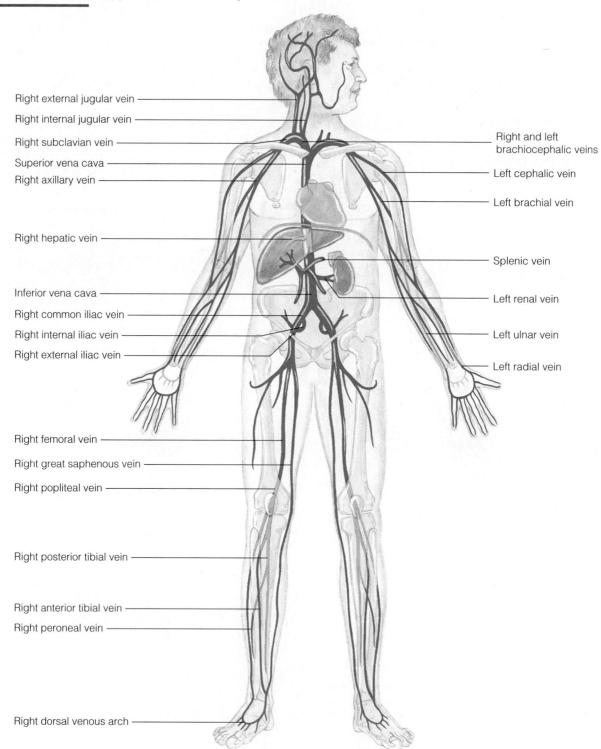

Right external jugular vein

Right internal jugular vein

Right subclavian vein

Superior vena cava

Right axillary vein

Right hepatic vein

Inferior vena cava

Right common iliac vein

Right internal iliac vein

Right external iliac vein

Right femoral vein

Right great saphenous vein

Right popliteal vein

Right posterior tibial vein

Right anterior tibial vein

Right peroneal vein

Right dorsal venous arch

Right and left brachiocephalic veins

Left cephalic vein

Left brachial vein

Splenic vein

Left renal vein

Left ulnar vein

Left radial vein

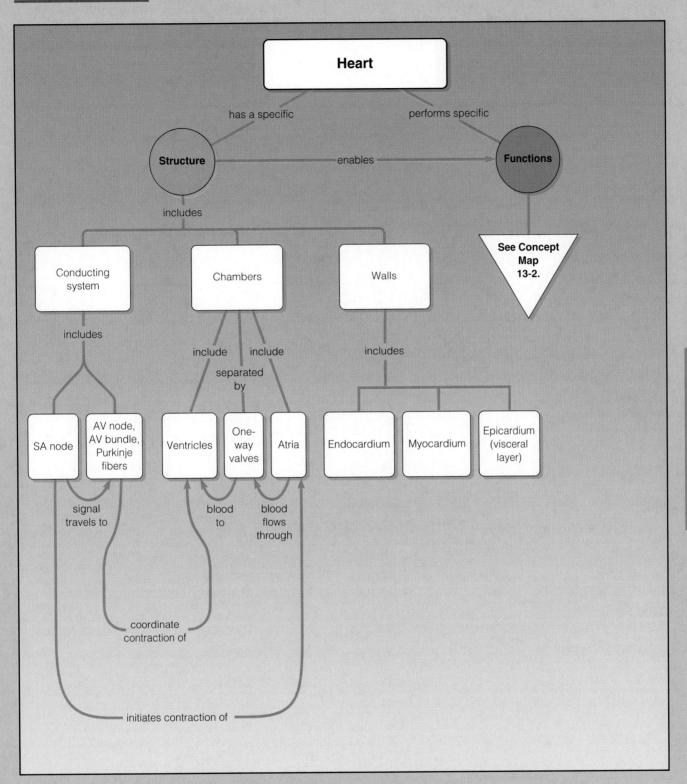

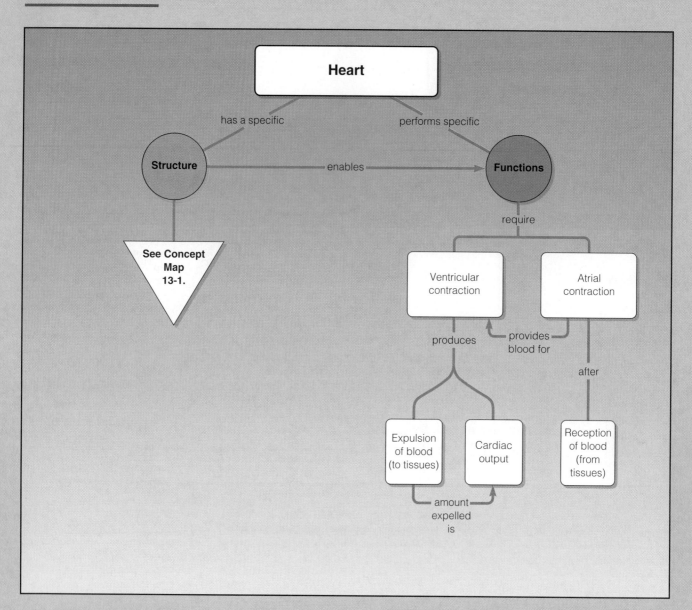

Heart

TERM WITH PRONUNCIATION	ANALYSIS	DEFINITION
arrhythmia ă-rĭth′-mē-ă	-ia = state of; condition a- = no; not rhythm/o = rhythm; steady beat	deviation from the normal heart rhythm **Note:** Double the "r" when spelling arrhythmia.
bradycardia brăd″-ē-kăr′-dē-ă	-ia = state of; condition brady- = slow card/i/o = heart	condition of a slow heart **Note:** In this application, both the "i" and "o" are dropped from card/i/o.
coronary kōr′-ō-nă-rē	-ary = pertaining to coron/o = crown	pertaining to the crown **Note:** The blood vessels that supply the heart sit on the heart like a crown.
electrocardiography ē-lĕk″-trō-kăr-dē-ŏ′-grăf-ē	-graphy = process of recording electr/o = electric card/i/o = heart	process of recording the electrical activity of the heart
epicardial ĕp″-ĭ-kărd′-ē-ăl	-al = pertaining to epi- = upon; above card/i/o = heart	pertaining to the epicardium
interatrial septum ĭn″-tĕr-ā′-trē-ăl sĕp′-tŭm	-al = pertaining to inter- = between atri/o = atrium	pertaining to the wall between the atria **Note:** Septum means wall.
myocardiorrhaphy mī″-ō-kărd″-ē-ōr′-ă-fē	-rrhaphy = suture my/o = muscle card/i/o = heart	suture of the muscular layer of the heart
pancarditis păn-kăr-dī′-tĭs	-itis = inflammation pan- = all card/i/o = heart	inflammation of all the heart layers, including the epicardium, myocardium, and endocardium
pericarditis pĕr″-ĭ-kăr-dī′-tĭs	-itis = inflammation peri- = around card/i/o = heart	inflammation of the pericardium
tachycardia tăk″-ē-kăr′-dē-ă	-ia = state of; condition tachy- = fast card/i/o = heart	condition of a fast heartbeat of usually greater than 100 beats per minute
valvuloplasty văl′-vū-lō-plăs″-tē	-plasty = surgical repair; surgical reconstruction valvul/o = valve	surgical repair of a valve

II—13

Blood Vessels

TERM WITH PRONUNCIATION	ANALYSIS	DEFINITION
angiectasis ăn″-jē-ĕk′-tă-sĭs	-ectasis = dilatation; stretching angi/o = vessel	dilatation of a blood vessel; vasodilatation
angiospasm ăn′-jē-ō-spăzm	-spasm = sudden, involuntary, violent contraction angi/o = vessel	sudden, involuntary, violent contraction of a blood vessel (synonymous with vasospasm)
aortostenosis ā-ōr″-tō-stĕn-ō′-sĭs	-stenosis = narrowing; stricture aort/o = aorta	narrowing of the aorta
arteriography ăr″-tē-rē-ŏg′-ră-fē	-graphy = process of recording; x-ray arteri/o = artery	x-ray of the arteries
arteriole ăr-tē′-rē-ōl	-ole = small arteri/o = artery	small artery
arteriosclerosis ăr-tē″-rē-ō-sklĕ-rō′-sĭs	-sclerosis = hardening arteri/o = artery	hardening of an artery
atherosclerosis ăth″-ĕr-ō-sklĕ-rō′-sĭs	-sclerosis = hardening ather/o = fatty debris	accumulation of fatty debris on the tunica intima of an artery
extravasation ĕks-trăv″-ă-sā′-shŭn	-ion = process extra- = outside vas/o = vessel	escape of fluid, such as blood, from a blood vessel
ischemia ĭs-kē′-mē-ă	-emia = blood condition isch/o = hold back	holding back of blood to a part
phlebothrombosis flĕb″-ō-thrŏm-bō′-sĭs	-osis = abnormal condition phleb/o = vein thromb/o = clot	abnormal condition of clots in a vein
thrombophlebitis thrŏm″-bō-flĕ-bī′-tĭs	-itis = inflammation thromb/o = clot phleb/o = vein	inflammation of a vein with clot formation
vascular văs′-kū-lăr	-ar = pertaining to vascul/o = vessel	pertaining to a vessel
vasoconstriction văs″-ō-kŏn-strĭk′-shŭn	-ion = process vas/o = vessel constrict/o = to draw together	process of drawing together the walls of a vessel; narrowing of the lumen of a vessel
vasodilation văs″-ō-dī-lā′-shŭn	-ion = process vas/o = vessel dilat/o = to expand	process of vessel expansion; widening of the lumen

TERM WITH PRONUNCIATION	ANALYSIS	DEFINITION
vasospasm văs′-ō-spăzm	-spasm = sudden, involuntary, violent contraction vas/o = vessel	sudden, involuntary, violent contraction of a vessel; vasoconstriction
venous vē′-nŭs	-ous = pertaining to ven/o = vein	pertaining to a vein

⬥ 13.6 ABNORMAL CONDITIONS

VASCULAR DISEASE	DESCRIPTION
aneurysm	abnormal bulging of the arterial wall **Note:** May be **fusiform**, where both sides of the artery expand; **saccular**, where one side of the artery dilates; or **dissecting**, where the blood seeps between the layers of the blood vessel. A burst aneurysm in the brain causes a **cerebrovascular accident**, commonly known as a stroke.

VASCULAR DISEASE	DESCRIPTION
coronary artery disease (CAD)	loss of oxygen and nutrients to the heart muscle caused by diminished blood flow through the coronary arteries

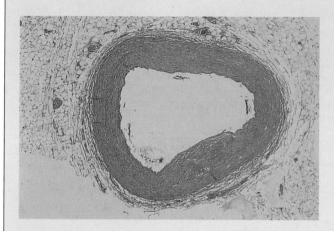 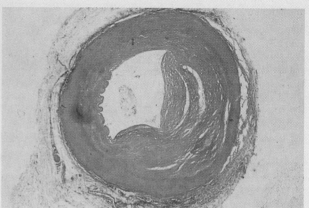

Note: Etiology includes atherosclerosis, in which fatty deposits (**atheroma**) gradually narrow the coronary artery lumen. Blood flow through the vessel is reduced resulting in **myocardial ischemia**.

Other coronary artery diseases that cause ischemia include a **thrombus** (thrŏm′-bŭs), an accumulation of blood components on the wall of a vessel; and an **embolus** (ĕm′-bō-lŭs), a blockage of a blood vessel from a foreign substance or blood clot. Emboli tend to move through the arterial system and can be fatal if an embolism becomes lodged in an artery leading to a major organ such as the heart or lungs.

Diagnostic investigations include electrocardiograms, coronary angiography, and radionuclide scanning with thallium.

Treatment includes nitroglycerin, angioplasty, and bypass surgery (all of these treatments are discussed later in this chapter).

hemorrhoids	persistent dilation of the veins in the rectum and anal region, caused by increased venous pressure
peripheral vascular disease	impairment of circulation in the extremities, caused by obstruction of the arterial lumen
Raynaud's disease (rā-nōz′)	disease of peripheral vascular system, characterized by spasmodic contraction of the arterioles of the fingers and toes in response to cold, cutting off circulation to these areas; more common in women than in men
cerebrovascular disease; stroke; cerebrovascular accident (CVA)	disturbance in the flow of blood to one or more parts of the brain

Note: With the loss of oxygen to parts of the brain, there is necrosis of nerve tissue. Disabilities depend on the part of the brain affected, but loss of speech and hemiplegia are common.

Types of cerebrovascular diseases include **hemorrhagic**, caused by bleeding into the brain, and **ischemic**, caused by occlusion of the blood vessel by a thrombus or embolus.

Diagnosis is made by computed tomography, brain scan, and a variety of laboratory and x-ray procedures. Included are angiography, electroencephalogram, and lumbar puncture (these are discussed later).

Improvement of cerebral circulation, which is of prime importance in treating CVA, is done by removing the embolus or thrombus, by repairing the aneurysm, or by bypass surgery (see under surgical treatment).

VASCULAR DISEASE	DESCRIPTION
transient ischemic attacks (TIA)	"little strokes"; temporary cessation of blood flow to a part of the brain, resulting in neurologic anomalies that may last from a few seconds to a number of hours
varicose veins	dilation of superficial veins, typically of the leg and usually of the saphenous vein
	Note: Results when incompetent valves fail to push the blood forward, causing backflow of blood. Veins become dilated and blood stagnates, creating unsightly clusters of protruding veins.

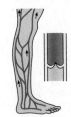

Valve closes, pushing the venous blood toward the heart.

Valves remain open, pooling the blood in the veins.

(a) Normal veins   **(b) Varicose veins**

DISORDERS OF THE HEART VALVE	DESCRIPTION
mitral valve stenosis	narrowing of the mitral valve, preventing the flow of blood through the heart
mitral valve incompetence; mitral valve insufficiency; mitral valve regurgitation	inability of the mitral valve to close tightly, resulting in a backflow of blood

ISCHEMIC HEART DISEASE	DESCRIPTION
myocardial infarction (MI)	**necrosis** of cardiac muscle tissue caused by ischemia of the heart muscle

Note: Primary symptom is **angina pectoris** (see under symptoms).

Diagnosis is by ECG, cardiac enzyme studies, echocardiography, and cardiac scans.

Treatment includes bed rest, angioplasty, bypass surgery, and drugs. Typical drugs used are **streptokinase** or **tissue plasminogen activator (TPA)**, thrombolytic agents used in the early stages of MI to dissolve the already present thrombus and restore blood flow to the heart muscle; **digoxin**, used to improve the strength of cardiac contractions; and **Inderal**, which reduces cardiac output, thereby reducing the stress on the heart.

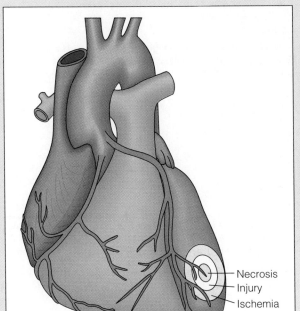

— Necrosis
— Injury
— Ischemia

II–13

HEART FAILURE	DESCRIPTION
congestive heart failure (CHF)	myocardial disease results in the failure of the heart to pump blood effectively through the blood vessels, resulting in congestion of the vascular system
	Note: The cause of heart failure may be valvular incompetence or damage to the left ventricle. The heart tries to compensate for its ineffectiveness by enlarging (**hypertrophy**) and pumping faster (**tachycardia**).
	These compensatory factors last for a while but, eventually, the heart again becomes unable to pump blood to the tissues. Blood backs up into the pulmonary system, causing respiratory difficulties.

DISORDERS OF THE CONDUCTION SYSTEM	DESCRIPTION
arrhythmia	abnormal rhythm of the heart beat
	Note: Examples include **fibrillation**, a very fast, irregular, uncoordinated heart beat, approximately 300–400 beats/minute, and **flutter**, a very fast, regular heart beat, approximately 160–250 beats/minute. Fibrillations and flutter can involve the atria and/or the ventricles.
cardiac arrest	sudden stoppage of the heart, usually caused by cardiac arrhythmia
heart block	interruption of the electrical impulses through the conduction system, resulting in failure of myocardial contractions
	Note: This condition is often idiopathic, although heart disease such as myocardial infarction or cardiomyopathy may be the cause.
	Types include **right bundle branch block (RBBB)** and **left bundle branch block (LBBB)**.
	Certain types are treated by the insertion of a pacemaker.

HYPERTENSIVE DISEASE	DESCRIPTION
hypertension	persistent, elevated blood pressure (greater than 140/90)
	Note: Two types of hypertension include **primary** (also known as **essential** or **idiopathic**), for which the cause is unknown; and **secondary**, which is caused by any number of conditions, including renal disease, peripheral vascular disease, and coronary artery disease, such as arteriosclerosis and atherosclerosis.
	Hypertension can also be described as **benign**, meaning that the onset is gradual and the duration prolonged; or **malignant**, meaning that the onset is abrupt and the duration short.
	If untreated, hypertension will affect the blood vessels of the brain and the kidney, producing strokes or kidney failure.
hypertensive heart disease (HHD)	heart disease secondary to hypertension

RHEUMATIC FEVER AND RHEUMATIC HEART DISEASE	DESCRIPTION
rheumatic fever	complication of a streptococcal infection causing inflammatory lesions primarily affecting the joints (arthritis) and the heart (carditis)
	Note: Usually occurs in children. Carditis or pancarditis is referred to as **rheumatic heart disease** and may lead to permanent dysfunction of the heart, particularly valvular insufficiency.

Inspection and **palpation** of the heart (abnormal vibration) may disclose **abnormal pulsations, extra heart sounds,** or **thrills.** Abnormal pulsations can be felt at different pulse points throughout the body (Figure 13–13). The **temporal** pulse is located on the temporal bone; the **brachial** pulse is located between the triceps and biceps muscles; the **radial pulse** is on the dorsum of the foot; the **popliteal pulse** is felt behind the knee; the **femoral pulse** is felt at the groin area; the **carotid pulse** is felt in the neck.

FIGURE 13–13

Peripheral Pulses

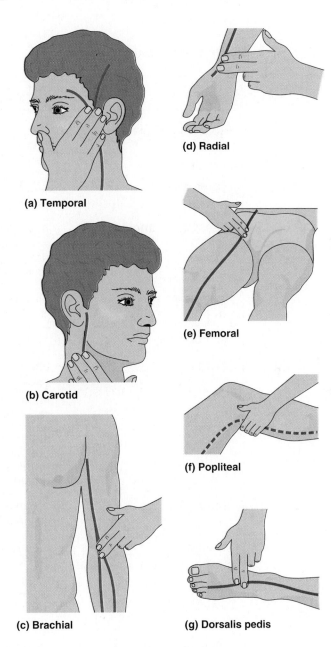

(a) Temporal

(b) Carotid

(c) Brachial

(d) Radial

(e) Femoral

(f) Popliteal

(g) Dorsalis pedis

Thrills are loud, vibratory sounds over the heart and may indicate an incompetent heart valve or stenosis of the pulmonary or aortic vessels.

Auscultation involves the use of a stethoscope for discerning whether the heart beat is normal or abnormal. The health care practitioner will listen for the S_1 and S_2. Abnormal sounds heard in auscultation are often referred to as **adventitious sounds** or **bruit** (brū'-ē). An example of an adventitious sound is the **murmur,** a blowing sound indicative of abnormal blood flow.

Percussion or **tapping** the area above the heart gives information on the size and position of the heart.

Signs and Symptoms

SIGN	DESCRIPTION
abnormal heart sounds	heart sounds other than the normal ones heard on closing of the cuspid and semilunar valves respectively; include **murmurs** and **bruits**
cardiomegaly	enlarged heart, particularly hypertrophied left ventricle
chest pain; angina	pain usually occurring in the epigastric area, which may or may not radiate down the left arm; can be substernal, retrosternal, or crushing
cyanosis	bluish discoloration of skin due to a reduction in oxygen to the tissues
diaphoresis	profuse sweating; feeling cool or clammy
dyspnea	difficulty in breathing; shortness of breath (SOB) Note: Various types include **exertional dyspnea**, where breathing becomes labored after moderate exercise; **orthopnea**, where the patient can breathe only when sitting up in bed; **paroxysmal nocturnal dyspnea**, which involves sudden attacks of difficult breathing occuring during the night.
edema	accumulation of excess fluid in the body tissues
effusion	the movement of fluid from the blood vessel into a part or tissue Note: **Hemopericardium** is the escape of blood into the pericardial space; **pericardial effusion** is the escape of fluid other than blood into the pericardial space.
hypertension	blood pressure higher than 140/90
intermittent claudication	pain in a limb, especially the leg, upon walking and the disappearance of the pain upon rest; seen in deep vein thrombosis
palpitations	unusually rapid heart beats of which the patient is consciously aware

SIGN	DESCRIPTION
pericardial tamponade	compression of the heart as a result of accumulation of fluid around the heart
purpura (ecchymoses, petechiae)	bleeding into the skin and mucous membrane
syncope	fainting

Laboratory Tests

PROCEDURE	DESCRIPTION
cardiac enzymes/ isoenzymes, blood	enzymes from the heart are released into the bloodstream following damage to the myocardium
	Note: High levels of these enzymes in the blood are good indicators of myocardial infarction.
	High levels of these enzymes do not signify cardiac dysfunction exclusively.
	AST, ALT, and LDH, for example, are elevated in certain liver dysfunctions. GGT levels are high in alcoholism and some urinary dysfunction. Important enzymes include: creatine kinase (CK), asparate, transaminase (AST, previously SGOT), alanine transaminase (ALT, previously SGPT), lactic dehydrogenase (LDH).

Radiology

PROCEDURE	DESCRIPTION
angiography	x-ray of the blood vessels following injection of a contrast medium
	Note: Often named after the structure being examined. For example **cardioangiography** is an x-ray of the vessels of the heart; **cerebroangiography** is an x-ray of the vessels of the brain.
digital subtraction angiography (DSA)	x-ray of the blood vessels utilizing intravenous contrast medium
	Note: Bone and soft tissue are deleted from the image by computer, allowing better examination of the vessels.
posteroanterior/lateral chest x-ray	See medical imaging, Chapter 18.
thallium scan	Following injection of thallium-201, a scan is obtained showing normal myocardial tissue taking up thallium, and diseased or necrosed tissue not taking up thallium.

II-13

Invasive Diagnostic Clinical Procedures

PROCEDURE	DESCRIPTION
cardiac catheterization	insertion of a catheter into a vein, sliding it upwards into the heart to obtain diagnostic information such as cardiac output, levels of oxygen and carbon dioxide, pressures inside the atria and ventricles, and valvular, arterial, and myocardial disease

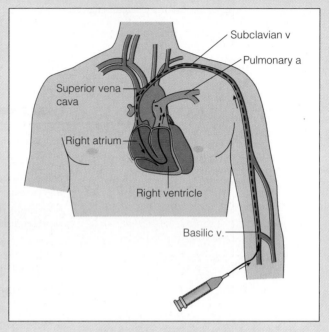

Subclavian v

Pulmonary a

Superior vena cava

Right atrium

Right ventricle

Basilic v.

Note: Angiocardiography is performed simultaneously to monitor the placement of the catheter as it is maneuvered into the heart.

electrophysiologic study (EPS)	used in the diagnosis of conduction system disorders; a catheter is used to insert intracardiac electrodes that stimulate the heart electrically to trigger the dysrhythmia that needs to be studied

Noninvasive Diagnostic Clinical Procedures

PROCEDURE	DESCRIPTION
stress test; exercise test	tests the heart's ability to adequately function when the patient is performing some type of physical exercise, usually walking on a treadmill or riding a stationary bike **Note:** The patient is simultaneously connected to an electrocardiographic device that monitors the heart's ability to function under stress.
telemetry	electronic device monitors heart function and rhythm, providing visual and audible record of the heartbeat
echocardiogram	high frequency sound waves are used to obtain an image of the anatomical structures of the heart and of the blood flow through the cardiovascular system; measures the strength of left ventricular contraction

PROCEDURE	DESCRIPTION
electrocardiogram (ECG; EKG)	See description earlier in this chapter.
Holter recording (monitor)	a miniature, portable electrocardiographic device that the patient wears for a 24–48 hour period to monitor the action of the heart as the patient goes through a normal daily routine

Treatment

Therapeutic Clinical Procedures

TREATMENT	DESCRIPTION
angioplasty	technique for increasing blood flow through a stenosed or blocked vessel by eliminating the plaque that has built up on the blood vessel wall
	Note: It is possible to obtain direct x-ray information of the procedure by angiography, which monitors the surgical instrument (catheter) as it is inserted into and maneuvered through a blood vessel to the site of occlusion. This procedure has been used as an alternative to coronary bypass surgery.
percutaneous transluminal coronary angioplasty (PTCA)	a balloon-tipped catheter, filled with water, placed into a stenotic vessel percutaneously and into the lumen of the blood vessel

Catheter threaded through the subclavian artery into the coronary artery

Balloon positioned in right coronary artery

(a)

(b) Balloon-tipped catheter in position.

(c) Balloon is inflated.

(d) The plaque is flattened against arterial wall.

(e) Previously obstructed artery is cleared.

Note: The balloon is inflated, flattening the plaque against the vessel wall and dilating the obstructed artery.

II–13

Therapeutic Clinical Procedures (continued)

TREATMENT	DESCRIPTION
laser angioplasty	a catheter equipped with a laser placed into the lumen of the stenosed or obstructed coronary artery
	Note: A light beam from the laser travels to the diseased site and vaporizes the fatty plaque.
valve angioplasty	a balloon-tipped catheter placed inside a stenosed valve
direct coronary atherectomy	a catheter equipped with a cutting device placed into the lumen of a stenosed or obstructed coronary artery
	Note: The catheter is activated and moved slowly forward. It shaves off the plaque and draws it into the tip of the catheter for removal.
centesis	surgical puncture of a cavity or space to remove fluid
	Note: Surgical puncture of the pericardial cavity to remove fluid is known as **pericardial centesis**.
defibrillation; cardioversion	the process of counteracting a fibrillating heart muscle by using an apparatus called a defibrillator

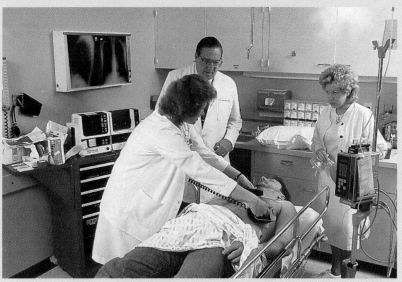

Note: An electric shock is applied to the heart muscle by placing the defibrillator on top of the chest wall. This electrical current momentarily stops the heart action so that the SA node can reestablish normal heart rhythm.

When a patient has dysrhythmias that are life threatening, such as ventricular tachycardia or fibrillation, an **automatic implantable cardioverter-defibrillator (AICD)** is placed directly into the heart to neutralize a fibrillating heart muscle.

| intra-aortic balloon pump (IABP) | a mechanical device implanted in the aorta that increases blood flow to the coronary arteries at the same time as it reduces ventricular workload |

Therapeutic Clinical Procedures (continued)

TREATMENT	DESCRIPTION
sclerotherapy	treatment for varicose veins requiring no hospital stay or anesthetic
	Note: A liquid solution is injected directly into a blood-free vein. The irritating solution causes fibrosis and hardening of the vein, resulting in obliteration of the vein due to adherence of the vessel walls to each other. The blood is then detoured through alternate veins.

Surgical Treatment

TREATMENT	DESCRIPTION
aortic root replacement	after excision of an aortic aneursym a tubular graft replaces the diseased portion
coronary artery bypass graft (CABG)	performed to reestablish adequate circulation to one or more segments of the heart when coronary artery disease diminishes blood flow

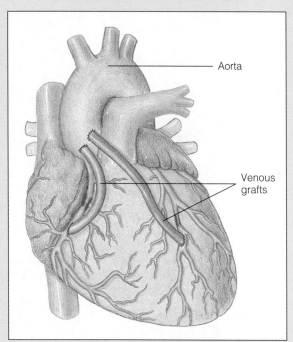

Aorta

Venous grafts

Note: A section of a vein is taken from another location, often the saphenous vein of the leg. The vein is reversed, so that the valves do not interfere with circulation, and attached from the aorta to below the blockage (anastomosis), rerouting the blood around the obstruction and restoring blood supply to the myocardium.

endarterectomy	removal of the atheroma from the inner layer of the arterial wall

II–13

TREATMENT	DESCRIPTION
insertion of cardiac pacemaker	insertion of a battery-operated apparatus that stimulates the heart by sending out electrical impulses; used in arrhythmias such as heart block and ventricular fibrillation

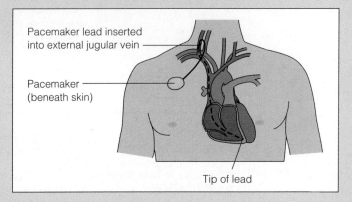

Pacemaker lead inserted into external jugular vein

Pacemaker (beneath skin)

Tip of lead

| **ligation and stripping of veins** | procedure for removing varicose veins, particularly the saphenous vein, which runs the length of the leg |

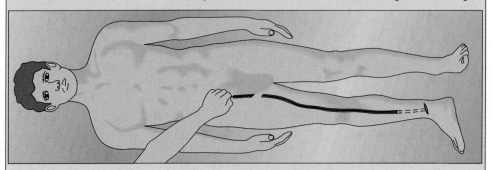

Note: The operation involves an incision at the ankle and groin. A long wire called a stripper is inserted at the ankle and manipulated until it reaches the groin incision. The vein at the ankle is tied to the stripper. The surgeon grasps the stripper at the groin and pulls, firmly removing the entire vein.

Because the saphenous vein is one of many superficial veins, the blood is rerouted, eventually returning to the heart.

| **heart transplants** | transfer of a heart from a donor to a recipient of the same species but not necessarily of the same genetic background |

Note: Recent advances have increased the long-term survival rate, with many patients living more than five years postoperatively and returning to active lives.

TREATMENT	DESCRIPTION
cardiopulmonary bypass	use of a mechanical device during open heart surgery, to redirect the blood away from the heart and lungs to obtain a clear, blood-free operative site with no cardiac motion
	Note: The device used is called the **heart-lung machine**. The process is called **extracorporeal circulation**.
	The heart-lung machine draws the blood from the aorta by means of a pump that acts as the heart. The blood travels into the lung portion of the machine, where carbon dioxide is given off and oxygen is brought on. The machine then circulates oxygenated blood through the body tissues.
	The heart must be artificially stopped before surgery is performed, usually by the infusion of **cardioplegics**.

Treatment Using Drugs

TREATMENT	DESCRIPTION
ACE inhibitors	elicits vasodilation, which improves cardiac function for patients with congestive heart failure; also acts as an antihypertensive
antianginal	relieves pain of angina pectoris by relaxing the muscular layers of the vascular wall (Nitroglycerin is the most common antianginal)
antiarrhythmics	counteracts abnormal heart rhythms by interfering with the transmission of neurotransmitters, the conduction pathway, and contraction of the myocardium (Quinidine is an example)
antihypertensive	used to reduce high blood pressure (Hydrodiuril is an example)
β blockers; beta adrenergic blockers	used for vasodilation, reduced heart rate, and cardiac output, thereby reducing the stress on the heart (Inderal is an example)
calcium blockers	interferes with the use of calcium at the neuromuscular junction, resulting in relaxation of the arterial walls and reducing oxygen consumption by limiting muscular contraction
	Note: Antiarrhythmics, antianginal, and antihypertensives are examples of calcium blockers.
inotropics; cardiotonics	sympathomimetic drugs used to increase the strength of ventricular contractions (common drugs in this classification are digitoxin and digitalis)
vasoconstrictors	narrows blood vessels; used in the treatment of cardiac arrest and atrioventricular heart block (Epinephrine is an example)
vasodilators	widens blood vessels for the treatment of angina or hypertension (Nitroglycerin is an example)

II—13

Heart		*Heart*	
ABBREVIATION	**DEFINITION**	**ABBREVIATION**	**DEFINITION**
AICD	automatic, implantable cardiovascular defibrillator	MI	myocardial infarction
AV	atrioventricular	RA	right atrium
ALT	alanine aminotransferase	RBBB	right bundle branch block
ASHD	arteriosclerotic heart disease	RV	right ventricle
AST	aspartate aminotransferase	SA	sinoatrial
		S_1	first heart sound
CABG	coronary artery bypass graft	S_2	second heart sound
		SGOT	serum glutamic oxaloacetic transaminase
CAD	coronary artery disease	SGPT	serum glutamic pyruvic transaminase
CCU	cardiac/coronary care unit		
CHF	congestive heart failure	*Blood Vessels*	
CK	creatine kinase	BP	blood pressure
CO	cardiac output	CVA	cerebrovascular accident
CPR	cardiopulmonary resuscitation	IVC	inferior vena cava
ECG; EKG	electrocardiogram	PTCA	percutaneous transluminal coronary angioplasty
HHD	hypertensive heart disease	PVD	peripheral vascular disease
IABP	intra-aortic balloon pump	SVC	superior vena cava
LBBB	left bundle branch block	TIA	transient ischemic attack
LA	left atrium	TPA	tissue plasminogen activator
LDH	lactic dehydrogenase		
LV	left ventricle		

Definitions

Definitions

Give the meaning for the following word parts.

Answers to the exercises are given in Appendix A.

1. brady- _____

2. angi/o _____

3. isch/o _____

4. phleb/o _____

5. vas/o _____

Give the word part for the following.

6. crown _____   10. valve _____

7. fast _____   11. stretching; dilation _____

8. above; upon _____   12. vein _____

9. all _____

Write definitions (or locations in the body) for the following terms.

13. arrhythmia _____

14. atrial _____

15. bradycardia _____

16. cardiomegaly _____

17. cardioplegic _____

18. coronary _____

19. electrocardiogram _____

20. epicardium _____

21. hemopericardium _____

22. infarction _____

23. interatrial _____

24. interventricular _____

25. myocardial infarction _____

26. pancarditis _____

27. pericarditis _____

28. tachycardia _____

29. valvuloplasty _____

30. angiography _____

31. angiospasm _____

32. aortostenosis _____

33. arterial _____

34. arteriostenosis _____

35. arteriole _____

36. arteriosclerosis _____

37. atheroma _____

38. atherosclerosis _____

39. brachiocephalic _____

40. endarterectomy _____

41. phlebothrombosis _____

42. sphygmomanometer _____

43. thrombophlebitis _____

44. tunica adventitia _____

45. tunica intima _____

46. tunica media _____

47. vascular _____

48. vasoconstriction _____

49. vasodilatation _____

50. vasospasm _____

51. venous _____

52. venule _____

Write the terms that correspond with the following abbreviations.

53. AV _____

54. ALT _____

55. ASHD _____

56. AST _____

57. CABG _____

58. CAD _____

59. CCU _____

60. CHF _____

61. CK _____

62. CO _____

63. CPR _____

64. EKG; ECG _____

65. HHD _____

66. IABP _____

67. LBBB _____

68. LV   _____

69. MI   _____

70. RBBB   _____

71. RV   _____

72. SA   _____

73. S$_1$ _____

74. S$_2$ _____

75. SGOT   _____

76. SGPT   _____

77. BP   _____

78. CVA   _____

79. TPA   _____

80. IVC   _____

81. PTCA   _____

82. PVD   _____

83. SVC   _____

84. TIA   _____

II–13

▶ **EXERCISE 13–2**   ## Word Building

Word Building

Build the medical words that mean the following.

1. without rhythm   _____

2. muscular structure of the heart   _____

3. inflammation of all the heart   _____

4. fast heart beat   _____

5. dilatation of a blood vessel   _____

6. narrowing of the aorta   _____

7. hardening of an artery   _____

8. pertaining to a vessel   _____

Practice Quiz

Briefly answer the following.

1. What body cavity houses the heart? _____

2. What is the name of the large, fluid-filled sac surrounding the heart? ____
_____

3. What separates the two sides of the heart? _____

4. What separates the atria? _____

5. Which side of the heart pumps blood to the lungs? _____

6. What is another name for the bicuspid valve? _____

7. What five terms are used to classify blood vessels? _____
_____
_____

8. What is the tunica adventitia? _____
_____

9. What is an anastomosis? _____
_____

▶EXERCISE 13-4   **Matching Terms with Meanings**

Matching

Match the term in Column A
with its meaning in
Column B.

Column A		Column B
1. arteriosclerosis	_____	A. impairment of circulation in the extremities
2. aneurysm	_____	B. narrowing of the mitral valve
3. Raynaud's disease	_____	C. inability of the mitral valve to close tightly
4. mitral valve stenosis	_____	D. shortness of breath
5. peripheral vascular disease	_____	E. fainting
6. mitral valve incompetence	_____	F. abnormal bulging of the arterial wall
7. dyspnea	_____	G. the movement of fluid from a blood vessel into tissue
8. edema	_____	H. degeneration of the muscular wall of an artery
9. effusion	_____	I. accumulation of fluid in body tissues
10. syncope	_____	J. disease of the peripheral vascular system

Diagrams

Place each of the names of major arteries listed below in the appropriate space on the diagram.

aortic arch
ascending aorta
brachiocephalic artery
common hepatic artery
descending aorta
left gastric artery
left internal iliac artery
left radial artery
left renal artery
left subclavian artery
left ulnar artery
right and left common
  carotid arteries
right anterior tibial
  artery
right axillary artery
right brachial artery
right common iliac
  artery
right dorsalis pedis
  artery
right external carotid
  artery
right external iliac artery
right femoral artery
right internal carotid
  artery
right peroneal artery
right popliteal artery
right posterior tibial
  artery
right subclavian artery
splenic artery

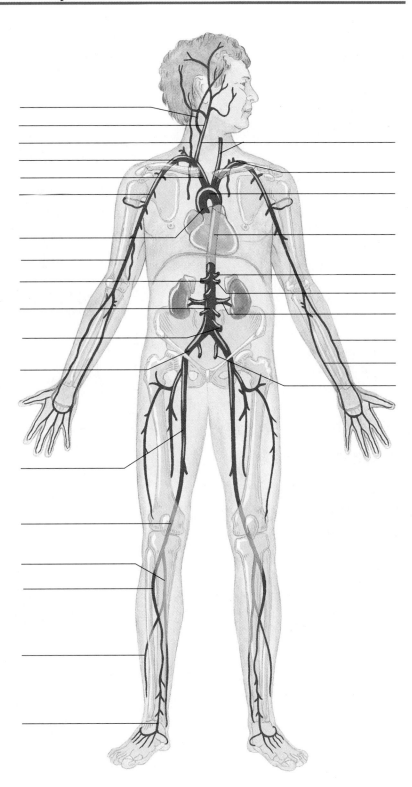

II–13

Place each of the names of major veins listed below in the appropriate space on the diagram.

inferior vena cava
left brachial vein
left cephalic vein
left radial vein
left renal vein
left ulnar vein
right and left
  brachiocephalic veins
right anterior tibial vein
right axillary vein
right common iliac vein
right external iliac vein
right external jugular
  vein
right femoral vein
right great saphenous
  vein
right hepatic vein
right internal iliac vein
right internal jugular
  vein
right peroneal vein
right popliteal vein
right posterior tibial vein
right subclavian vein
splenic vein
superior vena cava

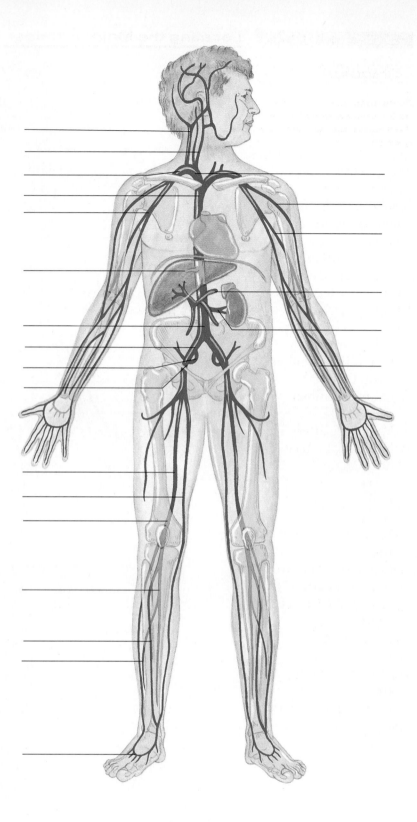

Spelling Practice

Place a check mark beside all misspelled words in the list that follows. Correctly spell those that you checked off.

1. aeorta ☐ _____

2. pericardeum ☐ _____

3. ventrical ☐ _____

4. atrium ☐ _____

5. myocardeum ☐ _____

6. bycuspid ☐ _____

7. semilunar ☐ _____

8. tunia media ☐ _____

9. cappilaries ☐ _____

10. anastomosis ☐ _____

11. anurysim ☐ _____

12. embulism ☐ _____

II–13

Medical Terms in Context

Define the underlined terms as they are used in context.

UNIVERSITY HOSPITAL ✚   ECHOCARDIOGRAPHY REPORT

ECHOCARDIOGRAPHY REPORT

Regular sinus rhythm. The left atrium is at the upper limits of normal. The other cardiac chamber dimensions are within the normal range. The aortic valve and tricuspid function normally. There is no evidence of significant regional wall motion abnormality. LV wall thicknesses are increased to 12 mm. The mitral valve is slightly thickened. There was mild mitral regurgitation detected. There was no evidence of intracardiac mass lesion or thrombus.

FINAL IMPRESSION: MITRAL VALVE THICKENING WITH MILD MITRAL REGURGITATION.

SIGNATURE OF DOCTOR IN CHARGE _____

1. echocardiography   _____

2. sinus rhythm   _____

3. atrium   _____

4. cardiac chamber   _____

5. aortic valve   _____

6. tricuspid   _____

7. LV   _____

8. mitral valve   _____

9. mitral regurgitation _____

10. intracardiac   _____

11. lesion   _____

12. thrombus   _____

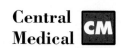
Central Medical CM

Mr. H. is a 42-year-old gentleman with known <u>coronary artery</u> disease who presented to the emergency room with <u>angina</u> on June 9. He previously had a <u>myocardial infarction</u> in January of 1994 and underwent <u>thrombolytic therapy</u> with <u>TPA</u>. His course was complicated by postinfarction <u>pericarditis</u> and <u>cardiac catheterization</u> revealed left <u>ventricular</u> dysfunction, minimal nonobstructive disease in the left coronary system and a total <u>thrombotic occlusion</u> of the right coronary artery. Today, the day of admission, he had again sudden onset of squeezing chest discomfort typical of his previous <u>MI</u> pain in 1994. He therefore immediately presented himself to the emergency room.

Authorized Health Care Practitioner _____

13. coronary artery   _____

14. angina   _____

15. myocardial infarction   _____

16. thrombolytic therapy   _____

17. TPA   _____

18. pericarditis   _____

19. cardiac catheterization _____

20. ventricular   _____

21. thrombotic occlusion   _____

22. MI   _____

II-13

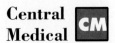

Central Medical CM

SUMMARY RECORD

On examination he was in some distress, <u>diaphoretic</u>, anxious with chest pain with a blood pressure of <u>167/104</u>. Head and neck were unremarkable. He had no <u>edema</u> and his <u>epigastrium</u> was quiet. Heart sounds were normal. His chest was clear with no <u>adventitious</u> sounds. The remainder of the exam was unremarkable.

FINAL DIAGNOSIS: ACUTE <u>INFEROLATERAL MYOCARDIAL INFARCTION</u>, QUERY RIGHT CORONARY ARTERY

Authorized Health Care Practitioner _____

23. diaphoretic _____

24. 167/104 _____

25. edema _____

26. epigastrium _____

27. adventitious _____

28. inferolateral myocardial infarction _____

Crossword Puzzle

Cardiovascular system

Across

2 Deviation from normal heart rhythm
4 Any disease of the innermost layer of the heart
6 Pertaining to the crown
7 Porcess of recording the heart's electrical activity
9 Vasospasm
10 Pertaining to a vessel
11 Vasodilation
12 Surgical repair of a valve

Down

1 Abnormally slow heart rate
3 Suture of the muscular layer of the heart
5 Abnormally fast heart rate
7 Pertaining to the epicardium
8 Inflammation of the pericardium

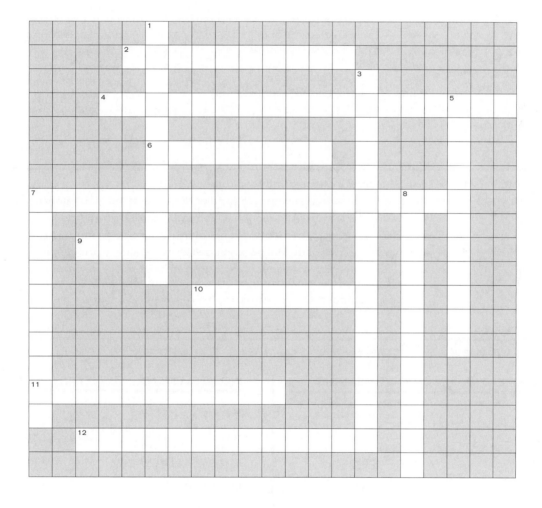

II—13

14 THE RESPIRATORY SYSTEM

CHAPTER OBJECTIVES

Upon successful completion of this chapter, the student will be able to do the following:

1. State the functions of the respiratory system.
2. Define the terms relating to the major divisions of the respiratory system.
3. Define the terms that describe the structures within the lungs.
4. Identify the major parts of the respiratory system by reference to a diagram.
5. Analyze, pronounce, define, and spell terms relating to the respiratory system.
6. List and define terms describing common respiratory disorders, signs and symptoms, diagnostic procedures, and treatment.
7. Define abbreviations common to the respiratory system.

WORD ELEMENTS PROMINENT IN THIS CHAPTER

WORD ELEMENT	TYPE	MEANING	WORD ELEMENT	TYPE	MEANING
adenoid/o	root	adenoids	pleur/o	root	side
alveol/o	root	lung	-pnea	suffix	breathing
bronch/i/o	root	bronchi	pneum/o; pneumon/o	root	air; lungs
glott/o	root	glottis	pulmon/o	root	lung
laryng/o	root	larynx	sinus/o	root	sinuses
lob/o	root	lobe of the lung	spir/o	root	breath
nas/o; rhin/o	root	nose	staphyl/o	root	uvula
pharyng/o	root	pharynx	thorac/o; steth/o	root	chest
phren/o	root	diaphragm	tonsill/o	root	tonsils
-phonia	suffix	sound; voice	trach/e/o	root	trachea

► 14.1 GENERAL ANATOMY AND PHYSIOLOGY OF THE RESPIRATORY SYSTEM

The respiratory system is composed of the **nose** and **nasal cavity**; the **pharynx, larynx**, and **trachea**; and the **bronchi** and **lungs**. See Figure 14–1. When one draws a breath, air enters through the nose and proceeds through the nasal cavity to the lungs by way of the pharynx, larynx, and bronchi. The two terms that describe the breathing process, also known as **external respiration** or **ventilation**, are **inspiration** and **expiration**. Inspiration refers to the inhalation of oxygen-rich air, and expiration refers to the expulsion of air that contains approximately 25 percent less oxygen than it did when it was inhaled. **Internal respiration**, which takes place within the body, is the exchange of gases between tissue cells and capillaries.

FIGURE 14–1   Structures of the Respiratory System

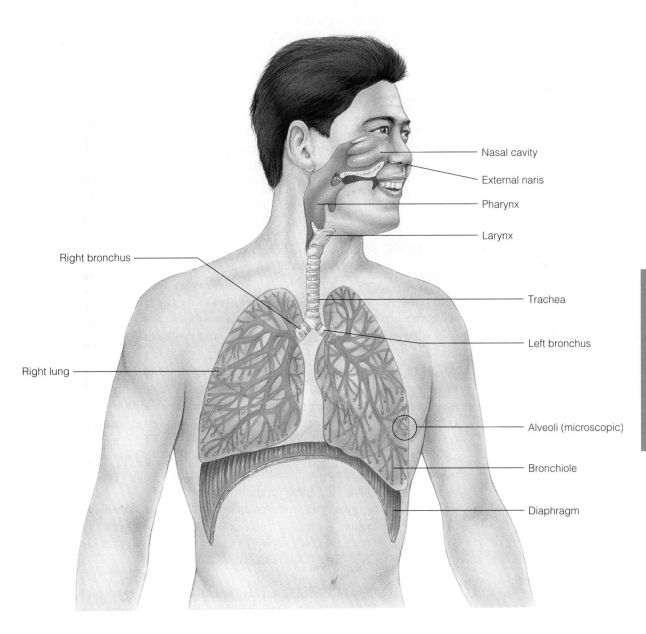

- Nasal cavity
- External naris
- Pharynx
- Larynx
- Right bronchus
- Trachea
- Left bronchus
- Right lung
- Alveoli (microscopic)
- Bronchiole
- Diaphragm

II–14

The respiratory system is essential in homeostasis, speech, and elimination of heat, water, and carbon dioxide, the latter playing a role in the regulation of pH (acid-base) balance.

Inspiration and Expiration

The **diaphragm** and the intercostal rib muscles enlarge the thoracic cavity to create a partial vacuum within the lungs; this vacuum draws air into the lungs, thus causing inspiration. When the muscles relax, the pressure gradient is reversed, and air is expelled from the lungs, thus effecting expiration. Since we can consciously control the muscles involved, we can inhale and exhale more deeply than we would in a passive state. When we consciously exhale, the muscles that control our breathing contract rather than relax.

Internal Respiration

Once inside the lungs, oxygen moves into the blood by way of the pulmonary capillaries and is carried by the red blood cells, specifically **hemoglobin**, into body tissue. The blood then transfers oxygen to the tissues while removing carbon dioxide from the tissues, both processes occurring by diffusion.

▶ 14.2 NOSE AND NASAL CAVITIES

The nose includes the **external nares** (nā'-rēz) (nostrils), which contain hair that filters dirt and other impurities from inhaled air. The nasal cavity, in which further filtering occurs, also warms and moistens the incoming air. The nasal cavity extends from the external nares to the pharynx and is divided in half by the **nasal septum.**

▶ 14.3 PHARYNX, LARYNX, AND TRACHEA

Pharynx

The pharynx, which is also referred to as the throat, connects the nasal cavity with the larynx. The pharynx has three parts: the **nasopharynx** (nā"-zō-fǎr'-ĭnks), the **oropharynx** (or"-ō-fǎr'-ĭnks), and the **laryngopharynx** (lǎr-ĭn"-gō-fǎr'-ĭnks).

The nasopharynx, which lies behind the nasal cavity, has four openings, two of which are called the **internal nares.** The internal nares open into the nasal cavity. The two other openings from the nasopharynx lead to the eustachian tubes (see Chapter 10). The nasopharynx contains the **pharyngeal** (fǎr-ĭn'-jē-ǎl) **tonsils,** also known as the **adenoids.**

The oropharynx, behind the oral cavity, contains the **palatine tonsils,** which are the tonsils we normally think of when we use the term, and the **lingual tonsils,** which lie at the base of the tongue.

The laryngopharynx, located behind the larynx, opens into the larynx and into the esophagus.

Larynx

The larynx, a boxlike structure commonly known as the voice box, is made of cartilage (see Figure 14–2). Consisting of nine cartilaginous pieces, it connects the pharynx and the trachea. The **thyroid cartilage**, which is a shield-shaped structure that forms the **laryngeal prominence** or **Adam's apple**, the **cricoid** (krī-koyd) **cartilage**, and the **epiglottis** (ĕp″-ĭ-glŏt′-ĭs) are each a single piece of cartilage. The epiglottis is attached to the thyroid cartilage inferiorly, and its superior end is unattached so that is can act as a lid, freely moving to cover the superior opening of the larynx on swallowing. The epiglottis prevents food from entering the respiratory tract. The other six pieces of cartilage are paired: the **arytenoid** (ăr″-ĭ-tē′-noyd), **corniculate** (kōr-nĭk′-ū-lāt), and **cuneiform** (kū-nē′-ĭ-form) cartilages.

FIGURE 14–2

The Larynx

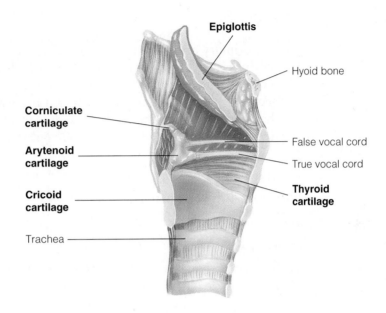

Two pairs of folds, one pair above the other, are formed by the mucous membrane lining the larynx. The upper folds are named **false vocal cords**. These cords do not function in voice production, while the lower folds, named **true vocal cords**, produce sound as air moves out of the lungs. The slit between the true vocal cords is the **glottis**. The tension and length of the vocal cords determine voice pitch. Males have a lower voice pitch than women do because their vocal cords are longer. See Figure 14–3.

FIGURE 14–3

Superior View of True Vocal Cords

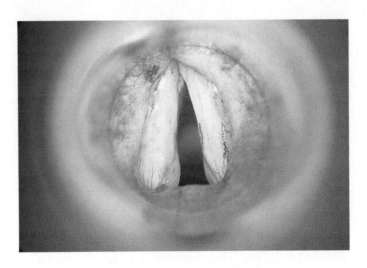

Trachea

The trachea, or windpipe, connects the larynx to the lungs via the bronchi. The trachea continues the filtering process, started by the nose, by collecting impurities from inhaled air and by preventing them from entering the lungs. The trachea is lined with ciliated mucous membrane that enables it to carry out this filtering function.

▶ 14.4 BRONCHI AND LUNGS

Bronchi

The **primary bronchi**, also called the right and left mainstream bronchi, are the two passageways extending from the trachea to the lungs, are connected to **secondary** and **tertiary bronchi** within the lungs. The tertiary bronchi are connected to **terminal bronchioles**, which branch into **respiratory bronchioles**. As the bronchi branch and rebranch, the structure resembles that of an inverted tree; hence the common name **bronchial tree** (see Figure 14–4).

FIGURE 14–4 Trachea, Bronchi, and Bronchioles (a) Anatomy of trachea and bronchial tree. (b) End of bronchial tree showing terminal bronchioles, alveolar duct, and alveoli.

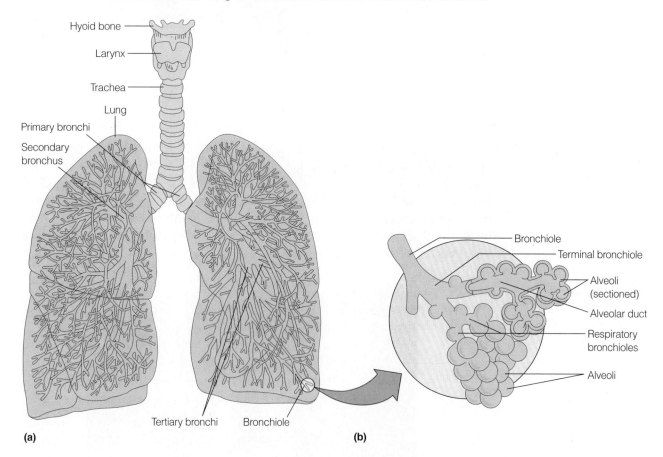

Lungs

Each lung is one of a pair of cone-shaped organs. Each has a narrow end called the **apex**, pointing upwards, and a wide end called the **base**. The **costal surface** of each lung faces the ribs. The surface facing toward the midline is the **mediastinal** (mē″-dē-ăs-tī′-năl) **surface**. The heart lies within the **cardiac notch** of the mediastinal surface of the left lung. Each lung attaches to the body at the **root**, which contains the **hilum** (hī-lŭm), an area through which the bronchus, blood vessels, nerves, and lymph vessels enter.

As its name implies, the **diaphragmatic surface** of the lung faces the diaphragm. The **lobes** of each lung are formed by **fissures** or grooves (see Figure 14–5).

FIGURE 14–5   **The Lungs** (a) Anatomical structures of the lung. (b) Capillary network surrounding the alveoli.

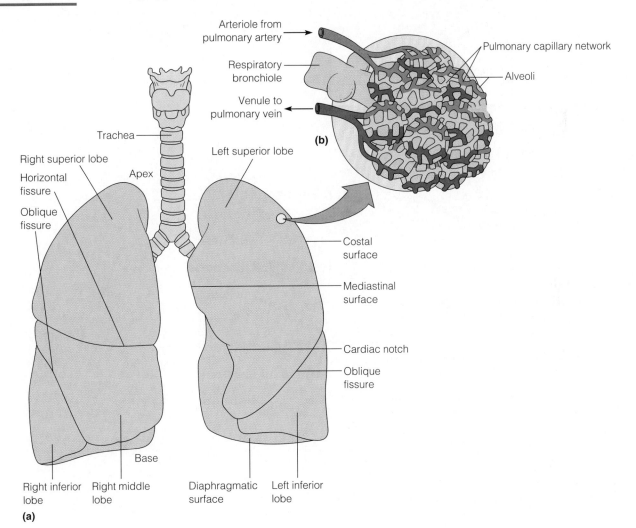

The lungs contain **alveoli** (ăl-vē′-ō-lī), which are connected to the bronchioles via the alveolar ducts. The alveoli, which are microscopic dead-end sacs, number about 300 million in each lung. The alveoli exhange oxygen and carbon dioxide.

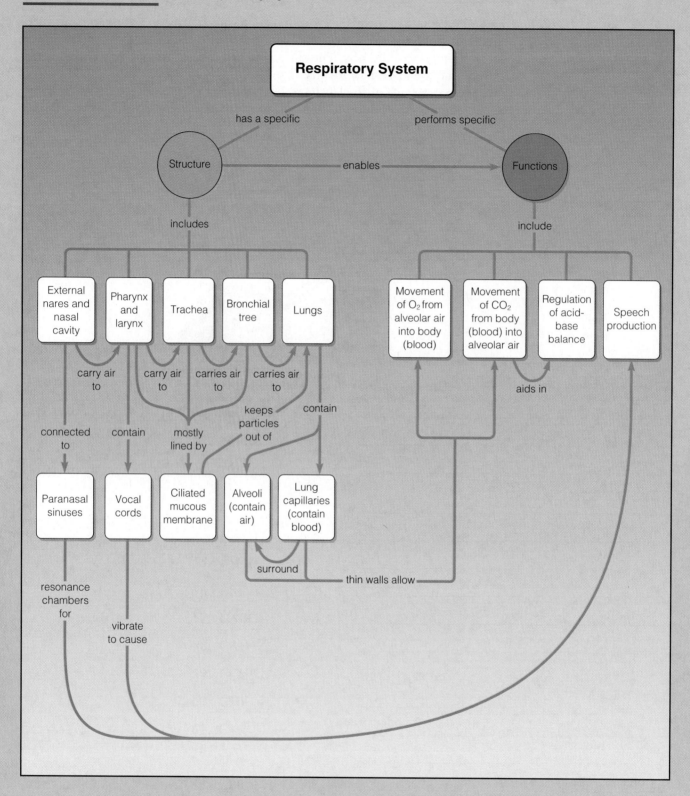

TERM WITH PRONUNCIATION	ANALYSIS	DEFINITION
adenoidectomy ăd″-ĕ-noyd-ĕk′-tō-mē	-ectomy = excision; removal adenoid/o = adenoid	excision of the adenoid
alveolar ăl-vē′-ō-lăr	-ar = pertaining to alveol/o = air sacs; saclike enlargement	pertaining to the air sacs
aphonia ă-fō′-nē-ă	-phonia = voice a- = no; not	no voice; loss of voice
bronchiectasis brŏng″-kē-ĕk′-tă-sĭs	-ectasis = dilatation; stretching bronch/i/o = bronchus	dilatation of the bronchus
bronchiolitis brŏng″-kē-ō-lī′-tĭs	-itis = inflammation bronchiol/o = bronchioles; little bronchi	inflammation of the bronchioles
bronchitis brŏng-kī′-tĭs	-itis = inflammation bronch/o = bronchus	inflammation of the bronchus
dysphonia dĭs-fō′-nē-ă	-phonia = voice dys- = difficult; bad; painful	difficulty in speaking
epiglottitis ĕp″-ĭ-glŏt-ī′-tĭs	-itis = inflammation epiglott/o = epiglottis	inflammation of the epiglottis
eupnea ūp-nē′-ă	-pnea = breathing eu- = normal; good	normal breathing
laryngotracheobronchitis lă-rĭng″-gō-trā″-kē-ō-brŏng-kī′-tĭs	-itis = inflammation laryng/o = larynx; voicebox trache/o = trachea; windpipe bronch/o = bronchus	inflammation of the larynx, trachea, and bronchus; also known as croup
oropharyngeal ŏr″-ō-făr-ĭn′-jē-ăl	-eal = pertaining to or/o = mouth pharyng/o = pharynx; throat	pertaining to the mouth and pharynx
pansinusitis păn″-sī-nŭs-ī′-tĭs	-itis = inflammation pan- = all sinus/o = sinus	inflammation of all the paranasal sinuses
phrenic frĕn′-ĭk	-ic = pertaining to phren/o = diaphragm	pertaining to the diaphragm
phrenoplegia frĕn-ō-plē′-jē-ă	-plegia = paralysis phren/o = diaphragm	paralysis of the diaphragm

II–14

TERM WITH PRONUNCIATION	ANALYSIS	DEFINITION
pneumonia nū-mō′-nē-ă	-ia = condition pneumon/o = lung	inflammation of the lung
pneumonitis nū″-mō-nī′-tĭs	-itis = inflammation pneumon/o = lung	inflammation of the lung
pulmonary pŭl′-mō-nĕ-rē	-ary = pertaining to pulmon/o = lung	pertaining to the lung
rhinorrhea rī″-nō-rē′-ă	-rrhea = flow; discharge rhin/o = nose	discharge from the nose
sinusotomy sī-nŭs-ŏt′-ō-mē	-tomy = process of cutting sinus/o = sinus; cavity	process of cutting into the sinus
staphylorrhaphy stăf″-ĭl-or′-ă-fē	-rrhaphy = suturing staphyl/o = uvula	suturing of the uvula; repair of a cleft palate
stethoscope stĕth′-ō-skōp	-scope = instrument used to examine steth/o = chest	instrument used to listen to chest sounds
thoracoplasty thō′-ră-kō-plăs″-tē	-plasty = surgical reconstruction; plastic repair thorac/o = chest	surgical reconstruction of the thorax
tonsillectomy tŏn-sĭl-ĕk′-tō-mē	-ectomy = excision; removal tonsill/o = tonsils	removal of the tonsils
tonsillitis tŏn-sĭl-ī′-tĭs	-itis = inflammation tonsill/o = tonsils	inflammation of the tonsils

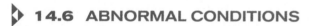

14.6 ABNORMAL CONDITIONS

ACUTE RESPIRATORY INFECTIONS	DESCRIPTION
allergic rhinitis; atopic rhinitis (atopic refers to diseases that are allergic in nature)	allergic response to inhaled allergens characterized by sneezing, rhinorrhea, ophthalmorrhea, nasal pruritus, and congestion **Note:** This disease category includes hay fever, a seasonal type of allergic rhinitis occurring in the spring, summer, or fall (caused by the inhalation of pollens or other allergens). Antihistamines effectively counteract the inflammatory response to the allergens.
bronchitis	acute inflammation of the bronchial tree caused by a virus, often following a cold
croup	viral disease of childhood, characterized by inflammation and obstruction of the upper and lower respiratory tracts; also called **laryngotracheobronchitis**

ACUTE RESPIRATORY INFECTIONS	DESCRIPTION
pleural effusion	the movement of any fluid out of the blood vessels and into the surrounding pleural cavity
	Note: The passage of fluid into the pleural cavity is called pleural effusion. There are different effusions, the terms for which depend upon the type of fluid effused. **Hemothorax** is blood in the pleural cavity; **pyothorax** or **empyema** is pus in the pleural cavity; **pneumothorax** is air in the pleural cavity; and **hydrothorax** is watery fluid in the pleural cavity.
pleurisy	inflammation of the pleura, characterized by pain and pleural effusion
	Note: Exudate may dry up, forming adhesions between the visceral and parietal layers that make breathing painful.
upper respiratory infection (URI)	infection of the noses, nasal cavity, pharynx, and larynx
	Note: The common cold (**coryza**) is the most common upper respiratory tract infection.

DISORDERS OF THE UPPER RESPIRATORY TRACT	DESCRIPTION
deviated nasal septum	shift of the nasal septum away from the midline, a condition that may be either congenital or traumatic, such as a blow to the nose
	Note: The condition is asymptomatic unless the deviation is severe enough to cause obstruction of the air through the nasal passages.
tracheoesophageal fistula	abnormal tubelike passage between the trachea and esophagus which may be caused by a congenital defect and resulting in the passage of food into the respiratory tract from the esophagus with subsequent choking

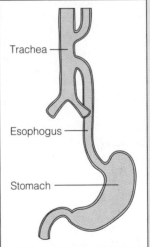

Trachea

Esophogus

Stomach

Note: In the normal newborn, the trachea is a separate structure located anterior to the esophagus.

II—14

ABNORMAL CONDITIONS OF THE LUNG	DESCRIPTION
asthma	reversible bronchospasm that obstructs the small airways and produces shortness of breath **Note: Status asthmaticus** is an unremitting bronchospasm occurring when the bronchus fails to relax following treatment with bronchodilators; the condition can be fatal.
atelectasis	inability of the alveoli to completely inflate, resulting in collapse of alveoli with no exchange of gases and with loss of oxygen to tissues; may be caused by occlusion of the airways by mucus, foreign bodies, lesions, or by inadequate ventilation
bronchiectasis	chronic dilation of the bronchi with destruction of the walls **Note:** The shape of the dilated bronchial walls can be **fusiform** (spindle-shaped), **saccular** (rounded), or **cylindrical** (column-shaped).

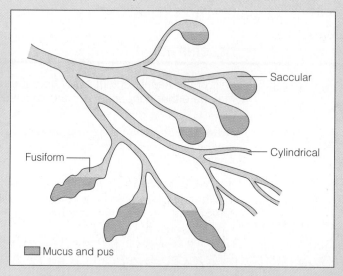

bronchitis, chronic	an inflammation of the bronchus, often characterized by mucopurulent secretions and a productive cough, in severe cases the airways are sometimes obstructed; considered chronic when, for at least two consecutive years, it persists for periods of at least two months **Note:** A productive cough refers to the coughing up of substances from the respiratory tract.

ABNORMAL CONDITIONS OF THE LUNG	DESCRIPTION
emphysema	dilatation of the alveoli with destruction of their walls, associated with a loss in pulmonary elasticity
	Note: The alveoli, once dilated, do not constrict; the air becomes trapped in the alveoli; the patient has difficulty exhaling the air and develops a characteristic barrel-shaped chest.
	A distention of the alveoli to a size greater than 2.5 inches (1 cm) in diameter is called a **bleb** or **bulla**. If a bulla ruptures, the air escapes into the surrounding lung tissue, causing pneumothorax.

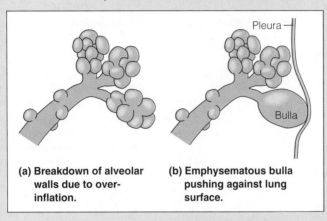

(a) Breakdown of alveolar walls due to over-inflation.

(b) Emphysematous bulla pushing against lung surface.

fungal infections	infection in the lungs caused by a fungus
histoplasmosis	The infectious condition **histoplasmosis**, caused by the fungus **Histoplasma capsulatum**, is manifested by a pulmonary lesion with the occasional infestation of other organs such as the spleen, liver, and lymph glands. Most prevalent in the Central United States, Mexico, and Central and South America.
coccidioidomycosis	Another infectious disease is **coccidioidomycosis,** or **valley fever**, caused by the fungus **Coccidioides immitis** and characterized by respiratory infection. Most common in the southwest United States, Mexico, and Central and South America.
hyaline membrane disease; respiratory distress syndrome (RDS)	atelectasis in the newborn; usually seen in premature births (before the 37th week of gestation) and newborns of diabetic mothers
	Note: The cause of this condition is a lack of **surfactant**, a substance produced by the lungs to keep the alveoli inflated. When there is deficiency of surfactant, the alveoli collapse and air entry is diminished, producing respiratory distress. The term **hyaline** refers to an abnormal, glassy membrane lining the alveoli and contributing to its collapse.
pneumoconiosis; black lung	accumuluation of dust particles in the lung from long exposure and inhalation of irritants, sometimes from an occupational environment
	Note: The various types of pneumoconioses are named for the type of dust inhaled. **Silicosis** is caused by the inhalation of silica dust found in quartz and sand; **anthracosis** is caused by the inhalation of coal dust; and **asbestosis** is caused by the inhalation of asbestos.

II–14

ABNORMAL CONDITIONS OF THE LUNG

DESCRIPTION

pneumonia
        inflammation of the lung, often impairing the exchange of gases

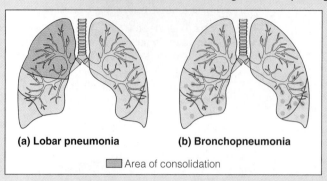

(a) Lobar pneumonia   (b) Bronchopneumonia

☐ Area of consolidation

Note: Two terms that refer to pneumonia are **consolidation**, filling of the alveoli with inflammatory exudate, and **resolution**, the disintegration of the exudate following treatment.

Pneumonia can be categorized by the etiologic agent or by the location of the consolidation (see Tables 14-1 and 14-2). Another type of pneumonia, **aspiration pneumonia**, is neither bacterial nor viral but rather is produced by aspiration of vomit into the lung.

TABLE 14–1   Etiologic Agents in Pneumonia

VIRUSES	BACTERIA	PARASITES	FUNGI
adenovirus	*Hemophilus influenzae*	*Pneumocystis carinii*	*Histoplasma capsulatum*
cytomegalovirus	*Klebsiella pneumoniae*		*Coccidioides immitis*
enterovirus	*Legionella pneumophila*		
Epstein-Barr virus	*Moraxella catarrhalis*		
influenza viruses	*Mycobacterium tuberculosis*		
(A, B, C)	*Neisseria meningitides*		
parainfluenza virus	*Staphylococcus aureus*		
	Streptococcus pneumonia		
	Streptococcus pyogenes		

TABLE 14–2   Site of Infection of Pneumonia

NAME	SITE
basal pneumonia	consolidation at the base of the lung
bronchopneumonia	consolidation along the bronchus
interstitial pneumonia	pneumonia involving tissue spaces within the lung
lobar pneumonia	partial or complete consolidation of a lobe of lung

ABNORMAL CONDITIONS OF THE LUNG	DESCRIPTION
pulmonary tuberculosis (TB)	caused by the Mycobacterium **tuberculosis bacteria**, which is carried through the air and inhaled into the lungs
	Note: Tuberculosis usually involves a specific area of the lung called a **focus**, where the initial reaction to the bacteria is inflammation and the formation of a **tubercle** or nodule. Later stages involve necrosis, fibrosis, **caseation** (the changing of necrotic tissue into a cheesy mass), and cavity formation when the cheesy mass liquefies. The tubercle bacilli can spread by the bloodstream to other organs.
	Diagnostic tests include the **Mantoux skin test** and **Ziehl-Neelsen stain** (acid-fast stain). See laboratory diagnostic tests.

MISCELLANEOUS ABNORMAL CONDITIONS	DESCRIPTION
cystic fibrosis (CF)	a genetic disease of the exocrine glands involving many organs, including the lungs, pancreas, liver, and sweat glands
	Note: Abnormal secretions of a viscid (glutinous) mucus in the bronchi results in bronchiectasis, bronchopneumonia, and lung abscesses. When the pancreas is involved, the thick mucus blocks the ducts affecting the secretion of pancreatic enzymes and, in turn, the digestive process. When the sweat glands are involved, they secrete a sweat high in salt concentration.

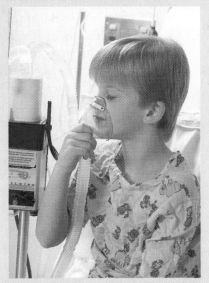

respiratory acidosis	pH imbalance (decrease) marked by abnormally high levels of acidity in the body tissues and fluid, caused by an increase in carbon dioxide
respiratory alkalosis	pH disturbance (increase) marked by abnormally high levels of base, caused by a decrease in carbon dioxide
sudden infant death syndrome (SIDS); crib death	unexpected death of a newborn, infant, or child usually between the ages of 3 weeks and 1 year.
	Note: The etiology is unknown, with death typically occurring when the child is sleeping, often without any apparent respiratory distress.

Chronic Obstructive Lung Disease and Allied Conditions

Chronic obstructive pulmonary disease (COPD) or **chronic obstructive lung disease (COLD)** may involve two or more chronic pulmonary conditions such as chronic obstructive bronchitis, chronic asthmatic bronchitis or emphysema in combination. If only one of these conditions exists, the name of the specific disorder is preferred.

▷ 14.7 PHYSICAL EXAMINATION, DIAGNOSIS, AND TREATMENT

Physical Examination

When inspecting the chest wall, the health care practitioner will note the rate, rhythm, and effort of breathing and any bony deformities of the chest, such as barrel chest (a long-term effect of emphysema.)

Palpation of the chest wall has a number of purposes. It helps identify areas of tenderness or abnormal masses; assesses **respiratory excursion**, the normal rhythmical movements of the chest wall as the patient inhales and exhales; and evaluates **fremitus** (frĕm′-ĭ-tŭs), the normal vibrations through the chest wall as the patient speaks. Increased and decreased fremitus occurs with abnormalities of the respiratory tract, particularly when airflow is obstructed.

Tissue underlying the chest wall can be filled with air or fluid, or it can be solid. Tapping the chest wall (percussion) reveals significant differences in the quality of sounds. Tone, intensity, and persistence can be clinically significant. There are five percussion notes that describe the intensity of the sound: **flatness**, a soft intensity; **dullness**, a medium intensity heard when the air normally in the lung is replaced by fluid or solid material; **resonance**, a loud sound typical of a normal lung; **hyperresonance**, a very loud sound characteristic of an **emphysematous lung**; and **tympany**, a bell-like sound characteristic of gas bubbles in the gastrointestinal tract.

Auscultation of the lungs produces sounds as the air flows through the trachea and bronchi to the lungs. A **stethoscope** is used to listen to the pulmonary sounds as the patient inhales and exhales normally. The quality of breath sounds is then described as follows: **vesicular** is a sound of low tone and low intensity; **bronchovesicular** is a sound of medium tone and medium intensity; **bronchial sounds** are of high pitch and high intensity. **Adventitious** (abnormal) breath sounds can also be described by the terms listed below:

TERM	DESCRIPTION
friction rubs	a sound resulting from two serous surfaces rubbing together, such as when parietal and visceral pleura rub together in pleurisy
rales	a crackling sound
rhonchi	a rattling sound
stridor	a hoarse, high-pitched sound characteristic of large or upper airway obstruction often heard in laryngotracheobronchitis
wheezing	a whistling sound characteristic of small or lower airway obstruction

ABNORMAL RESPIRATORY PATTERNS	DESCRIPTION
apnea; asphyxia	no breathing or respirations
ataxic (biotic respirations)	**irregular, unpredictable** breathing involving alternating periods of **hyperpnea**, **hypopnea**, and **apnea**
bradypnea	abnormally slow breathing
Cheyne-Stokes	**regular** and **rhythmic** breathing characterized by an alternating pattern of **hyperpnea** and **apnea**
dyspnea	difficult or painful respiration: can include **dyspnea on exertion (DOE)** (difficult breathing during physical exercise); **orthopnea** (difficult breathing except in the erect position); and **paroxysmal nocturnal dyspnea (PND)** (sudden attacks of difficult breathing occurring at night and waking the patient)
hyperpnea	abnormal increase in depth and rate of breathing
hyperventilation	abnormally prolonged deep and rapid breathing, increasing the amounts of oxygen entering the lungs and reducing the amounts of carbon dioxide
hypopnea	abnormal decrease in depth and rate of breathing
oligopnea	infrequent respirations
orthopnea	breathing only in the upright position
shortness of breath	insufficient supply of air resulting in brief respirations
tachypnea	abnormally fast respirations

ABNORMAL SECRETIONS	DESCRIPTION
hemoptysis	coughing up of blood
abnormal sputum	abnormal sputum (sputum is matter expectorated [coughed up] through the mouth from the air passages) contains bacteria, pus, and other material that may lead to a diagnosis
rhinorrhea	abnormal discharge from the nose

OTHER SIGNS	DESCRIPTION
bronchospasm	involuntary contractions of the bronchus
chest pain	thoracic pain during respiration
cyanosis	bluish discoloration of the skin and mucous membrane due to a lack of oxygen in the blood

II–14

OTHER SIGNS	DESCRIPTION
finger clubbing	soft tissue changes in the distal phalanges of the fingers and toes resulting in puffiness and reduced angle of the nail bed

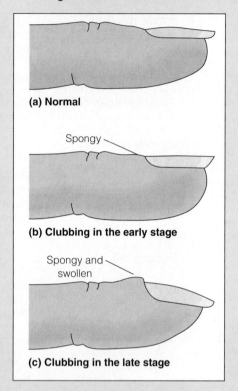

(a) Normal

Spongy

(b) Clubbing in the early stage

Spongy and swollen

(c) Clubbing in the late stage

Note: Causes of clubbing are varied.

hypercapnia	excessive carbon dioxide retention
hypoxia and anoxia	hypoxia is an abnormal decrease in the amount of oxygen in tissues; anoxia means tissues without oxygen (these terms are often used interchangeably)
respiratory failure	inadequate respiratory functions even at rest
respiratory insufficiency	inability of respiratory functions to meet body's demand on exertion
stridor	loud inspiratory sound heard as air tries to pass through an obstructed respiratory passage; audible without a stethoscope

Diagnosis

RADIOLOGY PROCEDURES	DESCRIPTION
chest radiology plain chest x-ray	anteroposterior (AP) and lateral view of the chest without use of any contrast medium
computed axial tomography (CAT) scan	provides a 3-dimensional view of an organ rather than the 2-dimensional view of conventional x-rays; a contrast medium may or may not be used
radionuclide scanning— the gallium scan	following injection of radioactive gallium, images are obtained of the respiratory and other organs **Note:** Gallium is readily taken up by inflamed tissue and some tumors.
bronchography	x-ray of the bronchial tree, including the trachea, following introduction of a contrast medium into the bronchus
pulmonary angiography	x-ray and fluoroscopy of the blood vessels of the lung following instillation of a contrast medium into the pulmonary artery or one of its branches
chest fluoroscopy	x-ray of the chest during respiration to monitor the chest while it functions

LABORATORY TESTS	DESCRIPTION
acid-fast stain; Ziehl-Neelsen (ZN) stain	staining techniques involve placing a dye onto a substance taken from the body, such as sputum and tissue samples, to aid in the identification of microorganisms **Note:** Acid-fast stain is a staining technique used to detect *Mycobacterium tuberculosis*. Once this stain penetrates the microorganism, it cannot be readily removed by acid and hence the name acid-fast stain.
arterial blood gases (ABG)	measures the amount of oxygen and carbon dioxide carried in the blood, indicating how effectively the lungs transfer oxygen to and remove carbon dioxide from the blood **Note:** The acid-base balance (pH level) is also monitored. It is necessary to have a balanced pH. Any deviation above or below the norm is life-threatening.

II—14

LABORATORY TESTS	DESCRIPTION
culture and sensitivity (C&S)	a method of identifying bacteria in a specimen taken from body fluids of a specific site and determining the best antibiotic to treat it
	Note: A sample is taken from the patient and put in an environment that fosters growth. The microorganism multiplies and thus is readily identifiable. Then, its sensitivity to various antibiotics is observed so that the most effective one can be prescribed.
Mantoux skin test; tuberculin skin test	test for *Mycobacterium tuberculosis* involving injection of an antigen extract of the bacteria within the skin; localized inflammation indicates infection
spirometry	process of measuring the flow and volume of air taken into the lung on inhalation and exhalation; the instrument used is called a spirometer
pulmonary function tests (PFT)	various tests of lung performance using a spirometer

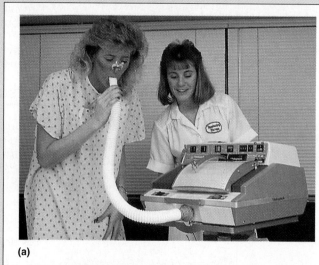

(a)

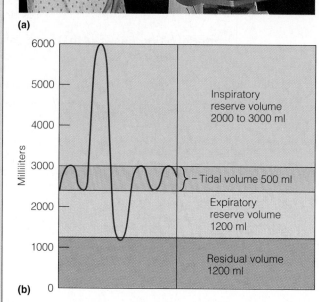

(b)

LABORATORY TESTS	DESCRIPTION
pulmonary function tests (continued)	**Note:** Pulmonary blood flow, acid-base balance, gas exchange, and pulmonary function are determined by measuring such quantities as **total lung capacity (TLC)** (the total volume of air that the lungs can hold). The TLC is the sum of four volumes described below: 1. **tidal volume (TV)**: the volume of air taken into the lungs on normal inspiration and expiration when the patient is at rest; normal TV is approximately 500 ml (a decrease may indicate any number of pulmonary dysfunctions including atelectasis, asthma, bronchiectasis, bronchitis, chronic obstructive lung disease, emphysema, and lung cancer). 2. **expiratory reserve volume (ERV)**: the volume of air that can be forced from the lungs above tidal expiration 3. **inspiratory reserve volume (IRV)**: the volume of air that can be forced into the lungs above tidal inspiration 3. **residual volume (RV):** the volume of air remaining in the lungs following maximal exhalation; after air has been forced out of the lungs, the air left is the residual volume
sweat test	used to determine the levels of salt (chloride) in a sample of sweat; high levels are seen in children with cystic fibrosis

CLINICAL PROCEDURES	DESCRIPTION
bronchoscopy	process of visually examining the bronchus with a bronchoscope
thoracocentesis	surgical puncture of the chest wall to remove fluid from the pleural cavity
percutaneous needle biopsy of pleura	following insertion of a needle through the skin into the pleura, a piece of tissue is excised or aspirated
thoracotomy	incision into the thorax

II—14

Treatment

MEDICAL TREATMENTS	DESCRIPTION
chest physical therapy	includes proper breathing techniques, coughing, exercises, and postural drainage; in the latter, the patient's position is changed to allow gravity to promote drainage to treat respiratory conditions characterized by increased secretions in the lungs
mechanical ventilator	device used to deliver air to the patient
continuous positive airway pressure (CPAP)	method of maintaining consistent respiratory pressure by use of a mechanical respirator
intermittent positive pressure breathing (IPPB)	method of inflating the lungs intermittently under positive pressure (pressure greater than that of the atmosphere)
positive end-expiratory pressure (PEEP)	method of increasing the volume of gas in the lung at the end of exhalation thereby improving gas exchange by use of a mechanical ventilator

PHARMACOLOGICAL AGENTS	DESCRIPTION
bronchodilators	agents that widen the bronchus to alleviate bronchospasm

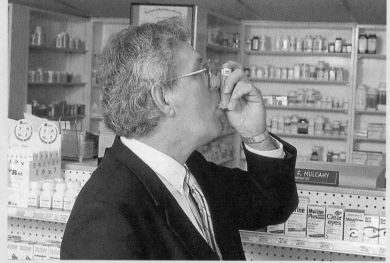

mucolytics	used to break down mucus so it can be expectorated (coughed up)
decongestants	used to reduce swelling of mucus membrane and congestion of nasal passages
expectorants	used to help in the coughing up of mucus from the trachea and bronchus

PHARMACOLOGICAL AGENTS	DESCRIPTION
antihistamines	used against histamines, which are natural body substances that produce redness, swelling, heat, and pain **Note:** Histamines are released from cells in an immune response to foreign substances such as pollens.
antitussives	substances used to stop coughing
isoniazid; INH	drug used to treat tuberculosis

SURGICAL TECHNIQUES	DESCRIPTION
antrostomy	operation to drain the paranasal sinus by approaching it through the nostril
Caldwell-Luc	surgery to drain the maxillary sinus of accumulated debris due to sinusitis; the maxillary sinus is entered through an incision in the gum, below the upper lip
endotracheal intubation	insertion of a tube into the trachea for the passage of air
lobectomy	excision of a lobe of the lung
nasal intubation	insertion of a tube through the nose and into the respiratory passages for the passage of air
phrenotomy	incision of the phrenic nerve
pneumonectomy	removal of the lung
rhinoplasty	surgical repair of the nose
tracheostomy	new opening into the trachea; may be temporary or permanent
tracheotomy	incision into the trachea

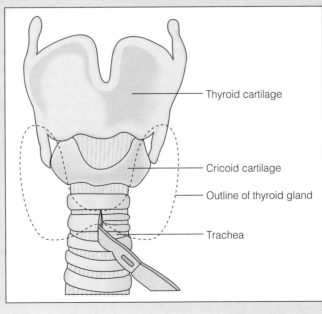

Thyroid cartilage

Cricoid cartilage

Outline of thyroid gland

Trachea

II–14

ABBREVIATION	DEFINITION	ABBREVIATION	DEFINITION
ABG	arterial blood gases	IRV	inspiratory reserve volume
AFB	acid-fast bacillus	MV	minute volume
ARDS	adult respiratory distress syndrome	O_2	oxygen
C&S	culture and sensitivity	PEEP	positive end expiratory pressure
CF	cystic fibrosis	PFT	pulmonary function test
CO_2	carbon dioxide	PND	paroxysmal nocturnal dyspnea
COLD	chronic obstructive lung disease	R	respiration
COPD	chronic obstructive pulmonary disease	RDS	respiratory distress syndrome
CPAP	continuous positive airway pressure	RV	residual volume
CXR	chest x-ray	SIDS	sudden infant death syndrome
DOE	dyspnea on exertion	SOB	shortness of breath
ERV	expiratory reserve volume	T&A	tonsillectomy and adenoidectomy
FEV	forced expiratory volume	TB	tuberculosis
FVC	forced vital capacity	TGV	thoracic gas volume
FRC	functional residual capacity	TLC	total lung capacity
IC	inspiratory capacity	TV	tidal volume
IPPB	intermittent positive pressure breathing	URI	upper respiratory infection
		VC	vital capacity
		ZN	Ziehl-Neelsen

Definitions

Definitions

Give the meaning for the following word parts.

1. alveol/o _____

2. -phonia _____

3. -capnia _____

4. laryng/o _____

5. phren/o _____

6. pneumon/o _____

7. pulmon/o _____

8. rhin/o _____

9. steth/o _____

10. thorac/o _____

Give the prefix, suffix, or word root for the following.

11. windpipe _____ 12. surgical puncture _____

13. uvula _____ 14. breath; breathing _____

15. bronchus _____ 16. adenoids _____

17. tonsils _____ 18. small bronchi _____

Write definitions (or locations in the body) for the following terms.

19. adenoidectomy _____

20. alveoli _____

21. aphonia _____

22. bronchiolitis _____

23. bronchiectasis _____

24. dysphonia _____

25. dyspnea _____

26. epiglottitis _____

27. eupnea _____

28. hypercapnia _____

29. laryngotracheo-
    bronchitis _____

30. lobectomy _____

31. pansinusitis _____

32. phrenic nerve _____

33. phrenoplegia _____

34. pneumonitis _____

35. pneumonia _____

36. pulmonary   _____

37. rhinoplasty   _____

38. sinusotomy   _____

39. spirometry   _____

40. staphylorrhaphy   _____

41. thoracocentesis; thoracentesis   _____

42. thoracoplasty   _____

43. tonsillectomy   _____

44. tonsillitis   _____

45. tracheostomy   _____

46. tracheotomy   _____

Write the terms that correspond with the following abbreviations.

47. ABG   _____

48. AFB   _____

49. ARDS   _____

50. C&S   _____

51. CF   _____

52. CO_2 _____

53. COLD   _____

54. COPD   _____

55. CPAP   _____

56. CXR   _____

57. DOE   _____

58. ERV   _____

59. FEV   _____

60. FVC   _____

61. FRC   _____

62. IC   _____

63. IPPB   _____

64. IRV   _____

65. MV   _____

66. O_2 _____

67. PEEP   _____

68. PFT   _____

69. PND _____

70. R _____

71. RDS _____

72. RV _____

73. SIDS _____

74. SOB _____

75. T&A _____

76. TB _____

77. TGV _____

78. TLC _____

79. TV _____

80. URI _____

81. VC _____

82. ZN _____

▶EXERCISE 14–2

Word Building

Word Building

Using the suffix -pnea, meaning breathing, build the medical word which means the following.

Example:
lack of breathing   apnea

Using the suffix -phonia, meaning voice, build the medical word which means the following.

Build the medical words that mean the following.

1. fast breathing _____

2. slow breathing _____

3. difficult breathing _____

4. rapid, deep breathing _____

5. breathing only in the upright position _____

6. normal breathing _____

7. no voice _____

8. difficulty in speaking _____

9. excision of the adenoids _____

10. dilatation of the bronchus _____

11. excessive levels of carbon dioxide in the blood _____

12. inflammation of all the paranasal sinuses _____

13. paralysis of the diaphragm _____

14. inflammation of the lung _____

15. suturing of the uvula _____

16. instrument used to listen to chest sounds _____

17. surgical reconstruction of the chest _____

18. inflammation of the tonsils _____

19. process of cutting into the trachea _____

20. process of measuring breathing capacity and volumes _____

▶EXERCISE 14–3

Short Answer

Briefly answer the following questions.

Practice Quiz

1. List the seven major divisions of the respiratory system. _____

2. What two terms describe external respiration? _____

3. What muscles help the diaphragm to draw air into and expel air from the lungs? _____

4. What is another term for nostril? _____

5. What is another term for throat? _____

6. Where are the palatine tonsils located? _____

7. What connects the pharynx to the trachea? _____

8. What are bronchioles? _____

9. What is the term used to describe the top part of the lung? _____

10. What is the term used to describe the bottom part of the lung? _____

11. Where is the hilum located? _____

12. What is the term that describes the lung surface facing the diaphragm? _____

Matching Terms with Meanings

Matching

Match the term in Column A with its meaning in Column B

Column A

1. allergic rhinitis _____
2. bronchitis _____
3. croup _____
4. pleural effusion _____
5. pleurisy _____
6. upper respiratory infection (URI) _____

Column B

A. acute inflammation of the bronchial tree due to a virus and often following a cold

B. allergic response to inhaled allergens characterized by sneezing, watery discharges from eyes and nose, nasal itchiness, and congestion

C. infection of the nose, nasal cavity, pharynx, and larynx

D. inflammation of the pleura

E. laryngotracheobronchitis

F. the movement of a fluid or gas from a blood vessel into a surrounding cavity

Match the term in Column A with its defintion in Column B.

Column A

7. rales _____
8. rhonchi _____
9. stridor _____
10. wheezing _____
11. friction rubs _____

Column B

A. a whistling sound

B. a crackling sound

C. the sound of serous surfaces rubbing together

D. a rattling sound

E. a hoarse, high-pitched sound

II-14

Match the term in Column A with its meaning in Column B.

Column A

13. apnea _____
14. ataxic respirations _____
15. bradypnea _____
16. Cheyne-Stokes _____
17. dyspnea _____
18. hyperpnea _____
19. hyperventilation _____
20. oligopnea _____
21. tachypnea _____

Column B

A. infrequent respirations

B. abnormally slow breathing

C. regular and rhythmic breathing characterized by an alternating pattern of hyperpnea and apnea

D. no breathing

E. difficult or painful breathing

F. abnormal increase in depth and rate of breathing

G. abnormally fast respiration

H. prolonged deep and rapid breathing

I. irregular and unpredictable breathing involving alternating periods of hyperpnea, hypopnea, and apnea

▶**EXERCISE 14–5**

Spelling

Place a check mark beside all misspelled words in the list that follows. Correctly spell those that you checked off

Spelling Practice

1. bronchiography ☐ _____
2. bradipnea ☐ _____
3. olegopnea ☐ _____
4. larynx ☐ _____
5. pharinx ☐ _____
6. trachiotomy ☐ _____
7. diagphram ☐ _____
8. crycoid ☐ _____
9. eppiglottus ☐ _____
10. medeastinul ☐ _____
11. rhinoitis ☐ _____
12. pleuresy ☐ _____
13. hyperapnea ☐ _____
14. tachyopnea ☐ _____
15. stridorr ☐ _____
16. anstrostomy ☐ _____
17. loboectomy ☐ _____
18. rhinoplasty ☐ _____
19. antitusive ☐ _____

Diagram

Identify each of the parts of the respiratory system indicated on the following diagram.

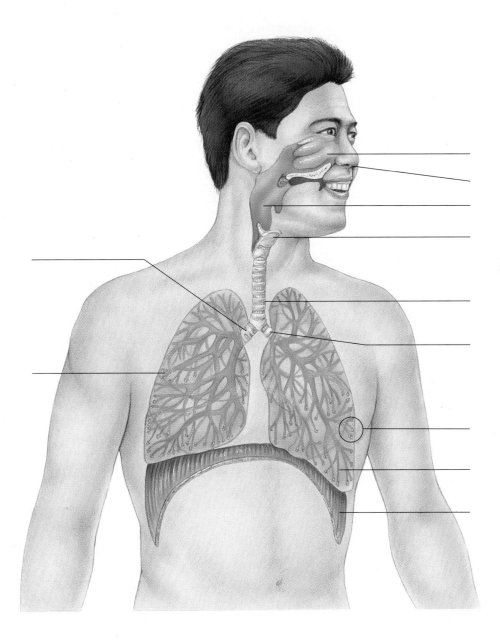

II–14

Medical Terms in Context

Define the underlined terms as they are used in context.

UNIVERSITY HOSPITAL ✚   SUMMARY RECORD

CHIEF COMPLAINT: Dyspnea and weight loss

HISTORY OF PRESENT ILLNESS:

Mr. B. is a 72-year-old male with advanced COPD who was admitted to the hospital with a 10-day history of increasing exertional dyspnea to the point that he was SOB at rest. He also complained of a productive cough. He had been started on outpatient antibiotics but the symptoms did not resolve.

PHYSICAL EXAMINATION:

On examination the patient was an elderly, frail-looking man. His vital signs were stable. He was afebrile. There was no clubbing or cyanosis. Chest was hyperinflated and kyphotic. Chest expansion was diminished. Breath sounds, however, were adequate, and there were no adventitious sounds with quiet breathing. Heart sounds were faint due to the hyperinflated chest.

INVESTIGATIONS:

Spirometry was markedly impaired with forced vital capacity of 1.1 liter, improving to 0.6 and 1.9 liters respectively prior to discharge. Right atrial enlargement was present on electrocardiogram. There was evidence of a right lower lobe pneumonia radiologically not present on previous outpatient film; otherwise the changes were compatible with COPD. Mantoux skin test was negative. Hemoglobin, white count, differential and electrolytes were normal. Mixed oropharyngeal flora were cultured from sputum. No acid-fast bacilli were present.

DISCHARGE DIAGNOSIS: 1. ACUTE EXACERBATION OF CHRONIC OBSTRUCTIVE PULMONARY DISEASE.

      2. CHRONIC RESPIRATORY FAILURE

      3. ANOREXIA WITH WEIGHT LOSS

SIGNATURE OF DOCTOR IN CHARGE _____

---

1. dyspnea _____

2. COPD _____

3. exertional dyspnea _____

4. SOB _____

5. antibiotics _____

6. afebrile _____

7. clubbing _____

8. cyanosis _____

9. hyperinflated _____

10. adventitious   _____

11. spirometry   _____

12. lobe pneumonia   _____

13. Mantoux skin test   _____

14. oropharyngeal   _____

15. acid-fast bacilli   _____

16. respiratory failure   _____

UNIVERSITY HOSPITAL   **RADIOLOGY RECORD**

CHEST X-RAY—ERECT POSTEROANTERIOR AND LATERAL

The lungs are <u>hyperinflated</u>. There is <u>bronchial dilatation</u>, with <u>peribronchial</u> thickening. The <u>hila</u> are mildly elevated, due to the presence of <u>parenchymal</u> disease. No new <u>consolidation</u> or collapse is seen.

IMPRESSION:

Appearances are consistent with advanced <u>cystic fibrosis</u>, with widespread <u>bronchiectasis</u> and parenchymal scarring, especially in the upper <u>lobes</u>. Overall, there has been no significant change since the previous examination, and no acute parenchymal changes are seen.

Authorized Health Care Practitioner _____

---

17. bronchial dilatation   _____

18. peribronchial   _____

19. hila   _____

20. parenchymal   _____

21. consolidation   _____

22. cystic fibrosis   _____

23. bronchiectasis   _____

24. lobes   _____

II—14

```
MEDICAL TERMINOLOGY USED IN SENTENCES

1. Percussion note was tympanic on both sides.

2. There was expiratory wheezing on both sides.

3. He has a long-standing history of COPD, asthma, with recurrent
   pneumonia.
```

25. percussion note _____

26. tympanic _____

27. expiratory wheezing _____

28. asthma _____

29. pneumonia _____

Crossword Puzzle

Respiratory Disorders

Across

1 Genetic predisposition to bronchospasms
4 Accumulation of inhaled irritants in the lungs
8 Inflamed nasal passage
9 Abnormal decrease in respiration rate
10 Inflammation of the pleura
12 The absence of breathing
13 Inflammation of the bronchi
15 Painful breathing
16 Abnormal increase in rate and depth of breathing
17 Excessive CO_2 retention

Down

1 Inability of the alveoli to inflate completely
2 Chronic dilation of the bronchi
3 Inflammation of the lung
5 Bluish coloration brought about by oxygen deficiency
6 Viral disease of childhood affecting the respiratory tracts
7 Rapid breathing
11 Overinflated alveolar walls caused by their reduced elasticity
13 Slow breathing
14 A shrill sound

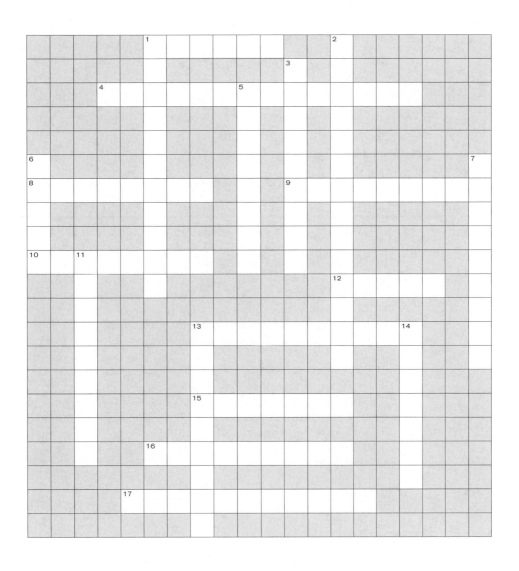

II–14

15

BLOOD, LYMPHATIC, AND IMMUNE SYSTEMS

CHAPTER OBJECTIVES

Upon successful completion of this chapter, the student will be able to do the following:

1. Name and describe the components of the blood.
2. Analyze, define, pronounce, and spell terms related to the blood.
3. Define common blood abnormalities.
4. Define common terms related to the diagnosis and treatment of abnormal blood conditions.
5. List and describe the organs of the lymphatic system.
6. List and describe primary and secondary organs of the immune system.
7. Analyze, define, pronounce, and spell terms related to the lymphatic and immune systems.
8. Define the terms related to the nonspecific defense system.
9. Define the terms related to the specific defense system.
10. Define the terms related to abnormalities of the lymphatic and immune systems.
11. Define the terms related to the diagnosis and treatment of conditions of the lymphatic and immune systems.
12. Define common abbreviations related to the blood and the lymphatic and immune systems.

BLOOD WORD ELEMENT	TYPE	MEANING
bas/o	root	base
chrom/o	root	color
-cytosis	suffix	slight increase in the number of cells
eosin/o	root	rosy-red
erythr/o	root	red
hem/o; hemat/o	root	blood
leuk/o; leuc/o	root	white
morph/o	root	shape; form
neutr/o	root	neutral
-phil	suffix	having an affinity for; attracted to
-phoresis	suffix	bearing
poikil/o	root	variation
sider/o	root	iron
thromb/o	root	clot

LYMPHATIC AND IMMUNE SYSTEMS WORD ELEMENT	TYPE	MEANING
immun/o	root	immunity
lipid/o	root	fat
lymph/o	root	lymph
lymphaden/o	root	lymph nodes
splen/o	root	spleen
-stitial	suffix	pertaining to a place
thym/o	root	thymus

15.1 BLOOD

Blood consists of approximately 45% cellular (or formed) elements, such as red blood cells, white blood cells, and platelets, suspended in liquid, or plasma, which makes up approximately 55% of blood. The red blood cells are called **erythrocytes** (ĕ-rĭth′-rō-sītz) and the white blood cells, **leukocytes** (loo′-kō-sītz). The **platelets** (plāt′-lĕts), so-named because of their shape (small, plate-like structures), are also called **thrombocytes** (thrŏm′-bō-sītz). There are 4.8 million to 5.4 million erythrocytes/cubic millimeter (or about 26 trillion erythrocytes in the body), 5,000 to 9,000 leukocytes/cubic millimeter (one white blood cell for every 500–900 red blood cell) and 250,000 to 400,000 thrombocytes/cubic millimeter.

All blood cells originate from undifferentiated stem cells or **hemocytoblasts** (hē″-mō-sīt′-tō-blăsts). As the cells differentiate, they mature into erythrocytes, thrombocytes, and leukocytes (see Figure 15–1).

II–15

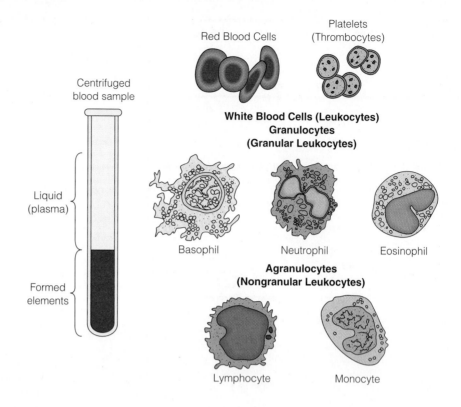

Erythrocytes distribute oxygen throughout the body while removing carbon dioxide. Each erythrocyte contains **hemoglobin** (hē″-mō-glō′-bǐn), an iron-containing protein that combines with oxygen and carbon dioxide and allows the cell to carry out its oxygen-transporting function.

A mature red blood cell is a biconcave disk with no nucleus. It has a life span of roughly 120 days. The production of red blood cells, called **hematopoiesis** (hē″-mă-tō-poy-ē′-sĭs), occurs in the red bone marrow. In adults, the red bone marrow is found in the skull, sternum, ribs, vertebrae, and pelvis.

Leukocytes protect the body from disease. Through a process called **diapedesis** (dī″-ă-pěd-ē′-sĭs), leukocytes move into tissue outside the blood vessels to carry out their disease-fighting function. Leukocytes are classified as either **granulocytes** (grăn′-ū-lō-sīts″) or **agranulocytes** (ā-grăn′-ū-lō-sīts) depending on the size and kind of granules they contain. Granulocytes (also called granular leukocytes) are further divided by staining properties into **neutrophils** (nū′-trō-fĭls), **eosinophils** (ē″-ŏ-sĭn′-ō-fĭls), and **basophils** (bā′-sō-fĭlz). Agranulocytes (also called agranular leukocytes) are divided into **monocytes** (mŏn′-ō-sīts) and **lymphocytes** (lĭm′-fō-sīts).

Thrombocytes help prevent blood loss through a broken vessel by collecting at the site of the break and forming a **platelet plug**. They also release chemicals that aid in coagulation. This action of thrombocytes is part of a process known as **hemostasis** (hē-mŏs′-tă-sĭs).

Plasma is 92 percent water. It carries nutrients and other essential products to the cells and removes waste products. Plasma proteins include **albumins**, **globulins**, and **fibrinogen**. The globulins are further divisible into alpha globulins, beta globulins, and gamma globulins. Gamma globulins are produced by the immune system.

Plasma carries fats such as triglycerides, cholesterol, and phospholipids. Triglycerides and cholesterol provide the body with energy, and phospholipids make up cell membranes. These fats are transported to the body tissues by attaching onto proteins; combined fats and proteins are called **lipoproteins**. The two common types of lipoproteins are **low density lipoproteins (LDL)**, which are often referred to as "bad cholesterol" because they form atheromatous plaques on the walls of arteries, and **high density lipoproteins (HDL)**, which are also called "good cholesterol" as they help the body break down and utilize excess cholesterol.

▷ 15.2 TERM ANALYSIS FOR BLOOD

TERM WITH PRONUNCIATION	ANALYSIS	DEFINITION
agranulocytosis ă-grăn″-ū-lō-sī-tō′-sĭs	-cytosis = slight increase in the number of cells a- = no; not granul/o = granules	slight increase in the number of agranulocytes
anisocytosis ăn-ī″-sō-sī-tō′-sĭs	-cytosis = slight increase in the number of cells an- = no; not is/o = equal	slight increase in the number of unequal sized cells
basophil bā′-sō-fĭl	-phil = affinity; to love bas/o = base	type of white blood cell that stains blue with a basic dye
elliptocytosis ē-lĭp″-tō-sī-tō′-sĭs	-cytosis = slight increase in the number of cells ellipt/o = ellipse	slight increase in the number of elliptical-shaped red blood cells
eosinophil ē″-ŏ-sĭn′-ō-fĭl	-phil = affinity; to love eosin/o = rosy-red	type of white blood cell that stains rosy-red with the acid dye eosin
erythremia ĕr″-ĭ-thrē′-mē-ă	-emia = blood condition erythr/o = red	abnormal increase in the number of red blood cells (also known as polycythemia vera)
erythroblast ĕ-rĭth′-rō-blăst	-blast = immature erythr/o = red	immature red blood cell
erythrocyte ĕ-rĭth′-rō-sīt	-cyte = cell erythr/o = red	red blood cell
erythrocytosis ĕ-rĭth″-rō-sī-tō′-sĭs	-cytosis = slight increase in the number of cells erythr/o = red	slight increase in the number of red blood cells
erythropenia ĕ-rĭth″-rō-pē′-nē-ă	-penia = deficiency; abnormal decrease erythr/o = red	deficiency in the number of red blood cells
erythropoiesis ĕ-rĭth″-rō-poy-ē′-sĭs	-poiesis = formation; manufacture erythr/o = red	manufacture of red blood cells
hematopoiesis hĕm″-ă-tō-poy-ē′-sĭs	-poiesis = formation; manufacture hemat/o = blood	manufacture of blood cells

TERM WITH PRONUNCIATION	ANALYSIS	DEFINITION
hemolysis hē-mŏl′-ĭ-sĭs	-lysis = destruction; breakdown; separate hem/o = blood	destruction of red blood cells
hemostasis hē-mŏs′-tă-sĭs	-stasis = stoppage; controlling hem/o = blood	stoppage of blood flow
hyperbilirubinemia hī″-pĕr-bĭl″-ĭ-roo-bĭn-ē′-mē-ă	-emia = blood condition hyper- = excessive; beyond; above normal bilirubin/o = bilirubin	excessive amount of bilirubin in the blood
hypercholesterolemia hī″-pĕr-kō-lĕs″-tĕr-ŏl-ē′-mē-ă	-emia = blood condition hyper- = excessive; beyond; above normal cholesterol/o = cholesterol	excessive amount of cholesterol in the blood
hyperchromia hī″-pĕr-krō′-mē-ă	-ia = condition; state of hyper- = excessive; beyond; above normal chrom/o = color	a term used to describe red blood cells that are overpigmented or excessively pigmented
hyperlipidemia hī″-pĕr-lĭp-ĭ-dē′-mē-ă	-emia = blood condition hyper- = excessive; beyond; above normal lipid/o = fat	excessive amount of fats in the blood
hypochromia hī″-pō-krō′-mē-ă	-ia = condition; state of hypo- = below normal; deficient; under chrom/o = color	a term used to describe red blood cells that are under-pigmented
leukemia loo-kē′-mē-ă	-emia = blood condition leuk/o = white	abnormal, excessive, uncontrollable increase in the number of white blood cells **Note:** For an explanation of the different types of leukemias, see abnormal conditions of the blood.
leukocyte; leucocyte loo′-kō-sīt	-cyte = cell leuk/o; leuc/o = white	white blood cell
leukocytosis loo″-kō-sī-tō′-sĭs	-cytosis = slight increase in the number of cells leuk/o = white	slight increase in the number of white blood cells usually due to infection or inflammation
leukopenia loo″-kō-pē′-nē-ă	-penia = deficiency; abnormal decrease leuk/o = white	deficiency in the number of white blood cells
lymphoblast lĭm′-fō-blăst	-blast = immature lymph/o = lymph	immature lymphocyte

TERM WITH PRONUNCIATION	ANALYSIS	DEFINITION
macrocytosis măk″-rō-sī-tō′-sĭs	-cytosis = slight increase in the number of cells macro- = large	slight increase in the number of macrocytes
microcytosis mī″-krō-sī-tō′-sĭs	-cytosis = slight increase in the number of cells micro- = small	slight increase in the number of microcytes
morphology mor-fŏl′-ō-jē	-logy = study of morph/o = form; shape	study of shape
myelogenous mī-ĕ-lŏj′-ĕn-ŭs	-genous = produced by myel/o = bone marrow	produced in the bone marrow
neutrophil nū′-trō-fĭl	-phil = affinity; to love; attraction for neutr/o = neutral	type of white blood cell that stains purple with neutral dyes
normochromia nor″-mō-krō′-mē-ă	-ia = state of; condition norm/o = normal chrom/o = color	normal colored red blood cells
pancytopenia păn″-sī-tō-pē′-nē-ă	-penia = deficiency pan- = all cyt/o = cell	deficiency of all types of blood cells
poikilocytosis poy″-kĭl-ō-sī-tō′-sĭs	-cytosis = slight increase in the number of cells poikil/o = variation	variation in the shape of red blood cells
polychromia pŏl-ē-krō′-mē-ă	-ia = condition; state of poly- = many chrom/o = color	red blood cells of many colors
polymorphonuclear pŏl″-ē-mor″-fō-nū′-klē-ăr	-ar = pertaining to poly- = many morph/o = shape; form nucle/o = nucleus	a type of neutrophil that has nuclei of many shapes
reticulocyte rĕ-tĭk′-ū-lō-sīt	-cyte = cell reticul/o = network	an immature red blood cell characterized by a network of granules within the cell membrane
sideropenia sĭd″-ĕr-ō-pē′-nē-ă	-penia = deficiency sider/o = iron	deficiency of iron in the blood
spherocytosis sfē″-rō-sī-tō′-sĭs	-cytosis = slight increase in the number of cells spher/o = spherical; rounded	slight increase in the number of rounded (spherical) red blood cells **Note:** Remember that a normal red blood cell is shaped as a biconcave disk.

TERM WITH PRONUNCIATION	ANALYSIS	DEFINITION
thrombocytopenia thrŏm″-bō-sī″-tō-pē-nē-ă	-penia = deficiency thromb/o = clot cyt/o = cell	deficiency in the number of clotting cells (thrombocytes or platelets)
thrombocytosis thrŏm″-bō-sī-tō′-sīs	-cytosis = slight increase in the number of cells thromb/o = clot	slight increase in the number of clotting cells
thrombolysis thrŏm-bŏl′-ĭ-sīs	-lysis = destruction; breakdown; separate thromb/o = clot	breakdown of a clot that is already formed
thrombosis thrŏm-bō′-sīs	-osis = abnormal condition thromb/o = clot	abnormal condition of clots; blood clot

▶ 15.3 ABNORMAL CONDITIONS OF BLOOD

Anemias

Anemia results from a reduction in the number of red blood cells or in the amount of hemoglobin, either of which decreases the ability of blood to carry oxygen. The causes include hemorrhage, hemolysis, and defective erythropoiesis.

ANEMIA	DESCRIPTION
deficiency anemia	lack of the essential ingredients for the manufacture of red blood cells, causing abnormalities in red blood cell color and morphology
iron deficiency anemia	most common type of anemia; caused by inadequate iron absorption or increased iron requirements
pernicious anemia	anemia due to a lack of vitamin B_{12}
hereditary hemolytic anemias	genetically based anemias where the reduction in the number of red blood cells is due to excessive destruction
sickle cell anemia	In sickle cell anemia, the red blood cells are sickle shaped rather than biconcave; the body's immune system recognizes these cells as abnormal and destroys them by phagocytosis, reducing the normal life span of a red blood cell.

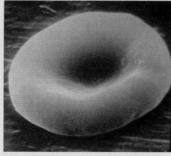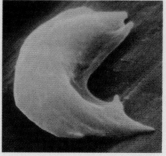

ANEMIA	DESCRIPTION
sideroblastic anemia	results from an inability to use iron in hemoglobin synthesis, even though an adequate supply is available
thalassemia	most commonly affects people of Mediterranean descent and is characterized by defective hemoglobin production
acquired hemolytic anemia	increased destruction of red blood cells leading to a reduction in the number of red blood cells due to causes other than those that are genetically based
erythroblastosis fetalis	hemolytic disease of the newborn results from an incompatibility of blood causing an antigen-antibody reaction between the maternal blood and that of the newborn or fetus, with subsequent destruction of fetal red blood cells

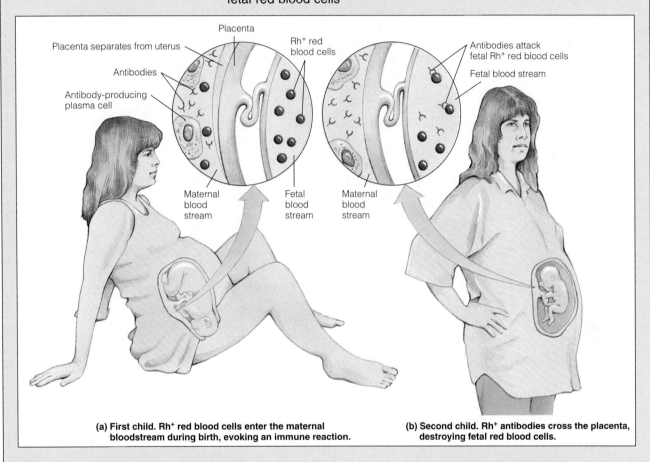

Placenta

Placenta separates from uterus

Antibodies

Antibody-producing plasma cell

Rh⁺ red blood cells

Antibodies attack fetal Rh⁺ red blood cells

Fetal blood stream

Maternal blood stream

Fetal blood stream

Maternal blood stream

(a) First child. Rh⁺ red blood cells enter the maternal bloodstream during birth, evoking an immune reaction.

(b) Second child. Rh⁺ antibodies cross the placenta, destroying fetal red blood cells.

Note: Symptoms in the newborn are jaundice, anemia, and brain damage. Immunization against this reaction is possible by injecting the mother with a drug such as **RhoGam**, which suppresses the production of antibodies against the fetal blood.

aplastic anemia	results from defective stem cells interfering with erythropoiesis, or from damage to the bone marrow, causing pancytopenia

II–15

Leukemias

Leukemias are malignancies, characterized by a massive proliferation of immature white blood cells and frequently by a decrease in red blood cells and platelets. Because of the proliferation of immature or substandard leukocytes, the white blood cells cannot defend the body against disease. If the number of red blood cells and platelets are decreased, oxygen content and the clotting mechanism are affected.

Different types of leukemia are named according to the white blood cells affected.

LEUKEMIA	DESCRIPTION
acute lymphoblastic leukemia (ALL)	excessive increase in the number of lymphoblasts, usually occurs in children
acute myelogenous leukemia (AML)	abnormal increase in the number of myeloblasts (neutrophils, eosinophils and basophils), can occur at any age with the average rate of survival being 1–2 years
acute monoblastic leukemia	proliferation in the number of monoblasts (immature monocytes), can occur in children or adults
chronic granulocytic leukemia; chronic myelogenous leukemia (CML)	abnormal increase in the number of immature granulocytes
chronic lymphocytic leukemia	proliferation of lymphocytes, usually occurs in middle or old age
hemophilia	genetic disorder characterized by dysfunction of the blood-clotting mechanism **Note:** One of the essential clotting factors, Factor VIII, is lacking. Thus thrombin formation, which is necessary for a blood clot to form, does not occur.
polycythemia vera	abnormal increase in the production of red blood cells causing a slowing of circulation and a thickening of blood (also known as erythremia)

LABORATORY TESTS	DESCRIPTION
bleeding time	a coagulation test which measures the bleeding time of a puncture wound to the surface of the skin
antiglobulin test (Coombs' test)	used to detect any antibodies on the surface of a patient's red blood cells and used in the diagnosis of hemolytic anemias and erythroblastosis fetalis.
complete blood count (CBC)	determination of the number of erythrocytes, leukocytes, and thrombocytes in the blood; also measures the percent of red blood cells and amount of hemoglobin
erythrocyte count; red blood cell count	calculation of the number of red blood cells in a sample of blood
erythrocyte sedimentation rate (ESR)	measures the time it takes for erythrocytes to settle out from a sample of blood to the bottom of a tube; during inflammation, the red blood cells have an increased tendency to form rouleaux and fall faster
hematocrit (HCT)	percentage of erythrocytes in a volume of blood
hemoglobin (Hb; Hgb)	measures the amount of hemoglobin in a sample of blood
lipid profile	determination of the levels of such blood lipids as cholesterol and triglycerides. **Note:** These fatty substances from food tend to accumulate on the walls of arteries, leading to obstruction of blood flow. High levels are considered a risk factor for coronary heart disease.

lipoprotein electrophoresis
  lipoproteins include:
    chylomicrons
    high density lipoprotein (HDL)
    low density lipoprotein (LDL)
    very low density lipoprotein (VLDL)
	lipoproteins are separated following the application of an electric field, allowing for careful analysis of the type and number of lipoproteins circulating in the blood

partial thromboplastin time (PTT)	a coagulation test which measures the time taken for a sample of blood to clot following the addition of thromboplastin (a blood-clotting agent)
platelet count	measures the amount of platelets in a sample of blood

II–15

LABORATORY TESTS	DESCRIPTION
prothrombin time (PT)	a coagulation test which measures the time taken for clot formation following the addition of a clot-forming agent
red blood cell indices	a collection of six different blood tests are performed to determine the volume of erythrocytes, hemoglobin concentration and hemoglobin content in red blood cells Included are: red blood cell count, hemoglobin, hematocrit, mean corpuscular volume (MCV), mean corpuscular hemoglobin (MCH), mean corpuscular hemoglobin, concentration (MCHC) Red blood cells of normal size are called **normocytic**; red blood cells of normal color are called **normochromic**.
red blood cell morphology	the study of red blood cells for abnormalities of size, shape, color, and structure
size abnormalities	macrocytosis, microcytosis, anisocytosis
shape abnormalities	spherocytosis, elliptocytosis, sickle cells (crescent-shaped) poikilocytosis
color abnormalities	hypochromia, hyperchromia, polychromia
rouleaux	a common abnormality where the erythrocytes look like a pile of coins. Although the presence of rouleaux is normal, increased or decreased rouleaux is abnormal.

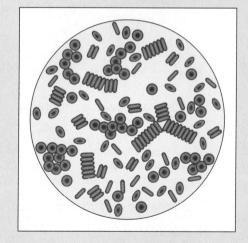

reticulocyte count	a determination of the percentage of reticulocytes to erythrocytes in a sample of blood (good indicator of bone marrow function)

LABORATORY TESTS	DESCRIPTION
Schilling test	tests the body's ability to absorb vitamin B_{12} from the digestive tract into the blood
serum folate; folic acid	measures the amount of folic acid in a sample of blood (folic acid is included in the vitamin B complex and is found naturally in liver and yeast)
white blood cell differential	measures the amount of each different type of white blood cell in a sample of blood
white cell count	measures the number of leukocytes in a sample of blood

ULTRASOUND	DESCRIPTION
Doppler ultrasound	measures the speed at which the blood flows through a blood vessel **Note:** Moving red blood cells are subjected to ultrasonic waves, which bounce back to a recording device that measures the velocity of blood flow. Slow flowing blood may indicate stenosis or occlusion.

CLINICAL PROCEDURES	DESCRIPTION
bone marrow biopsy, bone marrow aspiration	bone marrow is obtained for microscopic examination by placement of a needle through a bone, such as the sternum, into the bone marrow and withdrawing a sample for laboratory examination

PHARMACEUTICAL AGENTS	DESCRIPTION
antithrombotic therapy	prevents clot formation by inteferring with the clotting mechanism **Note:** These drugs do not lyse (break down) clots that have already formed. Heparin and aspirin are examples.
coagulants	agents used to aid in the clotting process (vitamin K is a common example)
thrombolytic agents	eliminates clot by breaking down fibrin (Streptokinase and tissue plasminogen activator [TPA] are examples)
lipid lowering agents; antihyperlipidemic agent	reduces the amounts of triglycerides and cholesterol in the blood (gemfibrozil is an example)

II—15

CLINICAL PROCEDURES	DESCRIPTION
blood transfusion	Following confirmation of blood compatibility, blood components from a donor are infused into a patient. Since a number of diseases can be transmitted through blood transfusion, tests are conducted on the donor's blood for such conditions as acquired immunodeficiency syndrome (AIDS) virus, hepatitis, syphilis and malaria.
bone marrow transplant	Bone marrow that has been suitably matched for tissue and blood type is harvested from a donor and infused into a patient suffering from conditions such as aplastic anemia, sickle-cell anemia, leukemia, or certain other malignancies.

▶ 15.5 ABBREVIATIONS FOR BLOOD

ABBREVIATION	DEFINITION	ABBREVIATION	DEFINITION
Ab	antibody	LDL	low density lipoprotein
Ag	antigen	MCH	mean corpuscular hemoglobin
ALL	acute lymphoblastic leukemia		
AML	acute myelogenous leukemia	MCHC	mean corpuscular hemoglobin concentration
baso	basophil	MCV	mean corpuscular volume
CBC	complete blood count	mono	monocyte
CML	chronic myelogenous leukemia	PMN	polymorphonuclear
		polys	polymorphonuclear leukocytes
diff	differential		
eosin	eosinophil	PTT	partial thromboplastin time
ESR	erythrocyte sedimentation rate	PT	prothrombin time
Hb, Hgb	hemoglobin	RBC	red blood cell
HCT	hematocrit	TPA	tissue plasminogen activator
HDL	high density lipoprotein	VLDL	very low density lipoprotein
		WBC	white blood cell

15.6 GENERAL ANATOMY AND PHYSIOLOGY OF THE LYMPHATIC SYSTEM

The lymphatic (lĭm-făt′-ĭk) system is made up of an extensive vascular system, a fluid called **lymph** (lĭmf), and the lymph organs. This vascular system is separate from but empties into the circulatory system. See Figure 15–2.

FIGURE 15–2

The Lymphatic System

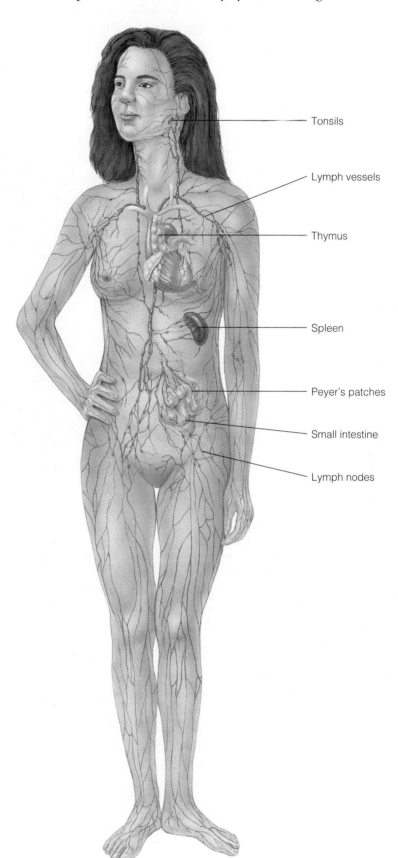

- Tonsils
- Lymph vessels
- Thymus
- Spleen
- Peyer's patches
- Small intestine
- Lymph nodes

Lymph Vessels

The vessels of the lymphatic system are divided into three categories according to size (Figure 15-3). The smallest vessels, the **lymphatic capillaries**, are components of all body tissue. The **lymphatics** are the next largest vessels. The largest lymph vessels are the two **lymph ducts**, which empty lymph into the bloodstream. As shown in Figure 15–4 on p. 450, the **right lymphatic duct** serves the right side of the head and neck, the right arm, and the right side of the chest. The remainder of the body is served by the **left** or **thoracic duct**.

FIGURE 15–3

Lymph Vessels

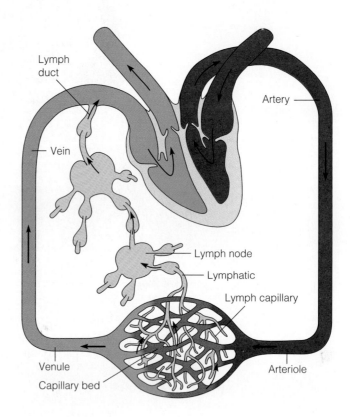

Lymph

The lymph vessels carry a fluid called **lymph**. This is a fluid that has passed from the blood into spaces around tissue cells (interstitial fluid). This fluid is similar to plasma except that it has no red blood cells, no platelets, and fewer proteins. Most of this fluid eventually returns to the circulatory system, but some of it enters the lymphatic system through the lymphatic capillaries before returning to the bloodstream. The major function of lymph is to transport white blood cells throughout the body as a means of fighting infection. Lymph also transports fat from the digestive system to the blood. The presence of fat gives lymph a milky appearance. Consequently, another name for the intestinal lymphatics that carry lymph from the intestines is **lacteals** (lăk′-tē-ălz) (lact/o = milk). Another name for the intestinal lymph is **chyle** (kīl).

The lymphatics are equipped with one-way valves that move the lymph in one direction only so that it empties into the two lymph ducts and returns through veins to the bloodstream. Lymph capillaries in body tissues merge into larger lymphatics, which merge into large lymph ducts. The lymph is drained back into the blood.

The other components of the lymphatic system are the lymph organs: the **lymph nodes**, which are located at intervals along the path of the lymphatics; the **thymus** (thī′-mŭs) **gland**, which processes lymphocytes; and the **spleen**, in which lymphocytes germinate and mulitply. **Peyer's** (pī′-ĕrz) **patches**, located in the small intestine, and the **tonsils**, located in the throat, are composed of lymphatic tissue and are also part of the lymphatic system.

Lymph Nodes

Located at intervals along the route of the lymphatics are the **lymph nodes**, as shown in Figure 15–4. The lymph nodes are grouped in specific regions. Included are the submandibular, cervical, axillary, and inguinal nodes. The lymph nodes are sites of residence and proliferation of leukocytes. White blood cells called **phagocytes** (făg′-ō-sīts) are found in the lymph nodes. As lymph flows through the lymph nodes, phagocytes engulf and destroy bacteria in the lymph. This process is known as **phagocytosis** (făg″-ō-sī-tō′-sĭs).

Thymus Gland

The thymus gland is located in the thoracic cavity close to the heart (Figure 15–2). As well as being a lymph organ, the thymus gland is an endocrine organ that secretes a hormone called **thymosin** (thī′-mō-sĭn). Thymosin stimulates red bone marrow to produce **T-lymphocytes** (lĭm′-fō-sīts), whose function is important in the immune system as described below. The thymus gland atrophies or involutes with age.

Spleen

The **spleen**, located in the left side of the abdominal cavity (Figure 15–2), stores blood cells and removes substances from it that are not functional, such as old red blood cells and invasive microorganisms. It is also important in hematopoiesis and B-lymphocyte multiplication.

FIGURE 15–4

**Body Areas Served By
the Two Lymph Ducts**

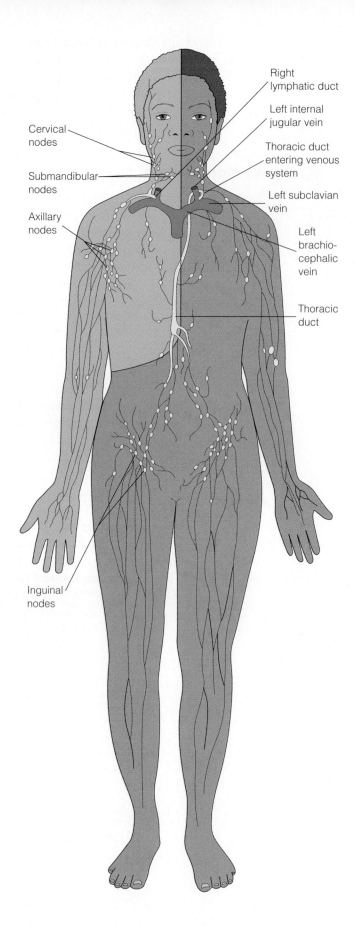

Cervical
nodes

Submandibular
nodes

Axillary
nodes

Inguinal
nodes

Right
lymphatic duct

Left internal
jugular vein

Thoracic duct
entering venous
system

Left subclavian
vein

Left
brachio-
cephalic
vein

Thoracic
duct

Tonsils and Peyer's Patches

Three pairs of tonsils, composed of lymphatic tissue, are located in the throat. The **pharyngeal** (făr-ĭn′-jē-ăl) **tonsils** in the nasopharynx are also known as **adenoids** (ăd′-ĕ-noydz). The **lingual** (lĭng′-gwăl) **tonsils** are located near the base of the tongue. The **palatine tonsils**, located in the oral cavity where it meets the pharynx, are usually referred to simply as "tonsils." The tonsils help fight microorganisms that may enter the body through the throat.

Peyer's patches are concentrations of lymphatic tissue located in the small intestine. This tissue contains lymphocytes that destroy infectious agents that may have entered the digestive tract.

▶ 15.7 IMMUNE SYSTEM

The primary organs of the immune system are red bone marrow, where **B-lymphocytes (B cells)** mature, and the thymus gland, where **T-lymphocytes (T cells)** mature.

The secondary organs of the immune system are the spleen, which removes foreign agents from blood, and the lymph nodes, which remove foreign agents from lymph.

The body is protected against invasion from infectious agents by two lines of defense known as the nonspecific defense system and the specific defense system.

Nonspecific Defense System

The nonspecific defense system protects the body against infection in a generalized way. The nonspecific defense system includes the **skin**, which protects body organs against invasion from foreign matter, and the **mucous** (mū′-kŭs) **membrane** linings of the digestive, respiratory, urinary, and reproductive tracts.

If foreign organisms such as bacteria succeed in crossing the skin or the mucous membranes, phagocytes are attracted to the infected region to destroy the invaders by the process of phagocytosis. When cancerous cells or virus-infected cells are involved, **natural killer cells** are called to destroy the invader. Natural killer cells attack body cells rather than foreign cells. Since viruses work inside the body's own cells, they are attacked by natural killer cells rather than by phagocytes.

Two other elements in the nonspecific defense system are proteins called **interferon** (ĭn-tĕr-fēr′-ŏn) and **complement**. Interferon is released by cells that are infected by a virus. This action signals nearby healthy cells to resist viral replication. Complement, so named because it "complements" the body's defense system, assists in the process of phagocytosis and in some cases acts directly to rupture bacteria cells.

Specific Defense System

When the generalized protection of the nonspecific defense system fails to halt foreign invaders, the specific defense system comes into play. The specific defense system utilizes white blood cells that have specialized roles in fighting particular invaders. These specialized cells are the T-lymphocytes and B-lymphocytes, both of which have been genetically programmed to recognize specific invaders and to either destroy them directly or to mark them for destruction by the cells of the nonspecific defense system.

Specific virus-infected cells and cancerous cells are combated by a process called **cell-mediated immune response** in which mature **T-lymphocytes** destroy the infected cells directly. These mature T-lymphocytes are called **killer** or **cytotoxic** (sī″-tō-tŏks′-ĭk) **T-lymphocytes**. They destroy infected cells by disturbing the cell's plasma membrane.

Specific bacterial cells are combated by **B-lymphocytes**, which produce proteins called **antibodies**. Antibodies are released into the body fluids (blood, lymph, and interstitial fluid). Since these body fluids are also known as "humors," the release of antibodies is called the **humoral immune response**.

Foreign invaders that activate the body's specific defense system are referred to by the term **antigen** (ăn′-tĭ-jĕn), which is shorthand for "antibody generator." It is important to note, however, that not all invaders are combated by antibodies. Some invaders are combated by lymphocytes directly, as described previously. "Antigen" is a general term that refers to both bacteria and viruses, as well as to plant pollen and to red blood cells in transplanted tissue.

In humoral immune response, an antibody binds to the particular antigen that it is specifically designed to combat. This process activates the release of complement, which in turn, attracts phagocytes to the site. Additionally, phagocytosis is accelerated by the process of **agglutination** (ă-gloo″-tĭ-nā′-shŭn); in agglutination, one antibody molecule binds to antigens from more than one cell at a time. This accumulation of antigen cells into clumps speeds up the process of phagocytosis.

Antibodies belong to a group of proteins called **gamma globulins** (glob′-ū-lĭnz). The gamma globulins are divided into five categories of **immunoglobulins (Ig)** (ĭm″-ū-nō-glŏb′-ū-lĭnz): immunoglobulin **M (IgM)**, **immunoglobulin G (IgG)**, **immunoglobulin E (IgE)**, **immunoglobulin A (IgA)**, and **immunoglobulin D (IgD)**. Most antibodies are type IgG.

The specialized role of lymphocytes and antibodies in combating specific antigens is made possible by the fact that each lymphocyte and each antibody has its own particular **antigen-binding site** or **antigen receptor**. Each receptor has a shape that is complementary to one particular antigen and is capable of recognizing and binding to that antigen only. During lymphocyte development, the genes that carry the code for antigen receptors are shuffled and recombined in a process called **natural genetic recombination**. In this way, millions of different antigen receptors, each having its own particular specificity, are produced, which allows the immune system to deal with an almost infinite number of antigens, including new mutations of viruses.

Any B-lymphocyte or T-lymphocyte that encounters an antigen for which it is specific quickly produces multiple copies of itself in a process called **cloning** (klō′-nĭng). Such cloned cells are called **effector** cells. Some of the cloned cells, however, are called **memory** cells. The effector cells die within a few days, but memory cells remain in circulation for many years. A subsequent exposure to the same antigen stimulates the memory cells to rapidly produce more effector cells, which destroy the antigen before it causes disease. The term **immunity** (īm-mūn′-ĭ-tĭ) refers, in its strictest sense, to the activity of these memory cells, which provide the body with resistance to any disease to which it has previously been exposed. Immunization against poliomyelitis, for example, is simply exposure to enough antigen to produce the memory cells that will make the body immune to the disease during future exposures.

Both the humoral and the cell-mediated immune responses are activated by specialized cells called **helper T-lymphocytes**, which rely on an intricate system of chemical messages. Phagocytes doing battle with bacteria in the nonspecific defense system secrete a protein called **interleukin-1**. This signals the helper-

T lymphocytes to secrete proteins called **lymphokines** (lĭm′-fŏ-kīnz). Lymphokines then, in turn, stimulate the multiplication of both B-lymphocytes and T-lymphocytes. For an overview of nonspecific and specific defense systems, see Figure 15–5.

FIGURE 15—5 Overview of the Body's Defense Mechanisms

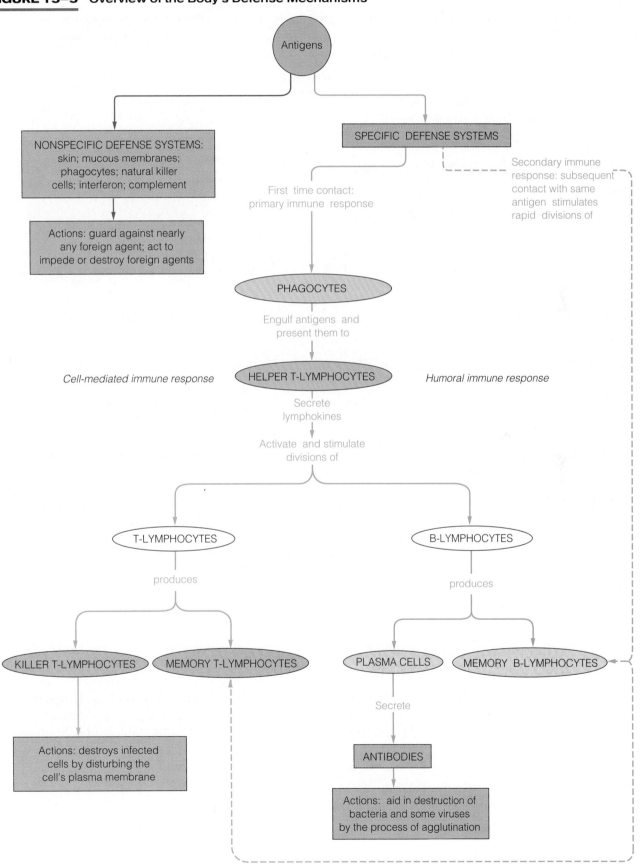

15.8 **TERM ANALYSIS FOR THE LYMPHATIC AND IMMUNE SYSTEMS**

TERM WITH PRONUNCIATION	TERM ANALYSIS	DEFINITION
autoimmune aw″-tō-ĭm-mūn′	-immune = immunity; safe; resistance to disease auto- = self	immunity against one's own body tissues
interstitial fluid ĭn″-tĕr-stĭsh′-ăl	-stitial = pertaining to a place inter- = between	fluid placed or lying between the tissue spaces
lymphadenopathy lĭm-făd″-ĕ-nŏp′-ă-thē	-pathy = disease lymphaden/o = lymph nodes	disease or enlargement of the lymph glands; disease of the lymph nodes
lymphangitis; **lymphangiitis** lĭm″-făn-jī′-tĭs	-itis = inflammation lymphangi/o = lymph vessels	inflammation of the lymph vessels
lymphedema lĭmf-ĕ-dē′-mă	-edema = accumulation of interstitial fluid lymph/o = lymph	accumulation of interstitial fluid leading to obstruction of the lymph in the lymph vessels
lymphocyte lĭm′-fō-sīt	-cyte = cell lymph/o = lymph	a lymph cell (a type of white blood cell)
lymphoma lĭm-fō′-mă	-oma = tumor or mass lymph/o = lymph	tumor of the lymphatics (often refers to malignant lymphoma)
lymphopenia lĭm-fō-pē′-nē-ă	-penia = deficiency lymph/o = lymph	deficiency in the number of lymphocytes in the blood
phagocyte făg′-ō-sīt	-cyte = cell phag/o = eating	cell that can engulf and digest unwanted material
splenorrhaphy splē-nor′-ă-fē	-rrhaphy = suture splen/o = spleen	suturing of the spleen
thymectomy thī-měk′-tō-mē	-ectomy = excision; removal thym/o = thymus gland	removal of the thymus gland

15.9 **ABNORMAL CONDITIONS OF THE LYMPHATIC AND IMMUNE SYSTEMS**

The following table lists some of the abnormal conditions of the lymphatic and immune systems. One of these conditions, acquired immunodeficiency syndrome (AIDS), is too complex to discuss briefly in the table and is discussed in detail below.

Acquired Immunodeficiency Syndrome (AIDS)

The **human immunodeficiency virus** (HIV-1) is the agent that attacks the immune system and causes **acquired immunodeficiency syndrome (AIDS)**. It may also attack the central nervous system, producing irreversible damage. The virus has an incubation period of from one to fourteen years. Diagnosis of HIV infection is generally made through the identification of antibodies to parts of the HIV-1 virus. Antibodies produced by the body to combat HIV, while effective in the short term, eventually are overwhelmed, and the immune system eventually becomes weakened and incapacitated. The primary effect of AIDS on the immune system is the infection and destruction of the helper T-lymphocytes. As discussed above, both the humoral and the cell-mediated immune responses are rendered inoperable without the action of the helper T-lymphocytes. Symptoms of AIDS include lymphadenopathy, fatigue, fever, weight loss, opportunistic infections, and splenomegaly. There is no cure for AIDS at the present time.

Following the breakdown of the specific defense system, numerous opportunistic diseases such as cancers and infections are able to attack the body. The most common diseases that afflict patients with AIDS are pneumonia, tuberculosis, and a cancer called **Kaposi's sarcoma**. These particular AIDS-related diseases are discussed in more detail below.

Current treatment is focused on life extension and symptom reduction. A drug known as azidothymidine (AZT) has been shown to prolong the lives of patients. AZT has a number of side effects, including anemia, leukopenia, and thrombocytopenia. Dideoxyinosine (ddI) is another drug used in AIDS treatment.

AIDS is transmitted through contaminated body fluids that have been exchanged through close or intimate contact. There is no evidence that HIV-1 is transmitted through casual social contact. Sexual contact (both heterosexual and homosexual) with a person who is HIV positive is the primary mode of transmission. Drug users frequently contract the virus by using contaminated syringes and needles. Contaminated blood products used in blood transfusions and contaminated donor organs can transmit the disease. The virus can also be communicated from the mother to the fetus or her newborn baby.

CONDITION	DESCRIPTION
anaphylaxis	acute hypersensitivity reaction to an antigen
	Note: For example, the patient may suddenly develop the symptoms of anaphylaxis following repeated exposure to bee stings or drugs such as penicillin. Symptoms may include hives, dyspnea, shock, and gastrointestinal symptoms that may be severe, even life-threatening.
autoimmune diseases	diseases in which the body's own cells instead of foreign cells are attacked by the immune system
	Note: Autoimmune diseases include rheumatoid arthritis, Graves' disease, multiple sclerosis, and systemic lupus erythematosus.

CONDITION	DESCRIPTION
Hodgkin's disease	neoplasm of the lymphatic tissue characterized by enlargement of the lymph nodes and spleen
	Note: Hodgkin's disease starts in one lymph node region and progresses to adjacent lymph nodes and finally to distant lymphatic regions and organs. Although Hodgkin's disease may be fatal, new methods of treatment have made this disease curable.
hypersensitivity; allergies	allergies and hyersensitivities are side effects of the defense system's response to an antigen; antigens that cause these undesirable side effects are called **allergens** and include some drugs, plant pollens, and insect venom.
	Note: These allergens are not in themselves a threat to the body. The defense system's excessive inflammatory response, as for example in hay fever, is more harmful to the body than is the allergen itself.
Kaposi's sarcoma	a rare form of cancer of the lining of the blood capillaries

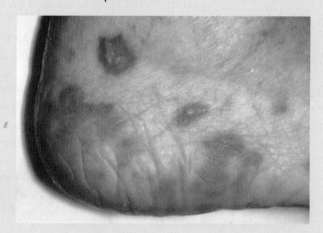

	Note: Kaposi's sarcoma is an opportunistic disease sometimes found in AIDS patients. A usual characteristic is congestion of tissues with blood, which causes purple discoloration of the skin. The bleeding can be fatal.
Mycobacterium avium complex infection	an opportunistic infection among AIDS patients
non-Hodgkin's lymphoma	malignant tumor of the lymphatic tissues with enlargement of the lymph nodes; cellular histology of the malignant lymphocytes is different than in Hodgkin's disease
Pneumocystis carinii parasite	This parasite causes an opportunistic type of pneumonia
	Note: Antibiotic treatment is sometimes successful, but recurrence is common.
tuberculosis	a common opportunistic disease among AIDS patients

RADIOLOGY	DESCRIPTION
lymphangiography	x-ray of the lymph vessels and lymph nodes following injection of a contrast dye usually through the feet

LABORATORY TESTS	DESCRIPTION
cytomegalovirus antibody	detection of the antibody to the cytomegalovirus (the cytomegalovirus is an opportunistic infection seen in AIDS patients)
human immunodeficiency virus (HIV) antibody detection	tests blood for antibodies to the human immunodeficiency virus that causes AIDS
enzyme-linked immunosorbent assay (ELISA)	blood test used to screen patients for antiboides to HIV
immunoelectrophoresis	separation of immunoglobulins IgA, IgM, IgG, IgD, and IgE by an electric current in a sample of blood or urine
T and B lymphocyte subset enumeration	tests for B and T cell deficiency
Western blot	an antibody detection test for HIV in the blood

◆ **15.11 ABBREVIATIONS FOR THE LYMPHATIC AND IMMUNE SYSTEMS**

ABBREVIATION	DEFINITION	ABBREVIATION	DEFINITION
AIDS	acquired immunodeficiency syndrome	Ig	immunoglobulin
ddI	dideoxyinosine (drug used to treat AIDS)	KS	Kaposi's sarcoma
HIV	human immunodeficiency virus	ZDV or AZT	zidovudine or azidothymidine (drug used to treat AIDS)

Definitions

Definitions

Give the meaning for the following term elements.

Answers to the exercises in this chapter are found in Appendix A.

1. thym/o _____

2. phag/o _____

3. -stitial _____

4. auto- _____

5. -blast _____

6. -phil _____

7. is/o _____

8. thromb/o _____

Give the prefix, suffix, or word root for the following.

9. immunity _____ 10. spleen _____

11. lymph vessels _____ 12. lymph _____

Write definitions (or locations in the body) for the following terms.

13. lymph _____

14. thoracic duct _____

15. thymosin _____

16. hematopoiesis _____

17. phagocyte _____

18. pharyngeal tonsils _____

19. Peyer's patches _____

20. lymph nodes _____

21. spleen _____

22. thymus gland _____

23. natural killer cells _____

24. cytotoxic T-lymphocytes _____

25. helper T-lymphocytes _____

26. nonspecific defense system _____

27. complement _____

28. interleukin-1 _____

29. interferon _____

30. cell-mediated immune response _____

31. anisocytosis _____

32. agglutination _____

33. gamma globulins _____

34. antibody _____

35. antigen _____

36. antigen receptor _____

37. humoral immune response _____

38. natural genetic recombination _____

39. clone _____

40. immunity _____

41. specific defense system _____

42. effector cells _____

43. lymphokines _____

44. memory cells _____

Write the terms that
correspond with the
following abbreviations.

45. KS _____

46. Ag _____

47. Ig _____

48. ZDV _____

49. Ab _____

50. HIV _____

51. HCT _____

52. MCV _____

► EXERCISE 15–2

Practice Quiz

Short Answer

Briefly answer the following
questions.

1. List the primary and secondary organs of the immune system. _____

_____

_____

2. List two functions of lymph. _____

_____

3. Where do B-lymphocytes mature? _____

4. List six components of the nonspecific defense system. _____

_____

_____

5. What is the definition of an antigen? List four specific antigens. _____

_____

_____

II–15

6. What is the process that ensures the production of antigen receptors that will recognize mutant viruses? _____

_____

7. What is the role of helper T-lymphocytes? _____

_____

8. What is the composition of lymph? _____

_____

9. Name the lymph organs. _____

_____

10. What organ combats infectious agents that enter the digestive tract?

_____

▶EXERCISE 15–3

Medical Term Building

Word Building

The suffix -penia means deficiency. Add -penia to a root to obtain a medical term for each of the following definitions.

Example: deficiency of iron sideropenia

1. deficiency in the number of thrombocytes _____

2. deficiency in the number of white blood cells _____

3. deficiency in the number of red blood cells _____

4. deficiency in all the cells _____

The suffix -cytosis means slight increase in the number of cells. Add -cytosis to a root to obtain a medical term for each of the following definitions.

Example: slight increase in the number of thrombocytes thrombocytosis

5. slight increase in the number of spherical cells _____

6. slight increase in the number of white blood cells _____

7. slight increase in the number of red blood cells _____

8. slight increase in the number of agranulocytes _____

9. slight increase in the number of unequally sized cells _____

The suffix -emia means blood condition. Use -emia to build a medical term for each of the following definitions.

10. excessive amounts of bilirubin in the blood _____

11. excessive amounts of cholesterol in the blood _____

12. excessive amounts of fat in the blood _____

13. malignant increase in the number of white blood cells   _____

14. holding back of blood to a part   _____

Matching Terms with Meanings

Matching

Match the term in Column A with its meaning in Column B.

COLUMN A	COLUMN B
1. spleen _____	A. genetically designed component of a lymphocyte or an antibody that is complementary to the shape of an antigen
2. natural killer cells _____	
3. T-cells _____	
4. antigen-binding site _____	
5. interleukin-1 _____	B. stimulates the production of T-lymphocytes
6. memory cells _____	C. white blood cells that release antibodies
7. B-lymphocytes _____	
8. thymosin _____	D. secreted by helper T-lymphocytes
9. lymphokine _____	E. removes foreign agents from the blood
10. complement _____	
	F. active in cell-mediated immune response
	G. clones of T cells or B cells that provide for future immunity
	H. attack the body's own cells
	I. attracts phagocytes to infected region
	J. secreted by phagocytes engaged in battle

Beside each of the following terms, place an "S" for terms that refer to the specific defense system or an "N" for terms that refer to the nonspecific defense system.

11. cell-mediated immune response   _____

12. interferon   _____

13. immunoglobulin M   _____

14. interleukin-1   _____

15. skin   _____

16. complement   _____

17. antibody   _____

18. agglutination   _____

19. B-lymphocytes   _____

20. natural killer cells   _____

21. effector cells   _____

22. lymphokines   _____

II–15

Medical Terms in Context

Define the underlined terms as they are in context.

UNIVERSITY HOSPITAL ✚

PATHOLOGY REPORT

MORPHOLOGY REPORT—PERIPHERAL BLOOD

The red cells are <u>normochromic</u> with moderate <u>anisocytosis</u>. Occasional <u>microcytes</u> are seen. There is reduction in <u>platelets</u>.

The white cell count is markedly elevated with many <u>blast</u> forms present showing scanty cytoplasm. An occasional blast shows folded nuclei. Occasional <u>nucleated red cells</u> are noted. Occasional <u>neutrophils</u> are also present.

CONCLUSION: This is a marked <u>leukocytosis</u> with many blast forms present that <u>morphologically</u> appear <u>lymphoblastic</u>.

SIGNATURE OF DOCTOR IN CHARGE _____

---

1. normochromic   _____

2. anisocytosis   _____

3. microcytes   _____

4. platelets   _____

5. blast   _____

6. nucleated red cells _____

7. neutrophils   _____

8. leukocytosis   _____

9. morphologically   _____

10. lymphoblastic   _____

MEDICAL TERMINOLOGY IN CONTEXT

1. An ultrasound guided needle biopsy was performed that revealed findings consistent with a <u>non-Hodgkin's lymphoma</u>.

2. A 28-year-old gentleman who is <u>HIV</u> positive, has a previous history of <u>Pneumocystis carinii pneumonia</u> infection in September, 1993. He was diagnosed as having <u>Mycobacterium avium intracellulare</u> in November, 1993.

3. The patient's pathology report from the biopsy revealed <u>Hodgkin's disease with lymph node involvement</u>.

4. Prior to admission to the hospital, the patient underwent a chest x-ray and a CT of the chest and abdomen, which revealed a <u>supraclavicular node</u> that was not <u>palpable</u>.

11. non-Hodgkin's lymphoma _____

12. HIV _____

13. Pneumocystis carinii pneumonia _____

14. Mycobacterium avium intracellulare _____

15. Hodgkin's disease with lymph node involvement _____

16. supraclavicular node _____

17. palpable _____

II–15

Crossword Puzzle

Terms Related to the Blood

Across

5 Slight increase in number of agranulocytes
10 Red blood cell
11 Stoppage of blood flow

Down

1 Polycythemia vera
2 White blood cell that stains blue with a basic dye
3 Slight increase in number of elliptically shaped red blood cells
4 White blood cell that stains red with eosin
5 Slight increase in number of unequal size cells
6 Iron deficiency
7 Slight increase in number of red blood cells
8 Deficiency of red blood cells
9 Destruction of red blood cells

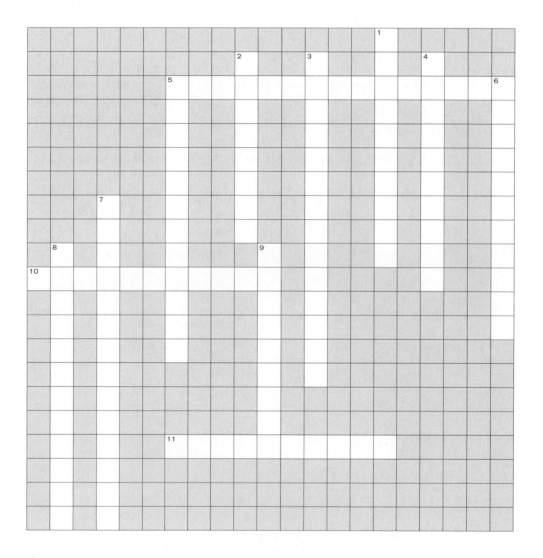

II—15

16 THE URINARY AND MALE REPRODUCTIVE SYSTEMS

CHAPTER ORGANIZATION

This chapter has been designed to help the student learn terms and abbreviations related to the urinary and male reproductive systems.

CHAPTER OBJECTIVES

Upon successful completion of this chapter, the student will be able to do the following:

1. State the function of the urinary system.
2. Name the organs of the urinary system.
3. Describe glomerular filtration.
4. Describe the paths of blood, filtrate, and urine flow through the kidney.
5. Describe tubular reabsorption and tubular secretion.
6. Define the terms describing the nephron.
7. Name the endocrine secretions of the kidney and describe their functions.
8. Pronounce, analyze, define, and spell terms related to the urinary system.
9. Describe common abnormalities of the urinary system.
10. List and define terms describing common urinary signs and symptoms, diagnostic procedures, and treatment.
11. Define the terms describing the male reproductive system.
12. Pronounce, analyze, define, and spell terms related to the male reproductive system.
13. Describe common abnormalities of the male reproductive system.
14. List and define common terms related to the physical examination, diagnosis, and treatment of abnormalities of the male reproductive system.
15. Define abbreviations common to the urinary system and male reproductive systems.

URINARY SYSTEM WORD ELEMENT	TYPE	MEANING
calic/o	root	calyces
cortic/o	root	cortex
crypt/o	root	hidden
cyst/o; vesic/o	root	bladder
glomerul/o	root	glomerulus
juxta-	prefix	near
lith/o	root	stone
medull/o	root	medulla
nephr/o; ren/o	root	kidney
pyel/o	root	renal pelvis
-sclerosis	suffix	hardening
trigon/o	root	trigone
ureter/o	root	ureter
urethr/o	root	urethra
-uria	suffix	urine
urin/o; ur/o	root	urinary tract; urine; urination

MALE REPRODUCTIVE SYSTEM WORD ELEMENT	TYPE	MEANING
andr/o	root	male
balan/o	root	glans penis
orchid/o; orch/o; testicul/o	root	testicle
prostat/o	root	prostate
sperm/o; spermat/o	root	sperm
vas/o	root	vessel; vas deferens

▶ 16.1 GENERAL ANATOMY AND PHYSIOLOGY OF THE URINARY SYSTEM

The survival of all body cells constantly depends on the volume and composition of extracellular fluid being maintained within quite strict limits. This maintenance of the blood plasma and interstitial fluid, which together constitute extracellular fluid, is the function of the organs of the urinary system: the kidney, the ureters, the urinary bladder, and the urethra (see Figure 16–1).

FIGURE 16–1 Anatomy of the Urinary System

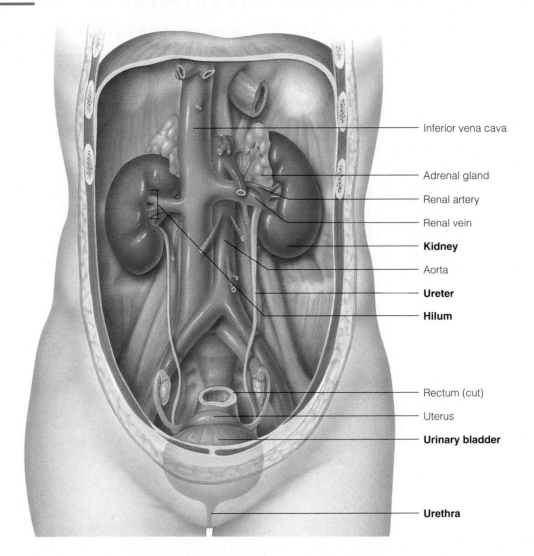

- Inferior vena cava
- Adrenal gland
- Renal artery
- Renal vein
- **Kidney**
- Aorta
- **Ureter**
- **Hilum**
- Rectum (cut)
- Uterus
- **Urinary bladder**
- **Urethra**

Kidneys

External Anatomy The kidneys are located beneath the diaphragm, one on each side of the lumbar spine. They are behind the peritoneal membrane and are therefore called **retroperitoneal** (rĕt″-rō-pĕr″-ĭ-tō-nē′-ăl). Each kidney is shaped like a bean. The indented region of the "bean" is called the **hilum** (hī′-lŭm) and is the site at which nerves and blood vessels enter and leave the organ. The covering of the kidney is called the **renal capsule**. Surrounding it is a thick layer of adipose tissue called **perirenal** or **perinephric fat** encased in a thin layer of connective tissue, the **renal** or **Gerota's fascia**. These layers keep the kidney firmly in position. Substantial loss of perirenal fat may cause **floating kidney**, a condition in which the kidney is out of its normal position.

Internal Anatomy   The first internal layer in the kidney is the **cortex**. Beneath it is the **medulla**, composed of triangular tissues called **renal pyramids**, which are separated by projections called **renal columns** (see Figure 16–2). The tip of each pyramid, the **renal papilla**, is directed into a cavity called a **minor calyx** (kā′-lǐks). Urine from the pyramids collects in a minor calyx, and several calyces drain into a **major calyx**. Urine is carried by ducts from the major calyces to the **renal pelvis**, a cavity that opens into the ureter.

FIGURE 16–2   Internal Anatomy of the Kidney

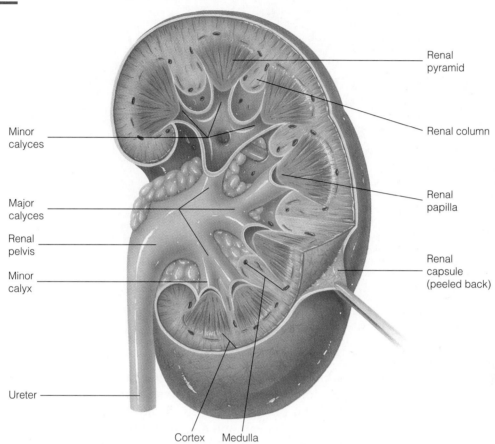

Renal pyramid

Renal column

Renal papilla

Renal capsule (peeled back)

Minor calyces

Major calyces

Renal pelvis

Minor calyx

Ureter

Cortex   Medulla

Ureter, Urinary Bladder, and Urethra

The functional aspect of fluid maintenance takes place in the kidneys. The ureters, urinary bladder, and urethra serve merely as a storage and transport system for urine.

A **ureter** (ū′rĕ-ter) is a foot-long tube that leads from each kidney to the urinary bladder. Urine is moved through the ureter by a process of muscular contractions called **peristalsis**.

The **urinary bladder** is an expandable sac located in the pelvic cavity. The bladder is simply a storage vessel in which urine collects so that it can be excreted periodically rather than constantly. The **trigone** (trī′-gōn) region of the bladder is so named because the two openings from the ureters, along with the opening to the urethra, form three points of a triangle (see Figure 16–3). The area outside the trigone is covered with the **detrusor muscle**, which contracts when the bladder is full and forces urine into the urethra.

FIGURE 16–3

Urinary Bladder, Anterior View

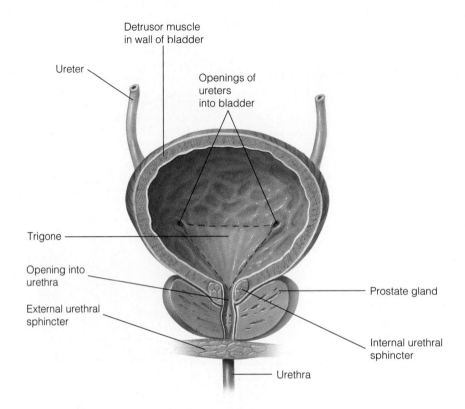

Detrusor muscle in wall of bladder

Ureter

Openings of ureters into bladder

Trigone

Opening into urethra

External urethral sphincter

Prostate gland

Internal urethral sphincter

Urethra

The **urethra** (ū-rē′-thră) is the tube that carries urine out of the body from the urinary bladder. The external opening of the urethra is called the urinary meatus. In females, the urethra is 1.6 inches (4.1 cm) long. In males, it runs along the length of the penis and also serves as part of the reproductive system for the transport of semen. The male urethra is also surrounded by the prostate gland (see Figure 16–3). The **internal urethral sphincter** leads from the bladder to the urethra and is controlled involuntarily. Excretion of urine (urination) is also known by the term **micturition** (mĭk-tū-rĭ′-shŭn), or **voiding**. The **micturition reflex** triggers the **external urethral sphincter** to open. This sphincter, however, can be controlled voluntarily.

Nephrons

Maintaining the composition and volume of extracellular fluid is carried out by microscopic structures called **nephrons** (see Figure 16–4), which are located within the kidney. Each kidney contains approximately 1 million nephrons. Each nephron is composed of two capillary networks located in the kidney cortex:

1. the **glomerulus** (glō-mĕr′-ū-lŭs), which is a clump of **glomerular capillaries** (see Figure 16–5), and
2. the **peritubular capillaries**.

FIGURE 16–4

Nephron Consists of the glomerulus, glomerular capsule, juxtaglomerular apparatus, proximal convoluted tubule, loop of Henle, distal convoluted tubule, collecting duct, and peritubular capillaries.

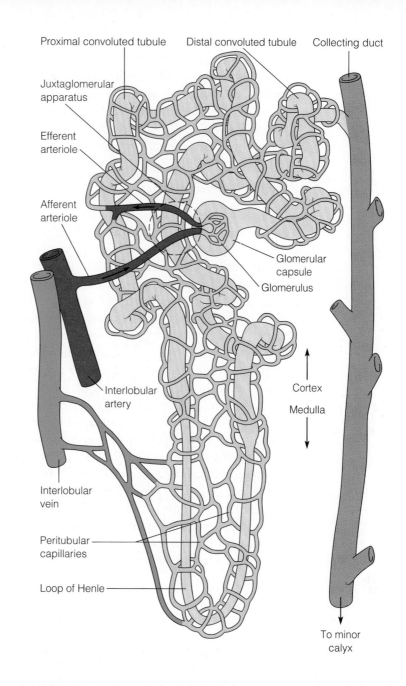

Proximal convoluted tubule   Distal convoluted tubule   Collecting duct

Juxtaglomerular apparatus

Efferent arteriole

Afferent arteriole

Glomerular capsule

Glomerulus

Interlobular artery

Cortex

Medulla

Interlobular vein

Peritubular capillaries

Loop of Henle

To minor calyx

FIGURE 16–5

Scanning Electron Micrograph of Glomerular Capillaries
From *Tissues and Organs: A Text-Atlas of Scanning Electon Microscopy* by Richard G. Kessel and Randy H. Kardon (W.H. Freeman and Company, 1979). Reprinted with permission.

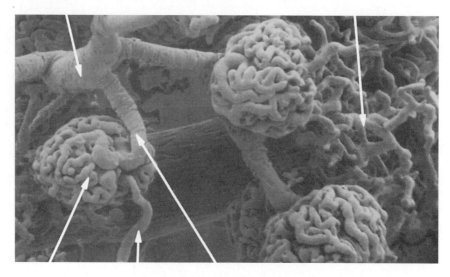

II–16

The third component of the nephron is the **renal tubule**, which is composed of the **glomerular capsule**, the **proximal convoluted tubule**, the **loop of Henle**, and the **distal convoluted tubule**. Attached to the end of the distal convoluted tubule is a **collecting duct** (see Figure 16–4).

The cup-shaped glomerular capsule at the beginning of each renal tubule is also known as **Bowman's capsule**. The glomerulus sits within this capsule. The glomerulus and capsule together are known as the **renal corpuscle**.

Urine Formation

Urine is formed by means of three distinct processes: **glomerular filtration, tubular reabsorption,** and **tubular secretion**.

Glomerular Filtration   The fluid that enters the lumen of the glomerular capsule is fluid from the glomerular capillaries that has had blood cells and proteins filtered out of it. This fluid, called **filtrate**, is therefore initially identical in composition to the blood plasma in the capillaries except that it lacks proteins. This filtrate fluid is formed by a process called **glomerular filtration,** in which three layers of tissue in the renal corpuscle filter the blood on its path from the glomerular capillaries to the lumen of the glomerular capsule. The first layer of tissue, making up the thin wall of the glomerular capillaries, is permeable to water and small proteins, but its pores strain out blood cells and large proteins. The second layer of tissue, situated between the capillary wall and the inner wall of the glomerular capsule, is made up of **basement cells**, which strain out the smaller proteins. The third layer of tissue, making up the inner wall of the capsule, is composed of cells called **podocytes** (pŏd′-ō-sīts), or "foot cells." These foot cells have projections called **foot processes**, or **pedicels**. Pedicels from a number of podocytes interlace with each other to form **filtration slits** (see Figure 16–6). It is through these slits that the filtered fluid enters the lumen of the capsule and empties into the proximal convoluted tubule, moving then through the loop of Henle and into the distal convoluted tubule.

FIGURE 16–6

Tissue Layers of Renal Corpuscle

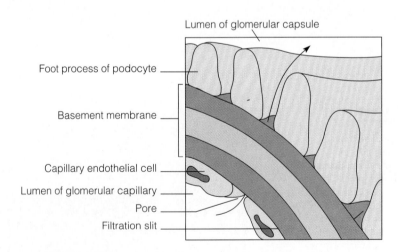

Lumen of glomerular capsule

Foot process of podocyte

Basement membrane

Capillary endothelial cell

Lumen of glomerular capillary

Pore

Filtration slit

Blood is supplied to the kidney through a branch of the aorta called the **renal artery** (see Figure 16–7), which enters the kidney at the hilum. The renal artery divides into a series of progressively smaller arteries as it travels toward the cortex. The artery entering the glomerulus is called the **afferent** (ăf'-ĕr-ĕnt) arteriole. Twenty percent of the blood entering the glomerulus is filtered into the glomerular capsule as filtrate. The remainder continues on through the glomerular capillaries and leaves the glomerulus through the **efferent** (ĕf'-ĕr-ĕnt) **arteriole**. The efferent arteriole branches into the nephron's second network of capillaries, the peritubular capillaries. The rate at which blood moves through the glomerulus is called the **glomerular filtration rate (GFR)**.

FIGURE 16–7

Blood Route Through the Kidney

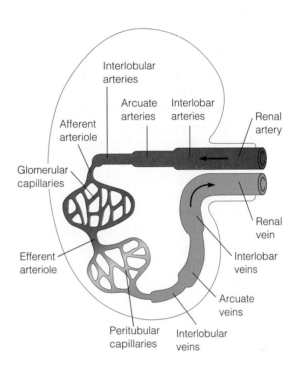

The peritubular capillaries are twined around the proximal convoluted tubule, the loop of Henle, and the distal convoluted tubule of the renal tubule, as shown in Figure 16–4.

The close proximity of the peritubular capillaries to the renal tubule allows materials to move back and forth between the tubule and capillaries in processes called **tubular reabsorption** and **tubular secretion** (see Figure 16–8).

FIGURE 16–8   **Tubular Reabsorption and Tubular Secretion**

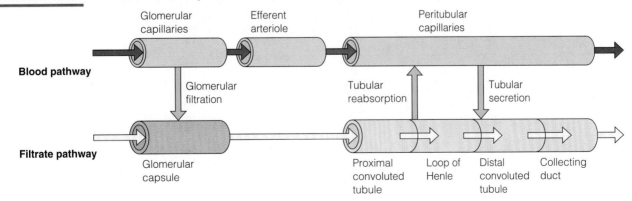

Tubular Reabsorption   In tubular reabsorption, all the glucose in the filtrate is absorbed back into the blood, as is most of the water. The amount of water reabsorbed varies to help maintain the body's internal fluid volume. Variable amounts of other materials, such as sodium, chloride, potassium, and calcium, are selectively reabsorbed according to the needs of the body at any given time. Some metabolic wastes, such as **urea** (ū-rē′-ă), are only partially reabsorbed. Other waste materials, such as **creatinine** (krē-ăt′-ĭn-ĭn), are left in the filtrate.

Tubular Secretion   In tubular secretion, materials are selectively transferred from the blood into the filtrate to be excreted in the urine. These materials include substances that were unable to pass through the filtering tissues of the renal corpuscle, as well as substances that may be present in the blood in excess amounts. Excess potassium, for example, is transferred from the blood into the filtrate under stimulation from aldosterone, which is released by the adrenal cortex when blood potassium levels are too high. Excess hydrogen is another example of material that is transferred from the blood into the filtrate. The tubular secretion of excess hydrogen contributes to the maintenance of the pH balance (acid-base balance) of extracellular fluid.

When the filtrate flows out of the collecting duct at the end of the distal convoluted tubule, its composition is no longer alterable, and it travels on to the pyramids as urine and collects in the calyces. As explained above, the composition of urine varies according to the amount of materials selected for reabsorption into the blood and secretion from the blood.

The blood in the peritubular capillaries, having been adjusted by tubular reabsorption and tubular secretion, travels from the capillaries into a system of small veins that drain into a single **renal vein** and is carried away from the kidney through the hilum.

It should be noted that the term *secretion*, when used in the context of tubular secretion, refers to the active transfer of materials from the blood to the filtrate and does not refer to glandular secretion. There are, however, two important endocrine secretions in the kidney: the hormones **erythropoietin** (ĕ-rĭth″-rō-poy′-ĕ-tĭn) and **renin** (rĕn′-ĭn). Erythropoietin helps in the production of red blood cells, and renin helps maintain blood pressure.

Juxtaglomerular Apparatus

Contributing to the kidney's endocrine control as well as to GFR control are two groups of specialized cells located in the region where the distal convoluted tubule runs between the afferent and efferent arterioles (see Figure 16–9). These cells are known collectively as the **juxtaglomerular** (jŭks″-tă-glō-mĕr′-ū-lăr) **apparatus**. The names of the specialized cells in the apparatus are the **juxtaglomerular cells**, in the wall of the afferent arteriole, and the **macula densa** (măk′-ū-lă dĕn′-să), in the wall of the distal convoluted tubule.

FIGURE 16–9 Juxtaglomerular Apparatus

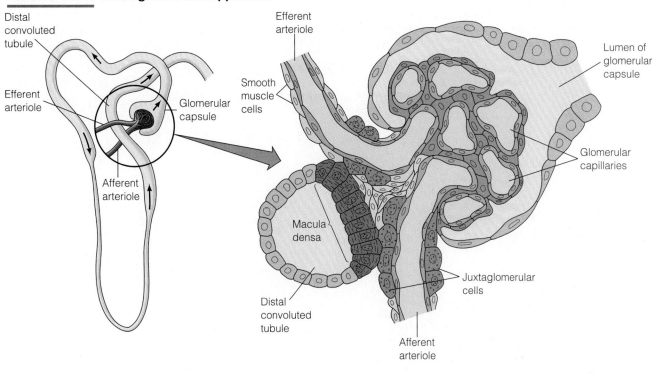

When the GFR needs to be increased, the macula densa send chemical signals that cause the afferent arteriole to dilate. The macula densa also send chemical signals that trigger the secretion of renin by the juxtaglomerular cells when GFR is low. Renin, in turn, leads to the secretion of **angiotensin** (ăn″-jē-ō-těn′-sĭn), which causes the efferent arteriole to constrict. This action, too, increases GFR. The macula densa are capable of sensing sodium and chloride levels in the fluid flowing through the renal tubule. Changing the GFR is another way (in addition to tubular reabsorption) of regulating sodium and chloride levels.

_____

_____

_____

_____

_____

_____

_____

_____

_____

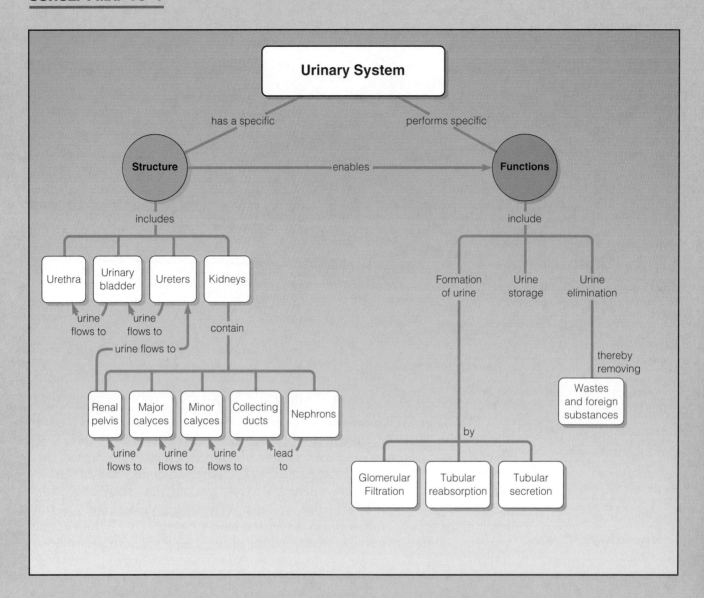

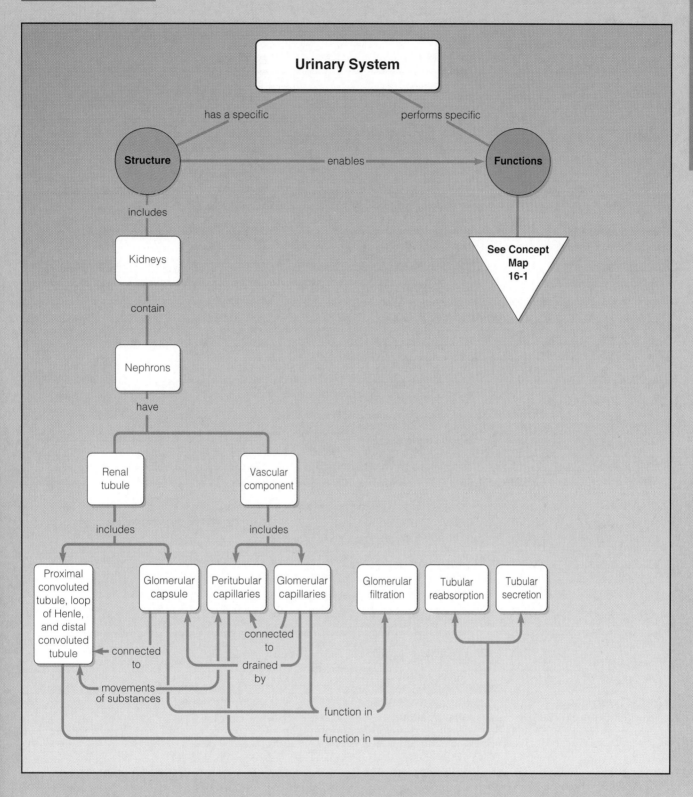

TERM WITH PRONUNCIATION	ANALYSIS	DEFINITION
cortical kor′-tĭ-kăl	-al = pertaining to cortic/o = cortex; outer layer	pertaining to the outer layer or cortex of the kidney
caliceal kăl″-ĭ-sē′-ăl	-eal = pertaining to calic/o = calyx	pertaining to the calices (calices can also be spelled calyces)
cystojejunostomy sĭs″-tō-jē-jū-nŏs′-tō-mē	-stomy = new opening cyst/o = bladder jejun/o = jejunum	new opening or an **anastomosis** between the bladder and the jejunum
extracorporeal ĕks″-tră-kor-por′-ē-ăl	-al = pertaining to extra- = outside corpor/o = body	pertaining to outside the body
glomerulonephritis glō-mĕr″-ū-lō-nĕ-frī′-tĭs	-itis = inflammation glomerul/o = glomerulus nephr/o = kidney	an inflammation of the glomerulus and the kidney
glomerulosclerosis glō-mĕr″-ū-lō-sklĕ-rō′-sĭs	-sclerosis = hardening glomerul/o = glomerulus	hardening of the glomerulus
lithotripsy lĭth′-ō-trĭp-sē	-tripsy = crushing lith/o = stones; calculi	crushing of stones
medullary mĕd′-ū-lār-ē	-ary = pertaining to medull/o = medulla	pertaining to the medulla
nephrolithiasis nĕf-rō-lĭth-ī-ă-sĭs	-iasis = abnormal condition nephr/o = kidney lith/o = stone	abnormal condition of stones in the kidney
nephropexy nĕf′-rō-pĕks-ē	-pexy = surgical fixation nephr/o = kidney	surgical fixation of the kidney
nephroptosis nĕf″-rŏp′-tō′-sĭs	-ptosis = drooping; falling; prolapse nephr/o = kidney	drooping kidney
proteinuria prō″-tē-ĭn-ū′-rē-ă	-uria = urine protein/o = protein	increased amounts of protein in the urine (also known as **albuminuria**)
pyelogram pī′-ĕ-lō-grăm	-gram = record pyel/o = renal pelvis	record of the renal pelvis
renal hypoplasia rē′-năl hī″-pō-plā′-zē-ă	-al = pertaining to ren/o = kidney -plasia = development; formation hypo- = below normal; under	underdeveloped kidney
trigonitis trĭg″-ō-nī′-tĭs	-itis = inflammation trigon/o = trigone	inflammation of the trigone of the bladder
ureteral ū-rē′-tĕr-ăl	-al = pertaining to ureter/o = ureter	pertaining to the ureters
ureterolith ū-rē′-tĕr-ō-lĭth	-lith = stone ureter/o = ureter	stone in the ureters

TERM WITH PRONUNCIATION	ANALYSIS	DEFINITION
urethrorrhagia ū-rē″-thror-ā′-jē-ă	-rrhagia = bursting forth of blood urethr/o = urethra	hemorrhage from the urethra
urethrostenosis ū-rē″-thrō-stěn-ō′-sĭs	-stenosis = narrowing; stricture urethr/o = urethra	narrowing of the urethra
urinary ū′-rĭ-nǎr-ē	-ary = pertaining to urin/o = urinary tract; urine; urination	pertaining to urine or the urinary tract
urogram ū′-rō-grǎm	-gram = record ur/o = urinary tract; urine; urination	record of the urinary tract
vesicosigmoidostomy věs″-ĭ-kō-sĭg″-moy-dŏs′-tō-mē	-stomy = new opening vesic/o = bladder sigmoid/o = sigmoid colon	surgical creation of a new opening between the bladder and sigmoid colon; anastomosis between the bladder and sigmoid colon

◊▸ 16.3 ABNORMAL CONDITIONS OF THE URINARY SYSTEM

Kidney

CONDITION	DESCRIPTION
acute renal failure	sudden loss of kidney function caused by a deficiency of blood flowing through the kidneys as a result of shock or dehydration or by cardiovascular or renal disease, or by toxins or obstruction
acute poststreptococcal glomerulonephritis (APSGN)	an immunologic reaction in which antigen/antibody complexes become trapped in the glomerulus producing inflammation and glomerular dysfunction; usually follows a streptococcal infection elsewhere in the body
hydronephrosis	accumulation of fluid in the renal pelvis caused by an obstruction of the normal urinary pathway
	Note: This obstruction can be caused by stenosis, calculus, or tumor. Urine continues to be produced but cannot pass the blockage, resulting in a dilation of the renal structures proximal to the obstruction.
nephroblastoma; Wilms' tumor	malignant neoplasm of the kidney containing embryonic material, usually occurs in children

CONDITION	DESCRIPTION
nephrolithiasis; renal calculi	formation of stones in the kidney

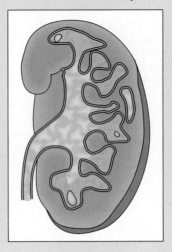

Note: These stones are crystals, many of which contain calcium phosphate or calcium oxalate. Size varies from very small, which are often termed **sand** or **gravel**, to giant **staghorn** calculi filling up the entire renal pelvis.

Once the stones are formed, they can lodge anywhere along the urinary tract.

polycystic kidneys	congenital disorder that causes multiple grapelike cysts to form on the kidney; these cysts eventually replace functional renal tissue, resulting in loss of renal function and leading to renal failure

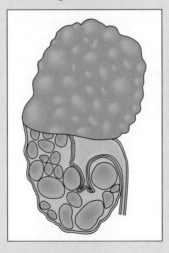

pyelonephritis	inflammation of the kidney and renal pelvis due to bacterial infection

Note: If left untreated, results in reduced renal function and eventual renal failure as scar tissue, and abscesses replace normal kidney tissue.

Ureters

CONDITION	DESCRIPTION
ureteral stricture	narrowing of the ureters, resulting in a blockage of urine as it flows through the urinary tract

Bladder

CONDITION	DESCRIPTION
cystitis	inflammation of the bladder usually caused by bacterial infection that travels to the bladder from the outside **Note:** More common in women than in men because the shorter urethra in women makes the bladder more easily accessible to bacteria from the exterior of the body.
neurogenic bladder	dysfunction of the urinary bladder due to disorders of the nervous system, including spinal cord injuries and brain disorders that alter nervous impulses to the bladder
vesicoureteral reflux	backward flow of the urine from the bladder to the ureter

Effects on the Kidney from Extrarenal Disorders

DISORDER	EFFECT
cardiac disease	heart conditions affecting cardiac output reduce the amount of blood delivered to the kidneys and reduces the amount of urine formed; over time, there is a loss of glomerular filtration, and renal dysfunction results
diabetic nephropathy; Kimmelstiel-Wilson syndrome	degeneration of the glomerular function following long-term diabetes mellitus; this condition leads to renal failure
hypertension	long-term, uncontrolled hypertension results in arterial damage to the kidney and leads to a reduction in kidney function (the reverse can also happen, with kidney disease resulting in hypertension)

◗ 16.4 PHYSICAL EXAMINATION, DIAGNOSIS, AND TREATMENT OF ABNORMAL CONDITIONS OF THE URINARY SYSTEM

An examination of the urinary system includes the typical examination procedures of inspection, palpation, percussion, and auscultation to check for abnormal swellings, abnormal growths, discharges, and abnormalities in structure. Some symptoms are listed first, followed by laboratory procedures used in diagnosing urinary disorders and radiologic diagnostic procedures. Computed tomography (CT), radioisotope studies, and ultrasound, which are discussed in Chapter 18, can also be used for diagnosis.

SIGNS AND SYMPTOMS	DESCRIPTION
albuminuria	albumin in the urine
anuria	absence of urine production
bacteriuria	accumulation of bacteria in the urine
dysuria	painful urination
enuresis	involuntary bedwetting

SIGNS AND SYMPTOMS	DESCRIPTION
frequency	increased urges to micturate or void but with a reduced volume of urine output
hematuria	blood in the urine
incontinence	loss of control of urinary excretion
	Note: Involuntary micturition when there is pressure on the bladder from coughing, laughing, and so forth, is called **stress incontinence**. The inability to stop the flow of urine once the urge to micturate has been felt is called **urge incontinence**.
nocturia	frequency of urination at night
oliguria	diminished urine output
polyuria	excretion of large amounts of urine
pyuria	pus in the urine
retention	inability to micturate; the kidney continues to produce urine
suppression	inability of the kidney to form urine
uremia	accumulation of waste products (urine) in the blood due to loss of renal function
urgency	sudden need to micturate or void

LABORATORY STUDIES	DESCRIPTION
blood urea nitrogen (BUN)	measures the amount of urea nitrogen in the blood; increased amounts indicate glomerular dysfunction
clearance studies	tests the ability of the kidney to clear or filter certain substances from the blood (also known as renal function test)
phenolsulfonphthalein (PSP)	urine samples taken following injection of a dye known as PSP indicate whether PSP is completely filtered and excreted by the kidney
creatinine clearance	tests the kidney's ability to clear creatinine from the blood
urinalysis	one of the most common tests performed to evaluate the general health of a person; macroscopic and microscopic observations of color, pH, presence of white or red blood cells, casts (molded cellular debris that has accumulated and then eliminated in the urine in a variety of pathological conditions), proteins, ketones, bilirubin, blood, sugar, pus, and other substances (the amount of wastes in the urine is also measured by specific gravity test)

LABORATORY STUDIES	DESCRIPTION
urine culture and sensitivity	identifies bacteria in a sample of urine and determines the best antibiotic to treat it
uric acid	measures the amount of uric acid in the blood and urine
	Note: Uric acid is a waste product of protein metabolism that is removed from the body by being excreted through the urine.

RADIOLOGIC STUDIES	DESCRIPTION
cystourethrography	x-ray of the bladder and urethra following injection of a contrast medium into the bladder through a catheter
intravenous urogram (IVU); intravenous pyelogram (IVP); excretory urogram	examination of the urinary tract to observe size, shape, and location of kidney, ureters, and bladder following intravenous injection of a contrast medium
kidney, ureters, and bladder (KUB); flat plate of the abdomen	x-ray of kidney, ureters, and bladder without contrast medium; sometimes called flat plate of abdomen as abdominal organs are also visualized
renal angiography	x-ray of the renal blood vessels following injection of a contrast medium into the renal vasculature
retrograde urography; retrograde pyelogram	examination of the size, shape, and location of the urinary structures following injection of a contrast medium into the renal pelvis by catheter; this procedure is a follow-up to IVP when IVP is inconclusive

MEDICAL TREATMENT	DESCRIPTION
anticholinergics	antispasmodic drugs to control bladder spasms
cholinergics	drugs to stimulate the bladder
sulfonamides	a type of antibiotic used to treat bacterial urinary tract infections

SURGICAL TREATMENT	DESCRIPTION

lithotripsy — procedure for the destruction of renal calculi

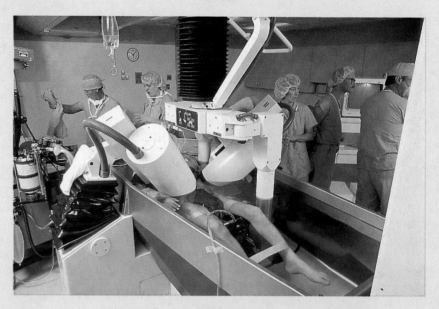

Note: Percutaneous lithotripsy and extracorporeal shock wave lithotripsy break up the renal stones for easy removal or spontaneous passage.

percutaneous lithotripsy — specialized surgical equipment is used to manually remove stones through a cystoscope

A new method utilizing methyl tert-butyl ether (MTBE) has been tried with some success. This procedure involves the percutaneous instillation of MTBE directly into the kidney via a catheter dissolving the renal calculi.

extracorporeal shock wave lithotripsy (ESWL) — utilizes high frequency sound waves to break up the stones into smaller pieces, thereby facilitating their passage through the urinary tract

meatotomy — incision of the urinary meatus

nephrolithotomy — invasive procedure for the removal of renal calculi through an incision into the kidney

sphincterotomy — incision of the urinary sphincter

uretero-ileostomy — anastomosis (surgical connection between two parts not normally attached) of the ureter and ileum

ureterocystostomy — anastomosis of the ureter and bladder

CLINICAL PROCEDURES	DESCRIPTION
dialysis	a procedure that replaces normal kidney function when kidney disease results in failure of the kidney to filter, secrete, and excrete substances from the blood

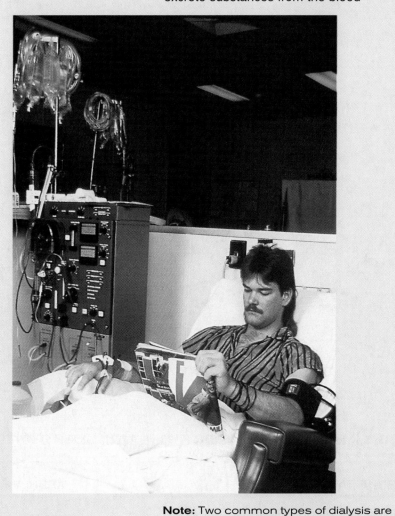

Note: Two common types of dialysis are **peritoneal dialysis** and **hemodialysis**.

peritoneal dialysis	waste products are removed via fluid instilled into the peritoneal cavity, either continuously or intermittently
hemodialysis	removal of waste products from the blood by passing the blood through a machine which selectively filters the blood of wastes
renal biopsy	excision of a piece of tissue from the kidney for microscopic examination
catheterization	insertion into the bladder of a flexible tube called a catheter for withdrawal of urine

CLINICAL PROCEDURES	DESCRIPTION
cystoscopy	direct visual examination of the bladder with a cystoscope

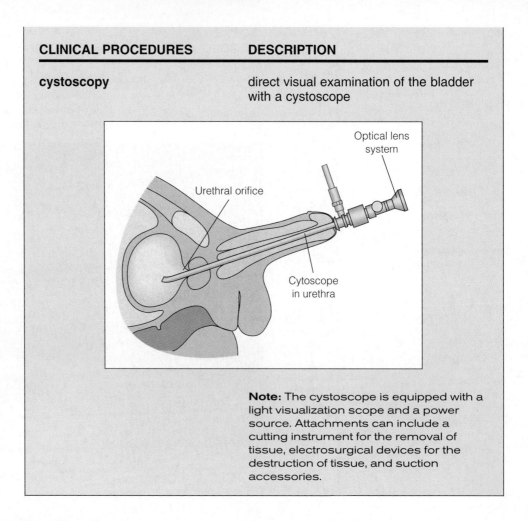

Optical lens system

Urethral orifice

Cytoscope in urethra

Note: The cystoscope is equipped with a light visualization scope and a power source. Attachments can include a cutting instrument for the removal of tissue, electrosurgical devices for the destruction of tissue, and suction accessories.

◆ 16.5 ABBREVIATIONS FOR THE URINARY SYSTEM

ABBREVIATION	MEANING
APSGN	acute poststreptococcal glomerulonephritis
ARF	acute renal failure
BUN	blood urea nitrogen
CAPD	continuous ambulatory peritoneal dialysis
CRF	chronic renal failure
ESWL	extracorporeal shock wave lithotripsy
GFR	glomerular filtration rate
IVP	intravenous pyelogram

ABBREVIATION	MEANING
IVU	intravenous urogram
K	potassium
KUB	kidney, ureter, bladder
KV	kilovolts (measurement for shockwaves in lithotripsy)
MTBE	methyl tert-butyl ether
Na	sodium
PSP	phenolsulfonphthalein
sp.gr.	specific gravity

◆ 16.6 GENERAL ANATOMY AND PHYSIOLOGY OF THE MALE REPRODUCTIVE SYSTEM

The male reproductive system (see Figure 16–10) is made up of male **gonads** (sex organs) called **testes** (tĕs′-tēz) or **testicles** (tĕs′-tĭ-klz), the male reproductive tract, accessory reproductive glands, and external genitalia.

FIGURE 16–10   Anatomy of the Male Reproductive System

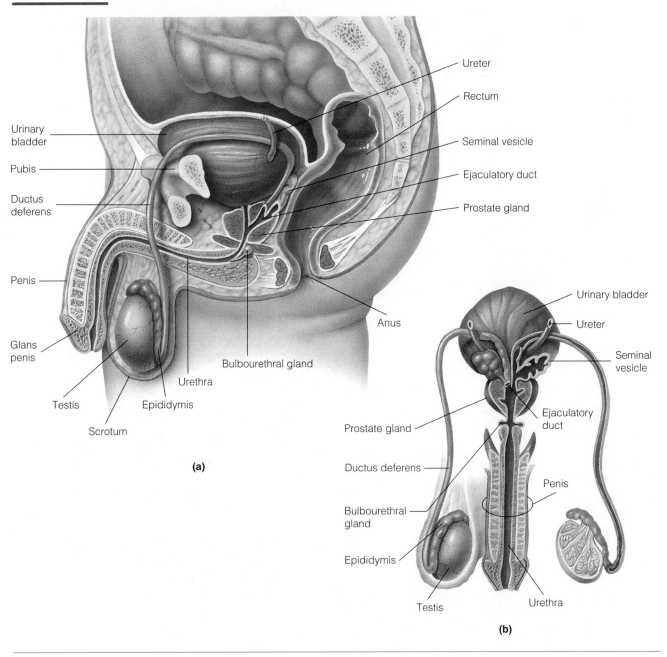

(a)

(b)

The testes are contained within a sac called a **scrotum** (skrō'-tum), located between the thighs. The function of the testes is twofold. The primary function is production of gametes (reproductive cells) called **sperm** or **spermatozoa** (spĕr"-măt-ō-zō'-ă), and the secondary function is production of the hormone, testosterone by the interstitial cells in the testes.

Producing sperm is called **spermatogenesis** (spĕr"-măt-ō-jĕn'-ĕ-sĭs); the production of sperm occurs in the seminiferous tubules located within the testes.

The sperm cell (Figure 16–11) is composed of a head, which carries the cell nucleus, a midpiece, and a tail called the **flagellum** (flă-jĕl'-ŭm), which whips back and forth to provide propulsion for the cell. The nucleus contains 23 chromosomes instead of the 46 chromosomes found in all other body cells. The female gamete likewise contains 23 chromosomes. When the male and female gametes unite, the resulting cell carrying genetic information for a new individual has 46 chromosomes.

FIGURE 16–11

Sperm Cell

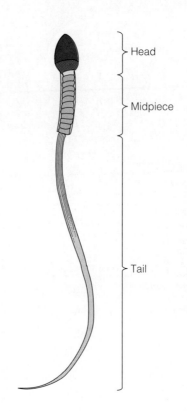

Head

Midpiece

Tail

Testosterone (tĕs-tŏs'-tĕr-ōn) is required for spermatogenesis. The production and secretion of testosterone is controlled by the hypothalamus and the anterior pituitary glands, as discussed in Chapter 12. Testosterone also contributes to the development of secondary sexual characteristics in the male including beard growth and enlargement of the larynx, which causes deepening of the voice at puberty.

The male reproductive tract is a system of ducts that not only serve as a storage site and passageway for gametes, but also contribute to the maturation of the gametes as they pass through it. The names of the respective ducts are the **epididymis** (ĕp"-ĭ-dĭd'-ĭ-mĭs), the **ductus deferens** (dĕf'-ĕr-ĕnz) (also known as the **vas deferens**), the **ejaculatory** (ē-jăk'-ū-lă-tō-rē) **duct**, and the **urethra**. The latter duct transports urine as well as sperm.

The accessory reproductive glands are two **seminal** (sĕm′-ĭ-năl) **vesicles,** the **prostate** (prŏs′-tāt) **gland,** and two **bulbourethral** (bŭl″-bō-ū-rē′-thrăl) or **Cowper's** (kow′-pĕrz) **glands.** Secretions from these glands, along with sperm, form a fluid called **semen** (sē′-mĕn). The secretions serve to nourish the sperm and to assist its movement.

The external genitalia includes the scrotum and the **penis** (pē′-nĭs), through which the urethra passes to transport sperm and urine outside the body. The distal tip of the penis is called the **glans penis** and is covered by excess skin called **foreskin** or **prepuce.**

A tough, fibrous cord, the **spermatic cord,** extends from the abdominal inguinal ring to the testis. It wraps around the vas deferens, testicular artery, veins, and nerves and contains blood vessels and nerves leading to and from the testicles and the vas deferens.

In summary, the route sperm travels is as follows:

seminiferous tubules of testes

↓

epididymis

↓

vas deferens

↓

ejaculatory duct

↓

urethra

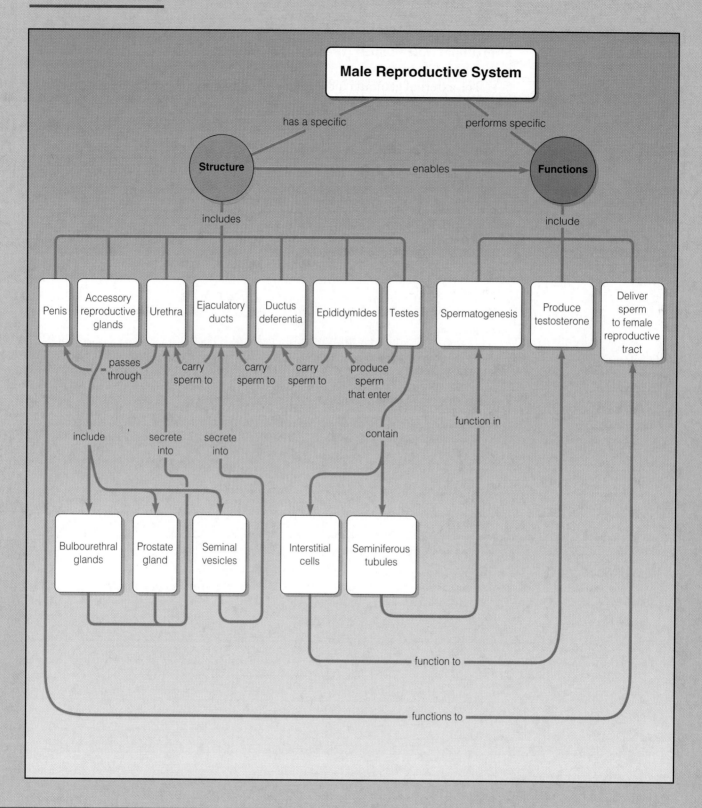

TERM WITH PRONUNCIATION	ANALYSIS	DEFINITION
androgenic ăn″-drō-jĕn′-ĭk	-genic = producing andr/o = male	producing masculinization
aspermatogenesis ă-spĕr″-mă-tō-jĕn′-ĕ-sĭs	-genesis = production; formation a- = no; not spermat/o = spermatozoa; sperm	no production of spermatozoa
balanitis băl-ă-nī′-tĭs	-itis = inflammation balan/o = glans penis	inflammation of the glans penis
circumcision sĕr″-kŭm-sĭ′-zhŭn	-ion = process circum- = around cis/o = to cut	removal of the prepuce or foreskin
cryptorchidism krĭpt-or′-kĭd-ĭzm	-ism = process crypt/o = hidden orchid/o = testicles; testes	undescended testicles
gynecomastia gī″-nĕ-kō-măs′-tē-ă	-ia = condition gynec/o = woman mast/o = breast	overdevelopment of the male mammary glands
oligospermia ŏl″-ĭ-gō-spĕr′-mē-ă	-ia = condition oligo- = scanty; deficient; few sperm/o = spermatozoa; sperm	deficient amounts of spermatozoa in the semen
orchidopexy or′-kĭd-ō-pĕk″-sē	-pexy = surgical fixation orchid/o = testicles; testes	surgical fixation of the testicles
orchitis or-kī′-tĭs	-itis = inflammation orch/o = testicles; testes	inflammation of the testicles
prostatitis prŏs″-tă-tī′-tĭs	-itis = inflammation prostat/o = prostate	inflammation of the prostate
resectoscope rē-sĕk′-tō-skōp	-scope = instrument used to visually examine re- = back sect/o = to cut	instrument used to remove tissue
spermaticidal spĕrm″-ăt-ĭ-sīd′-ăl	-cidal = to kill spermat/o = spermatozoa; sperm	pertaining to an agent used to kill spermatozoa
testicular tĕs-tĭk′-ū-lăr	-ar = pertaining to testicul/o = testicles	pertaining to the testicles
vasectomy văs-ĕk′-tō-mē	-ectomy = excision; removal vas/o = vas deferens	partial bilateral excision of the vas deferens for the purposes of sterilization

CONDITION	DESCRIPTION
benign prostatic hypertrophy (BPH)	benign enlargement of the prostate usually occurring in men over 50 years of age; etiology is unknown but hormonal imbalance as a consequence of old age has been implicated
	Note: As the prostate enlarges, it squeezes the urethra, thus obstructing the passage of urine. Urinary retention may result.
	Diagnostic tests include rectal examination, excretory urogram and blood, urine, and renal function tests. (See diagnostic investigations below.)
	Treatment includes alpha blocker medication to relax the bladder outlet, anti-androgens such as finasteride, **transurethral resection of the prostate (TURP)**, and infrequently, **suprapubic prostatectomy** (see treatment below).
	Symptoms which manifest themselves due to BPH and the subsequent urinary obstruction are known collectively as prostatism.
cryptorchidism	a common condition where there is failure of the testicle or testicles to descend from the abdominal cavity into the scrotum
	Although hormonal activity is not usually affected, spermatogenesis is, as the production of sperm depends on a cool environment. If the testicles remain in the abdominal cavity, the warm surroundings inhibit the production of sperm.
epispadias	congenital abnormality where the meatal opening is on the dorsum (top side) of the penis

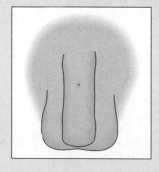

hematocele	accumulation of blood into the tunica vaginalis, a serous membrane covering the front and sides of the testes
hydrocele	accumulation of fluid into the tunica vaginalis

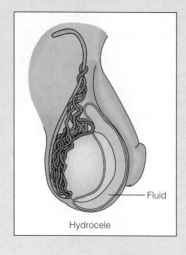

Fluid

Hydrocele

CONDITION	DESCRIPTION
hypospadias	congenital abnormality where the meatal opening is on the ventral (underside) of the penis

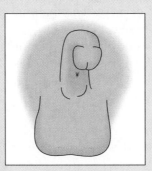

impotence	sexual dysfunction characterized by the inability to maintain an erection required for normal intercourse
phimosis	tightened foreskin that cannot be pulled back
seminoma	malignant tumor of the testicles
spermatocele	accumulation of a milky fluid containing spermatozoa in the epididymis
teratoma	a congenital tumor of the testicles composed of different types of tissues such as bone, teeth, hair, and skin (may also affect the ovaries)
testicular torsion	twisting of the spermatic cord causing ischemia to the testicles

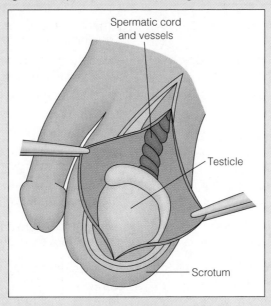

varicocele	dilatation of testicular veins inside the scrotum

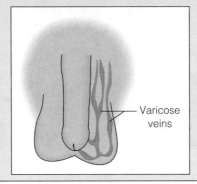

Routine physical examination of the genital organs involves inspection and palpation to identify any inflammatory lesions, abrasions, phimosis, abnormal masses, or tenderness. The inguinal and femoral areas are also inspected and palpated for hernias.

Prostate abnormalities, including cancer, can be identified through a rectal examination. A normal prostate feels solid and smooth. A prostate that is soft and spongy is referred to as **boggy**. One that is excessively hard is referred to as **indurated**.

Diagnostic Procedures

LABORATORY TESTS	DESCRIPTION
serum acid phosphatase	acid phosphatase is an enzyme found in the prostate and its secretions; increased amounts occur with prostatic cancer
prostate specific antigen (PSA)	an antigen contained in prostate tissue and measured by a blood test; increased levels found in prostate cancer and prostatitis

CLINICAL PROCEDURES	DESCRIPTION
biopsy	removal of piece of tissue for microscopic examination
punch biopsy	utilizes a sharp circular instrument to remove a piece of tissue
surgical excision biopsy	removal of an entire lesion by surgical excision

SURGICAL TREATMENT	DESCRIPTION
orchidopexy	surgical fixation of the testicles to the scrotum because of undescended testicles (cryptorchidism)
suprapubic prostatectomy	removal of the prostate through an abdominal incision above the pubis
transurethral resection of prostate	treatment for benign prostatic hypertrophy **Note:** The surgery involves the insertion of a resectoscope through the urethra and the resection of the enlarged prostatic tissue. The pressure on the urethra is reduced and normal urinary outflow in returned. No abdominal incision is made.

SURGICAL TREATMENT	DESCRIPTION
vasectomy	partial excision of the vas deferens bilaterally through an incision in the scrotum
	This procedure is usually done in 15 minutes under local anesthetic. A vasectomy results in sterilization. Following removal of the exised tissue, the free ends of the vas deferens are cauterized (sealed off using heat or electricity) or ligated (tied), thereby blocking the passage of sperm. There is no effect on testosterone production, sex drive, or penile erection.
	Vasectomies have been reversed with some success.

Vas deferens

▶ 16.10 ABBREVIATIONS FOR THE MALE REPRODUCTIVE SYSTEM

ABBREVIATION	MEANING
BPH	benign prostatic hypertrophy
PSA	prostate specific antigen
TUR	transurethral resection
TURP	transurethral resection of the prostate

Definitions

Definitions

Give the meaning for the following medical term elements.

Answers to the exercises in this chapter are found in Appendix A.

1. balan/o _____

2. orchid/o _____

3. vas/o _____

4. prostat/o _____

5. cyst/o _____

6. nephr/o _____

7. -plasia _____

8. pyel/o _____

9. -uria _____

10. ureter/o _____

11. -stenosis _____   15. ur/o _____

12. -gram _____   16. -rrhagia _____

13. corpor/o _____   17. andr/o _____

14. extra- _____

Give the prefix, suffix, or word root for the following.

18. below _____

19. drooping _____

20. stone _____

21. crushing _____

Define the following terms.

22. calyces _____

23. urethra _____

24. nephron _____

25. glomerulus _____

26. podocytes _____

27. efferent arteriole _____

28. tubular reabsorption _____

29. afferent arteriole _____

30. pedicels _____

31. filtrate _____

32. basement cells _____

33. glomerular filtration rate (GFR) _____

34. tubular secretion _____

35. creatinine _____

36. urea _____

37. renal vein _____

38. macula densa _____

39. juxtaglomerular apparatus _____

40. juxtaglomerular cells _____

41. trigone _____

42. renal capsule _____

43. renal corpuscle _____

44. renal pelvis _____

45. renal tubule _____

46. detrusor muscle _____

47. proximal convoluted tubule _____

48. peritubular capillaries _____

49. loop of Henle _____

50. distal convoluted tubule _____

51. collecting duct _____

52. Bowman's capsule _____

53. urine _____

54. filtration slits _____

55. erythropoietin _____

56. renin _____

57. urinary bladder _____

▶EXERCISE 16–2

Word Building

Build the word that means the following.

Word Building

1. hardening of the glomerulus _____

2. inflammation of the kidney _____

3. increased amounts of protein in the urine _____

4. underdeveloped kidney _____

5. inflammation of the trigone _____

6. stone in the ureters _____

7. narrowing of the urethra _____

8. pertaining to the kidney _____

1. What is the function of the bladder? _____
   _____

2. What is the composition of urine? _____
   _____

3. At what point does filtrate become inalterable? _____
   _____

   What is the filtrate called at this point? _____

4. What is the process that determines the water content of urine? _____
   _____

5. What is the process that helps regulate pH balance in extracellular fluid?
   _____

6. Name the tissues and cells involved in glomerular filtration. _____
   _____
   _____
   _____

7. Describe two mechanisms that change the GFR. _____
   _____
   _____

8. What is the micturation reflex? _____
   _____

9. What is the composition of filtrate when it enters the renal tubule? _____
   _____

10. What is the name of the blood vessel that connects the two capillary networks of the glomerulus?
    _____

Matching Terms with Meanings

Matching	COLUMN A	COLUMN B

Match the term in Column A with its meaning in Column B.

COLUMN A

1. glomerulus _____
2. efferent arteriole _____
3. tubular secretion _____
4. macula densa _____
5. calyx _____
6. trigone _____
7. distal convoluted tubule _____
8. filtrate _____
9. creatinine _____
10. tubular reabsorption _____
11. renin _____
12. Bowman's capsule _____

COLUMN B

A. part of the renal tubule

B. fluid in the renal tubule

C. transfer of material from renal tubule to peritubular capillaries

D. capillary system fed by afferent arteriole

E. waste material in urine

F. endocrine secretion in the nephron

G. artery carrying blood to peritubular capillaries

H. part of the renal corpuscle

I. transfer of material from peritubular capillaries to renal tubule

J. cavity in which urine collects

K. triangular region of the bladder

L. part of the juxtaglomerular apparatus

► EXERCISE 16–5   **Spelling Practice**

Spelling

Place a check mark beside all misspelled words in the list that follows. Correctly spell those that you checked off.

1. caylces ☐ _____
2. hilum ☐ _____
3. urether ☐ _____
4. micturition ☐ _____
5. glomerulus ☐ _____
6. loop of Helne ☐ _____
7. pedocytes ☐ _____
8. creatinine ☐ _____
9. musculka densa ☐ _____
10. detrusor muscle ☐ _____

Blood, Filtrate, and Urine Paths

Trace the path of blood flow by numbering the following terms in the proper sequence.

a. afferent arteriole _____   d. efferent arteriole _____

b. renal vein _____   e. glomerular capillaries _____

c. peritubular capillaries _____   f. renal artery _____

Trace the path of filtrate flow through the nephron by numbering the following terms in proper sequence

a. proximal convoluted _____   e. collecting duct _____
    tubule

b. basement cells _____   f. Bowman's capsule _____

c. loop of Henle _____   g. pores in the wall of _____
                                  glomerular capillaries

d. filtration slits _____   h. distal convoluted _____
                                  tubule

Trace the path of urine flow by numbering the following terms in proper sequence.

a. renal pelvis _____   f. urethra _____

b. external urethral _____   g. major calyces _____
    sphincter

c. minor calyces _____   h. internal urethral _____
                                  sphincter

d. ureter _____   i. urinary bladder _____

e. pyramids _____

► EXERCISE 16-7

Use of Medical Terms in Context

Medical Terms in Context

Define the underlined terms as they are used in context.

UNIVERSITY HOSPITAL ✚   HISTORY RECORD

ADMISSION DIAGNOSIS: RIGHT <u>HYDROURETER</u> AND <u>HYDRONEPHROSIS</u>

HISTORY OF PRESENT ILLNESS:

A 78-year-old female with psychological problems was admitted with abdominal pain. She had been having this pain off and on for the past two years. She was admitted on June 24, 1995, where she was found to have <u>diverticulosis</u>. An <u>IVP</u> was performed that showed poor function on the right with a <u>hypoplastic</u> scarred kidney. The patient therefore underwent outpatient <u>cystoscopy</u> and <u>retrograde pyelography</u> revealing a <u>malrotated</u> right kidney with a <u>stricture</u> involving the <u>distal one-third</u> of the ureter. The patient was admitted at this time for consideration of <u>nephrectomy</u>.

SIGNATURE OF DOCTOR IN CHARGE _____

1. hydroureter _____

2. hydronephrosis _____

3. diverticulosis _____

4. IVP _____

5. hypoplastic _____

6. cystoscopy _____

7. retrograde pyelography _____

8. malrotated _____

9. stricture _____

10. distal one-third _____

11. nephrectomy _____

MEDICAL TERMINOLOGY IN CONTEXT

1. Following the diagnosis of <u>obstructive pyelonephritic</u> right kidney, the patient underwent a <u>renal</u> scan revealing an <u>atrophic</u> scarred kidney accounting for less than 14% of the total <u>GFR</u>.

2. <u>Histopathology</u> of the <u>resected</u> kidney revealed marked <u>hydronephrosis</u> and <u>hydroureter</u> with thinning of the <u>renal parenchyma</u> and chronic <u>pyelonephritis</u>.

3. The sections shows gross <u>renal atrophy</u> which tends to be <u>localized</u>. In the atrophic areas, the <u>glomeruli</u> and <u>tubules</u> are unrecognizable, the tissue is <u>chronically</u> inflamed. A <u>cortical cyst</u> is noted. The <u>renal pelvis</u> and ureter show nonspecific chronic inflammation and <u>edema</u>.

---

12. obstructive pyelonephritic _____

13. renal _____

14. atrophic _____

15. GFR _____

16. histopathology _____

17. resected _____

18. hydronephrosis _____

19. hydroureter _____

20. renal parenchyma _____

21. pyelonephritis _____

22. renal atrophy _____

23. localized   _____

24. glomeruli   _____

25. tubules   _____

26. chronically   _____

27. cortical cyst   _____

28. renal pelvis   _____

29. edema   _____

Central Medical   **OPERATION REPORT**

OPERATION PERFORMED: <u>TRANSURETHRAL RESECTION</u> OF THE PROSTATE

PROCEDURE: After spinal anesthesia was achieved, the patient was placed in the lithotomy position. The lower abdomen was prepared and draped in the usual manner. A <u>resectoscope</u> was passed per urethra. Twenty grams of <u>benign</u>-appearing <u>prostatic</u> tissue was resected from the prostate. Following the resection, bleeding was well controlled and a <u>catheter</u> was inserted per urethra.

DIAGNOSIS: BENIGN PROSTATIC HYPERPLASIA

Authorized Health Care Practitioner _____

---

30. transurethral resection   _____

31. resectoscope   _____

32. benign   _____

33. prostatic   _____

34. catheter   _____

Across

1 Pertaining to the outer layer of the kidney
7 Record of the urinary tract
8 Outside the body
9 Record of the renal pelvis
10 Inflammation of the trigone of the bladder
12 Kidney stones
13 Drooping kidney
14 Drugs to stimulate the bladder

Down

1 Pertaining to the calices
2 Hardening of the glomerulus
3 Surgical fixation of the kidney
4 Stone in the ureters
5 Albuminuria
6 Pertaining to the mudulla
11 A procedure sometimes used in treating patients with a renal malfunction

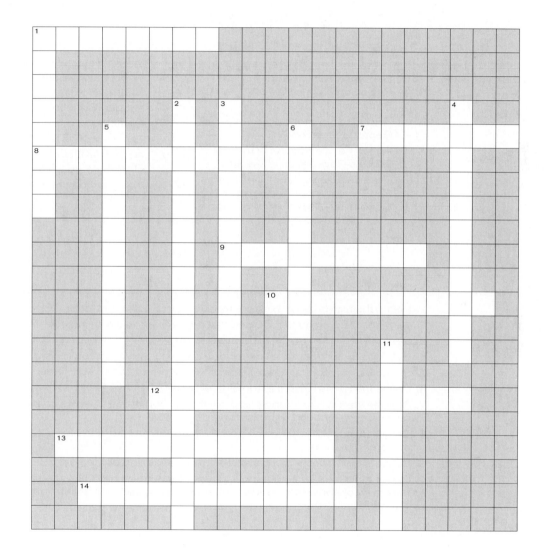

CHAPTER ORGANIZATION

This chapter has been designed to help the student learn terms and abbreviations related to the female reproductive system, human genetics, and obstetrics.

CHAPTER OBJECTIVES

Upon successful completion of this chapter, the student will be able to do the following:

1. Define the terms describing the female reproductive system.
2. Describe the hormonal patterns that regulate female reproduction.
3. Describe the processes of mitosis and meiosis.
4. Describe the process that determines variations in inherited traits.
5. Define the terms related to conception and prenatal development.
6. Define the terms related to the birth process.
7. Analyze, define, pronounce, and spell common medical terms of the female reproductive system, genetics, and obstetrics.
8. Define terms related to some common abnormalities of the female reproductive system.
9. Define abnormal conditions related to genetics and obstetrics.
10. Define the terms relating to physical examination, symptoms, diagnosis, and treatment of abnormal conditions related to genetics, obstetrics, and the female reproductive system.

WORD ELEMENTS PROMINENT IN THIS CHAPTER

FEMALE REPRODUCTIVE SYSTEM

WORD ELEMENT	TYPE	MEANING
all-	prefix	different
cervic/o	root	neck; cervix uteri
chori/o	root	chorion
colp/o	root	vagina
culd/o	root	cul-de-sac
di-	prefix	two
labi/o	root	lips
mamm/o; mast/o	root	breast
men/o	root	month
metri/o; metr/o; hyster/o; uter/o	root	uterus
oophor/o; ovari/o	root	ovaries
salping/o	root	fallopian tube; uterine tube; oviduct
thel/o	root	nipple
vagin/o	root	vagina
vulv/o; episi/o	root	external genitalia; vulva

OBSTETRICS

WORD ELEMENT	TYPE	MEANING
amni/o	root	amnion
-blast	suffix	in a preliminary stage of growth
-cyesis	suffix	pregnancy
galact/o; lact/o	root	milk
gen/o	root	producing
-gravida	suffix	pregnancy
gynec/o	root	female; woman
multi-	prefix	many
nat/i	root	birth
nulli-	prefix	none
o/o; ov/o	root	egg
oxy-	prefix	sharp; rapid; quick
-para	suffix	to give birth to a child
-partum	suffix	labor; delivery; childbirth
perine/o	root	perineum
primi-	prefix	first
secundi-	prefix	second
-tocia	suffix	labor
zyg/o	root	union

II—17

▶ 17.1 GENERAL ANATOMY AND PHYSIOLOGY OF THE FEMALE REPRODUCTIVE SYSTEM

The female reproductive system is made up of the female gonads called **ovaries** (ō′-vă-rēz), the **uterus**, the **uterine** or **fallopian tubes**, the **vagina**, and the external **genitalia** (see Figure 17–1). The **mammary glands** (măm′-ă-rē), which produce milk to nourish the newborn infant, are also considered part of the female reproductive system.

FIGURE 17–1   **Anatomical Structures of the Female Reproductive System** (a) The female reproductive organs in relation to the urinary and digestive tracts. (b) Uterus, ovaries, fallopian tubes, and related structures. (c) Reproductive organs in relation to the pelvis.

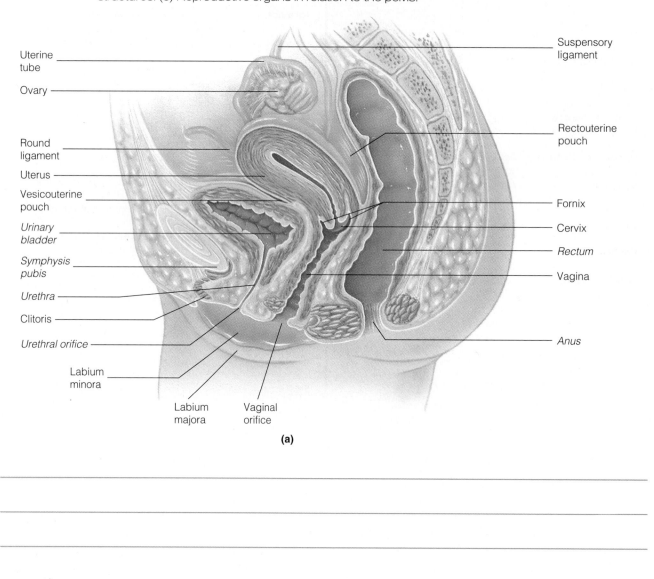

(a)

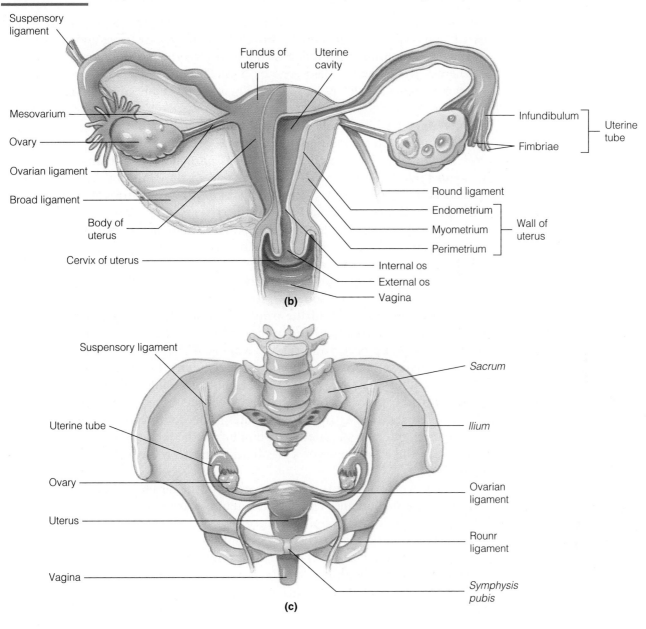

(b)

(c)

Ovaries

Two **ovaries**, one on each side of the vertebral column, are located in the pelvic cavity and are held in place by the **broad, mesovarian, ovarian,** and **suspensory ligaments**. The primary function of the ovaries is the development and release of the female gametes called eggs or **ova**. The process of ova production is known as **oogenesis** (ō″-ō-jĕn′-ĕ-sĭs). While the production of male gametes is a process that is continuous from puberty onwards, a lifetime supply of immature female gametes called **primary follicles** (fŏl′-ĭ-kl) are present in the female at birth. After female puberty, several primary follicles begin to mature each month. A fully mature follicle is called a **graafian** (grăf′-ē-ăn) follicle. One graafian follicle ruptures each month to release the ovum in a process called **ovulation** (ŏv″-ū-lā′-shun). Occasionally, two or more mature ova are released each month. If more than one egg is fertilized by sperm, a multiple birth (twins, triplets, etc.) results. Ovulation is regulated by **luteinizing hormone (LH)** secreted by the anterior pituitary. The mature ovum, like the sperm, contains only 23 chromosomes instead of 46. When an ovum becomes fertilized by a sperm, it is called a **zygote** (zī′-gōt), and the zygote then has a full package of genetic information in 46 chromosomes.

The second function of the ovaries is production of the female sex hormones, **estrogen** (ĕs′-trō-jĕn) and **progesterone** (prō-jĕs′-tĕr-ōn). The production of these hormones occurs in cycles averaging 28 days. Like the male sex hormones, female sex hormone secretions are regulated by the hypothalamus and anterior pituitary glands. Under stimulation from **follicle-stimulating hormone (FSH)** and LH, the developing follicle itself acts as an endocrine gland and secretes estrogen. The estrogen contributes to the continued development of the follicle itself and also stimulates the buildup of the lining of the uterus in preparation for the attachment of a fertilized ovum to the wall of the uterus (**implantation**).

After ovulation, the ruptured graafian follicle develops into a mass of cells called the **corpus luteum**. The corpus luteum secretes progesterone along with estrogen. Progesterone stimulates the growth of blood vessels in the uterus in preparation for the increased blood supply that will be needed to support a potential developing infant. If no fertilization by a sperm takes place, the corpus luteum degenerates within a few days, and its secretions of estrogen and progesterone thus cease. This cessation signals the hypothalamus and anterior pituitary to repeat the release of GnRH, FSH, and LH to start the monthly reproductive cycle again. If fertilization does takes place, the corpus luteum continues to secrete progesterone, which inhibits the hypothalamic secretions, and no further ovulation takes place during pregnancy.

If no implantation occurs, the buildup of tissue and blood vessels in the wall of the uterus is discharged in a process called **menstruation** (mĕn-stroo-ā′-shŭn). Between the ages of 45 and 55, all of a female's primary follicles have either degenerated or been expelled during ovulation. Consequently, estrogen secretion ceases to interact with the secretions of LH and FSH. The female reproductive cycles stops, and the female is in **menopause** (mĕn′-ō-pawz).

Two **uterine** or **fallopian** (fă-lō′-pē-ăn) **tubes** serve to transport the ova from the ovaries to the uterus. The proximal end of each tube is attached to the uterus. The distal ends are shaped like a funnel and are called the **infundibulum**. Fingerlike fingers called **fimbriae** at the end of each infundibulum move back and forth, sweeping the ovum into the tube.

Uterus

The **uterus** (ū′-tĕr-ŭs) is a hollow sac suspended and held in place in the pelvic cavity by the broad, round, uterosacral, and cardinal ligaments. It is roughly the size of a fist and shaped like an upside-down pear. The uterus comprises a **body, fundus,** and **cervix.** The body is a muscular wall surrounding the uterine cavity. The wall consists of the **perimetrium,** the outermost serous membrane layer; the **myometrium,** the middle layer of muscle; and the **endometrium,** the innermost layer, which is shed each month during menstruation. The fundus is the superior portion of the uterus; the cervix, the inferior portion. The uterine tubes and the ovaries, as well as the ligaments holding the uterus in place, are collectively called **adenxae,** as they are adjacent to the uterus and are considered accessory organs. The cervix projects into the **vagina** (vă-jī′-nă), which is a muscular tube connecting the uterus to the outside of the body and functions as the birth canal and receives the penis during sexual intercourse. The **hymen** (hī′-mĕn), a layer of mucous membrane, partially covers the **introitus** (ĭn-trō′-ĭ-tus), the entrance to the vagina. Contrary to popular belief, the absence of the hymen does not indicate the loss of virginity, nor does its presence confirm it.

External Genitalia

The external genitalia are known collectively as the **vulva** (vŭl′-va), and include the **clitoris** (klĭt′-ō-rĭs), the **labia majora** (lā′-bē-ă), the **labia minora,** the **mons pubis,** and **Bartholin's** (băr′-tō-lĭnz) **glands,** as shown in Figure 17–2. The Bartholin's glands secrete a fluid which lubricates the vagina, preparing it for intercourse.

FIGURE 17–2

Structures of the Female External Genitalia or Vulva

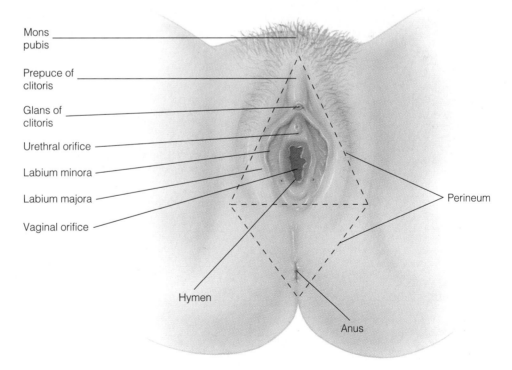

Mons pubis

Prepuce of clitoris

Glans of clitoris

Urethral orifice

Labium minora

Labium majora

Vaginal orifice

Hymen

Anus

Perineum

Breast

Each breast contains a mammary gland, which produces and secretes milk (lactation) after childbirth. Each gland consists of a number of lobes in which many little sacs called **alveoli** secrete the milk. The milk collects in the **lactiferous sinuses** and then travels through the **lactiferous duct** to one of a number of tiny openings in the **nipple** of the breast. The nipple is surrounded by a darker ring called the **areola**. After childbirth, glands in the areola produce oils that help prevent the skin of the nipple from drying out from breast feeding (see Figure 17–3).

FIGURE 17–3 **Mammary Glands** (a) Anterior view. Notice the difference between the lactiferous duct and lactiferous sinus. (b) Sagittal view. Notice the difference between lobes and lobules.

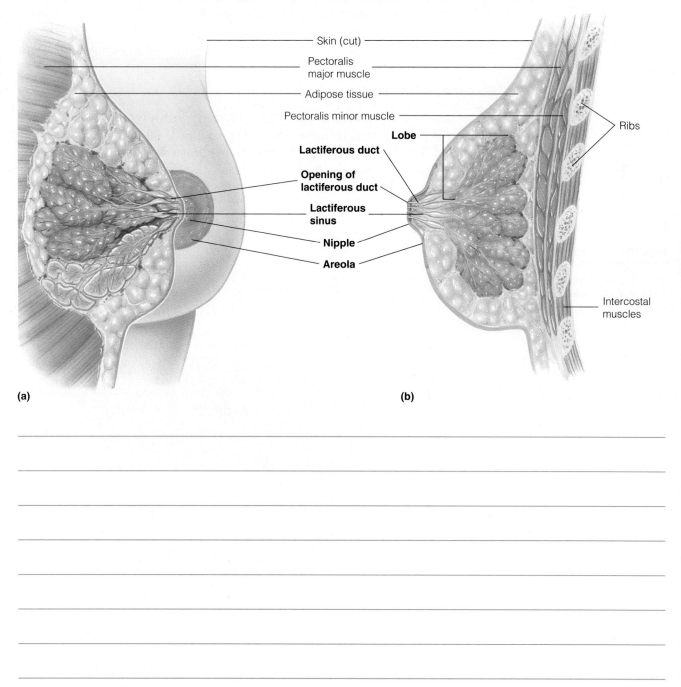

(a)   (b)

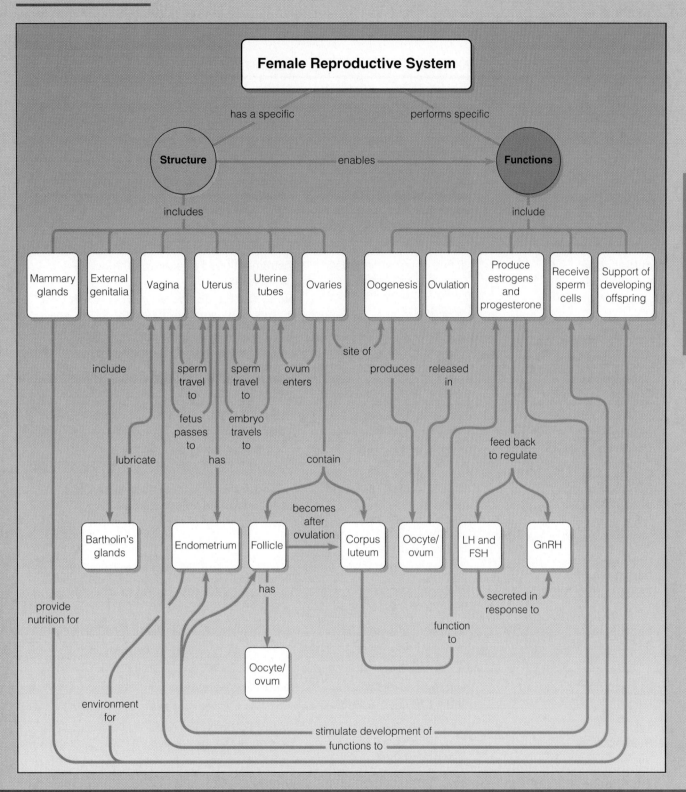

TERM WITH PRONUNCIATION	ANALYSIS	DEFINITION
cervicitis sĕr-vĭ-sī′-tĭs	-itis = inflammation cervic/o = cervix uteri	inflammation of the cervix uteri
colporrhaphy kŏl-por′-ă-fē	-rrhaphy = suture colp/o = vagina	suturing of the vagina
colpoperineoplasty kŏl″-pō-pĕr″-ĭn-ē′-ō-plăs″-tē	-plasty = surgical reconstruction; surgical repair colp/o = vagina perine/o = perineum	surgical reconstruction of the vagina and perineum
culdoscope kŭl′-dō-skōp	-scope = instrument used to visually examine culd/o = cul-de-sac (of Douglas)	instrument used to examine the cul-de-sac (of Douglas) **Note:** The cul-de-sac of Douglas is a pocket between the uterus and rectum. It is considered to be the lowest point in the abdominal cavity and can be a gathering place for fluid and microorganisms.
endometrium ĕn-dō-mē′-trē-ŭm	-ium = structure endo- = within; innermost metr/o = uterus	refers to the innermost structure (layer) of the uterus
galactorrhea gă-lăk″-tō-rē′-ă	-rrhea = flow; discharge galact/o = milk	discharge of milk from the breast at a time other than nursing a newborn or infant; excessive discharge of milk from the breast
gynecologist gī″-nĕ-kŏl′-ō-jĭst	-ist = specialist; one who specializes gynec/o = woman; female -logy = study of	a specialist in the study of diseases and treatment of the female genital tract
hematosalpinx hĕm″-ă-tō-săl′-pĭnks	-salpinx = uterine tube; fallopian tube; oviduct hemat/o = blood	accumulation of blood in the fallopian tube
hydrosalpinx hī-drō-săl′-pĭnks	-salpinx = uterine tube; fallopian tube; oviduct hydr/o = water	accumulation of water in the fallopian tube
hysterectomy hĭs-tĕr-ĕk′tō mē	-ectomy = excision; surgical removal hyster/o = uterus	removal of the uterus
hysterotomy hĭs-tĕr-ŏt′-ō-mē	-tomy = incision hyster/o = uterus	incision of the uterus
intrauterine in″-tră-ū′-tĕr-ĭn	-ine = pertaining to intra- = within uter/o = uterus	pertaining to within the uterus
labial lā′-bē-ăl	-al = pertaining to labi/o = lips	pertaining to the lips
lactogenesis lăk″-tō jĕn′-ĭ-sĭs	-genesis = production; formation lact/o = milk	production of milk

TERM WITH PRONUNCIATION	ANALYSIS	DEFINITION
mammary măm′-ă-rē	-ary = pertaining to mamm/o = breast	pertaining to the breast
mastectomy măs-těk′-tō-mē	-ectomy = excision mast/o = breast	removal of the breast
mastopexy măs′-tō-pěks-ē	-pexy = surgical fixation mast/o = breast	surgical fixation of the breasts to correct sagging breasts
menarche měn-ăr′-kē	-arche = beginning men/o = month	beginning of the regular menstrual cycle starting approximately at the age of 12
menopause měn′-ō-pawz	-pause = cessation; stoppage men/o = month	cessation of menstruation
myometrium mī″-ō-mē′-trē-ŭm	-ium = structure my/o = muscle metr/o = uterus	muscular structure of the uterus
oocyte ō′-ō-sīt	-cyte = cell o/o = egg	egg cell that develops into an ovum
oophoralgia ō″-ŏf-ō-răl′-jē-ă	-algia = pain oophor/o = ovary	pain in the ovary
ovariorrhexis ō-vā″-rē-ō-rěk′-sĭs	-rrhexis = rupture ovari/o = ovary	ruptured ovary
panhysterectomy păn″-hĭs-těr-ěk′-tō-me	-ectomy = excision; removal pan- = all hyster/o = uterus	removal of all the uterus
parametrium păr-ă-mē′-trē-ŭm	-ium = structure para- = near; beside metr/o = uterus	structures that are adjacent to or beside the uterus (refers to connective tissue located beside the uterus such as the ligaments holding the uterus in position)
perimetrium pěr-ĭ-mē′-trē-ŭm	-ium = structure peri- = around metr/o = uterus	structure around the uterus (refers to the outermost layer of the uterus)
perineorrhaphy pěr″-ĭ-nē-or′-ă-fē	-rrhaphy = suture perine/o = perineum	suturing of the perineum
polythelia pŏl″-ē-thē′-lē-ă	-ia = condition poly- = many thel/o = nipple	a condition of having more than two nipples
pyosalpinx pī″-ō-săl′-pĭnks	-salpinx = uterine tube; fallopian tube; oviduct py/o = pus	accumulation of pus in the fallopian tube
salpingopexy săl-pĭn′-gō-pěk″-sē	-pexy = surgical fixation salping/o = uterine tubes; fallopian tubes; oviduct	surgical fixation of the fallopian tubes
uterovesical ū″-těr-ō-věs′-ĭ-kăl	-al = pertaining to uter/o = uterus vesic/o = bladder	pertaining to the uterus and bladder

II–17

TERM WITH PRONUNCIATION	ANALYSIS	DEFINITION
vaginitis văj-ĭn-ī′-tĭs	-itis = inflammation vagin/o = vagina	inflammation of the vagina
vulvitis vŭl-vī′-tĭs	-itis = inflammation vulv/o = external genitalia	inflammation of the external genitalia

▶ 17.3 ABNORMAL CONDITIONS OF THE FEMALE REPRODUCTIVE SYSTEM

Breast

CONDITION	DESCRIPTION
fibroadenoma	benign rubbery tumor of the breast that can be removed leaving the breast intact
scirrhous carcinoma	hard, malignant tumor of the breast characterized by an overgrowth of fibrous tissue **Note:** Do not confuse scirrhous (meaning hard) with cirrhosis (meaning yellow).

Uterus, Tubes, Ovaries, and Other Adnexae

CONDITION	DESCRIPTION
cervical dysplasia, carcinoma in-situ, invasive carcinoma of the cervix	the appearance of abnormal changes (dysplasia) in cervical epithelium that can progress from minimal involvement of the cervical epithelial tissue (dysplasia), to moderate involvement (carcinoma in-situ), to invasive carcinoma **Note: Papanicolaou (Pap) smear** (see laboratory tests below) and tissue biopsy are used to detect abnormal cervical changes. Treatment depends on severity and will include drug therapy, radiation therapy, and surgery.
cervical polyps	benign tumor (papilloma) of the cervix

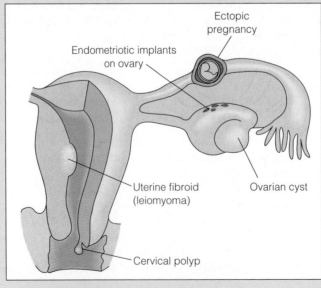

Ectopic pregnancy

Endometriotic implants on ovary

Uterine fibroid (leiomyoma)

Ovarian cyst

Cervical polyp

Note: Polyps are usually pedunculated and extend into the cervical cavity, where they can be surgically removed.

CONDITION	DESCRIPTION
cystocele and rectocele	a cystocele is a displacement of the urinary bladder onto the vaginal wall causing pressure and collapse of the vaginal wall into the vaginal canal a rectocele is a displacement of the rectum onto the vaginal wall causing collapse of the vaginal wall into the vaginal canal

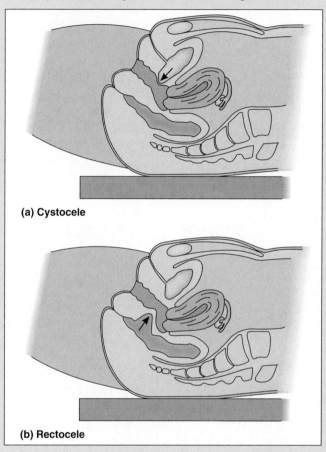

(a) Cystocele

(b) Rectocele

endometriosis	endometrial tissue found at sites other than the uterus, usually in the pelvic area
	Note: The ectopic tissue finds its way into the pelvic cavity through the open fallopian tubes. Abnormal sites where the endometrium can be found include the ovaries, tubes, parametrium, and portions of the peritoneum. Problems occur because the ectopic endometrium responds to the hormonal changes of the menstrual cycle and bleeds when there is no outlet for the old endometrium. A number of symptoms arise, such as inflammation, scarring, and adhesions. Infertility is a major complication because of the inability of the egg to reach the tube for fertilization.
leiomyoma; uterine fibroids	benign smooth muscle tumor of the uterus; also known as **fibroids**, **myomas**, and **fibromyomas**
	Note: Cause is unknown.
	May be asymptomatic. However, when symptoms do occur, the most frequent ones are painful and excessive menstruation. Other symptoms may result from the pressure a large tumor may have on the surrounding organs such as the back, urinary bladder, and colon.
	Treatment involves removal of the tumors. Hysterectomy is considered only in severe cases and take into consideration the size and location of the tumor, as well as the patient's age and number of children.

CONDITION	DESCRIPTION
malposition of uterus	abnormal displacement of the uterus from its normal, slightly anteverted position over the bladder

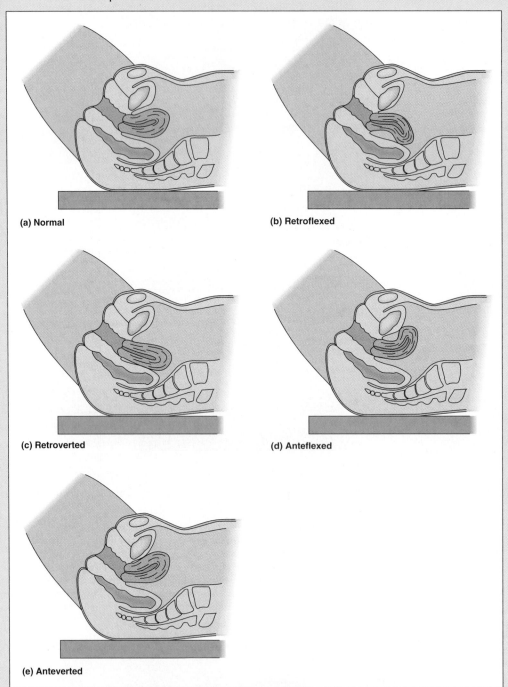

(a) Normal

(b) Retroflexed

(c) Retroverted

(d) Anteflexed

(e) Anteverted

Note: Because the uterus is freely movable, it may be displaced in one of several positions: **retroflexed**, the uterus bends backwards toward the rectum; **retroverted**, the uterus tips or tilts backwards toward the rectum; **anteflexed**, the uterus bends forward over the bladder; **anteverted**, the uterus is tipped or tilted forward over the bladder to a greater degree than normal.

CONDITION	DESCRIPTION
ovarian cysts	closed sac or cavity on the ovary containing fluid, semifluid, or solid material; these cysts can be described as **follicular cysts** involving the graffian follicle, **lutein cysts** involving the corpus luteum, and **polycystic ovaries** in which multiple cysts appear on the ovary **Note:** These cysts are usually benign.
pelvic inflammatory disease (PID)	bacterial infection of the uterus, cervix uteri, fallopian tubes, ovaries, or parametrium **Note:** Causative microorganisms include streptococci, staphylococci, gonococci, and Chlamydia. Responds well to antibiotic therapy, but if left untreated causes sterility.
uterine prolapse; metroptosis	protrusion or displacement of the uterus through the vaginal canal

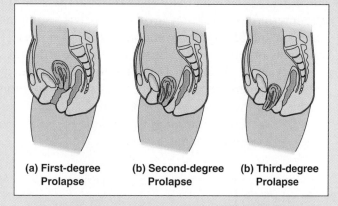

(a) First-degree Prolapse (b) Second-degree Prolapse (b) Third-degree Prolapse

Note: There are three stages of prolapse based upon the degree to which the uterus and cervix uteri are displaced through the entrance to the vagina.

first degree—the uterus and cervix project through the vaginal canal but not through the introitus.

second degree—the uterus is displaced further into the vaginal canal with the cervix protruding through the introitus.

third degree—the uterus and cervix project through the introitus. Also known as **procidentia**.

Vagina and External Genitalia

kraurosis	dry and wrinkled appearance of the external genitalia, especially the vulva; most frequently seen in postmenopausal or posthysterectomy women
pruritus vulvae	severe itchiness of the vagina

Disorders of Menstruation

amenorrhea	absence of menstruation **Note:** Called **primary amenorrhea** when the patient has never menstruated and **secondary amenorrhea** when menstruation has been absent for three or more consecutive months.
dysmenorrhea	painful menstruation due to strong uterine contractions; may be idiopathic
menorrhagia	excessive uterine bleeding during the menstrual period (menses)
metrorrhagia	excessive uterine bleeding during times other than the menstrual period
menometrorrhagia	excessive uterine bleeding at the time of menstruation and at variable intervals
oligomenorrhea	scanty uterine bleeding during menstruation

CONDITION	DESCRIPTION
premenstrual syndrome (PMS)	physical and emotional distress occurring in a cyclical pattern during the menstrual cycle; symptoms such as edema, fatigue, lethargy, irritability, and depression are usually present after ovulation and may occur with the menstruation

▶ 17.4 PHYSICAL EXAMINATION, DIAGNOSIS, AND TREATMENT OF ABNORMAL CONDITIONS OF THE FEMALE REPRODUCTIVE SYSTEM

A gynecologic examination includes an external and internal examination. The external examination includes a complete evaluation of the breasts, abdomen, and external genitalia. Any signs of tenderness or abnormal masses are noted. The internal examination involves a pelvic examination of the internal structures, including the cervix and uterus and a noting of the size, shape, position, and areas of tenderness. Masses of adnexal structures are also noted.

A vaginal speculum (see Chapter 22) is used during the internal examination to widen the vaginal openings so that any abnormal lesions are visible. At this time the cervix is also inspected.

During the examination, specimens are taken from the cervix, uterus, and vagina for cytologic examination.

SIGNS AND SYMPTOMS	DESCRIPTION
dyspareunia	pain on coitus (intercourse)
leukoplakia	white patches on the mucous membrane of the external genitalia
leukorrhea	whitish discharge from the uterus and vaginal canal
mittelschmerz	abdominal pain at time of ovulation
stress incontinence	involuntary micturition due to intra-abdominal pressure resulting from coughing, laughing, or straining
LABORATORY TESTS	**DESCRIPTION**
culture, cervical	identifies bacteria in a specimen of body fluids taken from the cervix uteri **Note:** The sample is taken from the patient and put in an environment that fosters bacterial growth. The microorganism multiplies and thus is readily identified.
smear, endometrial	a specimen for microscopic study is placed onto a glass slide, dried and stained to highlight the microorganism (the smear is named after the site from which the specimen is taken, in this case the endometrium)

LABORATORY TESTS	DESCRIPTION
exfoliative cytology Papanicolaou smear (Pap Smear) of the cervix uteri	cellular examination to differentiate normal cells from precancerous and cancerous cells of the cervix uteri
	Note: This test is based on the premise that normal and abnormal cervical cells fall from the lining of the cervix and pass into the cervical and vaginal secretions. The secretions are examined and any abnormalities can be identified before symptoms become apparent.
	The abnormal changes of the cervical epithelium are graded from mild, to moderate, to severe, to carcinoma in-situ as seen below.
	(CIN = cervical intraepithelial neoplasia)
	CIN I mild dysplasia
	CIN II moderate dysplasia
	CIN III severe dysplasia to carcinoma in-situ
	When the carcinoma progresses to carcinoma of the cervix, the cancer can be classified by the following stages:
	Stage 0 carcinoma in-situ
	Stage I carcinoma of the cervix with no adnexal involvement.
	Stage II carcinoma of the cervix with minimal adnexal invasion
	Stage III carcinoma of the cervix with involvement to the pelvic area
	Stage IV carcinoma of the cervix with involvement of structures outside the pelvic area
Schiller's test	test to diagnose cervical and vaginal neoplasia
	Note: An iodine stain such as Lugol's is painted onto the mucous membrane. Cancerous cells are easily identified, as they do not absorb the stain. Noncancerous cells absorb the stain and turn a brownish color.

RADIOLOGY	DESCRIPTION
mammography	a radiographic examination of the soft tissue of the breast; used to identify abnormal masses that would otherwise go undetected under physical examination
	Note: A method other than the common film mammography is **xeroradiography**, which is a dry process rather than the conventional wet process utilized in producing an x-ray. The process is similar to the image obtained by a photocopier.
hysterosalpingography (HSG)	x-ray of the uterus and fallopian tubes following injection of contrast medium into the uterus

II—17

CLINICAL PROCEDURES	DESCRIPTION
cervical punch biopsy and cautery	a sharp circular instrument is used to remove a piece of cervix for microscopic study (hemostasis may be maintained by cautery, the application of heat or electric current to the bleeding vessel)
cervical conization	a sharp instrument is used to remove a piece of cervix shaped like a cone for purposes of microscopic examination
colposcopy	process of visually examining the vagina, vulva and cervix uteri with a magnifying instrument called a colposcope. A biopsy may also be performed at the same time on any abnormal looking lesions. This procedure can be performed in the doctor's office with no anesthesia.
culdoscopy	process of visually examining the cul-de-sac of Douglas
culdocentesis	removal of fluid by surgical puncture of the cul-de-sac of Douglas for diagnostic purposes
Rubin test; insufflation of fallopian tubes	tests for the patency of the fallopian tubes by blowing (insufflation) carbon dioxide through the fallopian tubes via the uterus; if the fallopian tubes are open, the gas enters the abdominal cavity and shows up on x-ray **Note:** Used to rule out fallopian tube disease in cases of infertility.
laparoscopy	an instrument similar to a "telescope" is inserted into the abdomen through a small incision in the abdominal wall; through the laparoscope, the abdominopelvic organs can be seen

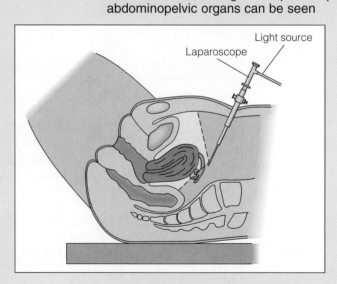

Light source

Laparoscope

Note: Laparoscopy may be exploratory when the patient complains of infertility or abdominal or pelvic pain; or it may be therapeutic for sterilization (see below), lysis of tubal adhesions, and other minor surgeries.

Laparoscopes are often equipped with lasers to allow destruction or removal of tissue without opening up the body cavity.

SURGICAL TREATMENT	DESCRIPTION
colporrhaphy	suturing of the vagina
dilation and curettage (D&C)	widening of the cervical opening with an instrument called a **dilator** and the insertion of a second instrument called a **curet (curette)** for the scraping out of the endometrial lining
hysterectomy	excision of the uterus **Note:** The uterus can be removed through the abdomen **(abdominal hysterectomy)** or through the vagina **(vaginal hysterectomy)**. Each of these can be further described as **total hysterectomy**, in which the entire uterus is removed; **subtotal hysterectomy**, in which all but the cervix is removed; and **radical hysterectomy**, in which the uterus and adjacent supporting structures and lymph glands are removed.
laparoscopic-assisted vaginal hysterectomy	following insertion of the laparoscope into the pelvic cavity, the ligaments that support the uterus are cut, freeing the uterus; the uterus is then removed through the vagina
laparoscopic hysterectomy	this is the same procedure as for laparoscopic-assisted vaginal hysterectomy except the uterus is removed through the laparoscope rather than through the vagina
lumpectomy	surgical removal of a malignant mass of tissue in the breast
mammoplasty	surgical reconstruction of the breast following mastectomy or for breast reduction or augmentation
salpingo-oophorectomy	excision of the fallopian tubes and ovaries, may be right-sided, left-sided, or bilateral
wedge resection	removal of a part of an organ or structure in the shape of a wedge

II–17

SURGICAL TREATMENT	DESCRIPTION

sterilization — the purpose of sterilization is to prevent pregnancy by blocking the route traveled by either the ovum or sperm

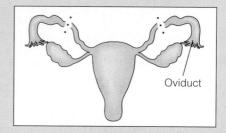

Oviduct

Note: Females can be sterilized by removing the uterus and/or ovaries. However, in most routine sterilizations, the method of choice is to destroy the lumen of the fallopian tube, thereby preventing the passage of sperm and ova.

Surgical procedures used to block the fallopian tubes are: **tubal ligation**, in which the lumen of the fallopian tube is blocked by constricting the tube with a threadlike material; **laparoscopy**, where a laparoscope is inserted through an incision into the abdominal wall, and the tube is grasped and tied (ligated) or sealed off using heat to destroy the tissue (electrocautery); **colpotomy** where the fallopian tube is grasped by an instrument placed through the vagina and uterus, and the tube is destroyed by excision of its distal end or by tubal ligation (there is no abdominal incision). In **culdoscopy** the tube is grasped by placing a culdoscope into the vagina. The tube is brought into the vagina, ligated, and excised, and clips are used in many instances.

Clips or bands block the lumen, making the sterilization potentially reversible in the future.

LASER TREATMENT	DESCRIPTION

Note: Lasers have a variety of general surgical applications, as explained in Chapter 22. The high energy source coming from the laser is also used to treat cancerous lesions of the female reproductive organs, cervical erosions, cervicitis, and some venereal diseases such as condylomata.

laparoscopic laser endometriosis vaporization — a laparoscope equipped with laser capabilities is inserted through a small incision into the pelvic cavity, and the powerful beam from the laser vaporizes the ectopic endometrium

endometrial ablation — used for menometrorrhagia

Note: A hysteroscope equipped with a laser is inserted into the uterus. Energy from the laser ablates (removes) the endometrium, stopping the excessive uterine bleeding.

lysis of adhesions — lasers with their direct energy source are able to destroy adhesions that cause infertility and pelvic pain

ABBREVIATION	MEANING	ABBREVIATION	MEANING
BSO	bilateral salpingo-oophorectomy	LH	luteinizing hormone
CIN	cervical intraepithelial neoplasia	LMP	last menstrual period
		Pap smear	Papanicolaou smear
CS	cesarean section	PID	pelvic inflammatory disease
D&C	dilation and curettage		
DUB	dysfunctional uterine bleeding	PMP	past menstrual period
		PMS	premenstrual syndrome
FSH	follicle-stimulating hormone	STD	sexually transmitted disease
GnRH	gonadotropin-releasing hormone	TAH	total abdominal hysterectomy
gyne; gyn	gynecology	vag	vaginal
HSG	hysterosalpingogram	VDRL	venereal disease research laboratories

◆ **17.6 HUMAN GENETICS**

Genetics (jĕ-nĕt′-iks) is the study of the development blueprint of individual persons. It is also the study of the parts of that blueprint that children inherit from their parents. Genetics is therefore closely related to the study of human reproduction.

Hereditary and developmental information are packaged in **genes** (jēnz), which are segments of threadlike structures called **chromosomes** that make up the nucleus of each body cell. Each chromosome is one molecule of **deoxyribonucleic** (dē-ŏk″-sē-rī″-bō-nū-klē′-ĭk) **acid (DNA)**.

Mitosis

For development to occur, body cells must divide and replicate themselves. All body cells except the reproductive cells divide by the process of **mitosis** (mī-tō′-sĭs) in which a parent cell divides into two daughter cells, each having 46 chromosomes like their parent. The 46 chromosomes in each of the daughter cells are genetically identical to one another and to the chromosomes in the parent cell. Cells having 46 chromosomes are called **diploid** (dĭp′-loyd) cells.

Meiosis

Reproductive cells (sperm and ova) divide by the process of **meiosis** (mī-ō′-sĭs). In meiosis, **reduction division** occurs. This results in daughter cells having only 23 chromosomes instead of 46. These 23-chromosome cells are called **haploid** (hăp′-loyd) cells.

Much confusion about genetic traits inherited through haploid cells can be avoided by keeping in mind that the original germ cells (**oogonia** [ō″-ō-gō′-nē-ă] and **spermatogonia** [spĕr″-măt-ō-gō′-nē-ă]) from which ova and sperm develop proliferate by mitosis. Thus the initial germ cells for sperm and ova are diploid cells having 46 chromosomes. It is only in later stages of their development that they divide by meiosis and become haploid cells.

Chromosomal Pairs and Inherited Traits

In diploid cells, the chromosomes are arranged in **chromosomal** (krō″-mō-sō′-măl) **pairs**, with each member of the pair having the same number of segments (genes) and with each gene being located at the same site (**locus**) on the chromosome. Thus, genes also occur in pairs. But genes may occur in alternative forms called **alleles** (ă-lēlz′). Some alleles are **dominant** (having a higher probability of being inherited by offspring), and some alleles are **recessive** (having a lower probability of being inherited by offspring). It is customary to represent dominant alleles by upper case letters and recessive alleles by lower case letters, as shown in Figure 17–4. Thus the gene that determines eye color, for example, may occur as allele C or c. In this example, the upper case C represents the dominant allele of brown eye color and the lower case c represents the recessive allele of blue eye color.

FIGURE 17–4

A Chromosomal Pair
(a) Illustrations of a single chromosome.
(b) Illustration of a pair of chromosomes.

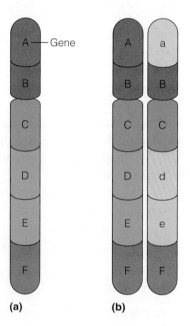

(a)   (b)

In haploid cells, only one half of a chromosomal pair is present, and the chromosomes in haploid cells are not identical to each other. These variations in cells, produced by meiosis, account for the variations in inherited traits among siblings.

As explained above, when a sperm unites with an ovum, the resulting zygote contains 46 chromosomes. The chromosomes of the zygote then fall into 23 pairs, with one member of each chromosomal pair coming from the mother's ovum and the other member of each chromosomal pair coming from the father's sperm, as shown in Figure 17–4. But notice (in the illustrated example) that while the genes of a zygote occur in pairs at the same locus on the two chromosomes, only the genes B, C, and F are identical (that is, the allele received from each of the respective parents is identical). In genes A, D, and E, on the other hand, dominant alleles are paired with recessive alleles. Either parent may contribute dominant alleles and either parent may contribute recessive alleles. The work of **geneticists** (jĕ-nĕt′-ĭ-sĭsts) includes predicting which alleles (each responsible for a specific trait) will be inherited by offspring.

Paired chromosomes in diploid cells are numbered by geneticists as pair 1 to pair 23. **Pair 23** is called the **sex chromosome** because it determines the sex of the offspring. In the female, the two chromosomes of pair 23 are both X chromosomes, and in the process of meiosis the ovum receives one X chromosome. In the male, pair 23 is made up of an X chromosome and a Y chromosome. Therefore, in the process of meiosis the sperm receives either an X chromosome or a Y chromosome but not both. When a sperm carrying an X chromosome unites with an ovum, the resulting zygote will have two X chromosomes in pair 23, and the offspring will be female. If the ovum is fertilized by a sperm carrying a Y chromosome, the zygote will have one X chromosome and one Y chromosome in pair 23, and the offspring will be male.

A **congenital** (kŏn-jĕn′-ĭ-tăl) disease or abnormality, as the name implies, is a condition that is present at the time of birth and is usually caused by irregularities in the chromosomes of the developing infant. **Down's syndrome**, for example, is caused by an extra chromosome in pair 21. Figure 17–5 shows a

FIGURE 17—5 Down's Syndrome (a) Karyotype of an individual with Down's Syndrome. (b) A photograph of a person with Down's Syndrome.

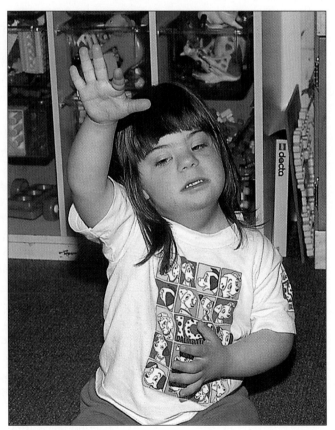

karyotype (kăr′-ē-ō-tīp) of an individual with Down's syndrome (a karyotype is made by staining and photographing a cell's chromosomal pairs).

▷ 17.7 OBSTETRICS

The branch of medicine dealing with **pregnancy** (prĕg′-năn-sē) and **labor** is called **obstetrics** (ŏb-stĕt′-rĭks).

Conception

The development of an infant (pregnancy) begins when a sperm cell unites with an ovum in **fertilization** or **conception** (kŏn-sĕp′-shun), which occurs in the fallopian tube after sperm have moved through the vagina and the uterus to meet the ovum.

The condition known as **infertility** (difficulty in conceiving) is often simply due to insufficient knowledge of the life span of the reproductive cells. An ovum lives for only 12 to 24 hours after ovulation, and sperm cells live for a maximum of three days after leaving the male. Furthermore, sperm cannot survive at all without the presence of a **cervical mucus**, which is secreted by the female cervix. Ovulation is signaled by the mucus becoming wet and slippery approximately three days prior to ovulation. The presence of this mucus then becomes clearly evident as it is discharged from the female's vagina, and it is only while it is in this state that it supports the life of the sperm. Research into this phenomenon by Dr. John Billings and his wife Dr. Lyn Billings in the 1960s led to the **ovulation method**, which is a form of **natural family planning (NFP)**. Conception is achieved by planning for sexual intercourse to occur during the **fertile days**, that is, the days of the reproductive cycle when the presence of fertile cervical mucus is plainly evident. In cases where circumstances require that pregnancies be prevented or postponed, women can restrict sexual intercourse to the **infertile days** of the reproductive cycle, that is, the days when the fertile mucus is absent.

Artificial contraception methods require surgical, hormonal, or mechanical methods as a means of preventing pregnancy. Such measures include surgical procedures on either the male or the female reproductive organs and affecting the female hormone cycles through the use of synthetic estrogen and progesterone in birth control pills. These pills are sometimes called **antiovulants** (ăn″-tē-ŏv′-ū-lănt), because they are intended to suppress ovulation by using synthetic estrogen to inhibit the secretion of LH, which is needed to stimulate ovulation. **Abortion** is the termination of a pregnancy before the embryo or fetus is viable outside the uterus. **Spontaneous abortion**, as distinguished from induced abortion, is usually referred to in lay terms as **miscarriage**.

For conception to take place, the thick covering of the ovum, the **zona pellucida** (pĕl-lŭ′-sī-dă), must be dissolved and penetrated by a sperm. This dissolution is accomplished by the action of enzymes from many sperm attacking the zona pellucida at once. Only one sperm, however, actually penetrates the ovum to form a zygote containing 46 chromosomes, 23 from the ovum and 23 from the sperm. This penetration (conception) usually takes place in the fallopian tube, and the zygote then divides by the process of mitosis to the point at which 16 cells are present. This initial cell division is called **cleavage**. The ball of 16 cells is called a **morula** (mor′-ū-lă). The initial cells that develop during cleavage are called **blastomeres** (blăs′-tō-mērz). The blastomeres become arranged into a hollow ball called a **blastocyst** (blăs′-tō-sĭst).

Sometimes the blastomeres forming the morula become separated into two groups of cells, both of which continue to develop and both of which implant in the uterus. The developing infants are in this case **identical twins**. Identical twins look exactly alike because a developing blastocyst divides by mitosis. As explained above, cells that divide by mitosis are genetically identical to one another and to the parent cell. **Fraternal twins**, on the other hand, do not have identical genetic information in their chromosomes because they are the result of two separate ova being fertilized by two separate sperm.

Embryonic Development

From the time of conception to the end of the eighth week of pregnancy, the developing offspring is referred to as an **embryo** (ĕm'-brē-ō). Approximately four days are required for the embryo to travel to the uterus through the fallopian tube. During these four days cleavage occurs. Eight days after conception, the embryo embeds itself in the uterine wall in the process of implantation. The embryo is at the blastocyst stage when it implants.

The **inner cell mass** of the blastocyst develops into an **embryonic disc**, from which the new infant is formed. The outer layer of the blastocyst is called the **trophoblast** (trŏf'-ō-blăst), which develops into an embryonic membrane called the **chorion** (kō'-rē-ŏn).

Three additional embryonic membranes are the **amnion** (ăm'-nē-ŏn), which grows along with the embryo; the **yolk sac**, which produces the first blood cells; and the **allantois** (ă-lăn'-tō-ĭs), which develops into the **connecting stalk** and eventually becomes the **umbilical cord**. The chorion and the amnion eventually form the **amniotic sac**, which is filled with **amniotic fluid** (ăm-nē-ŏt'-ik)— the infant lives in this fluid until birth—and the **placenta**. The embryo is connected to the placenta by the umbilical cord, which serves to transport nutrients and gases back and forth between the developing infant and the mother via the placenta.

The placenta also serves as an endocrine organ and secretes the hormones **human chorionic gonadotropin (hCG)**, **progesterone**, and **estrogen**, all of which ensure the proper maintenance of the uterine wall. The hormone **relaxin** (rē-lăk'-sĭn), also secreted by the placenta, softens the cervix in preparation for birth.

The time between conception and birth is divided into three segments called **trimesters**. Each trimester is approximately three months long. The first eight weeks of development are known as the **embryonic** (ĕm"-brē ŏn'-ĭk) **period**. Rapid development occurs during the embryonic period and includes the development and functioning of the heart, production of red blood cells and development of the circulation system, development of forebrain and hindbrain, and development of limbs, fingers, and toes.

Fetal Development

The period from the ninth week until birth is known as the **fetal period**, and the developing infant is called a **fetus**. Early in the fetal period, the liver, kidneys, and spleen begin to function, most of the lung structure is completed, and the external genitalia are completely developed. In the female fetus, ovaries and oogonia form (Figure 17–6). Fetal movements, known as **quickening**, can be felt by the mother, and reflex actions such as sucking of the thumb occur in the infant. Early in the last trimester, in the seventh month, the lungs become capable of gas exchange, and premature babies born at this stage are capable of surviving outside the uterus.

FIGURE 17–6

Fetus at Three Months

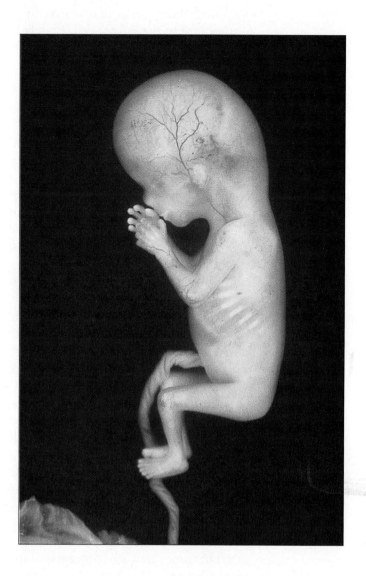

Parturition

The birth process is known as **parturition** (păr-tū-rĭsh′-ŭn). As discussed in Chapter 12, the hormone oxytocin, produced by the hypothalamus and released by the posterior pituitary, stimulates uterine contractions or **labor**, which is the beginning of parturition. The first stage of labor is known as **cervical dilation**. The cervix dilates to approximately 4 inches (10.2 cm) in diameter during this stage. The second stage, called **fetal delivery**, consists of uterine contractions that move the infant through the cervix and vagina to the outside world. The umbilical cord connecting the infant to the placenta is severed once the baby is out. In the last stage of labor, **placental delivery**, the placenta is expelled from the uterus (Figure 17–7).

In circumstances where the fetus is too large for a vaginal delivery or is in a **breech** position (with the buttocks instead of the head presenting itself into

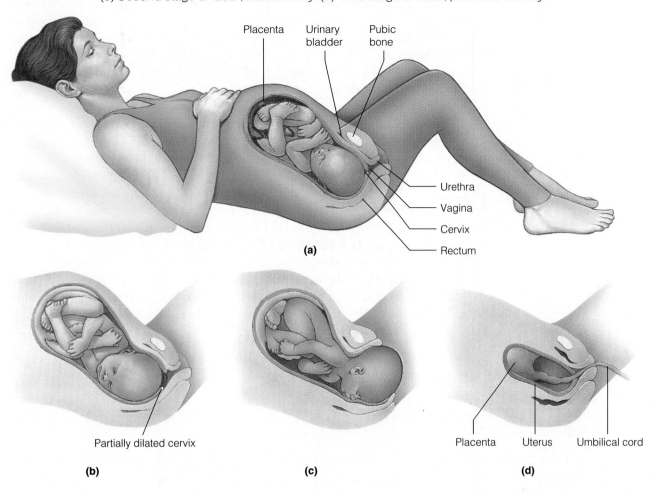

Placenta   Urinary   Pubic
            bladder   bone

Urethra
Vagina
Cervix
Rectum

(a)

Partially dilated cervix

(b)

(c)

Placenta   Uterus   Umbilical cord

(d)

II–17

the vagina) fetal delivery may be by **cesarean section (CS)**. This is a procedure in which the fetus is removed from the uterus surgically after an incision is made in the abdomen and uterus.

An **Apgar score** is a numerical expression of the condition of the newborn, determined one minute and fifteen minutes after birth. Heart rate, respiration, muscle tone, reflex response, and color are monitored and graded from 0–2 with "0" indicating absence and "2" indicating the highest rating. The best Apgar score a newborn can attain is 10.

Apgar Score

PHYSIOLOGICAL FACTORS	RATINGS (0–2)
Heart Rate	2
Respirations	2
Muscle Tone	2
Reflex Response	2
Color	2
Total Rating	10

The six to eight weeks following parturition are known as the **postpartum** period. During this time, the hormone prolactin is secreted from the anterior pituitary to stimulate the production of milk, called **lactation**, by the mammary glands. The hormone oxytocin regulates the flow of milk through the mammary glands. During the first few days following parturition, the mammary glands produce **colostrum** (kō-lŏs′-trŭm), a yellowish fluid that contains proteins and antibodies that nourish and protect the newborn infant. During the postpartum period, the reproductive organs return to normal size.

A woman's obstetrical history is often explained by using the terms **gravida** (grăv′-ĭ-dă), meaning the number of times the woman has been pregnant, and **para**, which refers to the number of past pregnancies that have resulted in viable births, regardless of the number of children born. For example, if a woman gives birth to twins, she has only given birth once despite producing two newborns. A woman pregnant for the first time is known as a **primigravida**, which is expressed as **gravida I, para 0 (G I P 0)**. When she delivers her first baby, she is described as **gravida I, para I (G I P I)**. When this woman delivers her second child, she is known as a **secundigravida (G II P II)**. If the same woman becomes pregnant with triplets, she is described as **gravida III**, and when the triplets are delivered, she is described as **gravida III, para III**. If the same woman becomes pregnant for the fourth time, she is **gravida IV, para III**. If she aborts the child, she is described as **gravida IV, para III, Ab 1**.

▷ 17.8 TERM ANALYSIS FOR OBSTETRICS

TERM WITH PRONUNCIATION	ANALYSIS	DEFINITION
amniocentesis ăm″-nē-ō-sĕn-tē′-sĭs	-centesis = surgical puncture amni/o = amnion	surgical puncture of the amnion (also called the amniotic sac or bag of waters) to remove amniotic fluid for examination
antepartum ăn-tē-păr′-tŭm	-partum = labor; delivery; childbirth ante- = before	period before the onset of labor, referring to the mother
chorionic kō-rē-ŏn′-ĭk	-ic = pertaining to chorion/o = chorion	pertaining to the chorion
dystocia dĭs-tō′-sē-ă	-tocia = labor dys- = difficult; bad; painful	difficult labor
episiorrhaphy ĕ-pĭs″-ē-or′-ă-fē	-rrhaphy = suture episi/o = vulva	suturing of the vulva
episiotomy ĕ-pĭs″-ē-ŏt′-ō-mē	-tomy = incision episi/o = vulva	incision of the vulva
multigravida mŭl″-tĭ-grăv′-ĭ-dă	-gravida = pregnancy multi- = many	a woman who has been pregnant two or more times (written gravida II, gravida III, gravida IV, etc., or as GII, GII, GIV, etc.)
multipara mŭl-tĭp′-ă-ră	-para = to bear; giving birth; part with a child multi- = multiple	a woman who has given birth two or more times (written as para II, para III, para IV, etc., or as PII, PIII, PIV, etc.)
neonatal nē-ō-nā′-tăl	-al = pertaining to ne/o = new nat/i = birth	pertaining to the first four weeks after birth

TERM WITH PRONUNCIATION	ANALYSIS	DEFINITION
nullipara nŭl-ĭp′-ă-ră	-para = to bear; giving birth; part with a child nulli- = none	a woman who has never given birth
nulligravida nŭl″-ĭ-grăv′-ĭ-dă	-gravida = pregnancy nulli- = none	a woman who has never been pregnant
oxytocia ŏk″-sē-tō′-sē-ă	-tocin = birth oxy- = rapid; quick; sharp	rapid birth
postnatal pōst-nā′-tăl	-al = pertaining to post- = after nat/i = birth	pertaining to after birth with reference to the newborn
postpartum pōst-păr′-tŭm	-partum = labor; delivery; childbirth post- = after	after delivery with reference to the mother
prenatal prē-nā′-tăl	-al = pertaining to pre- = before nat/i = birth	pertaining to before birth with reference to the fetus
primigravida prī-mĭ-grăv′-ĭ-dă	-gravida = pregnant primi- = first	a woman who is pregnant for the first time (also written as gravida I or G1)
primipara prī-mĭp′-ă-ră	-para = to bear; giving birth; part with a child primi- = first	a woman who has given birth for the first time (also written as para I or PI)
pseudocyesis soo″-dō-sī-ē′-sĭs	-cyesis = pregnancy pseudo- = false	false pregnancy **Note:** Cyesis can also be used by itself to mean pregnancy.
secundigravida sē-kŭn″-dĭ-grăv′-ĭd-ă	-gravida = pregnancy secundi- = second	a woman pregnant for the second time
secundipara sē″-kŭn-dĭp′-ă-ră	-para = pregnancy secundi- = second	a woman who has given birth to two viable offspring

▷ 17.9 ABNORMAL CONDITIONS RELATED TO OBSTETRICS AND GENETICS

CONDITION	DESCRIPTION
abruptio placenta	premature detachment of the placenta from the uterine wall resulting in hemorrhage and premature labor and ending in termination of the pregnancy **Note:** Risk to the fetus depends on amount of hemorrhage and fetal age. Maternal risk is minimal if bleeding is controlled.
acquired immunodeficiency syndrome (AIDS)	a disease caused by the human immunodeficiency virus (HIV), which attacks the immune system leaving the patient vulnerable to opportunistic infection (for further discussion of AIDS see Chapter 15, Blood, Immune and Lymphatic Systems)

CONDITION	DESCRIPTION
cephalopelvic disproportion	pelvic outlet is smaller than the size of the fetus; often indicates a reason for cesarean section
Down's syndrome	a condition caused by three chromosomes instead of two in pair 21 **Note:** Symptoms may include heart malformation and mental retardation. Some cases are fatal in infancy, but most persons with this condition live to adulthood.
ectopic pregnancy	implantation of the embryo in a uterine tube rather than in the uterus; the tube is unable to support the embryo, which dies within the first trimester **Note:** In some cases the tube ruptures after implantation, and the bleeding can be life-threatening to the mother.
erythroblastosis fetalis	see anemia, Chapter 15, Blood, Lymphatic, and Immune Systems
hepatitis B	a sexually transmitted disease that affects the liver and can be fatal
hyperemesis gravidarium	excessive and persistent vomiting during pregnancy accompanied by exhaustion and weight loss; may require hospitalization but is not fatal
placenta previa	in **placenta previa**, the placenta, which is normally placed high up on the uterine wall, is attached near the cervix uteri and may tear when the cervix dilates as the head of the fetus pushes against the cervical wall; the result is hemorrhaging and premature labor **Note:** The risk to the fetus depends on the amount of hemorrhage and fetal age. Maternal risk is minimal if bleeding is controlled.
sexually transmitted diseases (STD)	a variety of diseases transmitted by sexual contact; includes syphilis, genital herpes, chlamydia, pelvic inflammatory disease (PID), and gonorrhea **Note:** Syphilis, gonorrhea, chlamydia, and PID can be cured by antibiotics; treatment is available but no cure exists for genital herpes. Chlamydia and PID are inflammations of the female reproductive tract, and PID can result in sterility caused by scar tissue in the uterine tubes.
spontaneous abortion; miscarriage	discharge of the embryo or fetus before it is viable outside the uterus (approximately 50 percent of miscarriages are caused by chromosomal abnormalities)
subinvolution	failure of the uterus to return to its normal size following pregnancy
toxemia; preeclampsia; eclampsia	potentially life-threatening toxemia, involves a group of symptoms, including excessive edema, high blood pressure, and albuminuria, which together make up what is called **preeclampsia** **Note:** If preeclampsia goes untreated, convulsions and coma may result and the condition is then called **eclampsia**.
uterine inertia	loss of or lethargic uterine muscle contractions **Note:** When labor seems to have slowed down or ceased, uterine contractions may be induced using an injection of oxytocin or its synthetic counterpart, Syntocinon, to reestablish uterine contractions.

CLINICAL PROCEDURES RELATED TO OBSTETRICS

DESCRIPTION

amniocentesis — puncture of the amniotic sac through the abdominal wall to withdraw a sample of amniotic fluid; the fluid is examined to diagnose any fetal abnormality, especially genetic, such as Down's syndrome

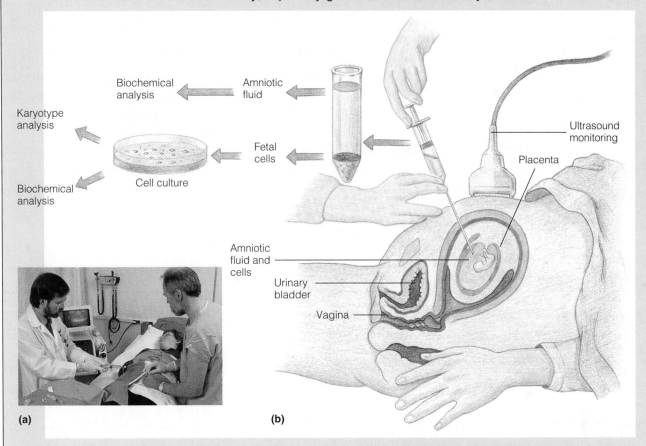

Biochemical analysis ← Amniotic fluid ←

Karyotype analysis ←

Fetal cells ←

Biochemical analysis ← Cell culture

Ultrasound monitoring

Placenta

Amniotic fluid and cells

Urinary bladder

Vagina

(a) (b)

chorionic villus sampling (CVS) — samples of fetal tissue are taken from the chorionic villi (fingerlike projections from the chorion) for the purpose of diagnosing fetal abnormalities

fetoscopy — examination of the fetus using a fetoscope (used to diagnose normal and abnormal fetal development)

Note: The fetoscope is placed through the abdominal wall of the mother and into the amniotic sac. The fetus is visualized and any malformations noted.

forceps delivery — use of an instrument shaped like tongs (forceps) to grasp the fetus by the head and remove it from the birth canal

artificial rupture of membranes (ARM) — the manual rupture of the amniotic sac to assist in delivery of the fetus

ABBREVIATION	MEANING
Ab	abortion
AIDS	acquired immunodeficiency syndrome
ARM	artificial rupture of membranes
CS	cesarian section
CVS	chorionic villus sampling
DNA	deoxyribonucleic acid
EDC	expected date of confinement
G	gravida
hCG	human chorionic gonadotropin

ABBREVIATION	MEANING
HIV	human immunodeficiency virus
IUCD	intrauterine contraceptive device
IUD	intrauterine device
MSAFP	maternal serum alpha-fetoprotein
NFP	natural family planning
P	para
STD	sexually transmitted disease
VDRL	Venereal Disease Research Laboratories (test for syphilis)

◗ EXERCISE 17–1

Definitions

Give the prefix, suffix, or word root for the following.

Answers to the exercises are found in Appendix A.

Give the meaning for the following word parts.

Definitions

1. cervix uteri _____
2. external genitalia _____
3. uterus (3) _____
4. fallopian tube _____
5. ovary (2) _____
6. breast (2) _____

7. gynec/o _____
8. oligo- _____
9. ante- _____
10. colp/o _____
11. culd/o _____
12. galact/o _____
13. thel/o _____
14. para- _____
15. peri- _____
16. lact/o _____
17. labi/o _____

18. DNA _____

19. FSH _____

20. GnRH _____

21. Ab _____

▶**EXERCISE 17–2**

Word Building

Using the suffix -rrhagia, meaning excessive bleeding, build the following medical terms.

Example:
  excessive bleeding from the ovaries   oophorrhagia

Using the suffix -rrhea, meaning flow or discharge, build the following medical terms.

Build the medical words that mean the following.

Word Building

1. excessive uterine bleeding at varying intervals _____

2. excessive uterine bleeding during menstruation _____

3. excessive uterine bleeding during menstruation and at varying intervals _____

4. painful menstruation _____

5. absence of menstruation _____

6. scanty menstruation _____

7. structures beside the uterus _____

8. structure around the uterus _____

9. removal of all the uterus _____

10. prolapsed uterus _____

11. removal of the breast _____

12. incision of the uterus _____

13. pertaining to within the uterus _____

14. suturing of the vagina _____

15. pain in the ovary _____

▶**EXERCISE 17–3**

Short Answer

Briefly answer the following questions.

Practice Quiz

1. What causes female reproductive cycles to cease at menopause? _____

_____

2. What process produces diploid cells? _____

_____

3. What is the composition of haploid cells? _____

_____

4. How is the zona pellucida dissolved? _____

_____

5. Describe the process of cleavage. _____

_____

6. What embryonic membranes form the placenta? _____

_____

7. What are the three stages of labor? _____

_____

8. When does implantation occur? _____

_____

9. Describe a chromosomal pair. _____

_____

10. When does oogenesis begin? _____

_____

11. Describe the difference in the processes that produce identical twins and fraternal twins. _____

_____

12. Name two endocrine organs (or glands) that secrete estrogen. _____

_____

13. How long do sperm live outside the male?

_____

Matching Terms with Meanings

Matching

Match the term in Column A with its meaning in Column B.

Column A

1. haploid cells _____
2. pair 23 _____
3. fertile mucus _____
4. zona pellucida _____
5. allantois _____
6. blastomeres _____
7. semen _____
8. corpus luteum _____
9. blastocyst _____

Column B

A. contains two X chromosomes in the female

B. composed partly of secretions from the prostate gland

C. dissolved by enzymes from sperm

D. first stage of the development of the umbilical cord

E. divides by mitosis

F. cells of the morula

G. primary follicle

H. made up of chromosomes that are not genetically identical

I. develops during cleavage

J. secreted by the cervix to support the life of sperm

▶EXERCISE 17–5

Spelling Practice

Spelling

Place a check mark beside all misspelled words in the list that follows. Correctly spell those that you checked off.

1. deoxyribonucleic acid ☐ _____
2. allele ☐ _____
3. morulla ☐ _____
4. amnion ☐ _____
5. oocite ☐ _____
6. colostrum ☐ _____
7. allantois ☐ _____
8. karyotype ☐ _____
9. zona pellucida ☐ _____

Medical Terms in Context

Define the underlined terms as they are used in context.

UNIVERSITY HOSPITAL ✚   SUMMARY RECORD

HISTORY:

This 33-year-old woman is a <u>gravida IV</u>, <u>para III</u> female who had severe <u>dysmenorrhea</u> and <u>menorrhagia</u>.

PAST HISTORY:

In 1989 she had a <u>tubal ligation</u>. Following this, she noticed significant worsening of her symptoms of dysmenorrhea. <u>Laparoscopy</u> in 1993 diagnosed <u>endometriosis</u>. She had a previous <u>lumpectomy</u> in 1990 for a benign <u>breast cyst</u> and a <u>D&C</u> in 1993 for <u>menometrorrhagia</u>.

COURSE IN HOSPITAL:

<u>Laser laparoscopy</u> was performed on March 29, 1994. Omental adhesions were <u>lysed</u>; some bowel adhesions were lysed. Conservative surgery for endometriosis was performed; however, it was noted that this patient had multiple <u>uterine leiomyomas</u>. The uterus itself was <u>retroverted</u>, <u>retroflexed</u>, somewhat fixed; and it was difficult to get all the endometriosis because the uterus was so large and bulky. It was obstructing to some degree the visibility and access down into the <u>cul-de-sac</u>. It was discussed with the patient postoperatively that the laser would not cure her <u>fibroids</u>.

DISCHARGE DIAGNOSIS: 1. ENDOMETRIOSIS

2. UTERINE LEIOMYOMATA

3. MENORRHAGIA

SIGNATURE OF DOCTOR IN CHARGE _Jan D. Kalsch_____

---

1. gravida IV   _____

2. para III   _____

3. dysmenorrhea   _____

4. menorrhagia   _____

5. tubal ligation   _____

6. laparoscopy   _____

7. endometriosis   _____

8. lumpectomy   _____

9. breast cyst   _____

10. D&C   _____

11. menometrorrhagia   _____

12. laser laparoscopy _____

13. lysed   _____

14. uterine leiomyomas _____

15. retroverted _____

16. retroflexed _____

17. cul-de-sac _____

18. fibroids _____

Central Medical `CM`   **OPERATIVE REPORT**

OPERATIVE REPORT

PREOPERATIVE DIAGNOSIS: MENORRHAGIA

ENDOMETRIAL POLYPS

Following standard preparation, the uterus was found to be
retroverted, mobile and small. No <u>adnexal</u> abnormality. The cervix
was <u>dilated</u> to admit the <u>endoscope</u>.

There were some endometrial polyps in the left cornual region;
otherwise the endometrium was pale, smooth, and symmetrical.
Electrocautery was performed over the entire surface and
particularly in the left cornual region just joining the <u>polypoid</u>
structures. This was brought down to the <u>endocervical</u> canal. Because
of the acute retroversion, some polyps were quite awkward to get to,
but with a struggle this was achieved. The patient tolerated the
procedure well with minimal blood loss.

POSTOPERATIVE DIAGNOSIS: ENDOMETRIAL POLYPS

Authorized Health Care Practitioner _____

---

19. endometrial polyps _____

20. adnexal _____

21. dilated _____

22. endoscope _____

23. polypoid _____

24. endocervical _____

Crossword Puzzle

Female Reproductive System

Across

1 Inflammation of the cervix uteri
3 Production of milk
4 Pertaining to the lips
5 Egg cell
6 Innermost layer of the uterus
12 More than two nipples
14 Pain in an ovary
15 Initial onset of menstruation

Down

1 Surgical reconstruction of the vagina and perineum
2 Ruptured ovary
7 Surgical fixation of fallopian tubes
8 Specialist in the diagnosis and treatment of female genital tract ailments
9 Excessive milk discharge
10 Suturing of the vagina
11 Cessation of menstruation
12 The outermost layer of the uterus
13 Structures adjacent to the uterus

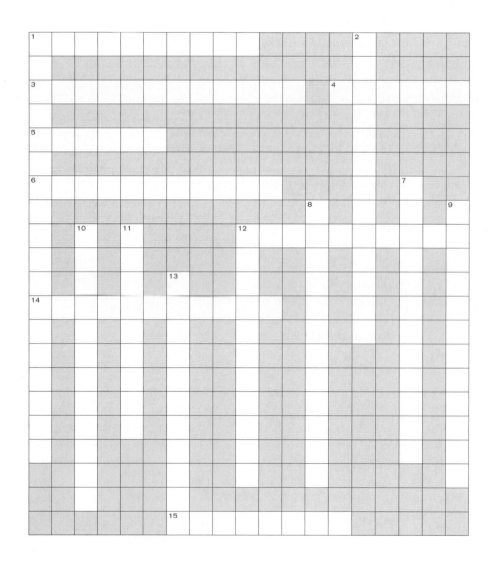

II–17

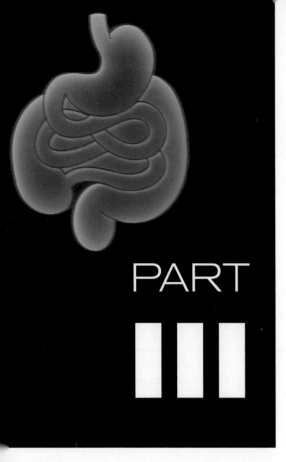

PART

III

MEDICAL

SPECIALTIES

CHAPTER

18 MEDICAL IMAGING

CHAPTER ORGANIZATION

This chapter has been designed to help you learn terms and abbreviations related to medical imaging.

18.1	What Is Imaging?
18.2	X-Ray Technology (Roentgenology)
18.3	Ultrasound

18.4	Nuclear Medicine
18.5	Magnetic Resonance Imaging
18.6	Term Analysis
18.7	Abbreviations

CHAPTER OBJECTIVES

Upon successful completion of this chapter, the student will be able to do the following:

1. Define terms related to x-ray technology.
2. Define terms related to ultrasound technology.
3. Define terms related to nuclear medicine.
4. Define terms and abbreviations applicable to imaging procedures.

WORD ELEMENTS PROMINENT IN THIS CHAPTER

WORD ELEMENT	TYPE	MEANING
-assay	suffix	to evaluate
axi/o	root	axis
-ducer	suffix	to lead
ech/o	root	sound
electr/o	root	electric
fluor/o	root	luminous
-gram	suffix	record
-graphy	suffix	process of recording; x-ray

WORD ELEMENT	TYPE	MEANING
-ide	suffix	binary compound
immun/o	root	safe
-lucent	suffix	to shine
nucle/o	root	nucleus compound
-opaque	suffix	dark
piez/o	root	to press
radi/o; roentgen/o	root	x-ray; electromagnetic radiation

WORD ELEMENT	TYPE	MEANING	WORD ELEMENT	TYPE	MEANING
-scan	suffix	to examine	tom/o	root	to cut; section
scint/i	root	spark	trans-	prefix	across
-scopy	suffix	process of viewing	ultra-	prefix	excess; beyond
son/o	root	sound	xer/o	root	dry

18.1 WHAT IS IMAGING?

Sometimes diagnosticians need to be able to look inside the human body to find out what is going on there. Two separate physical phenomena enable them to do so: electromagnetic wave theory and mechanical wave theory.

Electromagnetic Wave Theory

Electromagnetic radiation includes cosmic rays, nuclear radiation, x-rays, radio and television waves, microwaves, light, heat, and even electric current. We can understand some of the differences between these phenomena by considering their wavelengths. A broadcast radio wave travels in lengths measurable in yards, while an x-ray's wavelength is shorter than that of visible light, measuring approximately one one-hundred-millionth of an inch. This extremely short wavelength gives the x-ray the two characteristics that make it a valuable diagnostic tool: its ability to penetrate the human body and its ability to expose a photographic plate or a xerographic receptor in somewhat the same way that light does.

In 1895, Wilhelm Roentgen discovered x-rays; he called them "x" rays because he knew very little of their character. In the hundred years since Roentgen's discovery, the x-ray has found steadily increasing use as a medical tool. We still often refer to x-ray pictures as Roentgenography.

Nuclear radiation provides us with yet another tool for medical imaging. Since radioactive emissions can be detected accurately, they can be used to track the function of organs and tissues that have been infused with them.

Mechanical Wave Theory

The past decade has seen remarkable developments in ultrasound technology. Sound also travels in waves, but its character is different from that of an electromagnetic wave. That is to say, sound waves cannot travel through space.

A book on medical terminology is no place for a lengthy discussion of this phenomenon. However, a thorough understanding of the terms describing medical imaging systems requires us to acknowledge the essential character of a sound wave: a sound wave only exists inside the medium in which it travels, and the medium determines its wave characteristics.

As previously stated, x-rays can expose a photographic plate. As x-rays enter the human body, the density of the various body parts determines their diffraction rate. Therefore, placing the body part to be x-rayed between an x-ray source and a photographic plate yields a picture determined by the relative densities in that body area. The area of film behind a dense body area remains unexposed and thus shows up white on a negative. Such dense areas are called **radiopaque**. Bone is an example of a radiopaque substance. An x-ray picture of a broken bone would show the area of the break, since x-rays would pass through any separation in dense tissue. Soft tissue, called **radiolucent**, shows up as a dark area on the exposed negative, since it passes x-rays with greater ease than does dense tissue. In other words, x-rays expose the film behind a given body part if the x-rays reach the film's surface. Radiopaque areas, on the other hand, absorb x-rays and leave the film area behind them unexposed.

Photography is not the only method by which x-ray pictures can be made. Images can also be developed through **xerography** and **fluoroscopy**. Photographic and xerographic x-rays provide still pictures, while the fluoroscopic method provides moving pictures displayed on a cathode ray tube. The underlying principle, however, is exactly the same: x-ray penetration of tissue is inversely proportional to the density of the tissue.

X-rays can also show "slices" of the body through a process known as **tomography**. Most of us have heard the term **CT scan**. This is short for computerized axial tomography (CAT), and a CT scan gives a 3-dimensional view of the x-rayed part. The computer calculates body densities from the x-rays. It is coupled to a printer that responds to the calculations of each part of the scan and gives the diagnostician an accurate image of the body area scanned.

Some body parts are roughly the same density, and for this reason, radiologists sometimes order a **contrast medium** to be administered to the patient before x-rays are taken. Contrast media are used mostly to examine body cavities and passages. Specific x-ray procedures for which a contrast medium is required are presented in Table 18-1.

TABLE 18–1

Specific X-Ray Procedures for Which a Contrast Medium is Required

TERM	MEANING
angiography ăn″-jē-ŏg′-ră-fē	x-ray of the blood vessels
aortography ā″-or-tog′-ră-fē	x-ray of the aorta
arthrography ăr-thrŏg′-ră-fē	x-ray of the joints and their soft tissues
bronchography brŏng-kŏg′-ră-fē	x-ray of the bronchi
cholecystography kō″-lē-sĭs-tŏg′-ră-fē	x-ray of the gall bladder
cholangiography kō-lăn″-jē-ŏg′-ră-fē	x-ray of the biliary ducts
cholangiopancreatography kō-lăn″-jē-ō-pan″-krē-ă-tŏg′-ră-fē	x-ray of the biliary and pancreatic ducts

TERM	MEANING
hysterosalpingography his″-tĕr-ō-săl″-pĭn-gŏg′-ră-fē	x-ray of the uterus and fallopian tubes
upper gastrointestinal (GI) series găs-trō-ĭn-tĕs′-tĭ-năl	x-ray of the upper digestive tract, including the esophagus, stomach, and duodenum
lower gastrointestinal series	x-ray of the lower digestive tract, including the small and large intestines
excretory urography ĕks′-krĕ-tō-rē ū-rŏg′-ră-fē also called intravenous urography (IVU) and intravenous pyelography (IVP)	x-ray of the urinary system (contrast medium injected into a vein)
retrograde urography rĕt′-rō-grād ū-rŏg′-ră-fē	x-ray of the urinary system (contrast medium injected into the ureters)
voiding cystourethrography sĭs-tō-ū-rē-thrŏg′-ră-fē	x-ray of bladder and urethra during micturition
myelography mī-ĕ-lŏg′-rŭ-fē	x-ray of the spinal cord and its nerve roots
percutaneous transhepatic cholangiography (PTC) pĕr″-kū-tā′-nē-ŭs trăns-hĕ-păt′-ĭk kō-lăn″-jē-ŏg′-ră-fē	x-ray of the biliary ducts (contrast medium injected through the skin)
endoscopic retrograde cholangiopancreatography (ERCP) ĕn-dō-skŏp′-ĭk rĕt′-rō-grād kō-lăn″-jē-ō-păn-krē-ă-tŏg′-ră-fē	x-ray of the biliary and pancreatic ducts (contrast medium injected through the hepatopancreatic ampulla into the biliary ducts)

III–18

Fluoroscopy Fluoroscopy permits the observer to see a moving image. The image, which appears on a cathode ray tube, can be recorded either with or without the motion. Still pictures are recorded on what is called **spot film,** and motion pictures can be recorded in either videotape or on motion picture film. This latter process is called **cinefluorography.**

Digital Radiography The computer has made possible a new radiographic technique called digital radiography. Digitally stored information has several definite advantages over conventionally recorded analogue data. When information is stored as a series of numerical values, it can be enhanced by a computer. Furthermore, such information is devoid of all "noise." Just as the digitally recorded sound on a compact disk is noise-free, so are the images that digital radiography produces.

Diagnostic X-Rays for Specific Body Systems

Gastrointestinal System   Several radiographic procedures are routinely performed on the digestive system. The upper gastrointestinal tract includes the pharynx, esophagus, stomach, and duodenum. Several procedures may be performed: the esophagogram, upper GI series, small bowel series (SBS), and a small bowel follow-through (SBFT). The esophagogram is an x-ray of the pharynx and esophagus, and the upper GI series includes the distal esophagus, the stomach, and the proximal duodenum. The **small bowel series (SBS)** includes an examination of the duodenum, jejunum, and ileum. A combination of the upper GI series and small bowel series is referred to as a **small bowel follow-through (SBFT)**. The contrast medium used in these examinations is usually barium sulfate. Abnormalities that would be revealed in an upper GI series would be **reflux, ulcer craters, filling defects, foreign bodies,** and **varices.** (See table of definitions following the general discussion of body systems in this chapter.)

A lower GI examination also comprises several procedures. An x-ray examination of the large bowel is referred to as a **barium enema (BE)** or **lower GI series.** As in the upper GI series, filling defects and foreign bodies may be revealed in the examination.

Gallbladder and Biliary Ducts   As noted in an earlier chapter, the term **cholecystography** refers to an x-ray examination of the gallbladder. Since the contrast medium employed, **telepaque,** is administered orally, the procedure is also sometimes called an **oral cholecystogram (OCG).** The medium is absorbed into the blood stream, taken up by the liver, excreted into the bile, and concentrated into the gallbladder. In recent years, diagnosticians have come to rely more on ultrasound examination than on the oral cholecystogram.

The term **cholangiography** describes an x-ray of the biliary ducts, which include the hepatic, cystic, and common bile ducts. The three types of cholangiograms are the **operative, T-tube,** and **intravenous (IVC).** The first two are the most common, the first as a precautionary measure during surgery, and the second as a post-operative procedure.

Urinary System   An x-ray examination of the entire urinary system is called an **intravenous pyelogram (IVP)** or an **excretory urogram (IVU).** A contrast medium, injected into a vein and quickly picked up by the kidney, flows through the remaining urinary structures.

Antegrade urography is an x-ray of the urinary system following injection of a contrast medium through the skin into the renal pelvis. **Retrograde urography,** considered a surgical procedure, requires the contrast medium to be inserted through catheters into the ureter. It is done as a follow-up to the IVU when it is considered necessary.

Table 18–2 gives the general patient positions for x-rays.

TABLE 18–2

Patient Positions for
X-Rays

POSITION	DESCRIPTION
erect	standing or sitting in a upright position
prone	lying on the stomach
recumbent	lying on the back or sitting up in bed
supine	lying on the back
flexion	decrease of the angle at a joint (flexed position)
extension	return from flexion (unflexed position)
hyperextension	extension beyond the normal position
eversion	turning the ankle so that the sole of the foot faces outward (can be applied to other body joints as well)
inversion	turning the ankle so that the sole of the foot faces inward (can be applied to other body joints as well)
abduction	movement of a part away from the body
adduction	movement of a part toward the body
supination	turning a part upward

18.3 ULTRASOUND

Ultrasound refers to sound waves above the spectrum of human hearing, roughly those frequencies above 20 kHz or, more accurately, 20 cycles per second (as stated earlier, sound waves are mechanical, not electromagnetic). Since common practice permits labeling both classes of waves as Herzian, the practice in this book is to use Hz and kHz as the unit of measure for sound frequency.

Ultrasonography is a noninvasive technique. A **transducer**, a device that can convert one form of energy to another, is placed over the part of the body to be examined.

The energy forms transduced in ultrasonography are electrical impulses and sound waves. The transducer converts electrical impulses to sound waves, which then penetrate the organs being examined. The transducer senses the echoes from these organs and changes them back into electrical impulses, which are then processed to produce an image on a cathode ray tube.

Ultrasonographic transducers operate on the principle of **piezoelectricity**. This term refers to the properties of certain materials that flex when an electric current is applied to them (and conversely, generate an electric current when they are acted upon by a mechanical force such as a sound wave). Some of these materials, made of special ceramics, are **piezoceramic** materials, which are used in transducer design.

Doppler ultrasound is a special kind of ultrasound imaging. The Doppler Effect, named for its discoverer, Christian Johann Doppler, permits imaging that gives even more information than does conventional ultrasound. The Doppler Effect is an interesting physical phenomenon that almost everyone has experienced. Have you ever stood near a railroad crossing and listened while the engineer blew the horn as the train approaches? The sound from the horn lowers in pitch as the train passes. The Doppler Effect accounts for this change in pitch.

To understand why the pitch changes, let us imagine that the train's horn is blowing at 440 Hz, a perfect A above middle C. If we are standing still and the train is standing still, we will hear a 440 Hz sound wave, an A above middle C. If the train is moving toward us at 60 mph (approximately one-twelfth the speed of sound), one-twelfth of the 440 Hz sound (35 Hz) will be added to the frequency of the sound wave, and we hear a signal of 475 Hz (a note about halfway between a B-flat and a B). When the train passes and begins to travel away from us, we will hear 405 Hz (a note between G and A-flat) (see Figure 18–1).

FIGURE 18–1

The Doppler Effect

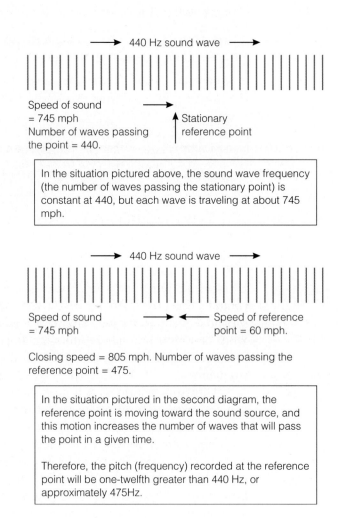

One can easily see that the Doppler Effect can be used in finding out flow rates and other relative motions. It is also the principle that allows the police to catch speeders in radar traps (the Doppler Effect is also observable in the electromagnetic spectrum).

Basic Concepts

Nuclear Medicine is a specialty which uses extremely small amounts of **radioactive substances** for diagnostic and therapeutic purposes. Before going on to study how these diagnoses and therapies are carried out, you must learn something about radioactivity itself. Most of us are familiar with the concept of materials being made up of atoms or elements. The elements, which have distinct chemical properties and physical characteristics, have been organized in a logical sequence in the **Periodic Table**. The Periodic Table identifies the more than 100 known elements and assigns each one a position based upon the number of **protons** found in its **nucleus**. Furthermore, the number of protons in the nucleus is equal to the total number of electrons contained within each atom. Electrons are organized around the nucleus in concentric shells or levels that are able to contain specific numbers of electrons. Once the closest level to the nucleus is filled, then the next level further away from the nucleus starts to fill. This arrangement continues until all the electrons an atom has are located in one of the shells. The chemical properties of an element are determined by the number of electrons occupying its outermost electron shell, the **valence shell**. The electrons in this outer shell are called valence electrons.

The nucleus of an atom contains not only protons, which are positively charged, but also **neutrons**, which are uncharged particles about the same size as protons. In a nonionized atom, the number of protons equals the number of electrons, a characteristic that keeps the atom electrically neutral. Since neutrons have no charge, their presence does not electrically affect the electrons, and thus they do not influence the chemical behavior of the atom. However, for any given element, different nuclear arrangements are possible. With its three forms, hydrogen is the simplest example.

In its most common form, hydrogen has one proton in its nucleus; however, a small amount of the hydrogen found in our immediate environment has a neutron and a proton. In this form, hydrogen is called deuterium or simply hydrogen-2. A still smaller portion of our immediate world's total hydrogen has two neutrons and a proton in its nucleus. This form is known as tritium or hydrogen-3. Each of the three forms of hydrogen has a single electron to balance the charge of its single proton. However, the masses of these hydrogen forms vary by nearly 300% because of the neutrons. Since all forms of hydrogen have only one electron, the differences in their chemical and physical properties are only those that relate to mass.

To specifically identify each of the possible versions of an element (**nuclides**), scientists use both the element name and the total number of neutrons and protons making up its nucleus (mass number). Thus, hydrogen is hydrogen-1, deuterium is hydrogen-2, and tritium is hydrogen-3. These forms of hydrogen may also be referred to as ^{1}H, ^{2}H, and ^{3}H.

Often the ratio of neutrons to protons is too great or too small and the nucleus becomes unstable and tends to rearrange itself so that stability returns. Unstable nuclei may achieve a more favorable neutron-to-proton ratio by emitting energetic particles such as beta and alpha particles, along with electromagnetic radiation in the form of gamma radiation (also called gamma photons or rays). This spontaneous emission of energy from the nucleus is called **radioactivity**.

The diagnostician can use radioactive substances because radioactive emissions can be accurately detected and displayed in the form of planar or tomographic clinical images. The time needed for one half of a sample of any specific radioactive substance to emit its excess energy is known as its half-life, which may range from seconds to thousands of years. This information, along with the energy and type of emission(s) for each radioisotope, is clearly laid out in a special chart called the **Trilinear Chart.**

Nuclear Concepts Used in Medicine

Diagnostic Uses Our bodies are made up of cells in which chemical processes of one form or another constantly occur. Whenever we suffer from injury or disease, the affected part of our body cannot properly carry out its chemical functions. In such instances, the diagnostician can introduce a radioactively labeled chemical called a **radiopharmaceutical** into the affected area, where it will take part in certain of these chemical activities. By detecting the gamma emissions from the radiopharmaceutical employed, we are able to produce useful information about the function and health of the organs that we are studying.

While most of the studies done in clinical nuclear medicine require the radiopharmaceutical to be injected into a vein (normally in the antecubital region), they may on occasion be inhaled, ingested, or injected through a catheter or other implanted device. Once the radiopharmaceutical has been administered to the patient, it travels through the body as though it were normally present. Since our bodies cannot distinguish a radiopharmaceutical from a normally present chemical, it handles it in the same way as it would a nonradioactive chemical. The only difference and advantage offered by the radiopharmaceutical is that the administered chemical can be detected externally.

A scintillation camera, which is able to map the distribution of the radiopharmaceutical within the patient's body, provides the images. These images, called **scintigraphs** or **scintiscans**, are produced when the gamma rays spontaneously emitted from the radiopharmaceutical escape from the patient's body. Each scintiscan is made up of hundreds of thousands of individual gamma ray interactions with the camera, and these many interactions are displayed as individual dots of light which are added together to form a single image.

Typically, images are recorded every 2 seconds immediately following the injection of the radiopharmaceutical. These initial images provide information on the arterial supply, capillary transit, and venous drainage of the organ or tissue of interest. After a period of time sufficient to permit the tissues to extract the radiopharmaceutical from the circulation, more images are recorded. These first images are called **dynamic images,** and the latter ones are called **statics** or **delayed images.**

The radiopharmaceutical used in the study of a particular organ must be chosen for its ability to accumulate in that particular organ. The choice also depends on the isolation of a chemical pathway or function that is peculiar to the organ that is to be imaged. For the most part, the **label** (the radioactive part of the pharmaceutical) used as a tag within the pharmaceutical doesn't affect its localization, and so materials are often labeled with **gamma emitters** that have the best combination of availability, energy, and half-life. A radionuclide called **technetium-99m** is frequently used because it can be produced onsite from a system called a **generator.**

The process of generation of Technetium-99m is a simple one: molybdenum-99 (^{99}Mo) decays to form Technetium-99m. Since technetium-99m is chemically different from molybdenum, it is easy to separate the two. A small amount of molybdenum can produce enough technetium each day to meet the needs of a typical nuclear medicine department. Also, technetium-99m emits gamma radiation at an acceptable energy level of 140 KeV. Although this level is higher than most X-rays, human tissue can tolerate it since gamma rays escape the body while x-rays tend to irradiate body tissues. The final reason for the popularity of this radionuclide is that it has a 6-hour half-life—long enough to allow the radiopharmaceuticals to accumulate in the tissues of interest and short enough to permit repeat studies within a day or so. The combination of the low energy (by gamma ray standards) and short half-life also gives the patient an acceptably low radiation dose.

The radioactivity principle can also be used to detect and measure substances in blood or urine, substances that may be present in such small concentrations that conventional methods cannot detect them. This technique, termed **radioimmunoassay (RIA)**, involves the production of antibodies specific to the substance being measured, the isolation of a pure extract of this substance (termed the antigen), and the radioactive labeling of the antigen. By mixing known amounts of these substances with the patient sample and allowing the whole to come to equilibrium in a test tube, one can separate the unreacted antigen (both from the patient and the labeled antigen) from that which has bound to the antibody provided for that purpose. The ratio of free-to-bound antigens permits a calculation of the amount of material present in the patient's original sample. Tests performed on blood or urine samples requiring that the radioactive chemical be added to the sample but not the patient are termed **in vitro** tests. Those procedures requiring a radioactive chemical to be administered to the patient are called **in vivo** tests. In vitro techniques are commonly used to measure various hormone levels, drug levels, and concentrations of other compounds of medical interest.

Some of the more common studies are described briefly in the following paragraphs.

Regular Brain Scan   Following the intravenous injection of technetium-99m-labeled glucoheptonate (a sugarlike material), a series of dynamic images is obtained that demonstrates the arterial blood supply to the brain, its capillary communications with the venous structures, and the venous drainage. Typically, these images are obtained in an anterior projection (i.e., the face is against the camera). After 1 to 2 hours, static images are taken of the front, back, and both sides of the head. In a healthy person, the material injected does not enter the brain tissue itself, but remains in the large vessels, venous sinuses, and areas that have profuse blood supplies (such as facial muscles). The reason for the exclusion of the glucoheptonate from the normal brain tissue is that the blood-brain-barrier (BBB) does not permit the radiopharmaceutical to enter the brain parenchyma. Disease, injury, and other pathologies cause the BBB to fail, and the glucoheptonate can enter the damaged tissues, thereby creating an abnormal region of uptake of the radiopharmaceutical on the image (see Figure 18–2).

FIGURE 18–2

Single Photon Emission
Computed Tomography
of the Brain

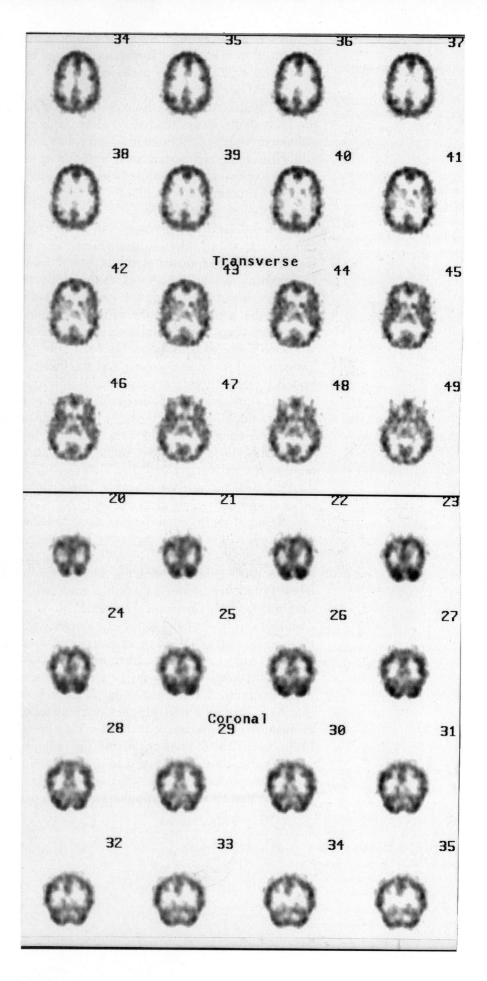

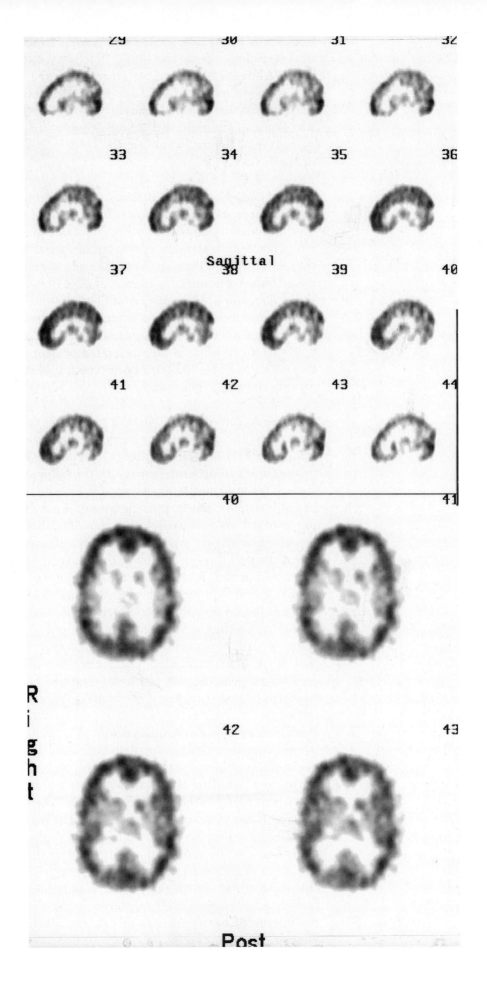

Functional Brain Scan Unlike a regular study in which the radiopharmaceutical is excluded from the brain, functional studies use materials that are metabolized by the brain and therefore cross the BBB. Images obtained from these radiopharmaceuticals reflect the regional metabolism of the brain at the time the material was injected (the images are like "snap-shots" of what the brain was doing at the time the radiopharmaceutical arrived). Functional brain imaging is used for studying mental disorders, epilepsy, and degenerative diseases of the brain.

Thyroid Studies Thyroid studies were among some of the earliest done in nuclear medicine. In vitro procedures are used extensively in the assessment of thyroid function, as well as other endocrine glandular investigations. Two different but complementary in vivo studies are also often ordered on patients with thyroid disorders: the thyroid uptake and the thyroid scan. The thyroid uptake measures the amount of a given oral dose of radioactive iodine that the thyroid accumulates in a 24-hour period. The thyroid scan is obtainable through the use of a number of different isotopes of iodine, or by using Technetium-99m. The images obtained are useful because they show which parts of the gland might be functioning at an accelerated or depressed rate. Treatment of thyroid disease is far more likely to be successful when the physician can specifically identify the abnormal tissue.

Cardiac Applications Nuclear techniques can reveal two major types of information crucial in the treatment of heart patients. By injecting a labeled substance that stays in the circulatory system, one can make images of the heart as it beats and can accurately measure the volumes of blood moved by each ventricle. This information is obtained by means of a computer linked to an electrocardiograph connected to the patient during the imaging. The computer output is based on a comparison of the data obtained to specified mathematical models. The second type of information that nuclear medicine can provide is the identity of those portions of the heart (if any) that are ischemic and those that are infarcted. A return to a normal blood supply will not repair an infarcted muscle, but it will greatly benefit ischemic tissue. A material called Thallium-201 has the unique ability to enter viable heart muscle (myocardium) in proportion to the blood flow to the region, and to then redistribute if that supply changes (such as occurs during strenuous exercise). By imaging a patient at rest and again after marked physical exertion, one can determine which heart regions are ischemic and which are infarcted. This test identifies those patients who will benefit from coronary by-pass surgery.

Respiratory System Applications Nuclear medicine can provide studies to demonstrate the distribution of air within the lungs (ventilation studies) and the distribution of blood around the alveoli (perfusion studies). Since the lungs do not supply blood to alveoli that are not normally supplied with air, it is important to perform the ventilation and the perfusion studies together. This approach shows whether perfusion is caused by chronic lung disease or whether a lack of blood supply is caused by vascular obstruction (pulmonary embolism, for example). The ventilation study requires that the patient breath in a radioactive gas or a labeled aerosol. Both are supplied through a closed system that delivers the material to the patient through a mask. In perfusion studies, extremely small radioactively labeled particles that are too large to pass through the microscopic arterioles supplying the alveoli are injected. These particles lodge in the arterioles and produce an image representing their distribution in the lungs (see Figure 18–3).

FIGURE 18–3 Perfusion Lung Scan

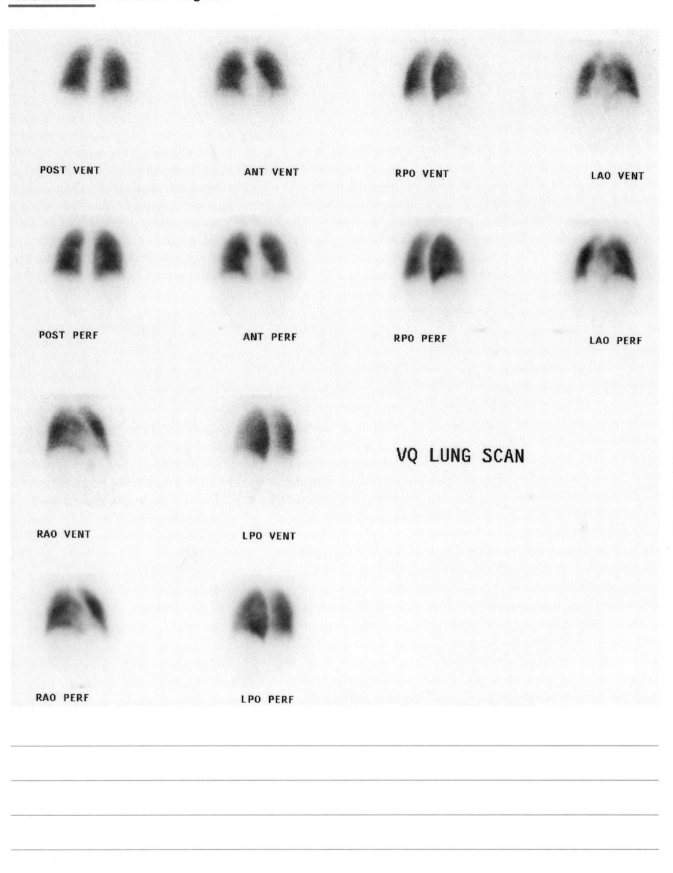

Gastrointestinal Tract   Applications of nuclear medicine to the GI system include imaging of the liver and spleen, finding bleeding sites in the bowels, studying the gallbladder and its ability to empty appropriately, and assessing the function of the stomach and esophagus. While many other modalities (ultrasound, MRI, and radiology) offer tests for many of these same structures, nuclear medicine offers an advantage: the tests do not alter the normal function of the structures and tissues being studied. In fact, if a one-phrase description of nuclear medicine were given, it might be, "a technique of assessing bodily functions." Many of the procedures performed on the gastrointestinal system give quantitative information, as well as images. The emptying rates for liquids and solids from the stomach can be determined, the percentage of the bile contained in the gallbladder ejected during a contraction of the gallbladder can be calculated, and the presence and degree of gastroesophageal reflux can be measured. This system is also one in which in vivo nonimaging studies are prominent; that is, the radioactive material is administered to the patient, but no image is obtained. These studies typically assess the ability of the gastrointestinal tract to absorb specific substances, such as Vitamin B_{12}.

Skeletal System   The skeletal system may seem an odd area for nuclear medicine's investigations, since x-rays can quite easily give us images of bones. However, bony tissue is very metabolically active, and radiographs represent only density maps and not metabolic images. While the scintigraphs produced by nuclear medicine lack the fine anatomic detail of an x-ray, they provide a very sensitive picture of the rate of regional remodeling going on in the skeleton. By using a radiopharmaceutical that is taken up by bone in proportion to regional blood flow and metabolic activity (i.e., in proportion to how actively the bone is functioning), nuclear medicine can detect, localize, and follow bony injury, pathology, and repair, often before any radiographic changes are apparent. Bone scans are also useful in detecting the spread of a number of primary tumors that tend to metastasize to bone and in distinguishing between osteomyelitis and cellulitis (see Figure 18–4).

FIGURE 18–4

Typical Normal Whole Body Scan

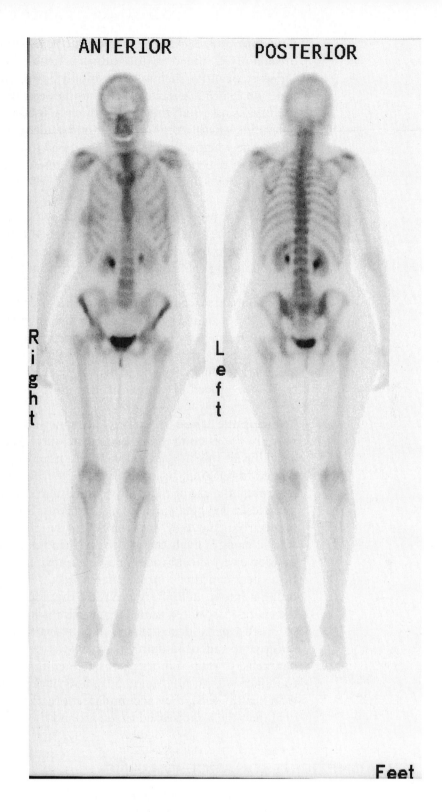

ANTERIOR   POSTERIOR

Right   Left

Feet

Genitourinary System   Nuclear medicine studies of the genitourinary system are mainly confined to the kidneys. Renal studies help assess masses in the kidneys, quantify their relative blood flows, and measure individual rates of function. Since nuclear medicine studies can be repeated without jeopardizing the organs assessed, they are frequently used to study transplanted kidneys to determine whether they are functioning adequately. If they are not, the tests can determine whether the problem is related to infection, mechanical obstruction, leakage, or rejection. These distinctions are valuable because each of these problems requires a different treatment.

Tumor and Infection   These two broad categories account for a large percentage of the studies done in nuclear medicine. A number of different radioisotopes have found specific niches in locating particular types of tumors and in pinpointing the sites of persistent infection. Many of these studies require that the patient be imaged as long as 96 hours following the administration of the radiopharmaceutical, since the rate at which the material accumulates in the tumor or in an infected site, combined with the small size of many of these lesions, means that we must wait longer for the radiopharmaceutical to concentrate adequately in the lesion. Notwithstanding the lengthy wait for the diagnosis, the sensitivity and ability of the scan to accurately locate the pathology makes the procedure well worth the effort.

Therapeutic Uses   Nuclear medicine has some therapeutic uses, although they are not as common as diagnostic ones. Although these techniques do play a significant role in the treatment of a number of diseases, they are not directly related to imaging. In most cases the mechanism by which therapy is possible is through the use of radioactive labels that decay by emitting energetic charged particles called beta particles or negatrons. Beta particles are equivalent in mass to electrons, but they are emitted by the nucleus with substantial amounts of kinetic energy. Even though these particles have a good deal of momentum, they have very short ranges in tissue (under 1 centimeter in most circumstances). If the beta-emitting source is delivered to a target tissue or organ by incorporating it into a radiopharmaceutical that localizes in the organ of interest, then the energy associated with the particles is lost within the target tissue. Having so much energy deposited in such a short distance often kills cells that are sensitive to radiation damage, or at least prevents them from dividing to form new cells. Certain tumors can be treated this way since they are more sensitive to radiation than nontumor cells, and since they are metabolically more active than healthy cells, they accumulate more of the administered radiopharmaceutical than the nondiseased tissue around the tumor.

▷ 18.5 MAGNETIC RESONANCE IMAGING

Magnetic Resonance Imaging (MRI) is also called **nuclear magnetic resonance (NMR)**. This technique relies on a strong magnetic field into which the patient is placed. A 3-dimensional record can be made of the area imaged through computer calculation of the responses of the body area's ion make-up.

All body tissues contain hydrogen atoms. When a patient is placed in a strong magnetic field, the hydrogen atoms in the tissues become aligned. In MRI techniques, this alignment is momentarily interrupted by an electromagnetic wave. When the electromagnetic wave is turned off, the hydrogen atoms return to their aligned state at a rate of speed that depends on the kind of body tissue in which they reside. The generated data is processed by a computer, which calculates the differences in realignment rates, thereby providing an image of the body area investigated.

▷ 18.6 TERM ANALYSIS

TERM WITH PRONUNCIATION	ANALYSIS	DEFINITION
angiocardiography ăn″-jē-ō-kăr-dēŏg′-ră-fē	-graphy = process of recording angi/o = vessel cardi/o = heart	x-ray examination of the heart and blood vessels
anteroposterior (AP) ăn-″tĕr-ō-pŏs-tē′-rē-or	-ior = pertaining to anter/o = anterior poster/o = posterior	the front-to-back direction an x-ray takes through a body (from anterior to posterior)
axial ăk′-sē-ăl	-al = pertaining to axi/o = axis	adjective meaning "around an axis"
bronchography brŏng-kŏg′-ră-fē	-graphy = process of recording bronch/i/o = bronchus	x-ray examination of the bronchi
cholecystography kō″-lē-sĭs-tŏg′-ră-fē	-graphy = process of recording chol/o = bile cyst/o = gall bladder	x-ray examination of the gall bladder
echogenic ĕk″-ō-jĕn′-ĭk	-genic = pertaining to producing ech/o = sound	refers to the body structures that reflect sound
echogram ĕk′-ō-grăm	-gram = record ech/o = sound	the image produced by ultrasound imaging
electrocardiograph ē-lĕk″-trō-kăr′-dē-ō-grăf	-graph = to write electr/o =	instrument used to record the electrical activity of the heart
electroencephalograph ē-lĕk″-trō-ĕn-sĕf′-ă-lō-grăf	-graph = to write en- = in electr/o = cephal/o = skull	instrument used to record the electrical activity of the brain
fluoroscopy floo-or-ŏs′-kō-pē	-scopy = process of viewing fluor/o = luminous	examination by means of a fluoroscope
generator		in nuclear medicine, a device for obtaining a radionuclide produced by another radionuclide as it decays radioactively
in vitro ĭn vē′-trō	in- = in; into vitr/o = glass	in a test tube or other artificial environment
in vivo ĭn vē′-vō	in- = in; into viv/o = life	in a living body
lymphangiography lĭmf″-ăn-jē-ŏg′-ră-fē	-graphy = process of recording lymph/o = angi/o = vessel	x-ray examination of the lymph vessels
myelography mī-ĕ-lŏg′-ră-fē	-graphy = process of recording myel/o = spinal cord or marrow	x-ray of the spinal cord

TERM WITH PRONUNCIATION	ANALYSIS	DEFINITION
nuclide nū′-klīd	-ide = binary compound nucle/o = nucleus	a species of an element characterized by the quantum state of its atom's nucleus
piezoelectric pī-ē″-zō-ē-lĕk′-trĭk	-ic = pretaining to piezo- = to press electr/o = electric	an adjective describing the characteristics of some crystalline materials, viz., the induction of an electric current as a result of the flexing of the material or the induction of a mechanical movement in the material as a result of the application of an electric current
posteroanterior pŏs″-ter-ō-ăn-tēr′-ē-or	-ior = pertaining to poster/o = posterior anter/o = anterior	the back-to-front direction an x-ray takes through a body (from posterior to anterior)
pyelography pī″-ĕ-lŏg′-ră-fē	-graphy = process of recording pyel/o = renal pelvis	x-ray examination of the kidney and ureter
radiogram rā′-dē-ō-grăm	-gram = record radi/o = x-ray; electromagnetic radiation	a record of an image produced on an x-ray film
radiography rā-dē-og′-ră-fē	-graphy = process of recording radi/o = x-ray; electromagnetic radiation	process of recording x-rays
radioimmunoassay (RIA) rā″-dē-ō-ĭm″-ū-nō-ăs′-ā	-assay = to evaluate radi/o = x-ray; electromagnetic radiation immun/o = safe	measurement of antigen-antibody interaction using a radiopharmaceutical
radioisotope rā″-dē-ō-ī′-sō-tōp	-tope = place radi/o = x-ray; electromagnetic radiation is/o = equal	a form of a radioactive element having an atomic weight different from that of the element itself
radiology rā-dē-ŏl′-ō-jē	-logy = study of radi/o = x-ray; electromagnetic radiation	the use of electromagnetic radiation in diagnosis and treatment
radionuclide rā″-dē-ō-nū′-klīd	-ide = binary compound radi/o = x-rays; electromagnetic radiation nucle/o = nucleus	an element that emits radioactivity
radiopaque rā-dē-ō-pāk′	-opaque = dark radi/o = x-ray; electromagnetic radiation	capable of blocking x-rays
radiopharmaceutical rā″-dē-ō-farm″-ă-sū′-tĭ-kăl	-al = pertaining to radi/o = x-ray; electromagnetic radiation pharmac/o = drug	a chemical carrying a radioactive substance used in nuclear medical diagnostic studies
roentgenology rĕnt″-jĕn-ŏl′-ō-jē	-logy = study of roentgen/o = x-rays	an alternate term for x-ray technology; refers to discoverer of x-rays, Wilhelm Roentgen
salpingography săl″-pĭn-gŏg′-ră-fē	-graphy = process of recording salpingl/o = tube	x-ray of the fallopian tubes
scintiscan sĭn′-tĭ-skăn	-scan = to examine scint/i = to spark	an image created by gamma radiation, showing its location and concentration within a given body area
sonogram sō′-nō-grăm	-gram = record son/o = sound	echogram

TERM WITH PRONUNCIATION	ANALYSIS	DEFINITION
sonolucent sō″-nō-loo′-sĕnt	-lucent = to shine son/o = sound	permitting the pasage of ultrasound
tomography tō-mŏg′-ră-fē	-graphy = process of recording tom/o = to cut; section	a method of x-ray examination in which the x-ray device is moved to "see" sections of the body
transducer trăns-dū′-sĕr	-ducer = to lead trans- = across	a device for converting energy from one form to another
Trilinear Chart trī-lĭn′-ē-ăr	-ar = pertaining to tri- = three line/o = line	a chart specifying the half-life, energy potential, and emission type of nuclides
ultrasonography ŭl-tră-sŏn-ŏg′-ră-fē	-graphy = process of recording ultra- = excess; beyond son/o = sound	imaging using sound waves above 20 Hz
xeromammography zē″-rō-măm-ŏg′-ră-fē	-graphy = process of recording xer/o = dry mamm/o = breast	xeroradiography of the breast
xeroradiography zē″-rō-rā″-dē-ŏg′-ră-fē	-graphy = process of recording xer/o = dry radi/o = x-ray; electromagnetic radiation	a dry process of obtaining x-ray images

◗ 18.7 ABBREVIATIONS

ABBREVIATION	MEANING
99Mo	molybdenum-99
99m Tc	technetium-99m
ant	anterior
AP	anteroposterior
Ba	barium
BE	barium enema
CAT	computed axial tomography
CCT	cranial computed tomography
CT	computed tomography
CXR	chest x-ray
decub	lying down
DSR	dynamic spatial reconstructor
ECRP	endoscopic retrograde cholangiopancreatography
FP	flat plate

ABBREVIATION	MEANING
IVP	intravenous pyelogram
IVU	intravenous urogram
keV	kilo electron volt
KUB	kidney, ureter, bladder
MRI	magnetic resonance imaging
NMR	nuclear magnetic resonance
PA	posteroanterior
PET scan	Positron emission tomography
PTC	percutaneous transhepatic cholangiography
RAI	radioactive iodine
RIA	radioimmunoassay
Tc	technetium
up	patient upright

III—18

Matching Terms with Meanings

Column A		Column B
1. angiography	____	A. x-ray of the blood vessels
2. aortography	____	B. x-ray of the aorta
3. arthography	____	C. x-ray of the joints and their soft tissues
4. cholecystography	____	D. x-ray of the gall bladder
5. cholangiography	____	E. x-ray of the biliary ducts
6. cholangiopancreatography	____	F. x-ray of the biliary and pancreatic ducts
7. bronchography	____	G. x-ray of the bronchi
8. hysterosalpingography	____	H. x-ray of the uterus and fallopian tubes
9. upper GI series	____	I. x-ray of the upper gastrointestinal tract, including the esophagus, stomach, and duodenum
10. lower GI series	____	J. x-ray of the lower digestive tract, including the small and large intestines
11. intravenous urography (IVU)	____	K. x-ray of the urinary system (contrast medium injected into a vein)
12. retrograde urography	____	L. x-ray of the urinary system (contrast medium injected into the ureters)
13. voiding cystourethrography	____	M. x-ray of the bladder and urethra during micturition
14. myelography	____	N. x-ray of the spinal cord and its nerve roots
15. percutaneous transhepatic cholangiography (PTC)	____	O. x-ray of the biliary ducts (contrast medium injected through the skin)
16. endoscopic retrograde cholangiopancreatography (ERCP)	____	P. x-ray of the biliary and pancreatic ducts (contrast medium injected through the hepatopancreatic ampulla into the biliary ducts)

Defining Terms

Give meanings for the
following terms.

1. abduction _____

2. supination _____

3. radiology _____

4. radiopaque _____

5. CAT scan _____

6. pyelography _____

7. myelography _____

8. fluoroscopy _____

9. Doppler Effect _____

10. transducer _____

11. radionuclide _____

12. axial _____

13. echogenic _____

14. anteroposterior _____

15. posteroanterior _____

16. roentgenology _____

17. xerocardiography _____

18. lymphangiography _____

19. piezoelectric _____

20. ant _____

21. AP _____

22. decub _____

23. CAT _____

24. CCT _____

25. BE _____

26. CT _____

27. IVP _____

28. IVU _____

29. DSR _____

30. CXR _____

31. FP _____

32. ECRP _____

Building Terms

Give medical terms for the
following phenomena,
processes, or procedures

1. x-ray examination of the bronchi _____

2. x-ray of the spinal cord _____

3. xeroradiography of the breast _____

4. x-ray examination of the kidney
   and ureter _____

5. x-ray of the uterine tubes _____

6. x-ray examination of the lymph
   vessels _____

7. x-ray of the heart and blood vessels _____

Spelling

Place a check mark beside
any misspelled word in the
following list. Correctly spell
those you checked off.

1. radology ☐ _____

2. salpinography ☐ _____

3. pyelography ☐ _____

4. lymphangography ☐ _____

5. flouroscopy ☐ _____

6. tranducer ☐ _____

7. radiosotope ☐ _____

8. radionuclide ☐ _____

9. mylogram ☐ _____

10. echoegenic ☐ _____

Crossword Puzzle

Terms Related to Imaging

Across

2 Around an axis
3 An element that emits radioactivity
4 The adjective describing a characteristic of some crystalline materials
6 An adjective describing body surfaces that reflect sound
8 X-Ray of the bronchi
10 Back-to-front
11 The opposite of radiolucent
12 X-Ray of the aorta
13 X-Ray of joints and associated soft tissues
14 X-Ray of the spinal cord and its nerve roots

Down

1 Front-to-back
2 X-Ray of the blood vessels of the heart
5 A device for converting energy from one form to another
7 Sonogram
9 X-Ray Technology

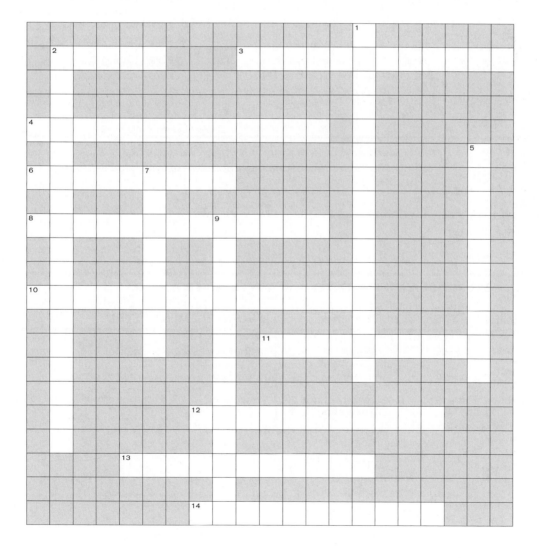

19 TERMS USED IN PSYCHIATRY

CHAPTER ORGANIZATION

This chapter has been designed to help you learn terms and abbreviations related to psychiatry.

CHAPTER OBJECTIVES

Upon successful completion of this chapter, the student will be able to do the following:

1. Differentiate between the various mental and emotional disorder categories.
2. Define the terms describing specific terms within the categories.

WORD ELEMENTS PROMINENT IN THIS CHAPTER

WORD ELEMENT	TYPE	MEANING	WORD ELEMENT	TYPE	MEANING
dys-	prefix	difficult	-phobia	suffix	fear
hypo-	prefix	beneath	psych/o	root or prefix	mind
mania; manic	root	unwarranted exhilaration	somat/o	root or prefix	the body (as opposed to the mind)

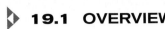

19.1 OVERVIEW

Like most other fields of medicine, psychiatry has its roots in ancient times. However, it was not until Benjamin Rush published his *Medical Inquiries and Observations upon the Diseases of the Mind* in 1812 that modern psychiatry was born. By 1844, the field had begun to develop rapidly, and the *American Journal of Insanity* began publication. The United States now has nearly 40,000 practicing psychiatrists.

Mental disorders can manifest themselves in a variety of ways. Some produce changes in the behavior of the patient; others cause abnormal sensations or create unusual emotional states. The causes of such disorders are sometimes psychological and sometimes biological. Symptoms can range from mild dysfunction to incapacitation.

The American Psychiatric Association has categorized mental disorders in its *Diagnostic and Statistical Manual of Mental Disorders*, which is often referred to simply as the *DSM*. First published in 1952, the *DSM* is currently available in a fourth edition. The definition of "mental disorder" given in this work allows the application of the term only if the condition. . .

". . . is associated with present distress (a painful symptom) or disability (impairment in one or more important areas of functioning) or with a significantly increased risk of suffering death, pain, disability, or an important loss of freedom."

Although this definition appears quite narrow in scope, the authors point out that behavioral and psychological manifestations lying outside it may nevertheless be treated by professionals in the field. Persons suffering the sudden loss of a loved one, for example, might find themselves in need of treatment. Those whose manifestations of distress exceed grief might be suffering from a mental disorder, but the cause of such a disorder, according to the definition, would lie beyond the loss that initiated the symptoms.

19.2 MULTIAXIAL SYSTEM OF CODING DISORDERS

Those diagnosing mental illnesses and those responsible for keeping medical records use a numbering system to indicate the results of mental disorder diagnosis. The five-axis method established for coding these results, shown in Table 19–1, comes from the *DSM*. Since no medical terminology is specifically associated with the system itself, no reason exists for its repetition here. Those persons needing to apply the system should refer directly to the current edition of *DSM*.

TABLE 19–1

Multiaxial Coding System

AXIS	NAME
I	clinical syndromes, V codes
II	developmental disorders, personality disorders
III	physical disorders and conditions
IV	severity of psychosocial stressors
V	global assessment of functioning

▶ 19.3 AFFECTIVE DISORDERS

Affective disorders are those associated with abnormal moods or mood swings. The two major divisions of mood disorders are the **bipolar** (bī-pō′-lăr) and the **depressive**. The **bipolar disorder** is characterized by one or more **manic** (măn′-ĭk) episodes associated with a history of major depressive episodes. **Cyclothymia** (sī″-klō-thī′-mē-ă) is a second kind of bipolar disorder comprising many **hypomanic** (hī″-pō-măn′-ĭk) episodes coupled with many depressive episodes. The terms **mania** (mā′-nē-ă) (a feeling of extreme euphoria) and **hypomania** (hī″-pō-mā′-nē-ă) (a feeling somewhere between normal optimism and mania) describe the level of elation the patient feels. Hypomanic episodes do not reach levels that cause significant functional impairment.

Depressive disorders also include two types: **major depression** and **dysthymia** (dĭs-thī′-mē-ă). Major depression, as its name suggests, includes one or more major episodes of depression lasting at least two weeks. Dysthymia describes chronic depression lasting for more than two years.

▶ 19.4 ANXIETY DISORDERS

Phobias

Anxiety disorders are common among the general population and include the various phobias with which most of us are familiar. A **phobia** (fō′-bē-ă) is an unreasonable fear of something. The definitions of common phobias are given in Table 19–2.

TABLE 19–2

Common Phobias

PHOBIA	DEFINITION
acrophobia	an unreasonable fear of heights
agoraphobia	an unreasonable fear of unfamiliar surroundings
ailuraphobia	an unreasonable fear of cats
algophobia	an unreasonable fear of pain
claustrophobia	an unreasonable fear of closed spaces
erythrophobia	a fear of blushing (such a fear often produces the symptom, which is also sometimes called erythrophobia)
mysophobia	an unreasonable fear of germs
panophobia	fear of everything
xenophobia	an unreasonable fear of foreigners

You may have noted that all but two of the definitions given in Table 19–2 include the word "unreasonable." Every normal person exercises caution to avoid falling from heights, feels less than comfortable in *some* crowds (a lynch mob, for example), does not enter a tiger's cage, avoids pain whenever possible, stays out of airless rooms whenever possible, and does not invite Martians for lunch. On the other hand, one who fears blushing or one who fears everything exhibits abnormal reactions unmarked by degree and unexplained by reason.

Post-Traumatic Stress Disorder

People who are subjected to particularly distressing experiences, those beyond the kind of conflict and difficulties we all encounter occasionally, sometimes relive such events either in dreams or while fully awake. Persons experiencing these episodes for more than a month after the actual experience are diagnosed with **post-traumatic stress disorder.**

Generalized Anxiety Disorder

Generalized anxiety disorder is characterized by unreasonable worry about several, or even many, things: financial security, performance in school, social acceptance, etc. Again, people who are facing a financial crisis based on real difficulty, people who must perform in school or face some terrible consequence, or people who hope to live healthy social lives probably do not suffer from generalized anxiety disorder. When such worries are groundless, however, or when they are accompanied by panic attacks or depression, the condition may be present.

▷ 19.5 DISSOCIATIVE DISORDERS

Dissociative (dĭs-sō″-sē-ă-tĭv) **disorders,** also called **hysterical neuroses,** affect the patient's identity, consciousness, or memory. It should be noted that many of the signs and symptoms of dissociative disorders can occur with other disorders, in which case the dissociative disorder may not be diagnosed.

Motion pictures and talk shows have brought a great deal of notoriety to the **multiple personality disorder,** an example of a dissociative disorder primarily affecting the patient's identity. **Psychogenic fugue** (sī″-kō-jĕn′-ĭk fūg) is another identity-focused disorder, which is characterized by the temporary assumption of a new identity, an inability to recall the original identity, and sudden and unexpected travel away from familiar people and surroundings. If the patient does not take on a second identity and leave familiar surroundings, the condition is called **psychogenic amnesia.**

A patient who has become socially or occupationally impaired because of a feeling of detachment, a mere observer of his own mental or bodily processes, suffers from **depersonalization disorder,** also sometimes called **depersonalization neurosis.** Patients may also feel as though they are in a robotic or dream state.

▷ 19.6 PSYCHOSEXUAL DISORDERS

Psychosexual disorders include two main types: **paraphilias** (pār″-ă-fĭl′-ē-ăz), also called **sexual deviations,** and **sexual dysfunctions.**

Paraphilias

Paraphilias are those mental disorders characterized by intense, unnatural sexual urges. These urges may be directed toward children or nonhuman objects, or they may direct one to satisfaction through the infliction or reception of pain, injury, or humiliation. Paraphilial symptoms sometimes result from **temporal lobe epilepsy (TLE),** a neurological condition.

The following specific disorders are defined in the succeeding paragraphs: exhibitionism, fetishism, transvestic fetishism, frotteurism, pedophilia, sexual masochism, sexual sadism, and voyeurism.

Exhibitionism   As the name implies, the sexual exhibitionist, nearly always a male, has recurring powerful urges to expose his genitals to strangers, nearly always women or female children.

Fetishism   A **fetish** (fĕt′-ĭsh) is any object, such as a rabbit's foot, to which one attributes magical powers. Most such objects represent nothing more than the superstitions of those who believe in them. **Sexual fetishism** (fĕt′-ĭsh-ĭzm), on the other hand, represents the disintegrative view of a person. Those exhibiting this disorder regard a body part or an item of clothing as an erotic object, sometimes to such an extent that only the fetish can lead to sexual arousal. A diagnosis of fetishism is made when the disorder lasts for more than six months or when the patient is distressed by or has acted on the urges. **Transvestic** (trăns-vĕs′-tĭk) **fetishism** is diagnosed when the articles of clothing used in "cross-dressing" have been identified as the fetish.

Frotteurism   The act is called **frottage** (frō-tŏzh′) and consists of touching a nonconsenting person. Perpetrators commit frotteurism because of the feeling of intimacy they gain, not by the coercive nature of the act. Since most acts of frottage are carefully planned and committed against strangers in public places (so that the perpetrator can escape arrest and prosecution), one might conclude that such acts are motivated by will rather than compulsion. Those who do not act on their urges, but rather acknowledge their disordered nature, may seek psychiatric help instead.

Pedophilia   As the etymology suggests, this disorder involves a sexual attraction to children. The mental disorder is usually chronic and often, although not always, begins in adolescence.

Sexual Masochism   Those who exhibit **sexual masochism** (măs′-ō-kĭzm) obtain sexual satisfaction by being made to suffer pain or humiliation. The term **infantilism** (ĭn-făn′-tĭl-ĭzm) is also used to describe the phenomenon of masochists who wish to be treated as helpless infants. **Hypoxyphilia** (hī-pŏx″-ĭ-fĭl′-ē-ă), another form of masochism, is characterized by the desire to be deprived of oxygen. The masochistic disorder, which is most often chronic, is sometimes accompanied by fetishism or sadism.

Sexual Sadism   **Sexual sadism** (sā′-dĭzm) is similar to masochism, except that the object of suffering and humiliation is someone other than the person suffering from the disorder. As the course of the condition progress, the sadist often finds it necessary to increase the level of violence meted out to the victim in order to achieve satisfaction.

Voyeurism   This disorder is characterized by an intense desire to watch unsuspecting people disrobe or engage in the sex act. Its first manifestations usually occur before the age of 15, and the disorder is often chronic.

Sexual Dysfunctions

Sexual dysfunction is, as the prefix dys- (difficult) suggests, difficulty in completing the sexual response cycle. No special terminology is associated with sexual dysfunction disorders.

19.7 SCHIZOPHRENIC DISORDERS

The schizophrenic disorder includes delusions and a reduction of one's ability to function normally. Some types of delusion are quite common, such as the belief that one's thoughts are controlled by an outside force or that one's thoughts are broadcast to the world at large.

Sometimes, the schizophrenic's thought processes become incoherent, and this condition is called **formal thought disorder**. Sufferers of this disorder often talk a great deal without conveying any real information.

Hallucinations are common in schizophrenia, the auditory type being the most often encountered.

When apparently schizophrenic signs and behavior are discovered to have organic causes, a diagnosis of schizophrenia is not applicable.

19.8 SOMATOFORM DISORDERS

Somatoform disorders include physical symptoms for which physical causes are unknown.

Body Dysmorphic Disorder

This disorder, also known as **dysmorphophobia** (dĭs-mor″-fō-fō′-bē-ă), is characterized by an excessive concern for one's physical appearance and by the belief that some minor defect (or even normal feature) is a disfigurement.

Conversion Disorder

Psychological distress is thought to cause **conversion disorder**, which can manifest itself in many ways, such as paralysis, blindness, etc. A diagnosis of this disorder is accurate only if some physical reason for the impairment cannot be found.

Hypochondriasis

This disorder, also known as **hypochondriacal** (hī″-pō-kŏn-drī′-ă-kăl) **neurosis** (or commonly, **hypochondria** [hī″-pō-kŏn′-drē-ă]), is the victim's conviction that he or she has a serious disease, despite medical assurances to the contrary.

Somatization Disorder and Somatoform Pain Disorder

Like the victim of hypochondriasis, the victim of **somatization** (sō″-mă-tī-zā′-shŭn) **disorder** seeks medical attention for imagined ailments or minor aches and pains that normal people would ignore. The somatization disorder appears almost exclusively in females.

Somatoform pain disorder occurs in both females and males, but it is more common in females. Although the condition may lead to extreme physical distress for the sufferer, physical treatment, including surgery, never successfully alleviates the pain.

Undifferentiated Somatoform (sō-mă′-tō-form) **Disorder** is diagnosed when a full clinical picture does not indicate somatization disorder.

▶ 19.9 PSYCHOACTIVE SUBSTANCE ABUSE DISORDERS

Psychoactive (sī″-kō-ăk′-tĭv) **substance dependence** is the primary disorder in this category. The presence of any three of the following criteria justifies diagnosis of dependence: increasing quantity of duration of use; lack of success in controlling use; persistent desire; interference with fulfillment of responsibilities or social and recreational activities; continued use in the face of negative social or physical response to the use; the need for increasing amounts of the substance to achieve the desired effect; withdrawal symptoms; substance use to avoid withdrawal symptoms.

Psychoactive substance abuse is a secondary category. It is diagnosed when substance use is maladaptive, but the criteria for dependence are not met.

The categories of psychoactive substances involved in dependence or abuse are as follows: alcohol; nicotine; inhalants; opiates; hallucinogens; amphetamines; cannabis; cocaine; phencyclidine (PCP); sedatives; hypnotics; and anxiolytics.

▶ 19.10 IMPULSE CONTROL DISORDERS

This group of disorders is characterized by the failure to resist an impulse to do something that is dysfunctional to the individual or harmful to others. Tension or arousal are experienced prior to committing the act, and pleasure or release of tension are felt during the act, sometimes followed by remorse or guilt. The types are **kleptomania** (klĕp″-tō-mā′-nē-ă) (uncontrollable stealing), **pathological gambling**, **pyromania** (pī″-rō-mā′-nē-ă) (uncontrollable fire-lighting), **explosive disorder** (intermittent and serious aggressive acts on persons or property), and **trichotillomania** (trĭk″-ō-tĭl″-ō-mā′-nē-ă) (persistent pulling out of one's hair).

▶ 19.11 PERSONALITY DISORDERS

Personality disorders are diagnosed when personality traits are dysfunctional to social or occupational goals or cause significant distress to the affected person. They are classified in three clusters.

Cluster A includes the **paranoid** (păr′-ă-noyd), **schizoid** (skĭz′-oyd), and **schizotypal** (skĭz″-ō-tī′-păl) **personality** disorders. The **paranoid disorder** is marked by unreasonable suspiciousness, jealousy, and persistent interpretation of others' actions as hostile, demeaning, or threatening. These people cannot accept criticism, usually look tense, are argumentative, and grossly exaggerate difficulties. They are typically humorless and insensitive, very defensive, revere power, and despise weakness. They can be moralistic and rigid and have grandiose ideas.

Persons with **schizoid personality** disorders are loners, usually lacking any sort of close relationship. They rarely express anger, joy, or aggressiveness, have no interest in sex with others, prefer solitary endeavours, are uninterested in others' opinion of them, and are socially cold. Occupationally, they succeed only in solitary, task-oriented positions requiring minimal social interaction.

Schizotypal disorder shares many characteristics with schizoid and paranoid disorder. However, schizotypal disorder is principally characterized by unusual or bizarre thinking patterns, quite often involving perceptual illusions such as a sense of clairvoyance or contact with a "spirit world." Speech patterns are typically odd and physical grooming is often lacking. Unusual or bizarre mannerisms are frequent. Schizotypals often talk to themselves in public and ordinarily are unresponsive to the social gestures of others.

Cluster B includes the **antisocial, borderline, histrionic** (hĭs″-trē-ŏn′-ĭk), and **narcissistic** (năr-sĭs-sĭst′-ĭk) personality disorders. Those with **antisocial personalities** begin displaying antisocial behavior in childhood or adolescence. Characteristic behavior (referred to as **conduct disorder**) involves persistent and frequent lying, stealing, physical and emotional aggression, vandalism, cruelty, running away from home, and academic failure. **Attention-deficit hyperactivity disorder** (ADHD) in childhood is also strongly associated with **adult antisocial disorder**. Typical adult behavior includes extreme irresponsibility with spouses, children, co-workers, and friends. They are promiscuous, physically violent, and often abusive to spouses, children, and other family members. They do not often sustain close or responsible relationships, but many are superficially charming. They are often substance abusers, thrill-seekers, feel no remorse, and have little anticipatory anxiety. Roughly 3% of males and 1% of females have the disorder. Both genetic and environmental factors are important in the development of the disorder. Although most with the disorder have poor earning capacity due to lack of academic success and adult irresponsibility, some antisocial personalities achieve significant success in business or politics, when their superficial charm, unscrupulousness, and easy dishonesty can overcome the deficit of their irresponsibility.

Borderline personality disorder is associated with suicide attempts, self-mutilation, impulsive and self-damaging behavior such as substance abuse, unstable but intense personal relationships, extreme mood shifts, uncertainty regarding life goals, sexual orientation, values, and life-style, and chronic boredom and emptiness. Aimlessness and hopelessness are hallmarks.

Persons with **histrionic personality** disorder need to be the center of attention at all times. They will constantly seek approval or praise and most frequently concentrate on being as physically or sexually attractive as possible to achieve this goal. Their emotional displays are excessive in relation to the occasion, and they constantly seek immediate gratification. In ordinary terms, such people would be described as shallow and self-absorbed.

The **narcissistic personality disorder** is very similar to the histrionic, with the addition of totally unrealistic, grandiose thoughts of themselves and extreme sensitivity to others' opinions of them. The exaggerated sense of self-importance frequently involves a fantasy life focusing on success and power. These people are envious of others' success. They will seek out compliments but show no empathy for others' desires or needs. They will expect special treatment and form friendships only where there is advantage to be gained. Depression is common, particularly with increasing age and decreasing physical attractiveness.

III–19

Cluster C of the personality disorders contains the **avoidant, dependent, obsessive compulsive, and passive aggressive** types. The **avoidant disorder** involves fear of negative assessment by others, social discomfort, and shyness. The chief concern of such persons is to be liked and accepted, but their fear of appearing foolish or stupid undermines their ability to fulfill this need, leading to distress, anxiety, and sometimes phobias relating to social situations.

The **dependent disorder** is exemplified by extreme submissiveness and dependence on others. Persons with this disorder therefore dislike being alone and fear abandonment. They are easily wounded by criticism and rejection and will often go to extremes to be accepted. They will depend on others to make their decisions for them and are devastated when relationships are ended.

Those with **obsessive compulsive** personality disorder are perfectionistic and rigid. They set their standards so high that they often achieve less than their ability would allow. In their own eyes, they never achieve enough. They are typically fixated on trivial rules and procedures, so that they cannot see the bigger picture. They are driven workers, usually sacrificing holidays for further productivity. They are stingy with their hearts and their money, and are often hoarders. They are indecisive, overconscientious, inflexible, and often moralistic.

Passive aggressive disorder involves habitual use of passive behaviors to resist external demands. It can therefore be occupationally and socially destructive. These persons can be extremely stubborn. They will be forgetful, procrastinate, or be purposely inefficient to avoid work demands. They are resentful of authority figures, lack self-confidence, and may abuse alcohol. They are vulnerable to depression.

▶ 19.12 EATING DISORDERS

There are four classified eating disorders: **anorexia nervosa** (ăn-ō-rĕk′-sē-ă nĕr-vō′-să), **bulimia** (bŭ-lĭm′-ē-ă) **nervosa, pica** (pī′-kă), **and rumination disorder of infancy.** Anorexia is characterized by refusal to maintain normal body weight. Its onset is normally in early to late adolescence. The person is preoccupied with being fat, and weight reduction is accomplished by restricted food intake, self-induced vomiting, excessive exercise, or abuse of laxatives or diuretics. It primarily affects females and results in death in 10–20% of cases. However, in many cases, normal body weight is achieved after a single episode.

Bulimia nervosa involves repetitive, uncontrollable eating, followed by purging by vomiting, or by the use of laxatives and diuretics. Guilt and depression follow eating episodes. Normal body weight is frequently maintained, but the person's life is essentially controlled by concerns related to eating.

Pica affects infants and children. It involves the consumption of non-nourishing substances such as wood, paint, cloth, hair, pebbles, or even animal droppings. It rarely persists into maturity.

Rumination disorder of infancy is rare. The infant repeatedly regurgitates food and either ejects it or chews it and reswallows it. The condition can result in severe malnutrition and death.

▶ 19.13 ABBREVIATIONS

ABBREVIATION	MEANING	ABBREVIATION	MEANING
ADHD	attention deficit hyperactivity disorder	MAOI	monamine oxidase inhibitor (antidepressant)
CA	chronological age	MDA	methylene dioxyamphetamine (hallucinogenic drug)
DMT	dimethyltryptamine (hallucinogenic drug)		
GAF Scale	global assessment of functioning scale (scale ranging from 1–100, where 1 refers to poor mental health and inability to function in society; 100 refers to good mental health and the ability to function well in society)	OCD	obsessive compulsive disorder
		PCP	phencyclidine (psychoactive drug)
		PDDNOS	pervasive developmental disorder not otherwise specified
		SAD	seasonal affective disorder
HCA	heterocyclic antidepressants	TCA	tricyclic antidepressants
IQ	intelligence quotient (measurement of intellectual functioning as obtained by a number of intelligence tests; normal IQ is between 90–110, subnormal IQ is below 70)	THC	delta-9-tetrahydrocannabinol (major psychoactive constitutent in marijuana)
		WAIS	Wechsler Adult Intelligence Scale
LSD	lysergic acid diethylamide (hallucinogenic drug)	WISC	Wechsler Intelligence Scale for Children
MA	mental age		

▶ EXERCISE 19–1

Short Answer

Briefly answer the following questions.

Answers to all exercise questions appear in Appendix A.

Practice Quiz

1. What is an affective disorder? _____

2. Name the two major divisions of affective disorders. _____

3. What is the difference between major depression and dysthymia? _____

4. What is a phobia? _____

5. What is post-traumatic stress disorder? _____

_____

6. What is another term for dissociative disorder? _____

_____

7. What is the distinguishing feature between psychogenic fugue and psychogenic amnesia? _____

_____

8. What is a fetish? _____

_____

9. What are the two types of psychosexual disorders? _____

_____

10. What is another name for hypochondriacal neurosis? _____

▶EXERCISE 19–2

Vocabulary Study

Definitions

Write definitions for the following terms.

1. acrophobia _____

2. agoraphobia _____

3. ailuraphobia _____

4. algophobia _____

5. bipolar disorder _____

6. body dysmorphic disorder _____

7. claustrophobia _____

8. conversion disorder _____

9. cyclothymia _____

10. depersonalization disorder _____

11. dysthymia _____

12. erythrophobia _____

13. exhibitionism _____

14. fetishism _____

15. frotteurism _____

16. generalized anxiety disorder _____

17. hypochondriasis _____

18. hypomania _____

19. major depression _____

20. mysophobia _____

21. panophobia _____

22. paraphilia _____

23. pedophilia _____

24. post-traumatic stress disorder _____

25. psychogenic fugue _____

26. sexual masochism _____

27. sexual sadism _____

28. somatization disorder _____

29. somatoform disorder _____

30. voyeurism _____

31. xenophobia _____

▶EXERCISE 19–3   Matching Terms and Abbreviations with Meanings

Matching

Match the term in Column A with its meaning in Column B.

Column A		Column B
1. acrophobia	_____	A. fear of cats
2. agoraphobia	_____	B. fear of strangers
3. ailuraphobia	_____	C. fear of blushing
4. claustrophobia	_____	D. fear of heights
5. erythrophobia	_____	E. fear of pain
6. mysophobia	_____	F. fear of everything
7. panophobia	_____	G. fear of closed spaces
8. xenophobia	_____	H. fear of unfamiliar surroundings
9. algophobia	_____	I. fear of germs
10. SAD	_____	J. an antidepressant
11. MA	_____	K. Diagnosis and Statistical Manual of Mental Disorders
12. MAOI	_____	
13. GAF Scale	_____	L. chronological age
14. DSM	_____	M. mental age
15. CA	_____	N. seasonal affective disorder
		O. global assessment of functioning scale

Crossword Puzzle

Psychiatric Terms

Across

1 An unreasonable fear of being closed in
3 An unreasonable fear of pain
5 A feeling somewhere between normal optimism and mania
9 The opposite of manic
11 A fear of blushing
12 An unreasonable fear of germs
13 An unreasonable fear of cats
14 A term used to indicate physical symptoms without apparent physical causes
15 A mental disorder characterized by unnatural sexual urges

Down

1 A kind of bipolar disorder
2 Touching a non-consenting person in an intimate way
4 Regarding a body part or an item of clothing as an object of sexual desire
6 Unreasonable fear of high places
7 An unreasonable fear of unfamiliar surroundings
8 An unreasonable fear of foreigners
9 Chronic depression lasting more than two years
10 Fear of everything

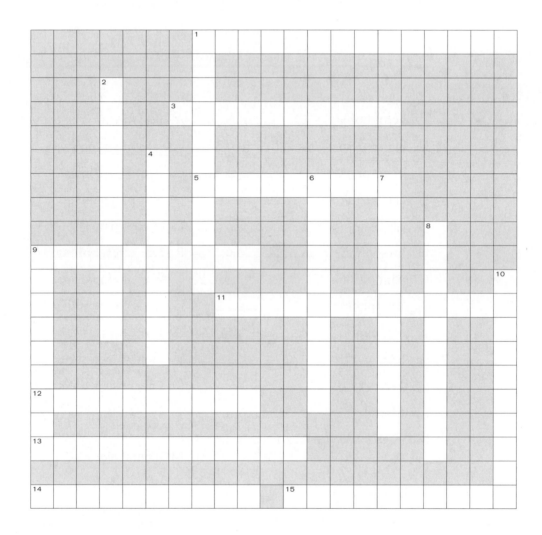

III–19

CHAPTER

20 PHARMACOLOGY

CHAPTER ORGANIZATION

This chapter has been designed to help the student learn terms and abbreviations related to pharmacology.

20.1 Drug Names

20.2 Classification of Drugs

CHAPTER OBJECTIVES

Upon successful completion of this chapter, the student will be able to do following:

1. Define the terms that identify major classes of drugs.
2. Spell generic names of some major drugs.

INTRODUCTION

Throughout history, mankind has searched for substances called **drugs** to alleviate pain, cure illness, and maintain good health. Through trial and error over many centuries, substances that would fulfill these needs were discovered. Native Americans, for example, discovered that pine needles boiled into a tea helped them maintain good health. Likewise, the Inuit of the Arctic considered the internal organs of hunted animals a "health food." The healthful substances discovered in these two instances are known today as Vitamin C and Vitamin A.

Natural substances that alleviated pain were similarly found by trial and error. But diseases caused by foreign invaders were difficult to combat before people were aware of the existence of germs. The first microscope was invented in The Netherlands in 1590 by Zacharias Janssen, but it was not until nearly 100 years later, in 1683, that a Dutch scientist named Antonie van Leeuwenhoek discovered bacteria while using a microscope. In the 19th century, Louis Pasteur demonstrated that germs cause disease, and research began on the development of agents that would combat germs without harming the body. Antibiotics were developed in the 20th century, beginning with Sir Alexander Fleming's discovery that a certain mold could kill bacteria. That mold was the source of the first penicillin.

Today, about half of the substances that cure disease and enhance good health are still obtained from natural sources such as plants, animals, and metals in soil and rocks. The other 50 percent of modern drugs are manufactured synthetically.

Professionals who research and develop new drugs are called **pharmacologists** (făr″-mă-kŏl′-ō-jĭsts). Those who dispense the drugs are called **pharmacists** (făr′-mă-sĭsts). These terms are derived from the Greek word *pharmacon*, which means both medicine and poison.

▶ 20.1 DRUG NAMES

Drugs are now systematically divided into **classes** according to their respective functions, such as alleviation of pain, elimination of foreign invaders, maintenance of body fluid levels, etc. In addition to classification name, all drugs have a **generic** (jĕn-ĕr'-ĭk) name derived from the main ingredient of the particular drug and a **brand** name assigned by the manufacturer. For example, **Bayer** is a brand name of the generic ingredient acetylsalicylic acid, or **aspirin**, which is classified as a pain killer or an **analgesic** (ăn″-ăl-jē'-zĭk). Any U.S. pharmaceutical company that develops a new drug is given a 17-year patent on the drug. When the patent expires, other companies may manufacture the drug and sell it under their own brand names. Thus, there are many brand names for each generic drug.

Drugs that are judged as being dangerous to patients when they are taken without medical supervision cannot be legally dispensed without orders from a physician. These are known as **prescription drugs**. Drugs that can be legally dispensed without a prescription are called **over-the-counter (OTC)** drugs.

Some of the major classes of drugs are listed below. Generic names and some typical brand names are also listed.

▶ 20.2 CLASSIFICATION OF DRUGS

Analgesics

Analgesics alleviate mild to moderate pain. Some typical generic names of analgesics are aspirin and acetaminophen. Some typical brand names are Anacin®, Tylenol®, Advil®, Motrin,® Bayer, Duoprin, and Goody's Headache Powders.

Narcotic Analgesics

Narcotic analgesics are habit-forming. They are sometimes prescribed as analgesics in combination with aspirin or acetaminophen. Some typical generic names of narcotic analgesics are codeine, morphine, and oxycodone. Typical brand names are Demerol, Percocet, and MS Contin.

Antianginal

Angina pectoris is a condition caused by a decreased blood supply to the heart. Antianginal (ăn″-tĭ-ăn-jī'-năl) drugs are administered in a variety of ways. One common method is **sublingual** (sŭb-lĭng'-gwăl) administration, in which a tablet is placed under the tongue to dissolve. Some generic names of antianginals are nitroglycerine, propranolol, and isosorbide dinitrate. Some typical brand names are Nitrostat, Isordil, and Inderal.

Antiarrhythmic

These drugs are used to treat irregular heart rhythms caused by abnormal electrical impulses in the heart. Some generic names of antiarrhythmics (ăn″-tĭ-ă-rĭth'-mē-ăks) are amiodarone, disopyramide, procainamide, and quinidine. Some brand names are Cordarone, Norpace, Pronestyl, and Quinaglute.

III—20

Antibiotics

Antibiotics (ăn″-tĭ-bī-ŏt′ĭks) are chemical compounds that destroy harmful organisms. They are sometimes produced by living cells such as bacteria, yeasts, or molds and can also be commercially synthesized. Some typical generic names of antibiotics are penicillin, amoxycillin, tetracycline, and erythromycin. Some typical brand names are Vibramycin, Biaxin, Ceclor, and E-mycin.

Antihistamines

Antihistamines (ăn″-tĭ-hĭs′tă-mēnz) are used to treat conditions such as hay fever in which histamines are released in response to certain allergens. Some generic names of antihistamines are doxylamine, diphenhydramine, and terfenadine. Some typical brand names are Alamine, Benadryl, Dimetapp, and Seldane.

Anticoagulants

A blood clot in the heart or blood vessels is called a **thrombus** (thrŏm′-bŭs), and the condition is known as **thrombosis** (thrŏm-bō′-sĭs). When a blood clot becomes detached from the vessel wall and moves through the blood stream, it is called an **embolus** (ĕm′-bō-lŭs), and the condition is known as **embolism** (ĕm′-bō-lĭzm). Some anticoagulants are used to prevent the formation of clots, and others are used to dissolve clots that have already formed. Typical generic names of anticoagulants are heparin and warfarin and a typical brand name is Coumadin.

Anticonvulsants

Anticonvulsants (ăn″-tĭ-kŏn-vŭl′-sănts) are used in the treatment of epilepsy to inhibit convulsions or seizures. Some generic names of anticonvulsants are valproic acid, carbamazepine, and phenytoin. Typical brand names are Tegretol, Depakote, and Dilantin.

Antidepressants

Antidepressants (ăn″-tĭ-dē-prĕs′-ănts) relieve symptoms of psychological depression by altering messages between brain cells. Some generic names of antidepressants are trazodone, imipramine, amitryptiline, and fluoxetine. Typical brand names are Desyrel, Sinequan, Elavil, and Prozac.

Anesthetics

Anesthetics (ăn″-ĕs-thĕ′-tĭks) are drugs that produce a loss of feeling or sensation. The loss of sensation may be partial, as in **local anesthesia** (aň″-ĕs-thē′-zē-ă), or a complete loss of sensation, as in **general anesthesia**. Anesthetics can be administered by injection or by inhalation of gaseous agents. Physicians who specialize in **anesthesiology** (ăn″-ĕs-thē″-zē-ŏl′-ō-jē) are called **anesthesiologists** (ăn″-ĕs-thē″-zē-ŏl′-ō-jĭsts). Topical anesthetics are used to treat such conditions as skin irritations and hemorrhoids. **Topical** administration of drugs refers to application on the skin. Some generic names of anesthetics are nitrous oxide, halothane, lidocaine (a topical anesthetic), and benzocaine. Benzocal and Xylocaine are two typical brand names.

(ACE) Angiotensin-Converting Enzyme Inhibitor

ACE inhibitors reduce resistance in arteries and strengthen the heartbeat. They are used to treat high blood pressure and congestive heart failure. Captopril is a typical generic name of an ACE inhibitor, and typical brand names are Prinivil and Capoten.

Cyclopegics

Cyclopegia (sī″-klō-pē′-jē-ă) is the term used for paralysis of the ciliary muscle. A mydriatic cyclopegic is an agent that dilates the pupil of the eye and blocks the response of the ciliary muscles during eye examinations. Some generic names of cyclopegics are homatropine, atropine, and scopolamine. Some typical brand names are Atropisol, Isopto, and Dispersa.

Diagnostic Aids

Many drugs fall into the class of diagnostic aids. One example is cholecysto-graphic agents used for gallbladder x-ray tests. Some generic names of **cholecystographic** (kō″-lĕ-sĭs″-tō-grăf′-ĭk) **agents**, which make the gallbladder visible on x-rays after having become absorbed into the blood and concentrated in the gallbladder, are iocetamic acid, ipodate, and tyropanoate. Typical brand names are Bilopaque and Telepaque.

Diuretics

Diuretics (dī′-ū-rĕt′-ĭks) reduce fluid retention in body tissues by enhancing fluid excretion by the kidneys. Some generic names of diuretics are indapamide, hydrochlorothiazide, and furosemide. Typical brand names are Diuril, Lozol, and Lasix.

Electrolyte Replenishers

Electrolytes (ē-lĕk′-trō-līts) in body fluids need to be replenished when they become deficient as a result of disease or as a result of dehydration following diarrhea. A generic name of an electrolyte replenisher is potassium phosphate, and typical brand names are K-Phos and Neutra-Phos.

Emetics

Emetics (ē-mĕt′-ĭks) are agents that induce vomiting. They are used to treat medication overdose and ingestion of some poisons. One generic name of an emetic is ipecac, and typical brand names include Ipecac Syrup and Queledrine.

III-20

Nutritional Supplements

Mineral and vitamin supplements aid in maintenance of health in cases where diets are deficient or in cases where absorption of nutrients is inhibited by disease. Some generic names and brand names of nutritional supplements are shown in Table 20–1.

TABLE 20–1

Nutritional Supplements

GENERIC NAMES	TYPICAL BRAND NAMES
iron	Geritol Tablets; Ferralyn
calcium	Mega-Cal; Oystercal
niacin (Vitamin B-3, Nicotinic Acid)	Nico-400; Niacor
Vitamin C (Ascorbic Acid)	Ascorbicap; Flavorcee
Vitamin B-12 (Cyanocobalamin)	Alphamin; Rubion

Sedatives

Sedatives known as **barbiturates** (băr-bĭt′-ū-rāts) depress the central nervous system and are used to treat nervousness and headaches. They are habit-forming. Some generic names of sedatives are phenobarbitol, diazepam, triazolam, and alprazolam. Typical brand names are Phrenilin, Valium, Halcion, and Xanax.

Sympathomimetics

Sympathomimetics (sĭm″-pă-thō-mĭm-ēt′-ĭks) are agents whose effect mimics the impulses of the sympathetic nervous system. They are used in the treatment of asthma and allergic reactions, and as decongestants. Some generic names of sympathomimetics are pseudoephidrine, albuterol, and epinephrine. Typical brand names include Ventolin, Epipen, and Sudafed.

▶ **EXERCISE 20–1**

Matching

Matching

Beside each of the following terms write a (C) if the term is a class name, a (B) if the term is a brand name, or a (G) if the term is a generic name.

Answers to the exercises in this chapter are found in Appendix A.

1. aspirin　_____
2. codeine　_____
3. antiarrhythmic　_____
4. scopolamine　_____
5. thiazide　_____

6. diuretic　_____
7. Oystercal　_____
8. penicillin　_____
9. erythromycin　_____

Column A

10. analgesic   _____

11. antianginal   _____

12. hemorrhoid treatment   _____

13. thrombosis treatment   _____

14. diuretic   _____

15. emetic   _____

16. general anesthetic   _____

17. cyclopegic   _____

Column B

A. heparin

B. furosemide

C. nitroglycerine

D. halothane

E. acetaminophen

F. ipecac

G. homatropine

H. benzocaine

▶EXERCISE 20–2

Short Answer

Briefly answer the following questions.

Short Quiz

1. What is the term used to describe drugs dispensed only on orders from a physician? _____

2. What is the term for a licensed drug dispenser? _____

3. What is a common method of administering antianginals? _____

_____

4. Explain the difference between a brand name and a generic name. _____

_____

_____

5. What are the natural sources of antibiotics? _____

_____

6. What class of drugs is used to treat an exaggerated response by the body to allergens? _____

7. What class of drugs is used to treat an embolism? _____

8. What generic drug is used to treat medication overdose? _____

9. What class of drugs would be administered by an ophthalmologist? _____

_____

10. What class of drugs alleviates the condition known as edema?

_____

Spelling

Place a check mark beside all misspelled words in the list that follows. Correctly spell those that you checked off.

1. acetaminaphen ☐ _____

2. nitroglycerine ☐ _____

3. erythromyacin ☐ _____

4. anasthetic ☐ _____

5. diuretic ☐ _____

6. ipecac ☐ _____

7. asorbic acid ☐ _____

8. acetylsalicylic acid ☐ _____

9. ephedrene ☐ _____

10. barbituate ☐ _____

Crossword Puzzle

Finding the Generic Name

Across

1 Bayer
4 Tridione
6 Cardioquin
7 Oystercal
8 Duracillin
9 Cordorone
12 Anthrombin-K
13 Mesatoin
15 Phrenilin
16 Omni-Tuss

Down

1 Duoprin
2 Inderal
3 Nitrol
5 Ferralyn
10 Peganone
11 Dilantin
14 Nico-400

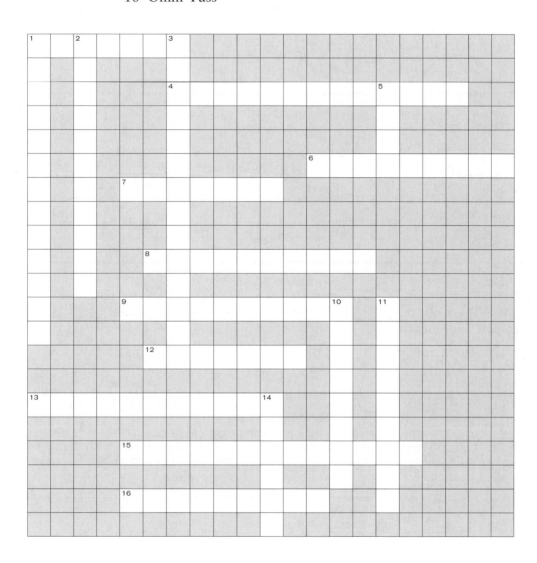

21 LABORATORY TERMINOLOGY

CHAPTER OBJECTIVES

Upon successful completion of this chapter, the student will be able to do the following:

1. Define terms related to the division of laboratory studies.

2. Define terms and abbreviations denoting miscellaneous laboratory tests and studies.

INTRODUCTION The body systems chapters in Part II often included laboratory terms as part of the sections labelled Physical Examination, Diagnosis, and Treatment. In this chapter, medical laboratory terms are covered more systematically.

Laboratory studies are divisible into **histopathology**(hĭs″-tŏ-pă-thŏl′-ō-jē), **clinical microbiology** (mī″-krō-bī-ŏl′-ō-jē), **immunohematology**(ĭ-mū-nō-hēm″-ă-tŏl′-ō-jē), **hematology** (hē″-mă-tŏl′-ō-jē), and **clinical chemistry**.

Histopathology

Histopathology departments process tissues that have been surgically removed. Before any processing can take place, a chemical solution known as a fixative is added to the tissue to keep it from deteriorating. The fixative kills bacteria and prevents chemical reactions from occurring in the tissues. The pathologist notes the size, shape, color, and texture and then cuts small samples from areas that appear diseased. These small samples are then processed for microscopic examination.

Processing for microscopic examination consists in the removal of the water in the sample and its replacement with wax. This provides a solid sample that can be sliced, a process called **microtomy** (mī-krŏt′-ō-mē). The slices, which can be less than one-cell thick, are placed on a slide and stained. Microscopic examination thus yields a view of all parts of the cell. For example, the glomerulus and renal tubules would be visible in a tissue sample from a kidney.

The entire process takes approximately 48 hours. A faster method, in which the tissue sample is frozen, is used when quick answers are needed for a surgical procedure already in progress.

Clinical Microbiology

The identification of infectious microorganisms is the job of those who work in a clinical **microbiology** (mī″-krō-bī-ŏl′-ō-jē) department. Disease-causing microorganisms include bacteria, viruses, yeasts, and fungi.

Most pathogenic bacteria can be cultured (grown artificially) within 48 hours. After the pathogen has been identified, it is tested against various **antimicrobials** (ăn″-tī-mī-krō′-bē-ălz), either antiobiotics or chemicals, that may be suitable for treatment of the patient.

A **Gram** stain is added to the material to be microscopically examined. This stain performs two jobs: it renders the body cells and bacteria visible under the microscope, and it helps divide bacteria into two large groups. Gram-positive bacteria appear purple, and Gram-negative bacteria appear pink. Each of these groups can then be further divided according to their shape. The shapes include **cocci** (kŏk′-sī), which are round, and **bacilli** (bă-sĭl′-ī), which are rod-shaped.

Bacteria may appear singly, in pairs (**diplococci** [dĭp″-lō-kŏk′-se], in clusters (**staphylococci** [stăf″-ĭl-ō-kŏk′-sē], or in long chains (**streptococci** [străep″-tō-kŏk′-sē], but most have no fixed arrangement.

The organism causing tuberculosis does not stain with the Gram stain. It requires a special stain called the *Ziehl-Neelsen* (zēl-nēl′-sĕn) stain.

Immunohematology

The primary function of an **immunohematology** department is the cross-matching of blood. Donated blood is mixed with a sample of the patient's blood before a transfusion so that potentially adverse reactions can be discovered. Reactions are determined to be adverse if either **agglutination** (ă-gloo″-tĭ-nā′-shŭn), which is the clumping together of blood cells, or **hemolysis** (hē-mŏl′-ĭ-sĭs), which is the rupture of blood cells, takes place.

The cross match is accompanied by a determination of the blood type and Rh blood group of the patient.

Hematology

Since the blood nourishes all the organs of the body and since it is so easily accessible for sampling, it is frequently examined as an indicator of the state of the body's various organs. Blood cells are evaluated in relation to their size and shape, and the numbers of each different type of cell are counted. The complete blood count (CBC) includes a hemoglobin, **hematocrit** (hē-măt′-ō-krĭt) (PCV), white cell count and differential, and calculations of the volume of red blood cells (MCV).

The test that determines the average amount of hemoglobin in each red blood cell is referred to as an MCHC. Since hemoglobin is the molecule that carries iron, the MCHC can detect anemia. Hematocrit refers both to the volume percentage of erythrocytes in whole blood and to the test used in its determination.

The white cell count, the ratio of white cells per volume, can indicate the presence of either an infection or a diminished capacity of the immune system. A high white cell count indicates infection, and a low count indicates immune deficiency. White cell differential is determined by a microscopic examination of white blood cell types. In viral infections, for example, an abnormal number of lymphocytes are present.

Coagulation studies help in the diagnosis of hemophilia and in the regulation of patients receiving certain kinds of therapy for heart conditions.

Clinical Chemistry

The chemical constituents of the body are determined in tests made by the **clinical chemistry** division of laboratory studies. The body's organs constantly process and produce chemicals. A change in the level of production can indicate that a particular organ is not functioning properly.

⧈ 21.2 MISCELLANEOUS LABORATORY TESTS AND STUDIES

Diagnostic tests to determine individual abnormal conditions are given in each of the anatomy and physiology chapters. Table 21–1 provides a broad look at some of the tests that may not have been already mentioned in connection with an anatomical system.

TABLE 21—1   Miscellaneous Laboratory Tests and Procedures

DEPARTMENT	TEST	PURPOSE
microbiology and serology	cultures of CSF	meningitis
	cultures of blood	subacute bacterial endocarditis
	C-reactive protein	inflammation and tissue destruction of any kind
	rheumatoid factors	rheumatoid arthritis
	serological test for syphilis	syphilis
	ANA	lupus erythematosis
	monospot	infectious mononucleosis
	rubella titers	rubella
clinical chemistry	bilirubin; alkaline phosphatase (ALP); serum proteins	liver profile
	creatinine kinase (CK); lactic dehydrogenase (LD); isoenzyme	cardiac profile
	immunoelectrophoresis	evaluation of the immune status
	urinalysis; urea; creatinine and clearance test	kidney function
	amylase	pancreas function
	ketosteroids; hydroxycorticosteroids	adrenal glands
hematology	erythrocyte sedimentation rate (ESR)	presence of infection
	red cell fragility	bone marrow function in red cell production
immunohematology	HIV	human immune deficiency virus
	hepatitis B & C	hepatitis B & C
histopathology and cytology	bronchial washings; bronchial brushings	diagnosis of lung disease
	fine needle aspirates	cancer diagnosis

The abbreviations most commonly used in laboratory terminology are given below:

ABBREVIATION	MEANING	ABBREVIATION	MEANING
ABO	blood types: A, B, and O	IgG, IgM, IgA, IgE, IgD	immunoglobulin: G, M, A, E, and D
ANA	antinuclear antibodies	L/S ratio	lecithin/sphingomyelin ratio
AST	aspartate aminotransferase	LDL	low-density lipoprotein
CBC	complete blood count	MBC	minimum bactericidal concentration
CIN	cervical intraepithelial neoplasia	MI	myocardial infarct
CIS	carcinoma in situ	MIC	minimum inhibitory concentration
CLL	chronic lymphocytic leukemia	PCV	packed cell volume
CML	chronic myologenous leukemia	Rh	Rh factor in the blood
CSF	cerebrospinal fluid	SBE	subacute bacterial endocarditis
ESR	erythrocyte sedimentation rate	STS	serological test for syphilis
HDL	high-density lipoprotein	VLDL	very-low-density lipoprotein
IEP	immunoelectrophoresis	VMA	vanillymandelic acid

Practice Quiz

Short Answer

Briefly answer the following questions.

Answers to the exercises in this chapter appear in Appendix A.

1. List the five major areas of laboratory study. _____

   _____

   _____

2. To what does the term microtomy refer? _____

   _____

3. What are the two advantages afforded by a Gram stain? _____

   _____

   _____

4. What is the term used to describe bacteria that appear in clusters? _____

   _____

5. What is the Ziehl-Neelsen stain used for? _____

   _____

6. What term refers to the rupturing of blood cells? _____

7. What term is used to refer to the clumping together of blood cells? _____

   _____

8. What is the purpose of cross-matching? _____

   _____

9. What is the name of the iron-carrying molecule? _____

10. What does a high white blood cell count indicate? _____

    _____

11. What does a low white blood cell count indicate? _____

    _____

12. What does hematocrit mean? _____

    _____

Matching Abbreviations and Meanings

Match the abbreviation in
Column A with its meaning
in Column B.

Column A

1. ABO _____
2. ANA _____
3. AST _____
4. CBC _____
5. CIN _____
6. CIS _____
7. CLL _____
8. CML _____
9. CSF _____
10. ESR _____
11. HDL _____
12. IEP _____
13. IgM _____
14. L/S ratio _____
15. LDL _____
16. MBC _____
17. MI _____
18. MIC _____
19. PCV _____
20. Rh _____
21. SBE _____
22. STS _____
23. VLDL _____
24. VMA _____

Column B

A. minimum inhibitory concentration

B. minimum bactericidal concentration

C. blood types

D. Rh factor in the blood

E. subacute bacterial endocarditis

F. serological test for syphilis

G. antinuclear antibodies

H. complete blood count

I. packed cell volume

J. chronic lymphocytic leukemia

K. chronic myologenous leukemia

L. cerebrospinal fluid

M. erythrocyte sedimentation rate

N. aspartate aminotransferase

O. myocardial infarct

P. immunoelectrophoresis

Q. immunoglobulin M

R. high-density lipoprotein

S. low-density lipoprotein

T. very-low-density lipoprotein

U. vanillymandelic acid

V. lecithin/sphingomyelin ratio

W. carcinoma in situ

X. cervical intraepithelial neoplasia

Crossword Puzzle

Laboratory Terminology

Across

2 Bacteria appearing in long chains
5 Minimum bactericidal concentration
7 The color of Gram-positive bacteria
8 Round-shaped bacteria
9 Bacteria appearing in pairs
12 Very-low-density lipoprotein
14 The clumping together of blood cells
15 Minimum inhibitory concentration

Down

1 Serological test for syphilis
2 Bacteria appearing in clusters
3 Erythrocyte sedimentation rate
4 Complete blood count
6 Rod-shaped bacteria
7 The color of Gram-negative bacteria
10 Packed cell volume
11 The rupture of blood cells
13 Subacute bacterial endocarditis
14 Blood types

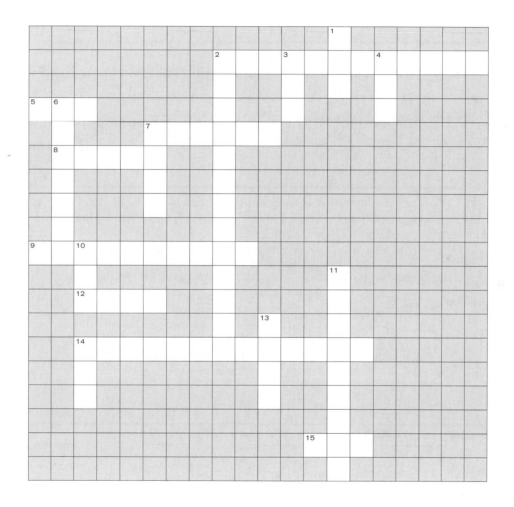

22 SURGICAL TERMINOLOGY

CHAPTER OBJECTIVES

Upon successful completion of this chapter, the student will be able to do the following:

1. Describe what is meant by perioperative care.
2. Differentiate between elective, urgent, and emergent admission.
3. Define a standard care plan and preoperative checklist.
4. Describe standard procedures in preoperative reception, patient identification, and chart preparation.
5. List and define common surgical supplies and equipment.
6. Differentiate between the following forms of anesthesia: general, local, spinal, epidural, and regional nerve block.
7. List and define common surgical positions, surgical incisions, suture material, and suturing techniques.
8. Define, pronounce, and spell common surgical terms.
9. Define abbreviations related to surgery.

WORD ELEMENTS PROMINENT IN THIS CHAPTER

ELEMENT	TYPE	MEANING	ELEMENT	TYPE	MEANING
a-; a (n) -	prefix	no; not	di-	prefix	two
-ana	prefix	again; upward	dia-	prefix	through; complete
bi/o	root	life	-ectomy	suffix	removal; excision
-centesis	suffix	surgical puncture	electr/o	root	electric
cis/o	root	to cut	endo-	prefix	within
cry/o	root	cold	epi-	prefix	upon; above
-desis	suffix	surgical binding or fusion	esthesi/o	root	sensation

ELEMENT	TYPE	MEANING		ELEMENT	TYPE	MEANING
ec-; ex-	prefix	out of		-scope	suffix	instrument used to view
filament/o	root	thread; filament		-scopy	suffix	process of viewing with the aid of an instrument
in-	prefix	in; into		sect/o	root	cut
intra-	prefix	within		-seps/o	root	infection
medi/o	root	middle		-stat	suffix	instrument used to hold something in a stable state
mono-	prefix	one				
multi-	prefix	many		-stomy	suffix	new opening
-opsy	suffix	vision		sub-	prefix	under; below
para-	prefix	beside; near		supra-	prefix	above
peri-	prefix	surrounding		-therapy	suffix	treatment
-pexy	suffix	surgical fixation		-thermy	suffix	heat
-plasty	suffix	surgical repair; reconstructive surgery		-tome	suffix	instrument to cut
post-	prefix	after		-tomy	suffix	to cut; incise
pre-	prefix	before		trans-	prefix	across
re-	prefix	back; again		-tripsy	suffix	to crush
-rrhaphy	suffix	suture				

▷ 22.1 CARE OF THE SURGICAL PATIENT

The organization of surgical departments varies greatly from hospital to hospital, but one common factor is the **surgical team,** which may include some or all of the following: medical doctors, registered nurses, operating room (OR) technicians, respiratory technologists, clerks, aides, and porters. Surgery can occur within hospitals, in outpatient settings, in emergency departments, and as day surgery. Regardless of the type of surgery or length of stay, there are three phases to the care provided: **preoperative** (prē-ŏp′-ĕr-ă-tĭv) (before surgery), **intraoperative** (ĭn″-tră-ŏp′-ĕr-ă-tĭv) (during surgery), and **postoperative** (pōst-ŏp′-ĕr-ă-tĭv) (after surgery). Together, these phases can be described as **perioperative** (pĕr″-ē-ŏp′-ĕr-ă-tĭv) patient care. Following is a brief description of common features of care for the surgical patient.

Admission

Patients requiring surgical treatment may be admitted to a health care facility on an elective, urgent, or emergency basis. An **elective admission** is preplanned, because the condition is not an emergency and the life of the patient is not in danger. An **urgent admission** is for patients requiring immediate treatment of a non-life-threatening condition. An **emergency admission** is for patients requiring immediate treatment of a condition involving risk of death or serious disability.

Standard Care Plan

Patient care follows certain standards, which are set out in a form called a **standard care plan.** This plan begins by describing all of the preoperative requirements for the patient. These requirements are set out in another form called a **preoperative checklist** (see Figure 22–1).

FIGURE 22–1

Preoperative Checklist

university hospital — **Pre-operative Checklist**

Allergies _____ Date _____ HT _____ Wt _____

Indicate with initials and a ✓ if completed:

_____ ☐ Consent to Diagnostic and Treatment Procedure form on chart

_____ ☐ Doctor's Orders record, Medication record, Patient Care record, TR record

_____ ☐ Report of History and Physical Examination

_____ ☐ Money and valuables secured

_____ ☐ Sensitivity Record on chart

_____ ☐ Consultant physicians' reports

_____ ☐ Addressograph plate with chart

_____ ☐ Patient identiband in place

_____ ☐ Nail polish, facial makeup removed

_____ ☐ Jewellery, hairpins removed

_____ ☐ Dentures and prosthetic devices removed (list prostheses)

Pre-operative assessment

_____ BP _____ T _____ P _____ R _____ (within 4 hours of surgery)

_____ Hgb result _____ Date drawn _____ (within 7 days of surgery)

_____ Cross-matched for _____

_____ Blood available in Blood Bank: ☐ Yes ☐ No Urinalysis report on chart: ☐ Yes ☐ No (within 3 days of surgery)

_____ Urine sugar _____ Urine protein _____

_____ Time and date patient last voided: _____ hr _____ (date)

_____ NPO since: _____ hr _____ (date)

Specific pre-operative orders

_____
_____
_____
_____

Special instructions to OR staff

_____
_____
_____

Initials	Signature	Initials	Signature

FIGURE 22–1

Preoperative Checklist
(concluded)

GUIDELINES FOR PRE-OPERATIVE CHECKLIST

1. Enter the current date.
2. Enter the patient's most recent height and weight.
3. Indicate completion of pre-operative routines with a checkmark (✓) in Section I of the form.
4. List any prosthetic devisces in Section I.
5. Enter pre-operative blood pressure, temperature, pulse, and respiratory rate in Section II.
6. Enter the most recent hemoglobin result, and the date it was drawn.
7. Enter the amount and type of blood products for which the patient was crossmatched.
8. Indicate the availability of blood in the blood bank by checking (✓) "Yes" or "No".
9. Indicate the presence of a urinalysis report on the chart, tested within 3 days of surgery.
10. If the urinalysis report is not available, enter the results of unit testing for Urine Sugar and Urine Protein.
11. Enter the date and time the patient last voided or indicated if urinary catheter in situ.
12. Enter the date and time the patient was placed npo (nothing by mouth).
13. List specific pre-operative orders in Section III, and indicate completion or incompletion of these orders-

    i.e. Fleet enema - given

    Shave prep - done

    NG tube - not inserted
14. Enter specific instructions to OR staff in Section IV, if applicable.
15. Sign the form, and place on patient's Chart.
16. Complete documentation of all procedures and patient responses on the Patient Care Record.

This form is a "check-off" list used to ensure that all necessary preoperative steps are performed and recorded. The checklist is retained with the patient record as a permanent summary and is utilized in the continuing assessment of the quality of care. The standard care plan also describes the requirements of the operating environment, how the patient will be transported and admitted to the operating room, the requirements of the surgical team in relation to anesthesia, the surgery to be performed, and immediate postoperative care. In all phases of perioperative care, proper aseptic guidelines must be followed to minimize the chance of wound infection. Any special requirements in this regard are recorded on the standard care form.

Preoperative Reception

The preoperative reception, or holding area, is the room the patient is taken to just prior to surgery. The patient is greeted, introduced to members of the surgical team, and made to feel comfortable. The operating room staff is aware that reassurance and support are important at this stage. The patient can derive much of the needed psychological support from simple things: not being left alone, being called by name, being asked simple questions that can be readily responded to, and given choices when possible.

Patient Identification

With patients coming and going, the possibility of the wrong surgical procedure being performed on a patient is very real unless patient identification procedures are carefully followed. Several methods of cross-checking identification are generally used. If patients are not too sedated, they are asked their name and often the name of their physician. The patient's bracelet is matched with the hospital admission form and the OR identification slip, which shows the hospital number, patient's name, and patient's physician. Patients are asked what surgery they are having to ensure that this corresponds with the information in the preoperative checklist.

Patient Chart

To ensure quality patient care and to avoid legal liability, hospitals maintain strict procedures for completing the patient chart. The preoperative checklist, which will become part of the patient chart, must be completed before the patient is admitted to the operating room. The chart accompanies the patient to the reception area. There, it is checked to ensure that all necessary items, such as laboratory reports, patient history, physical examination report, and required consent forms, are complete. The preoperative laboratory reports vary from hospital to hospital, but they usually include at least a urinalysis and blood work. The patient history and physical exam must be signed by the patient's physician. If this signature is missing, neither the patient nor the hospital have proper assurance that the intended operation is justified. Without such assurance, legal liability could result.

Consent forms (see Figure 22–2) are critically important. An operation is an assault if consent is not given and could result in criminal charges as well as liability for damages. The only exception to this rule is an emergency for which delay would increase risk. Consent means "informed consent." The patient must know the dangers of the operation in order to properly weigh the risks and benefits. Informed consent can be given only by a person who is fully aware and capable of judging the risks of an operation. A sedated patient may not be able to make such a judgment, so consent forms must be obtained by the physician before preoperative sedation is administered.

FIGURE 22–2

Consent Form

university hospital	Authorization and Consent to Diagnostic and Treatment Procedures

Patient: _____ Date: _____ Time (hours) _____

1. I hereby authorize Dr._____and/or such assistants as may be selected by that physician to perform the following procedure(s):

List procedure(s) _____

_____

on (name of patient or myself) _____

2. The procedure(s) listed in paragraph #1 have been explained to me by a physician and I understand the nature of the procedure(s).

3. I recognize that during the course of the procedure(s), unforeseen or unknown conditions may necessitate additional or different procedures than those set forth in paragraph #1. I, therefore, further authorize and request that the above named physician his/her assistants, or his/her designate, perform such procedures as are in his/her professional judgement, necessary and desirable.

4. I consent to the administration of anesthesia and to the use of such anesthetics as may be deemed advisable by the anesthetist.

5. I acknowledge that no guarantees have been made to me as to the results of the procedure(s).

Witness_____ Signature of patient _____

Second witness (if necessary) _____

See note below.

If the patient is unable to sign by reason of age, mental or physical disability, complete the following:

The patient's age is _____ years of age.

The patient is unable to sign because _____

As the parent, legal guardian (for patients under the age of majority) or legal guardian (for mentally incapacitated adults). I hereby sign on the patient's behalf.

Witness _____

Signature _____ Relationship _____

Note: indicate below the method of receiving consent, if received by telegram, letter or telephone. In case of letters or telegrams, please attach. In case of telephoned consent, there should be two witnesses' signatures obtained above.

Consent received by: letter   telegram   telephone, etc.

From (name) _____ Relationship to patient _____

Witness _____ Witness _____

III—22

22.2 COMMON SURGICAL SUPPLIES AND EQUIPMENT

Operative instruments include sharps, clamps, graspers or holders, retractors, and probes. A few examples of each are discussed below, and Table 22–1 summarizes these instruments.

TABLE 22–1 Summary of General Surgical Instruments

INSTRUMENT	DESCRIPTION	EXAMPLES
sharps	used to cut, incise, or separate tissue	scalpels, scissors, trocars, punches, chisels, osteotomes, curettes, rongeurs, dissectors, elevators, rasps, saws, drills, bone cutters
clamps	used to control bleeding and to grasp tissue	Kelly, Lower, Hemostat or snap, mosquito
graspers and holders	used to grasp or hold tissue	Kocker, Allis, Babcock, tenaculum, obstetrical forceps, iris forceps, sponge forceps, bone forceps, needle drivers
retractors and speculums	used to hold back tissue	Book-Walter, Senn, Parker, Deaver, Richardson, rake, malleable retractors, vaginal speculum, nasal speculum, rectal speculum
probes	used to explore pathological and anatomical structures	lacrimal duct probe, Hegar dilator, Hawkins dilator, Hanks dilator

Sharps

Sharps are instruments used to incise or separate tissue. Certain types of sharps are used exclusively for soft tissue, such as skin, subcutaneous tissue, muscle, and fat. Others are for tough tissue, such as bone or cartilage.

Sharps used to cut soft tissue include **scalpels** (scăl'-pĕlz), **scissors,** and **trocars** (trō-kărz). **Scalpels** and **scissors** (such as **Metzenbaum** [mĕt'-zĕn-bŏm]) cut. **Trocars** puncture a cavity.

Sharps used on bone include **chisels, osteotomes** (ŏs'-tē-ō-tōmz), **curettes** (kū-rĕts'), **rongeurs** (rŏn-zhŭrz'), **dissectors,** (dĭ-sĕk'-tŏrz) **elevators, raspatories** (răs'-pă-tō-rēz) **(rasps), bone cutters, saws,** and **drills.** Chisels are wedge-shaped, sharp-ended instruments that remove bony material. Osteotomes are bone cutters. Curettes are sharp, spoonlike instruments used to scrape out tissue. Rongeurs looks something like nutcrackers and bite into bone. Elevators are used to lift or retract bone (see Figure 22–3).

FIGURE 22–3

**Sharps (a) Metzenbaum
Scissors; (b) Curette;
(c) Rongeurs;
(d) Raspatory**

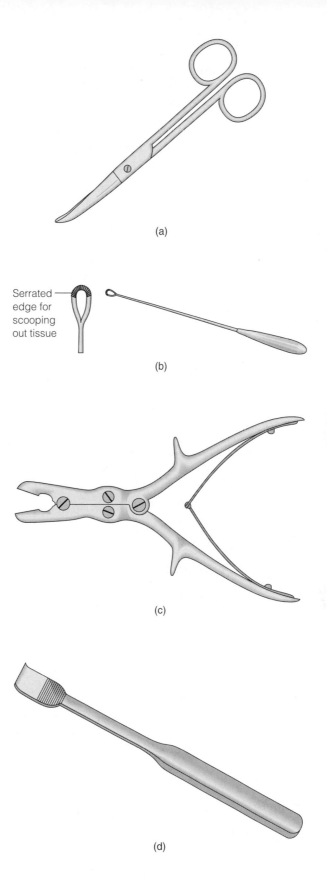

(a)

Serrated
edge for
scooping
out tissue

(b)

(c)

(d)

III–22

Clamps

Clamps are used to control bleeding and to grasp tissue. Those used to compress a blood vessel are called **hemostats** (hē'-mō-stăts) or **snaps.** A small hemostat is known as a **mosquito.** Other examples of clamps include **Kelly** and **Lower.**

Graspers or Holders

Forceps (for'-sĕps), also known as **fingers, tissues,** or **pickups,** are used to grasp or hold tissue. **Nontoothed** forceps handle delicate tissue, and **toothed forceps** handle thick or difficult-to-manage tissue. Some common forceps are **tenaculum** (tĕn-ăk'-ū-lŭm) (see Figure 22–4), **Babcock, Kocker, Allis,** and **obstetrical.** Forceps are often named for the structure they are intended to grasp. For example, iris forceps grasp the iris, sponge forceps hold sponges, needle drivers grasp and hold needles, and bone forceps grasp bone.

FIGURE 22–4

Teneculum

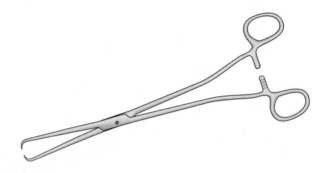

Retractors

Retractors (rē-trăk'-torz) hold back tissue from the operative site to provide a clear visual field (see Figure 22–5).

FIGURE 22–5

(a) Richardson Retractor

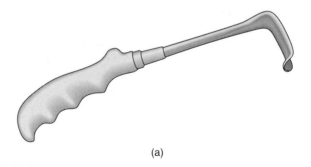

(a)

FIGURE 22–5 (concluded)

(b) Rake

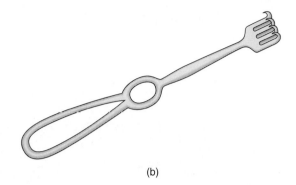

(b)

Some retractors are held in place by a member of the surgical team, while others are self-retaining, holding themselves in place by rachets, springs, or locks. Examples include **Book-Walter** (for cardiovascular procedures); **Senn** (for superficial procedures); **Parker** (for minor surgery); **Deaver** and **Richardson** (for inside the abdomen); **rake** (for minor and major surgery); and **malleable retractors,** also known as **ribbon retractors** (which can be bent into the desired shape by the surgeon and used in the abdomen and skull). A special type of retractor is the **speculum** (spĕk′-ū-lŭm), which is inserted into a body cavity. There are various types of speculums, each named after the organ into which it is inserted (vaginal speculum, rectal speculum, nasal speculum, etc.).

Probes

Probes, also known as **sounds,** are used to explore pathological and anatomical structures such as wounds and the lumen of a body part. They can also be used as **dilators** (dī′-lā-torz) to widen the diameter of an opening. Examples are lacrimal duct probes (used for stenosis of the lacrimal duct) and **Hegar** (hā′-găr), **Hawkins,** and **Hanks dilators** (used to widen the cervix uteri). See Figure 22–6.

FIGURE 22–6

Probe

Miscellaneous Surgical

See Table 22–2.

See Table 22–2.

TABLE 22–2

Miscellaneous Surgical
Equipment

TYPE OF EQUIPMENT	DEFINITION OR EXAMPLE
monitors used during anesthesia	**cardiac monitor** used to check heart function; **electrocardiograph** monitors the electrical activity of the heart; **sphygmomanometer** measures blood pressure; and **oxygen monitor analyzer** checks oxygen concentration in the blood
dermatomes	used to remove slices of skin for skin grafting; variations in the thickness of the donor skin can be obtained by adjusting the dermatome
electrosurgical units	uses an electric current to destroy tissue, to incise tissue, and to maintain hemostasis of cut blood vessels; common term is **cautery**
endoscopes	used to look inside a cavity; endoscopes are equipped with a light, scope, and power source; attachments can include a cutting instrument for the removal of tissue, electrosurgery, and suction accessories **Note:** Scopes are named after the structure being viewed. Some examples are cystoscope, arthroscope, laparoscope, bronchoscope, colonoscope, and culdoscope.
lasers	used for cutting, hemostatsis, and destruction of tissue by use of a light ray **Note:** Laser is an acronym that has been accepted as a word. It is short for light amplification by stimulated emission of radiation.
prosthetic devices	artificial devices used to temporarily or permanently replace important anatomical components **Note:** Examples of prostheses include pacemakers, arterial grafts, artificial ball and sockets for hip joints, and internal fixators such as pins, screws, and plates.
tourniquets	device used to compress an extremity, thereby temporarily stopping blood flow to it **Note:** The automatic tourniquet has a cuff connected to a supply of nontoxic, nonflammable gas that furnishes and maintains pressure.

22.3 ANESTHESIA

General anesthetics produce loss of consciousness, block pain sensation, and produce muscle relaxation. **Local anesthetics** block pain sensation to the operative site without inducing unconsciousness. **Spinal anesthetics** are injected into the subarachnoid space, blocking electrical impulses to nerve roots leading to the lower extremities, abdomen, and pelvis. **Epidural anesthesia** is often used in obstetrical surgery; the anesthesia is injected into the epidural space, acting on the abdomen and pelvis. A **regional nerve block** involves the injection of a local anesthetic into a nerve plexus, eliminating pain in a certain area. Table 22–3 lists anesthetics by classification.

TABLE 22–3 Drugs Used During Anesthesia

CLASSIFICATION	DESCRIPTION	EXAMPLES

analgesics	includes narcotics that reduce the patient's threshold of pain	narcotics:
		  morphine
		  meperidine (Demerol)
		  fentanyl (Sublimaze)
		  alfentanyl (Alfenta)
		  codeine

muscle relaxants	drugs that interfere with the transmission of nerve impulses at the myoneural junction	succinylcholine (Anectine) pancuronium (Pavulon) tubocurarine (Tubarine) atracurium (Tracrium) vecuronium (Norcuron) metocurine iodide (Metubine)
general anesthetic drugs and gases	drugs that produce analgesia, muscle relaxation, and unconsciousness; can be administered intravenously, intramuscularly, or by inhalation	**administered intravenously:** thiopental sodium (Sodium Pentothal) propofol (Diprivan) fentanyl and droperidol (Innovar) **administered intramuscularly:** ketamine hydrochloride (Ketalar) **Administered by inhalation:** nitrous oxide halothane (Fluothane) isoflurane (Forane)
local anesthetics	drugs that produce anesthesia of a localized area of tissue; the patient remains conscious	lidocaine hydrochloride (Xylocaine) bupivacaine (Marcaine) cocaine procaine hydrochloride (Novocain) tetracaine hydrochloride (Pontocaine)
spinal anesthesia	drugs injected into the subarachnoid or epidural space of the spinal cord resulting in blockage of nerve impulses at the nerve roots leading to the abdomen, pelvis, and lower extremities	bupivacaine (Marcaine) procaine hydrochloride (Novocain) tetracaine hydrochloride (Pontocaine) lidocaine hydrochloride (Xylocaine)

TABLE 22–3 Drugs Used During Anesthesia (concluded)

CLASSIFICATION	DESCRIPTION	EXAMPLES
epidural anesthesia	local anesthetic injected into the extradural space blocking pain sensation leading to the lower abdomen and pelvis; often used in obstetrical surgery	bupivacaine (Marcaine) procaine hydrochloride (Novocain) tetracaine hydrochloride (Pontocaine) lidocaine hydrochloride (Xylocaine)
regional nerve block	local anesthetic injected into the nerve plexus; covers a greater area than a localized injection to the operative site	bupivacaine (Marcaine) procaine hydrochloride (Novocain) tetracaine hydrochloride (Pontocaine) lidocaine hydrochloride (Xylocaine)

▶ 22.4 SURGICAL POSITIONS

Table 22–4 describes the various surgical positions.

TABLE 22–4

Surgical Positions

POSITION	DESCRIPTION
Fowler (sitting position)	patient in a seated position with back angle half way between vertical and horizontal (45°); **semifowler position** lowers the back to 30° angle from horizontal; used for some shoulder procedures and in the recovery room

lateral decubitus	lying on side with arms stretched out

TABLE 22–4

Surgical Positions
(concluded)

POSITION	DESCRIPTION
lithotomy position	lying face up with lower body in sitting position, knees supported or suspended by stirrups; used for hemorrhoidectomies and gynecological procedures

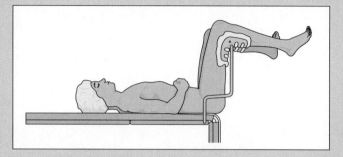

POSITION	DESCRIPTION
prone position	lying face down; used for back surgery and heel surgery

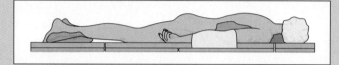

POSITION	DESCRIPTION
supine position; dorsal recumbent	lying face up, head straight; most common surgical position

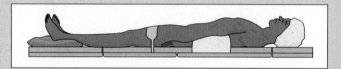

POSITION	DESCRIPTION
Trendelenburg	patient lying face up, knees slightly flexed, head and feet below height of knees

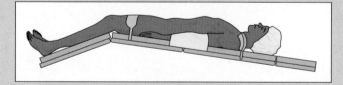

Note: Used for fallopian tube clipping and vaginal hysterectomies; this position is preferred as the gut is temporarily moved from the pelvis.

Types of incisions are shown in Figure 22–7.

FIGURE 22–7

Types of Incisions

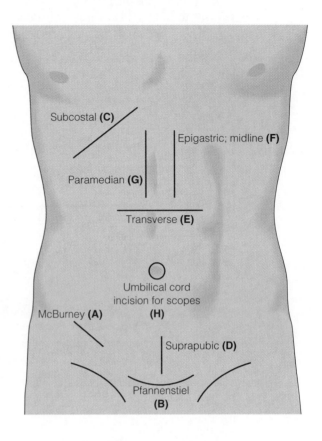

An incision is a cut. Several layers of tissue must be cut to get to an organ or cavity. For example, to reach the abdominal organs, the surgeon must cut through the skin, subcutaneous tissue, fascia, muscle, and peritoneum (See Figure 22–8).

FIGURE 22–8

Abdominal Wall Layers

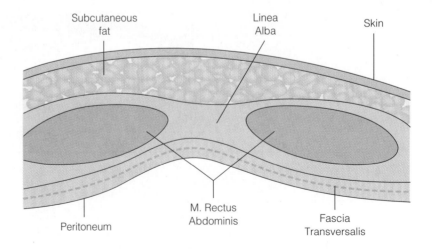

Different types of incisions are used for different operations. They include the following:

McBurney - incision above McBurney's point. Used to reach the appendix.

Pfannenstiel (făn'-ĕn-stēl) - curved abdominal incision just above the symphysis pubis. Used in gynecological surgery to reach the uterus, fallopian tubes, and ovaries.

right and left subcostal (sŭb-kŏs'-tăl) - incision below the ribs. The right subcostal is used to reach the gallbladder and biliary tract. The left subcostal is used to reach the spleen.

suprapubic (soo"-pră-pū-bĭk) - incision above the symphysis pubis.

transverse - incision across the abdomen.

epigastric (ĕp-ĭ-găs'-trĭk); **midline** - incision in the midline above the umbilicus, adjacent to the stomach. Used to reach the stomach, duodenum, and pancreas.

paramedian (păr"-ă-mē'-dē-ăn) - incision beside the midline. Used to reach pelvic structures and colon.

22.6 SUTURING

Sutures and Suture Material

As a noun, the term **suture** (sū'-chūr) refers to the material used to sew up a wound or tie a blood vessel. As a verb, it describes the sewing of a wound or tying of a blood vessel.

No single suture material is appropriate for all tissue, but all suture material should be easy to handle, strong for its caliber, low in irritation to the body, sterile, nonshrinking, nonconducting, not conducive to bacterial growth, and of consistent diameter and strength.

Sutures designed to be absorbed by the body over time are called **absorbable sutures**. Sutures that cannot be absorbed are referred to as **nonabsorbable**.

Some sutures consist of a single strand and are referred to as **monofilament** sutures. Others consist of several strands braided together and are referred to as **multifilament** sutures.

Among the types described are many varieties. No one variety is used by all surgeons for similar procedures. The variety chosen for a particular procedure depends on its suitability given the patient's condition and the surgeon's preference.

Absorbable Sutures   Absorbable sutures can be **natural** or **synthetic.** Natural absorbable sutures are called **catgut** and are made from the collagen of mammals. Strength varies with the amount of collagen used. Catgut can be treated with chromium salts to increase strength and prolong the absorption rate. Treated catgut is called **chromic catgut,** while untreated is called **plain catgut. Synthetic absorbable sutures** are made from nonanimal materials.

Nonabsorbable Sutures   Nonabsorbable sutures resist being broken down by the action of living tissue. They can be natural or synthetic. Natural nonabsorbable sutures include silk, cotton, linen, and stainless steel wires. Synthetic nonabsorbable sutures include nylon, polyester, and polypropylene.

Suture Size and Strength The caliber or diameter of the suture material is stated numerically as 3-0, 4-0, 5-0, etc. The bigger the first number is, the smaller the suture diameter. Therefore 5-0 is smaller than 4-0, and 4-0 is smaller than 3-0. Suture size can also be written as 3/0, 4/0, and 5/0.

Clips and Staples

Although suturing is essential for certain procedures, clips and staples are safe, effective, and fast alternatives in many cases.

Clips Clips are used to tie small structures such as veins, arteries, and nerves. Clips offer significant advantages over sutures in terms of speed and ease of use. Thus, when bleeding must be controlled quickly, or when the structure to be tied is deep or difficult to reach, clips are the method of choice.

Clips come in both absorbable and nonabsorbable forms. The absorbable types are made of synthetic, nonmetallic material designed to maintain strength until healing occurs. Over time, the clip dissolves. Absorbable clips are sterile and do not produce tissue irritation of any significance. They do not show up on x-ray or CT scans, which is advantageous in postoperative assessment.

Nonabsorbable clips are used when intended to be removed later or when a permanent clipping of a structure is desired. They are made of steel, titanium, or tantalum and thus do appear on x-rays and CT scans.

Staples Like clips, staples are advantageous because they can be used to close a wound quickly, thus reducing the time the patient is anesthetized. Their use can also minimize tissue damage because less handling of the tissue is required.

Staples are applied with a stapler and may be used on the skin for wound closure (see Figure 22–9).

FIGURE 22–9

Skin Stapler

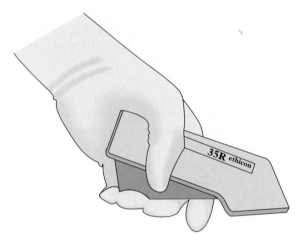

Staples can result in less scarring than suturing on certain wounds. They are also used for anastomosis (joining parts of an organ not normally joined). For example, when a section of intestine must be removed, staples are used to join the remaining intestine.

Staples in the skin are removed with an extractor, which is a device that has a small tongue that fits between the skin surface and staple top. When the handle of the extractor is squeezed, a small lever is pushed down on the top of the staple, indenting it so it looks like a "3." This indenting action pulls the bottom prongs of the staple out of the skin, allowing removal without tissue damage.

Common Suturing Techniques

Bringing the edges of a wound together is called **approximation.** This term refers to the sewing up of tissues such as skin, muscle, fat, etc. The term **ligate** (lī′-gāt) (to tie) refers to blood vessels. The blood vessel is said to be **ligated,** and the suture material used to tie the blood vessel is called a **ligature** (lĭg′-ă-chūr). There are various ways of ligating and approximating tissues.

Ligating can involve the tying of a blood vessel with a **free tie,** a solitary strand of suture material placed around the blood vessel, which is held by a Hemostat; the free tie is tightened and knotted, thus occluding the vessel. A **stick tie** is one in which a needle attached to suture material is used to secure the suture material to the tissue before occlusion of the blood vessel.

The sutures that hold the edges of an incision in approximation form what is called the **primary suture line.** Sometimes, a **secondary suture line,** also known as **retention sutures, tension sutures,** or **stay sutures,** is also needed. This secondary line of sutures, typically one to two inches on either side of the primary suture, lends support to the primary line. It eases the tension on the primary sutures, thus reducing the chance of a **dehiscence,** (dē-hĭs′-ĕns), the splitting open of the operative incision.

Suturing techniques are simply different ways of sewing together two edges of a wound, with different stitches used depending upon the need. Common suturing techniques include the **continuous, interrupted, mattress, purse-string, subcuticular,** (sŭb-kū-tĭk′-ū-lăr), and **retention.** Each describes the method in which two edges of the wound are approximated.

Continuous suture - single thread is used to close the entire wound. There is a knot at the beginning and end of the suture. The suture line is uninterrupted (see Figure 22–10).

FIGURE 22–10

Continuous Suture

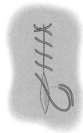

Interrupted sutures - each suture is separated and isolated by a knot (see Figure 22–11).

FIGURE 22–11

Interrupted Sutures

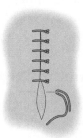

Mattress sutures - two types, horizontal and vertical. The horizontal involves stitches that run parallel to the wound, passing under the surface to be tied off on the other side. The vertical mattress passes beneath and over the surface of the wound in both deep and shallow bites (see Figure 22–12).

FIGURE 22–12

Mattress Sutures

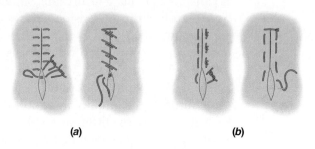

(a)　　　　　　　*(b)*

Over-and over sutures - the edges of the wound are approximated by piercing the skin an equal distance on either side of the wound. The needle is placed into the skin on one side and pulled out on the other. Can be continuous or interrupted.

Subcuticular sutures - following the line of the wound, the edges of the skin are approximated by placing the stitches just under the skin. Can be continuous or interrupted (see Figure 22–13).

FIGURE 22–13

Subcuticular Sutures

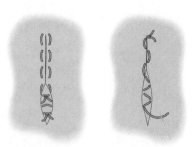

Purse-string sutures - continuous suture around a circular wound, acting like a draw-string (see Figure 22–14).

FIGURE 22–14

Purse-String Sutures

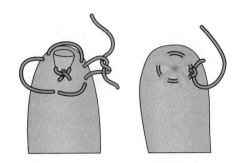

22.7 DRAINS, DRESSINGS, AND BANDAGES

Drains

Drains are used during or following an operation to remove air or fluids (serum, blood, lymph, pus, bile, intestinal secretions) from the operative site and to prevent a deep wound infection. The drain is inserted directly into the incision or into a separate wound, called a **stab wound,** near the incision.

Examples of drains are the **Levin's tube** (inserted into the stomach through the nose, to drain stomach contents); **Hemovac** and **Saratoga Sump** (drains blood); **Penrose drain** (drains blood or fluid); **T-tube** (drains bile following exploration of the commone bile duct); and the **Foley catheter** (drains the urinary bladder).

Dressings and Bandages

The simplest type of dressing is gauze held in place by tape. Other examples include Elastoplast, plaster of Paris, stockinette, teflon strips, skin tapes, flannel, and pads.

▶ 22.8 LIST OF COMMON SURGERIES

There are hundreds of surgeries performed on each system. The following list in Table 22–5 is only a partial list of the more common surgical procedures.

TABLE 22–5

Common Surgical Procedures

SYSTEM OR ORGAN	PROCEDURES
breast	simple mastectomy, radical mastectomy, lumpectomy, biopsy, reduction mammoplasty, augmentation mammoplasty
cardiovascular	mitral valvulotomy, valve replacement, coronary artery bypass, percutaneous transluminal coronary angioplasty, laparoscopy, endarterectomy, pacemakers, heart transplants
ears, nose, and throat	submucous resection, stapedectomy, tympanoplasty, tonsillectomy and adenoidectomy, myringotomy and insertion of tubes, Caldwell Luc
gynecological	abdominal and vaginal hysterectomy, salpingo-oophorectomy, colporrhaphy, cesarean section, laparoscopy, tubal ligation, tubal clipping, hysteroscopy, dilation of the cervix and curettage (D&C) of the uterus, laparoscopic assisted surgery
abdominal	laparotomy, laparoscopy partial gastrectomy, gastroenterostomy, pyloroplasty, pyloromyotomy, hemicolectomy, colostomy, hemorrhoidectomy, herniorrhaphy, cholecystectomy, choledochotomy, appendectomy
nervous	craniotomy, discectomy, neuroanastomosis
eye	strabismus repair, cataract extraction with lens implant, repair retinal detachment, corneal transplant, laser surgery
orthopedics	reduction of fractures, hip and knee replacements, arthroplasty, arthrodesis, arthroscopy, bunionectomy, meniscectomy, tenotomy, laminectomy, bone grafts
thoracic	tracheostomy, pneumonectomy, lobectomy
transplants	heart transplants, corneal transplants, bone marrow transplant, kidney transplant
urology	nephrectomy, pyelolithotomy, lithotripsy, nephrolithotomy, nephrostomy, ureterolithotomy, ureterosigmoidostomy, ureteroileostomy, ureterostomy, lithotripsy, cystoscopy, cystectomy, transurethral prostatectomy, circumcision, vasectomy, vas anastomosis, orchidopexy, orchiectomy

See Table 22–6

TABLE 22–6

Miscellaneous
Terminology

TERM	DESCRIPTION
ambulatory care	care provided to the patient without hospitalization
amputation	removal of a portion or all of the extremity
anastomosis	surgical joining of two structures that are normally separate, following removal of the part that formerly joined them
asepsis	free from infectious contamination
biopsy	removal of a piece of living tissue for microscopic examination
diathermy	use of an electric current to coagulate blood vessels and thus stop bleeding; it also destroys or cuts tissue (also known as **cautery**)
circulating nurse	usually a registered nurse **Note:** With the medical doctor, a circulating nurse is responsible for patient safety and for ensuring that supplies and equipment are ready perioperatively.
conization; cone biopsy	removal of a cone-shaped piece of tissue; often used to remove a piece of uterine tissue for biopsy
day surgery	a scheduled procedure on an outpatient basis; the patient is discharged on the same calendar day as admitted
decompression	release of pressure from a specific body area such as the brain or abdomen
dehiscence	splitting open of a surgical incision following closure (a retention suture is used to prevent this complication)
disarticulation	amputation through a joint
dissection	separation of body parts
draping	placement of a thick sheet (drape) over the operative site, with an opening over the incision for accessibility; the purpose of the drape is to reduce the chance of infection
emergency department	area in the hospital for treating patients who need immediate care for a life-threatening or potentially disabling condition

III–22

TABLE 22–6

Miscellaneous Terminology (continued)

TERM	DESCRIPTION
endoscopic surgery	surgery that utilizes an endoscope to allow visual examination of the internal cavities of the body; the endoscope is often equipped with accessories such as a light, knife, biopsy forceps, suction, electrosurgery devices, or a videocamera that provides a clear picture of the internal structures
	Note: One type of endoscope, a **laparoscope,** facilitates the visual examination of the abdominal cavity during surgery. A laparoscope may be used in the removal of the appendix, gallbladder, and bowel, and the procedures are called laparoscopic appendectomy, cholecystectomy, and bowel resection, respectively.
	Other endoscopic surgeries include bronchoscopy, gastroscopy, sigmoidoscopy, arthroscopy, ophthalmoscopy, otoscopy, cystoscopy, and culdoscopy.
	Advantages of this type of surgery includes a minimal length of stay of 1–2 days, reduced recovery period, less pain as a result of smaller incisions, and decreased risk of complication
	An enhancement to the laparoscopic surgery is the use of the laser for dissection and removal of normal and abnormal structures.
ennucleation	removal of the eyeball
evisceration	protrusion of viscera outside of the abdominal cavity, particularly through an operative incision
fulguration	electrical destruction of tissue
intraoperative	during surgery
laceration	an open wound with jagged edges
laser surgery	a narrow beam of light energy is absorbed by tissue, resulting in the tissue's vaporization without the destruction of adjacent tissue
	Note: The heat from the laser is used to coagulate, destroy, and dissect tissue and is employed in such surgery as abdominal, ophthalmic, orthopedic, gynecological, and urinary.
ligation and stripping	method of removing varicose veins in the legs in which the veins are cut, tied, and removed
minimally invasive surgery	an alternative to the traditional open cavity surgery, in which a procedure such as a hysterectomy, tubal ligation, cholecystectomy, or nephrectomy can be performed by insertion of a laparoscope through a single incision
operating room suite	surgical area of the hospital
	Note: The term includes operating room theaters, ancillary rooms for storage and supply, and the recovery room.
operating room theater	a room within the operating room suite where the surgery is carried out; also known as operating room (OR) or theater
outpatient department	provides treatment to patients who do not require an overnight stay

TABLE 22–6

Miscellaneous
Terminology (concluded)

TERM	DESCRIPTION
patient	an individual under treatment; may or may not be admitted to hospital
perioperative	before, during, and after surgery
postoperative	after surgery
preoperative	before surgery
punch biopsy	a circular piece of tissue taken for microscopic examination
scrub	a hand wash lasting a prescribed length of time of 3 to 5 minutes **Note:** Special cleansing products are used to scrub from finger tips to elbows.
scrub nurse	controls the instruments during a surgical procedure
skin preparations	procedure to reduce the chance of postoperative infection **Note:** The body hair near the surgical site is shaved or clipped as near to the surgical time as possible. The surgical site is then washed with an antibacterial solution.
resection	excision of all or a part of an organ or structure
transection	to cut across

III–22

22.10 ABBREVIATIONS

ABBREVIATION	MEANING	ABBREVIATION	MEANING
BSO	bilateral salpingo-oophorectomy	OR	operating room
C & D	cystoscopy and dilation	PARR	postanesthetic recovery room
D & C	dilation and curettage	preop; pre-op	preoperative
ECBD	exploration of common bile duct	prep	prepared
ECCE	extracapsular cataract extraction	postop; post-op	postoperative
endo	endoscopy	SMR	submucous resection
EUA	examination under anesthesia	S/R	suture removal
GA	general anesthesia	T&A	tonsillectomy and adenoidectomy
I & D	incision and drainage	TA	therapeutic abortion
IUD	intrauterine device	TAH	total abdominal hysterectomy
MUA	manipulation under anesthesia	TUR	transurethral resection
		TURP	transurethral resection of prostate

Defining Surgical Terms

Although you will not find the
following terms defined in
this chapter, you should be
able to write definitions for
those you encountered in
previous chapters. Write
simplified definitions for
unfamiliar terms by recalling
the meanings of the word
elements that make them
up.

*Answers to the exercises in this
chapter are found in Appendix A.*

1. abdominocentesis _____

2. adenoidectomy _____

3. adrenalectomy _____

4. aneurysmectomy _____

5. angioplasty _____

6. appendectomy _____

7. arthrodesis _____

8. arthroplasty _____

9. arthroscopy _____

10. blepharopexy _____

11. bronchoscopy _____

12. bursectomy _____

13. cecopexy _____

14. cheilorrhaphy _____

15. cholecystectomy _____

16. cholelithotomy _____

17. colectomy _____

18. colonoscopy _____

19. colostomy _____

20. colporrhaphy _____

21. culdocentesis _____

22. culdoscopy _____

23. cystoscopy _____

24. cystotomy _____

25. dermatoplasty _____

26. duodenorrhaphy _____

27. endarterectomy _____

28. enterocolostomy _____

29. enterostomy _____

30. episiorrhaphy _____

31. episiotomy _____

32. fasciectomy _____

33. funduscopy _____

34. ganglionectomy _____

35. gastrectomy _____

36. glossorrhaphy _____

37. hemicolectomy _____

38. hemihepatectomy _____

39. hemorrhoidectomy _____

40. herniorrhaphy _____

41. hypophysectomy _____

42. hysterectomy _____

43. hysteropexy _____

44. iliectomy _____

45. iridectomy _____

46. laminectomy _____

47. laparoscopy _____

48. laparotomy _____

49. laryngectomy _____

50. ligamentopexy _____

51. lithotripsy _____

52. lobectomy _____

53. lumpectomy _____

54. mammoplasty _____

55. mastectomy _____

56. maxillotomy _____

57. meatotomy _____

58. meniscectomy _____

59. metacarpectomy _____

60. myringotomy _____

61. nephrectomy _____

62. nephrolithotomy _____

63. nephropexy _____

64. nephrostomy _____

65. oophorectomy _____

66. oophoropexy _____

67. ophthalmoscopy _____

68. orchiopexy _____

69. otoplasty   _____

70. otoscopy   _____

71. ovariocentesis   _____

72. palatoplasty   _____

73. pancreatectomy   _____

74. parathyroidectomy   _____

75. patellectomy   _____

76. perineorrhaphy   _____

77. peritoneoscopy   _____

78. pleurocentesis   _____

79. pneumonectomy   _____

80. prostatectomy   _____

81. pyelolithotomy   _____

82. pyloromyotomy   _____

83. pyloroplasty   _____

84. rhinoplasty   _____

85. salpingectomy   _____

86. salpingo-oophorectomy   _____

87. salpingopexy   _____

88. sigmoidoscopy   _____

89. sinusotomy   _____

90. splenorrhaphy   _____

91. stapedectomy   _____

92. stomatoplasty   _____

93. tarsectomy   _____

94. tenodesis   _____

95. tenorrhaphy   _____

96. tenotomy   _____

97. thoracentesis; thoracocentesis _____

98. thoracoplasty   _____

99. thoracotomy   _____

100. thrombectomy   _____

101. thyroidectomy   _____

102. tonsillectomy   _____

103. tracheostomy _____

104. tracheotomy _____

105. tympanocentesis _____

106. ureteroileostomy _____

107. ureterolithotomy _____

108. ureterosigmoidostomy _____

109. ureterostomy _____

110. valvulotomy _____

111. vasectomy _____

112. venovenostomy _____

113. ventriculotomy _____

Write the terms that correspond with the following abbreviations.

114. BSO _____

115. C&D _____

116. D&C _____

117. endo _____

118. EUA _____

119. ECCE _____

120. GA _____

121. ECBD _____

122. I&D _____

123. IUD _____

124. MUA _____

125. OR _____

126. PARR _____

127. prep _____

128. preop; pre-op _____

129. postop; post-op _____

130. SMR _____

131. S/R _____

132. T&A _____

133. TA _____

134. TAH _____

135. TURP _____

136. TUR _____

III–22

Short Answer

Briefly answer the following questions.

1. What single term describes the preoperative, intraoperative, and postoperative phases of surgery? _____

2. What term describes the admission of a patient requiring immediate treatment of a non-life-threatening condition? _____

3. What is the purpose of an analgesic? _____

   _____

4. What three methods are available for administration of general anesthetics? _____

   _____

5. What term describes a sitting position for the surgical patient? _____

   _____

6. What term describes the incision used for an appendectomy? _____

   _____

7. Define suture. _____

   _____

8. What term describes the most common surgical position? _____

   _____

9. What term describes bringing the edges of a wound together? _____

   _____

10. What is a purse-string suture? _____

    _____

11. To what does dehiscence refer? _____

    _____

12. What is the purpose of draping? _____

    _____

Matching Terms with Meanings

Match the term in Column A with its meaning in Column B.

Column A		Column B
1. ambulatory care	_____	A. splitting open of a surgical incision following closure
2. anastomosis	_____	B. a scheduled procedure on an outpatient basis
3. asepsis	_____	C. removal of the eyeball
4. circulating nurse	_____	D. care provided to the patient without hospitalization
5. day surgery	_____	E. the person responsible for readying surgical supplies and equipment
6. decompression	_____	
7. dehiscence	_____	f. surgical joining of two structures normally separate
8. disarticulation	_____	G. during surgery
9. ennucleation	_____	H. free from infectious contamination
10. intraoperative	_____	I. release of pressure from a specific body area
		J. amputation through a joint

Match the items in Column A with the items in Column B. Use each letter as many times as required.

Column A		Column B
11. Senn	_____	A. sharps
12. osteotome	_____	B. graspers or holders
13. Hanks dilator	_____	C. retractors and speculums
14. trocar	_____	D. probes
15. Babcock	_____	E. clamps
16. curette	_____	
17. rake	_____	
18. mosquito	_____	
19. forceps	_____	
20. rongeur	_____	

Spelling Practice

Spelling

Place a check mark beside all misspelled words in the list that follows. Correctly spell those that you checked off.

1. interoperative ☐ _____

2. scapal ☐ _____

3. Metsenbaum ☐ _____

4. tenaculum ☐ _____

5. dilaters ☐ _____

6. curretes ☐ _____

7. dermotome ☐ _____

8. endasope ☐ _____

9. tournequet ☐ _____

10. Novocaine ☐ _____

11. Marcaine ☐ _____

12. Tendelburg ☐ _____

13. MacBurney ☐ _____

14. Pfanenstiel ☐ _____

15. monafilament ☐ _____

16. dehisence ☐ _____

17. angioplasty ☐ _____

18. ascepsis ☐ _____

19. disection ☐ _____

20. enucleation ☐ _____

Medical Terms in Context

Define the underlined terms as they are used in context.

UNIVERSITY HOSPITAL ✚   OPERATIVE REPORT

DATE: FEBRUARY 08, 1995

PREOPERATIVE DIAGNOSIS: RIGHT-SIDED <u>L4-5 HERNIATED NUCLEUS PULPOSUS</u>

OPERATION PROPOSED: RIGHT-SIDED L4-5 <u>DISCECTOMY</u>

OPERATIVE INDICATIONS:

This lady has had ongoing pain in the right leg that has failed to subside. <u>CT scan</u> showed a huge disk herniation. She was offered surgery.

OPERATIVE PROCEDURE:

Under <u>general anesthesia,</u> the patient in the <u>prone</u> position with appropriate padding. After <u>prepping</u> and <u>draping,</u> a <u>midline incision</u> was made and <u>dissection</u> carried down the right side of the <u>spinous processes</u> of L4-5. Small <u>laminotomy</u> was performed, and an extremely inflamed <u>nerve root</u> was identified sitting behind a detached piece of disc. This was removed and the disc space explored; there was no further disc material evident.

At this stage, the wound was irrigated, the nerve root was completely free. A sponge was placed over the laminotomy site, and the wound was closed in layers with <u>chromic catgut</u> to the <u>fascia</u> and <u>subcutaneous tissues</u> and <u>staples</u> to the skin. <u>Sterile</u> dressing was applied, and the patient returned to the recovery room in satisfactory condition.

POST-OPERATIVE DIAGNOSIS: BACK PAIN, RIGHT LEG <u>SCIATICA</u>

OPERATION PERFORMED: RIGHT-SIDED L4-5 DISCECTOMY

SIGNATURE OF DOCTOR IN CHARGE _____

---

1. L4–5 herniated nucleus pulposus _____

2. discectomy _____

3. CT scan _____

4. general anesthesia _____

5. prone position _____

6. prepping _____

7. draping _____

8. midline incision _____

9. dissection _____

10. spinous processes _____

11. laminotomy _____

12. nerve root _____

13. chromic catgut _____

14. fascia _____

15. subcutaneous tissues _____

16. staples _____

17. sterile _____

18. sciatica _____

Crossword Puzzle

Surgical Instruments

Across

3 Instruments used to hold back tissue
5 Instruments used to cut tissue
9 Instruments used to look inside cavities

Down

1 Instruments used to remove slices of skin
2 Instruments used to hold tissues
4 Instruments used to control bleeding
6 Sounds
7 Light amplification by stimulated emission of radiation
8 Devices used to temporarily stop blood flow to an extremity

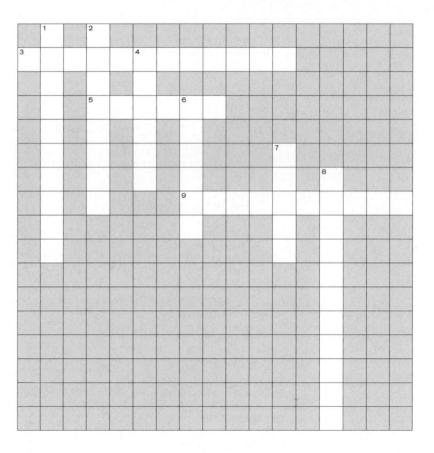

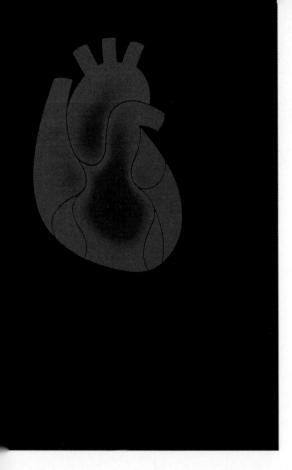

APPENDIXES

ANSWERS TO EXERCISES

CHAPTER 1

Exercise 1–1

1. root
2. prefix
3. -ous
4. pertaining to
5. around

Exercise 1–2

1. T
2. F
3. T
4. T
5. F

Exercise1–3

1. nares
2. psychoses
3. fundi
4. fungi
5. glomeruli
6. viruses
7. maxillae
8. diverticula
9. fornices
10. carcinomata, carcinomas
11. diagnosis
12. malleolus
13. sinus
14. os coxa
15. meatus
16. petechia
17. acetabulum
18. meniscus
19. ganglion
20. thorax

CHAPTER 2

Exercise 2–1

1. pain
2. hernia
3. pain
4. dilation
5. condition of the blood
6. condition
7. inflammation
8. stone
9. dissolution
10. enlargement
11. tumor
12. abnormal increase
13. disease
14. deficiency
15. unreasonable fear

Exercise 2–2

1. disease process
2. paralysis
3. prolapse
4. bursting forth
5. flow
6. rupture
7. -sclerosis
8. -stenosis
9. -rrhexis
10. any one of the following answers is acceptable: -emia;
    -iasis; -osis
11. -stenosis
12. -ptosis
13. -rrhagia
14. -rrhea

Exercise 2–3

1. a written record
2. surgical puncture to remove fluid
3. instrument used to produce a written record
4. process of making a written record
5. study
6. measure
7. -opsy
8. pcxy
9. -centesis
10. -plasty
11. -meter
12. -tome
13. -rrhaphy
14. -scope
15. -scopy
16. -stasis

Exercise 2–4

1. immature
2. cell
3. study
4. to eat or swallow
5. specialist
6. producing
7. -genous
8. -oid
9. -trophy
10. -pnea
11. -ac; -al; -ar; -ary; -eal; -ic; -ior; -ose; -ous; tic

Exercise 2–5

1. E	8. I	15. P
2. J	9. D	16. R
3. H	10. B	17. L
4. F	11. O	18. M
5. A	12. Q	19. N
6. G	13. S	20. T
7. C	14. K	

Exercise 2–6

1. -dynia, -algia
2. -itis
3. -cele
4. -oma
5. -oid
6. -phobia
7. -emesis
8. -plegia
9. -meter
10. -ptosis
11. -tome
12. -desis
13. -scope
14. -gram
15. -opsy
16. -plasty
17. -ectomy
18. -pexy
19. -centesis
20. -ostomy
21. abnormal condition

22. written record
23. formation; development
24. suture
25. process of writing
26. new opening
27. instrument used in making a written record
28. to eat or swallow
29. rupture
30. stopping or controlling
31. process of visual examination with an instrument
32. study of
33. process of incising
34. producing
35. a cutting instrument
36. stone
37. breathing
38. destruction; separation; breakdown
39. spitting
40. blood condition
41. through 55.
    Check marks should be next to 42, 44, 47, 48, 50, 53, and 55.

Exercise 2–7

1.	cardiopathy	disease
2.	gastralgia	pain
3.	cystocele	hernia
4.	otodynia	pain
5.	nephrectasis	dilation, stretching
6.	ischemia	blood condition
7.	nephrolith	stone
8.	hepatosplenomegaly	enlargement
9.	osteoma	tumor
10.	hyperplasia	development, formation
11.	hemostasis	stopping, controlling
12.	dysuria	urine
13.	carcinogenic	producing
14.	lithoid	resembling
15.	endogenous	produced by
16.	dermatosclerosis	hardening
17.	arthritis	inflammation
18.	electrolysis	destruction
19.	leukocytosis	abnormal increase
20.	leukopenia	deficiency
21.	quadriplegia	paralysis
22.	leukorrhea	discharge
23.	arteriostenosis	narrowing
24.	blepharoptosis	drooping
25.	odontorrhagia	bursting forth
26.	hypochondriasis	abnormal condition
27.	hypertrophy	development
28.	abdominocentesis	surgical puncture
29.	spondylodesis	surgical fusion

Exercise 2–8

1. cardiac
2. renal
3. tonsillar
4. mammary
5. pharyngeal
6. gastric
7. anterior

8. adipose
9. venous
10. necrotic

CHAPTER 3

Exercise 3–1

1. mamm/o; mast/o
2. (any two) cutaneo; dermo; dermato
3. cervic/o
4. cephalgia; cephalodynia
5. thorac/o
6. pertaining to the skin; pertaining to the nose
7. ophthalm/o

Exercise 3–2

1. Angi/o refers to any vessel; arteri/o refers specifically to artery.
2. Arthr/o means joint; oste/o means bone.
3. Cyst/o means bladder; cyt/o means cell.
4. Enter/o refers to the small intestine; col/o refers to the large intestine.
5. Gastr/o means stomach; abdomin/o means abdomen.
6. card/i/o
7. col/o
8. cost/o
9. cyst/o
10. cyt/o
11. enter/o
12. gastr/o
13. gloss/o; lingu/o

Exercise 3–3

1. Hem/o means blood; hepat/o means liver.
2. Hist/o means tissue; hyster/o means uterus.
3. My/o means muscle; myel/o refers to the spinal cord or bone marrow.
4. nephr/o
5. oste/o
6. neur/o
7. ven/o; phleb/o
8. pneumon/o; pulmon/o
9. oophor/o
10. blood tumor (contusion; bruise)
11. graphic representation of bone marrow (bone marrow x-ray)
12. pertaining to the vertebrae
13. pertaining to the internal organs
14. blood in the urine

Exercise 3–4

1. abdomen
2. head
3. neck
4. skull
5. skin
6. skin
7. breast
8. breast
9. nose
10. nose
11. ear
12. mouth
13. chest
14. gland
15. vessel
16. artery
17. joint
18. heart
19. brain
20. cartilage
21. large intestine
22. rib
23. bladder
24. cell
25. small intestine
26. stomach
27. tongue
28. blood
29. liver
30. tissue
31. uterus
32. spinal cord or bone marrow
33. kidney
34. nerve
35. ovary
36. bone
37. vein
38. lung
39. kidney
40. spinal column
41. testicles
42. vein
43. vertebrae
44. internal organs
45. nas/o; rhin/o
46. thorac/o
47. abdomin/o
48. cutane/o; derm/o; dermat/o
49. aden/o
50. arteri/o
51. cerebr/o
52. col/o
53. cyt/o
54. neur/o
55. hem/o
56. hist/o
57. oste/o
58. pneumon/o; pulmon/o
59. spin/o
60. myel/o
61. ven/o; phleb/o
62. vertebr/o
63. incision into the skull
64. instrument for incising the skull
65. discharge from the ear
66. device for visually examining the eye
67. process of visually examining the eye with an ophthalmoscope
68. inflammation of the nasal passages
69. pertaining to the chest
70. pertaining to the skin
71. inflammation of a vessel or vessels
72. tumor in a vessel
73. pertaining to the heart

74. pain in a joint
75. inflammation of the large intestine
76. breast x-ray
77. pain in a joint
78. pertaining to the mouth
79. pertaining to the skin
80. pertaining to the brain
81. surgical puncture of the chest cavity
82. pertaining to the ribs
83. inflammation of the breast
84. disease of a gland
85. process of visually examining the urinary bladder with a cystoscope
86. bursting forth (hemorrhage) from the eye
87. discharge (bleeding) from the eye
88. erythro   red (blood cells)
89. gastr   stomach
90. hem   blood
91. histo   tissue
92. leuko   white
93. neuro   nerve
94. oophor   ovary
95. osteo   bone
96. ven   vein
97. myelo   bone marrow

Exercise 3–5

1. M	7. P	12. G
2. J	8. C	13. O
3. N	9. F	14. K
4. A	10. L	15. I
5. E	11. D	16. H
6. B		

Exercise 3–6

1. hepatitis
2. cardiology
3. cervical
4. abdominal
5. adenoma
6. angiography
7. arterial
8. arthritis
9. otitis
10. chondromalacia
11. cephalgia; cephalodynia
12. mastectomy
13. thoracotomy
14. dermatitis
15. angiogram
16. myelocele
17. ophthalmoscopy
18. colonic
19. costovertebral
20. thoracocentesis; thoracentesis
21. arthroscopy
22. cytology
23. nasal
24. enteritis

Exercise 3–7

Mispelled words (correct spellings in parentheses):
4 (hypoglossal), 5 (hemolysis), 7 (ophthalmoscope), 9 (myelogram), and 10 (vertebral)

CHAPTER 4

Exercise 4–1

1. E	7. F	13. B
2. C	8. I	14. D
3. J	9. G	15. C
4. A	10. B	16. E
5. D	11. A	17. F
6. H	12. G	

Exercise 4–2

1. two
2. half
3. under
4. outside
5. around
6. within
7. in; into
8. self
9. apart; backward; up
10. bad
11. tri-
12. contra-
13. con-
14. peri-
15. brady-
16. tachy-
17. sub-
18. ad-
19. ab-
20. multi-; poly-

Exercise 4–3

1. immature
2. contralateral
3. antenatal
4. abduction
5. tachycardia
6. synarthrotic
7. pancarditis
8. monocyte
9. indigestible
10. microencephaly

CHAPTER 5

Exercise 5–1

1. B	13. K	25. E
2. D	14. I	26. D
3. I	15. E or I	27. C
4. B	16. H	28. A
5. K	17. J	29. H
6. G	18. K	30. K
7. G	19. K	31. E
8. I	20. H	32. G
9. E or K	21. I	33. E
10. E or I	22. E	34. G
11. A	23. H	35. J
12. K	24. G	36. J

Exercise 5–2

1. Anatomy, a branch of biology, includes the study of plant, animal, and human structures.
2. Physiology is the study of bodily function.
3. A cell is composed of a plasma membrane, cytoplasm, and nucleus.
4. epithelial, connective, nerve, and muscle
5. homeostasis
6. metabolism
7. dorsal and ventral
8. dorsal
9. the anatomical position
10. transverse, sagittal, and frontal
11. inspection, palpation, percussion, and auscultation

Exercise 5–3

1. C
2. J
3. G
4. B
5. I
6. A
7. D
8. F
9. H
10. E
11. abdominopelvic
12. thoracic
13. thoracic
14. spinal
15. cranial
16. abdominopelvic
17. thoracic
18. abdominopelvic
19. abdominopelvic
20. H
21. L
22. D
23. G
24. I
25. B
26. K
27. J
28. F
29. M
30. A
31. E
32. O
33. C
34. N

Exercise 5–4

Misspelled words (correct spellings in parentheses):
2 (axillary), 3 (balanitis), 4 (anatomy), 6 (cervicitis), 8 (coccygeal), 10 (epididymitis), 11 (femoral), 12 (fibular), and 15 (laryngitis)

CHAPTER 6

Exercise 6–1

1. stratum basale, stratum spinosum, stratum granulosum, stratum lucidum, and stratum corneum
2. stratum basale
3. outermost layer
4. The epidermis receives oxygen from the blood supply in the dermis.
5. The epidermis contains epithelial tissue; the dermis and subcutaneous tissue are composed of connective tissue.
6. thermoregulation, nutritive supply, skin sensation, and glandular secretions
7. padding, shock absorption, and insulation
8. The lunula is found at the base of the nail; the nail bed lies beneath the nail.
9. Eccrine glands secrete in response to heat and exercise; apocrine glands secrete in response to emotional stress.
10. Sebaceous gland secretions keep hair pliable and skin soft and waterproof; sudoriferous gland secretions help cool the body; ceruminous gland secretions protect the ear from bacteria.

Exercise 6–2

1. a condition characterized by a lack of pigment in the skin, hair, and eyes
2. sweat glands that respond to emotional stress
3. yellow, exogenous skin pigment
4. a waxy substance secreted within the external ear
5. glands that secrete a waxy substance called cerumen
6. a protein, produced by fibroblasts in the dermis, that provides strength and stability
7. another name for the dermis
8. bedsores
9. the skin layer between the epidermis and the subcutaneous tissue
10. sweat glands that respond to heat and exercise
11. a transparent substance believed to be formed from keratin in the stratum granulosum
12. the outermost skin layer
13. the cells covering the body's surface and lining its cavities
14. cuticle
15. a cell that produces collagen
16. a tube surrounding the root of a hair
17. an anticoagulant produced by mast cells in the dermis
18. a substance important in inflammatory reactions
19. abnormal condition characterized by a hard overgrowth of epithelial tissue
20. a protein that infiltrates dead skin cells and makes the skin tough, waterproof, and resistant to bacteria
21. the white, half-moon-shaped base of the nail
22. white blood cells of the dermis responsible for phagocytosis
23. the producer of heparin and histamine
24. dark pigment
25. dead tissue
26. an antibody producer
27. pus-producing
28. glands that secrete an oily substance called sebum
29. the bottom layer of the epidermis
30. collective name of the stratum basale and stratum spinosum
31. the third-to-the-bottom layer of epidermis
32. the fourth-to-the-bottom layer of epidermis
33. the second-to-the-bottom layer of epidermis
34. connective tissue layer separating the dermis from underlying organs and muscles
35. sudoriferous glands; eccrine and apocrine glands

Exercise 6–3

1. D	10. I	19. K
2. J	11. A	20. C
3. A	12. D	21. J
4. F	13. L	22. H
5. G	14. F	23. C
6. C	15. G	24. D
7. H	16. I	25. A
8. B	17. B	26. E
9. E	18. E	27. B

Exercise 6–4

1. carbuncle	6. hirsutism	11. cryotherapy
2. exfoliation	7. HSV 1	12. Moh's surgery
3. atopic	8. plantar warts	13. curettage
4. tinea capitus	9. nevus	14. debridement
5. psoriasis	10. electrolysis	15. PUVA

Exercise 6–5

Mispelled words (correct spellings in parentheses):
1 (carotene), 2 (germinativum), 3 collagenous,
5 (ceruminous), 7 ecchymosis, 9 (dehiscence),
11 (impetigo), 12 (pityriasis), and 13 (psoriasis)

Exercise 6–7

Exercise 6–6

1. malignant tumor of the melanocytes
2. colored
3. small node that can be detected be palpation
4. indication of a disease
5. bleeding
6. inflammation of joints
7. throat
8. disease of lymph glands
9. pertaining to the armpit
10. pertaining to the groin
11. pertaining to the heart and circulation
12. pertaining to the abdomen
13. enlargement of an organ
14. benign skin lesion
15. moles
16. having to do with breathing
17. assessment of patient condition
18. second degree burns
19. first degree burns
20. both sides
21. shedding
22. fluid samples taken from the wounds
23. bacteria
24. bacteria
25. cleaning of the affected area
26. skin grafts of varying thicknesses

[crossword puzzle with answers: exogenous, adipose, ichthyosis, acanthosis, carotenoderma, anhidrosis, epidermis, filiform, dermatology, avascular, and others including anthocyanins, collagen, dermatitis, diaphoretic, cyanosis, carotene, cicatrix, carbuncle]

CHAPTER 7

Exercise 7-1

1. hip socket
2. heel
3. tailbone
4. collarbone
5. thighbone
6. bone in the upper arm
7. lower jaw bone
8. upper jaw bone
9. elbow
10. kneecap
11. breastbone
12. shoulder blade
13. chest
14. bone in the lower leg
15. acromyoclavicular
16. antinuclear body
17. ankylosing spondylitis
18. cervical
19. cervical vertebrae
20. calcium
21. congenital dislocation of hip
22. developmental dysplasia of hip
23. distal interphalangeal
24. fracture
25. interphalangeal joint
26. lumbar
27. lumbar vertebrae
28. metacarpophalangeal
29. musculoskeletal system
30. osteoarthritis
31. orthopedics
32. phosphorus
33. proximal interphalangeal
34. rheumatoid arthritis
35. rheumatoid factor
36. range of motion
37. serum alkaline phosphatase
38. thoracic
39. thoracic vertebrae

Exercise 7-2

1. arthralgia; arthrodynia
2. arthrodesis

Exercise 7-3

1. support, protection, movement, mineral storage, and formation and development of blood cells
2. long, short, flat, and irregular
3. They are two of the seven parts of a long bone.
4. blood cell production
5. the sphenoid bone
6. sutures

7. turbinates
8. temporomandibular joint or TMJ
9. the hyoid bone
10. 33
11. 7
12. C1

Exercise 7-4

1. H	17. F	33. E
2. A	18. G	34. H
3. F	19. G	35. J
4. E	20. B	36. K
5. G	21. A	37. I
6. I	22. C	38. A
7. D	23. C	39. D
8. C	24. B	40. P
9. B	25. A	41. M
10. A	26. B	42. B
11. C	27. A	43. N
12. D	28. B	44. O
13. B	29. C	45. L
14. H	30. B	46. F
15. E	31. C	47. G
16. E	32. C	

Exercise 7-5

Mispelled words (correct spellings in parentheses):
1 (osteoblast), 3 (humerus), 4 (sternum), 6 (cartilage), 7 (hematopoiesis), 8 (tubercle), 10 (fossa), 11 (condyle), 12 (sella turcica), 17 (phalanges), 18 (olecranon), 19 (supination), and 20 (osteomyelitis)

Exercise 7-6

1. disease of a joint
2. shoulder joint
3. hyaline cartilage covering the end of a bone at a joint
4. hardening in the rib area
5. high
6. projection on the humerus
7. lower
8. the lateral tip of the shoulder
9. acromioclavicular joint
10. producing inflammation
11. manipulation of the ends of the fractured bone after making an incision into the injured area
12. immobilizing the bone pieces by means of pins or other mechanical fasteners
13. a broken bone
14. the part of the fibula that articulates with the talus
15. outwards
16. downwards
17. the adjective form of the noun fibula
18. escape of fluid
19. displacement of bones forming a joint

Exercise 7–7

Crossword solution

Across:
- 1. adduction
- 4. flexion
- 7. hyperextension
- 8. supination
- 9. eversion
- 10. depression
- 11. retraction
- 12. protraction

Down:
- 1. abduction
- 2. circumduction
- 3. inversion
- 5. extension
- 6. pronation
- 9. elevation

CHAPTER 8

Exercise 8–1

1. Cardiac muscle tissue, located in the heart, is striated, involuntary muscle; visceral muscle tissue, located in the other organs, is non-striated, but is also involuntary; skeletal muscle tissue makes up striated, voluntary muscle.
2. the positioning, alignment, and movement of body parts
3. long and slender
4. muscle fibers
5. fasciculi
6. deep fascia
7. An origin is the attachment point of a muscle to a bone that does not move when the muscle contracts; the insertion is the attachment point of a muscle to a bone that does move when the muscle contracts.
8. an aponeurosis
9. ligament
10. abductor muscles

Exercise 8–2

1. D	3. A	5. F
2. G	4. J	6. B

7. I
8. C
9. H
10. E
11. H
12. A
13. H
14. A
15. B
16. H
17. C
18. B
19. E
20. G

Exercise 8–3

Mispelled words (correct spellings in parentheses):

1 (buccinator), 2 (platysma), 3 (pectoralis major), 5 (biceps femorus), 7 (dystrophy), 8 (ligamentous), 11 (mysitis), 16 (tendon), 17 (ligament), and 18 (muscle fibers)

Exercise 8–4

1. absence of muscle tone
2. decrease in size
3. impaired movement
4. disorder caused by lack of nutrition
5. adjective form of fascia
6. excision of the fascia
7. inflammation of fascia
8. excessive movement
9. study of movement
10. instrument used for measuring movement

11. tumor of smooth muscle
12. malignant tumor of smooth muscle
13. adjective form of ligament
14. adjective form of muscle
15. muscular pain
16. rapid contraction and relaxation cycle
17. replacement of muscle tissue with fibrous tissue
18. muscle inflammation
19. inability of muscle to relax after contraction
20. inflammation of many muscles
21. destruction of striated muscle tissue
22. tumor of striated muscle
23. malignant tumor of striated muscle
24. adjective form of tone
25. inflammation of a tendon
26. adjective form of tendon
27. inflammation of the tendon sheath
28. cutting of a tendon

Exercise 8–5

1. shortening of the palmar fascia
2. excision of the fascia
3. finger
4. contraction of a tendon
5. metacarpaophalangeal joint
6. proximal interphalangeal joint
7. decreased angle between articulating bones
8. an abnormal condition characterized by the wasting away of the muscles
9. creatine kinase
10. removal and examination of tissue
11. able to walk
12. increase in size
13. abnormal shortening of muscle
14. fibrous tissue connecting muscle to bone

Exercise 8–6

Across / Down solution grid:

- 1 (down) a
- 2 (across) a — 3 t e n o s y n o v i t i s — s
- 4 (across) a b d u c t o r
- 3 (down) t o o p h y ...
- 6 (across) h y p e r k i n e s i a
- 7 (across) t o n i c
- 8 (across/down) d y s t r o p h y
- 10 (across) b r a d y k i n e s i a
- 13 (across) f l e x i o n
- 14 (across) m y a l g i a

Down words:
- abduction (4 down): a d d u c t ...
- contractility (3 down): t o o p h y ...
- 2 down: a t o n l c y
- 6 down: h y k l n e s i a
- 8 down: d y s t k l n e s i a
- 9 down: r o p h a b d o m y o s i s
- 5 down: m y a s t h e n i a
- 10 down: b r a d y k i n e s i a
- 11 down: d y s t o n i a
- 12 down: k i n e s i o l o g

CHAPTER 9

Exercise 9–1

1. brain
2. nerve root
3. myelin sheath
4. cortex; outer layer
5. glue
6. gray
7. bridge
8. membrane; meninges
9. nerve
10. thick
11. nerve root
12. sleep
13. seizure
14. crush
15. bone marrow; spinal cord
16. progressive motor neuron disease
17. an abnormality caused by damage to the CNS before, during, or soon after birth
18. an example of a partial seizure
19. acute encephalopathy and fatty degeneration of the viscera
20. acute, progressive polyneuritis
21. progressive weakening of skeletal muscles caused by abnormalities of the neuromuscular junction
22. incomplete closure of the neural arch
23. a fast-growing intracranial brain tumor within the brain's substance
24. chronic, progressive disorder characterized by bradykinesia, muscular rigidity, and resting tremors
25. inflammation of the myelin sheath leading to demyelination around the axon
26. inherited disease producing degeneration of the basal ganglia and cerebral cortex
27. epilepsy
28. IV motor: eye movements
29. XII motor: tongue movements
30. VII sensory: taste; motor: facial movements, saliva secretion
31. XI motor: shoulder and head movements, voice production
32. VI motor: eyeball movement
33. V motor: mastication; sensory: sensations of head and face, muscle sense
34. carpal tunnel syndrome
35. cerebral palsy
36. central nervous system
37. electromyogram
38. Huntington's disease
39. electroencephalography
40. autonomic nervous system
41. acetylcholine
42. acute encephalopathy and fatty degeneration of viscera
43. blood-brain barrier

Exercise 9–2

1. ventricul/o
2. cortic/o
3. gangli/o; ganglion/o
4. lept/o
5. myelin/o
6. myel/o
7. gli/o
8. -lepsy
9. pachy-
10. neur/o
11. cerebr/o; encephal/o
12. medull/o
13. pont/o
14. radicul/o; rhiz/o
15. -tripsy
16. cerebellitis
17. cortical
18. demyelination
19. encephalomyelitis
20. epidural
21. ganglionectomy
22. intramedullary
23. menigoencephalocele
24. myelogram
25. neuromuscular
26. neurolysis
27. neurotripsy
28. poliomyelitis
29. radiculopathy
30. thalamic

Exercise 9–3

1. C	13. B	25. G
2. B	14. I	26. B
3. G	15. C	27. L
4. H	16. A	28. E
5. A	17. J	29. N
6. D	18. E	30. O
7. J	19. G	31. M
8. E	20. H	32. K
9. I	21. C	33. A
10. F	22. J	34. I
11. D	23. I	35. F
12. F	24. E	36. D

Exercise 9–4

1. the central nervous system (CNS) and the peripheral nervous system (PNS)
2. connect, support, and protect neurons
3. sensory (afferent) neurons, motor (efferent) neurons, and interneurons
4. A synapse acts as a switching mechanism between two neurons or between a neuron and a muscle.
5. cerebrum
6. the bones of the skull
7. 12
8. Sally Said Meet Me By My Boat So Bob Brought Mackerel Munchies.
9. an involuntary response to a stimulus
10. sympathetic and parasympathetic systems

Exercise 9–5

1. astrocytes
2. axon
3. white matter of the cerebrum

4. midbrain, the pons, and the medulla oblongata
5. corpus callosum
6. cauda equina
7. choroid plexus
8. spinal canal
9. Babinski's reflex
10. sympathetic system
11. lumbar

Exercise 9–6

Mispelled words (correct spellings in parentheses)
1 (neuroglial), 2 (synapse), 4 (norepinephrine), 6 (parietal lobe), 7 (diencephalon), 8 (hypothalamus), 10 (cerebellum), 11 (filum terminal), 12 (subdural space), 14 (lateral ventricles), 17 (glossopharyngeal), and 19 (sciatic nerve)

Exercise 9–7

1. water on the brain
2. lack of muscular coordination
3. computerized axial tomography
4. an imaging technique employing a strong magnetic field for measuring the body's ion makeup
5. bleeding between the arachnoid and the pia mater
6. inflammation of the meninges
7. the study of the nervous system
8. a shunt between the ventricles and peritoneum
9. a vertical cut that divides the skull into equal right and left portions
10. below the xiphoid
11. white line
12. a crown saw used in removing bone
13. side opening
14. cerebrospinal fluid
15. adjective relating to the ventricles and peritoneum

CHAPTER 10

Exercise 10–1

1. fibrous tunic
2. choroid, ciliary body, and iris
3. ciliary muscles
4. pupil
5. malleus, incus, and stapes
6. aqueous humor
7. orbital cavity
8. ABR
9. pinna
10. oval window
11. perilymph and endolymph

Exercise 10–2

1. c	5. d	8. a
2. a	6. d	9. c
3. a	7. d	10. d
4. d		

Exercise 10–3

1. phac/o; phak/o
2. aque/o; hydr/o
3. -ptosis
4. dacryocyst/o
5. -opia
6. mi/o
7. ocul/o; ophthalm/o
8. vitre/o; vitr/o
9. bar/o
10. stapedi/o
11. auditory brainstem response
12. air conduction
13. right ear
14. left ear
15. bone conduction
16. decibel (metric symbol; not an abbreviation)
17. electronystagmography
18. ear, nose, and throat
19. dacryocystorhinostomy
20. intracapsular cataract extraction
21. pupils equal, react to light and accommodation
22. extraocular movement
23. idoxuridine
24. eyes, ears, nose, and throat
25. dimness of vision not caused by organic defect or refractive error
26. a watery fluid produced by the ciliary processes
27. a focusing disorder brought about by an irregular surface of the lens or cornea
28. measurement of one's hearing acuity across the range of audible frequencies
29. collective name of the malleus, incus, and stapes
30. the part of the outer ear that is referred to as the ear in non-technical conversation
31. normal vision; seeing one object instead of two while both eyes are open
32. a thin layer of mucous membrane covering the surface of the eyeball
33. an abnormal condition characterized by opaque areas in the lens of the eye
34. a cyst of the eyelid; a meibomian cyst
35. a cyst of the middle ear or mastoid region
36. the dark colored inner lining of the sclera
37. the collective name for the ciliary muscles and ciliary processes at the anterior edge of the choroid
38. the muscles that adjust the shape of the lens
39. the part of the inner ear that houses the cochlear duct, a membranous structure
40. inflammation of the conjunctiva
41. the mucous membrane lining the part of the eye exposed to air; includes the palpebral conjunctiva and the bulbar conjunctiva
42. a reflex action in which the two eyeballs move medially when focusing on a near object
43. the anterior outer layer of the eyeball
44. double vision
45. process of recording the electrical activity of the cochlea
46. process of recording the electrical impulses of the retina following stimulation by light
47. fluid that fills the membranous labyrinth

48. auditory tube connecting the middle ear and the throat
49. removal of the contents of the eyball, except for the sclera
50. outward protrusion of the eyeball
51. part of the external ear
52. six muscles attaching to the sclera of each eye
53. the outer layer of the eyeball
54. depression in the macula lutea
55. an eye condition caused by increased intraocular pressure
56. examination of the anterior chamber of the eye
57. a sty with pustular lesions
58. farsightedness
59. bleeding into the anterior eye chamber
60. an auditory ossicle (the anvil)
61. flat, circular structure in the middle layer of the inner eye
62. the glands that produce tears
63. yellowish area near the center of the retina
64. an auditory ossicle (hammer)
65. condition of the inner ear causing dizziness, hearing loss, and a sensation of pressure in the middle ear
66. nearsightedness
67. incision into the tympanic membrane
68. rapid, involuntary eye movement
69. gonococcal infection of a newborn baby
70. disease of the eye
71. the area of the retina where the optic nerve begins
72. receptor organ in the inner ear for hearing
73. inflammation of the middle ear
74. a device for viewing the parts of the ear
75. surgical reconstruction of the ear
76. transmits sound from the stapes to the inner ear
77. eyelids
78. accumulation of fluid in the optic disc
79. fluid filling inner ear passageways
80. intolerance or sensitivity to light
81. the opening in the center of the iris
82. the inner layer of the eyeball
83. inflammation of the retina
84. disease of the retina
85. a pigment that increases rods' responsiveness to light
86. a comparison of air conduction and bone conduction
87. photoreceptor cells in the retina
88. white posterior portion of the fibrous tunic
89. an area of depressed vision within the visual field
90. removal of the stapes
91. an inner ear muscle
92. an auditory ossicle (stirrup)
93. drooping of the eyelid
94. absence of directional control of both eyes
95. adhesion of the eyeball and eyelid
96. adhesions of surfaces
97. a middle ear muscle
98. measurement of intraocular pressure
99. bacterial infection causing chronic conjunctivitis
100. conversion of energy from one form to another
101. inflammation of the uvea

102. middle layer of the eyeball
103. a gel-like glassy substance
104. a test to compare the equality of hearing in both ears

Exercise 10–4

1. tympanoplasty
2. otomycosis
3. presbycusis
4. otitis media
5. otalgia
6. otorrhea
7. barotitis media
8. ophthalmologist
9. optician
10. optometrist

Exercise 10–5

1. B	8. F	15. E
2. D	9. J	16. A
3. G	10. E	17. A
4. A	11. A	18. B
5. C	12. A	19. E
6. I	13. C	20. A
7. H	14. D	

Exercise 10–6

Mispelled words (correct spellings in parenthesis)
1 (eustachian), 2 (otitis), 4 (audiometry), 7 (ophthalmologist), 8 (optician), 9 (optometrist), 10 (choroid), 13 (auditory), 14 (acoustic), 15 (conjunctivitis), 17 (organ of Corti), 18 (endolymph), and 19 (myopia)

Exercise 10–7

1. inflammation in both ears with watery exudate
2. drugs that prevent disease and infection by inhibiting or destroying microorganisms
3. puncture
4. incisions in both tympanic membranes
5. insertion of tubes to drain the ear
6. lying on the back
7. a device for viewing objects too small to be seen with the naked eye
8. waxy substance secreted within the ear
9. retracted eardrum
10. escape of fluid
11. incision into the front upper part of the eardrum
12. an opaque spot
13. removal
14. eyesight
15. able to see at 20 feet what a person with normal vision would see at 70 feet
16. emulsification of the lens
17. insertion of an artificial lens into the posterior chamber of the eye

Exercise 10–8

```
                e                                   o p t i c i a n
a n i s i c o r i a                                             y
p     o     h           q                                      c
h     t     o                   l           c           l      v
a     r     r   b l e p h a r o p t o s i s
k     o     i   l o         c       r               p          t
i     p     o   e u         r       e               l          r
a     i     r   p s         i       o               e          e
      a     e   h           m       m               g          o
      t     a               m       e               i          u
      i     r               l       t               c          s
      n     o                       e           p
      i     s   e x o t r o p i a               a
      t     p                                   l
      i     a                                   p
      s     s                                   e
      m y d r i a s i s                         b
                                                r
                                                a
                                                l
```

CHAPTER 11

Exercise 11–1

1. mouth
2. salivary gland
3. saliva
4. colon
5. relaxation
6. fusion of parts; stiff
7. cheek
8. rectum
9. patch
10. flank; abdomen
11. emesis
12. gastr/o
13. gluco/o; glyc/o
14. enter/o
15. hepat/o
16. labi/o
17. gloss/o; lingu/o
18. dent/o; odont/o
19. nasogastric
20. barium enema
21. nausea and vomiting
22. gastroesophageal reflux
23. intravenous cholangiogram
24. hepatitis A virus
25. common bile duct
26. stomach and duodenum
27. small bowel series
28. an adjective used interchangeably with digestive
29. hollow centre of digestive tract
30. a muscular tube connecting the pharynx and the stomach
31. throat
32. innermost layer of tissue lining the digestive tract
33. outermost layer of tissue lining the stomach and intestines
34. outermost layer of tissue lining the esophagus
35. an adjective describing the abdominal and pelvic regions
36. small organ that hangs into the throat and closes off the nasal passages during swallowing
37. an adjective describing the palate and tongue
38. an adjective describing the palate and pharynx
39. papillae at the back of the tongue that contain taste buds
40. temporary
41. the gum
42. around the tooth

43. the mouth
44. mucous membrane connecting the lips to the gums
45. mucous membrane connecting the tongue to the bottom of the mouth
46. projections forming the rough surface of the tongue
47. section of the pharynx behind the nasal cavity
48. one of the two sections of the pharnyx through which food passes
49. one of the two sections of the pharynx through which food passes
50. circular muscle that relaxes and contracts to control passage of material
51. the upper sphincter of the esophagus
52. one of the four regions of the stomach
53. one of the four regions of the stomach
54. folds in the inner surface of the stomach that permit the stomach wall to stretch
55. a digestive enzyme produced by gastric glands in the stomach
56. an adjective describing the rectum
57. mixture of food and secretions in the stomach
58. one of the three sections of the small intestine
59. one of the three sections of the small intestine
60. one of the three sections of the small intestine
61. valve connecting the ileum and large intestine
62. folds on the surface of the small intestine
63. fingerlike projections projecting from plicae circularcs
64. hairlike projections projecting from villi
65. glands in the small intestine that produce water, ions, and mucus
66. visual examination of the colon
67. excision of the ileum
68. an adjective describing the region under the tongue

Exercise 11–2

1. cecopexy
2. cheilorrhaphy
3. cholangiogram
4. cholecystolithasis
5. ileostomy
6. colitis
7. endodontist
8. gastrospasm
9. gluconeogenesis
10. hepatocytes
11. labioglossopharyngeal
12. laparoscope
13. odontalgia
14. leukoplakia
15. peritonitis

Exercise 11–3

1. fungiform and circumvallate
2. oropharynx and laryngopharynx
3. sphincter
4. folds on the inner surface of the stomach
5. mucus, hydrochloric acid, instrinsic factor, and pepsinogen.
6. enzymes and sodium bicarbonate
7. hepatocytes

8. abnormal pockets in the mucous membrane of the digestive tract
9. a muscle that regulates the flow of pancreatic juice into the duodenum
10. in the duodenum

Exercise 11–4

1. F	5. D	9. C
2. H	6. I	10. K
3. E	7. B	11. J
4. G	8. A	

Exercise 11–5

Misspelled words (correct spelling in parentheses)
2 (salivary), 5 (biliary), 6 (peristaltic), 13 (cecum), 14 (ileectomy), 16 (absorption), 19 (palate)

Exercise 11–6

1. sensation of the need to vomit
2. ejection of stomach contents through the mouth
3. inflammation of the wall of the digestive tract
4. the intestine
5. fluoroscopic x-ray of the pharynx and esophagus, the distal esophagus, stomach, and proximal duodenum following oral intake of barium sulfate
6. opening in the throat for passage of food
7. tube between pharynx and stomach
8. a J-shaped sac into which food passes from the esophagus
9. the upper region of the small intestine
10. the contrast medium used in UGI
11. visual examination of the colon using an endoscope
12. large intestine
13. the lower section of the large intestine below the spleen
14. visual examination of stomach interior with an endoscope
15. inflammation of the stomach
16. inflammation of the duodenum
17. open sores on the lining of the digestive tract
18. removal of gallbladder with laparascope
19. failure of contents of digestive tract to move toward rectum. Causes include intussusception, volvulus, paralytic ileus, ashesions, and hernias.
20. the upper and middle region of the abdomen
21. stones that form in the gallbladder from cholesterol and bile components
22. the navel
23. a band of tissue found in various muscles and organs
24. below the xiphoid process
25. fibrous scar tissue
26. excision of the stomach
27. duct carrying bile to and from the gallbladder
28. body plane
29. x-ray of a bile vessel
30. the nearest duct and the most remote duct from point of reference (in this case the gallbladder)
31. cut apart
32. duct which drains into the duodenum from the gallbladder
33. chronic inflammation of the gallbladder

```
                        1s  t  o  m  a  t  i  t  i  s       2s
                                                            u
                                                            b
                  3p   4c  h  e  i  l  o  s  i  s           l
                   t    e                                   i
                   y    l              5c                   n
   6a  c  h  7a  l  a   s  i  a         h        8c         g
    n     n    l  a     o               o         h         u
    k     o    i  9c 10h o  l  a  11g   i  o  g   r  a  m
    y     d    s    e   e               n         i  l      l
    l     o    m    p   c               g         e  c
    o     n         a   y               i         y
    g     t         t   s               v         s
    l     i         o   t               o         t
    o     a         c   i               b         e
    s               y   t               u         c
    s               t   i               c         t
    i               e   s               c         o
    a                                   c         o
       12o  d  o  n  t  o  r  r  h  a  g  i  a    m
                                         l         y
```

CHAPTER 12

Exercise 12–1

1. gland
2. cortex
3. urea
4. secrete
5. female
6. potassium
7. thirst
8. milk
9. sharp; quick
10. body
11. endo-
12. ex-
13. -megaly
14. eu-
15. calc/o
16. acr/o
17. andr/o
18. -tocin
19. home/o
20. pituitar/o
21. natr/o
22. pan
23. gynec/o
24. -trophic; -tropic
25. gonadotrophin-releasing hormone
26. corticotrophin-releasing hormone
27. prolactin-inhibiting hormone
28. thyroid-stimulating hormone
29. luteinizing hormone
30. prolactin
31. adrenocorticotrophic hormone
32. triiodothyronine
33. diabetes insipidus
34. follicle-stimulating hormone
35. growth hormone (GH)
36. T3
37. hydrocortisone

Exercise 12–2

1. polydipsia
2. thyroiditis
3. thyrotrophin

4. oxytocin
5. panhypopituitarism
6. hypocalcemia
7. hypokalemia
8. euthyroid
9. exophthalmia
10. endocrinology

Exercise 12–3

1. hypothalamus
2. Exocrine secretions are transported by ducts; endocrine secretions are secreted directly into the extracellular fluid and transported by the blood stream.
3. substances that provide a chemical signal to the body
4. adrenal, thyroid, parathyroid, pineal
5. oxytocin, produced by the hypothalamus and released by the posterior pituitary (neurohypophysis)
6. triiodothyronine (T_3) and thyroxine (T_4)
7. calcitonin
8. mineralocorticoid
9. When released by the chromaffin, adrenaline enters the blood stream and is carried to all body cells. When released by the brain cells, adrenaline acts upon specific muscle cells or upon other glands.
10. corticotrophin, somatotrophin, GHIH.

Exercise 12–7

11. Trophic hormones secreted by the hypothalamus regulate the release of the following hormones from the anterior hypophysis: somatotrophin (GH), thyroid-stimulating hormone (TSH), corticotrophin (ACTH), follicle-stimulating hormone (FSH), luteinizing hormone (LH), prolactin (PRL), and melanocyte-stimulating hormone (MSH).
12. in the andenohypophysis itself

Exercise 12–4

1. G	4. E	7. G
2. A	5. C	8. B or D
3. E	6. F	9. B or D

Exercise 12–5

Misspelled words (correct spellings in parentheses)
1 (hypothalamus), 2 (somatotrophin),
5 (triiodothyronine), 7 (endocrine), 11 (diabetes),
12 (luteinizing)

Exercise 12–6

1. hyposecretion of adrenal glands
2. decreased secretion of the pituitary gland
3. tumor of the chromaffin cells
4. diagnostic procedure using ultrasonic waves
5. visual examination of the stomach with an endoscope
6. a benign tumor of glandular cells

CHAPTER 13

Exercise 13–1

1. slow
2. vessel
3. hold back
4. vein
5. vessel
6. coron/o
7. tachy-
8. epi-
9. pan-
10. valvul/o
11. -ectasis
12. phleb/o
13. abnormal heart rhythm
14. adjective form of atrium and atria
15. abnormally slow heartbeat
16. enlargement of the heart
17. chemical used to stop the heart during surgery
18. pertaining to a crown
19. a recording of heart activity
20. outer layer of the heart's middle wall
21. pertaining to blood in the pericardium
22. the formation of necrotic tissue
23. between the atria
24. between the ventricles
25. heart attack
26. diffuse inflammation of the heart
27. inflammation of the pericardium
28. rapid heartbeat
29. surgical repair of a heart valve
30. x-ray of blood vessels
31. involuntary contraction of a blood vessel
32. constricted aorta
33. adjective form of artery
34. constricted artery
35. small artery
36. hardening of an artery
37. fatty deposit in an artery
38. accumulation of fatty deposits in an artery
39. pertaining to the arm and head
40. removal of atheroma
41. clots in a vein
42. instrument for measuring blood pressure
43. inflammation of a vein with clot formation
44. the outermost layer of a wall of an artery or vein
45. the innermost layer of a wall of an artery or vein
46. the middle layer of a wall of an artery or vein
47. pertaining to a vessel
48. constriction of a vessel
49. expansion of a vessel
50. spasm of a vessel
51. pertaining to a vein
52. small vessel
53. atrioventricular
54. alanine aminotransferase
55. arteriosclerotic heart disease
56. aspartate aminotransferase
57. coronary artery bypass graft
58. coronary artery disease
59. cardiac/coronary care unit
60. congestive heart failure
61. creatine kinase
62. cardiac output
63. cardiopulmonary resuscitation
64. electrocardiogram
65. hypertensive heart disease
66. intra-aortic balloon pump
67. left bundle branch block
68. left ventricle
69. myocardial infarction
70. right bundle branch block
71. right ventricle
72. sinoatrial
73. first heart sound
74. second heart sound
75. serum glutamic oxaloacetic transaminase
76. serum glutamic pyruvic transaminase
77. blood pressure
78. cerebrovascular accident
79. tissue plasminogen activator
80. inferior vena cava
81. percutaneous transluminal coronary angioplasty
82. peripheral vascular disease
83. superior vena cava
84. transient ischemic attack

Exercise 13–2

1. arrhythmic
2. myocardium
3. pancarditis
4. tachycardia
5. vasodilation
6. aortostenosis
7. arteriosclerosis
8. vascular

Exercise 13–3

1. thoracic
2. pericardium
3. interventricular septum
4. interatrial septum
5. right side
6. mitral valve
7. arteries, arterioles, veins, venules, and capillaries
8. the outermost layer of a vessel wall
9. an alternate blood vessel connection around a blocked area

Exercise 13–4

1. H	5. A	8. I
2. F	6. C	9. G
3. J	7. D	10. E
4. B		

Exercise 13–5

Refer to Figures 13–11 and 13–12.

Exercise 13–6

Misspelled words (correct spellings in parentheses)
1 (aorta), 2 (pericardium), 3 (ventricle), 5 (myocardium), 6 (bicuspid), 8 (tunica media), 9 (capillaries), 11 (aneurysm), and 12 (embolism)

Exercise 13–7

1. the process of recording heart function by reference to echoes from ultrasound waves directed through the chest cavity
2. absence of sinoatrial arrhythmia
3. the left upper heart chamber
4. chamber of the heart
5. semilunar valve between the aorta and left ventricle
6. valve between the right atrium and right ventricle
7. left ventricle
8. valve between the left atrium and left ventricle
9. backflow of blood
10. within the heart
11. discontinuity of tissue
12. injury
13. the arteries branching from the ascending aorta
14. acute pain in the chest caused by reduced blood supply to the heart muscle
15. heart attack
16. therapy to dissolve a thrombus
17. tissue plasminogen activator
18. inflammation of the pericardium
19. insertion of a catheter
20. pertaining to a ventricle
21. blockage
22. myocardial infarction
23. perspiring
24. systolic/diastolic
25. accumulation of fluid
26. upper abdomen
27. abnormal
28. heart attack with infarct formation on the lower side

Exercise 13–8

Crossword solution:

- 1 Down: **b** a...
- 2 Across: **arrhythmia**
- 2 Down: **a r a a y c a** (arcady... — vertical letters: a, r, a, a, y, c, a)
- 3 Down: **m y o c a r d i o g r a p h** → myocardiograph
- 4 Across: **endocardiomyopathy**
- 5 Down: **t a c h c a r d i a** (tachycardia)
- 6 Across: **coronary**
- 7 Across: **electrocardiography**
- 7 Down: **e p i c a r d i a l** (epicardial)
- 8 Down: **p e r i c a r d i t i s** (pericarditis)
- 9 Across: **angiospasm**
- 10 Across: **vascular**
- 11 Across: **angiectasis**
- 12 Across: **valvuloplasty**

CHAPTER 14

Exercise 14–1

1. air sacs
2. voice
3. carbon dioxide
4. larynx
5. diaphragm
6. lung
7. lung
8. nose
9. chest
10. chest
11. trache/o
12. -centesis
13. staphyl/o

14. spir/o; -pnea
15. bronch/i/o
16. adenoid/o
17. tonsill/o
18. bronchiol/o
19. removal of adenoids
20. air sacs
21. without voice
22. inflammation of the bronchioles
23. dilation of the bronchus
24. difficulty in speaking
25. difficult breathing
26. inflammation of the epiglottis
27. normal breathing
28. excessive carbon dioxide retention
29. croup
30. removal of a lobe of a lung
31. inflammation of all paranasal sinuses
32. diaphragm nerve
33. paralysis of the diaphragm
34. inflammation of the lung
35. inflammation of the lung
36. pertaining to the lung
37. surgical repair of the nose
38. incision of a sinus
39. measurement of flow and volume of air inhaled and exhaled
40. surgical correction of a cleft palate
41. surgical puncture of chest wall
42. surgical repair of the thorax
43. removal of the tonsils
44. inflammation of the tonsils
45. new opening into the trachea
46. incision of the trachea
47. arterial blood gases
48. acid-fast bacillus
49. adult respiratory distress syndrome
50. culture and sensitivity
51. cystic fibrosis
52. carbon dioxide
53. chronic obstructive lung disease
54. chronic obstructive pulmonary disease
55. continuous positive airway pressure
56. chest x-ray
57. dyspnea on exertion
58. expiratory reserve volume
59. forced expiratory volume
60. forced vital capacity
61. functional residual capacity
62. inspiratory capacity
63. intermittent positive pressure breathing
64. inspiratory reserve volume
65. minute volume
66. oxygen
67. positive end-expiratory pressure
68. pulmonary function test
69. paroxysmal nocturnal dyspnea
70. respiration
71. respiratory distress syndrome
72. residual volume
73. sudden infant death syndrome
74. shortness of breath

75. tonsillectomy and adenoidectomy
76. tuberculosis
77. thoracic gas volume
78. total lung capacity
79. tidal volume
80. upper respiratory tract infection
81. vital capacity
82. Ziehl-Neelsen

Exercise 14–2

1. tachypnea
2. bradypnea
3. dyspnea
4. hyperpnea
5. orthopnea
6. eupnea
7. aphonia
8. dysphonia
9. adenoidectomy
10. bronchiectasis
11. hypercapnia
12. pansinusitis
13. phrenoplegia
14. pneumonia; pneumonitis
15. staphylorrhaphy
16. stethoscope
17. thoracoplasty
18. tonsillitis
19. tracheotomy
20. spirometry

Exercise 14–3

1. nose, nasal cavity, pharynx, larynx, trachea, bronchi, and lungs
2. inspiration and expiration
3. diaphragm and intercostal rib muscles
4. external nare
5. pharynx
6. in the oropharynx
7. the larynx
8. small bronchi
9. apex
10. base
11. in the root
12. diaphragmatic surface

Exercise 14–4

1. B	8. D	15. C
2. A	9. E	16. E
3. E	10. A	17. F
4. F	11. C	18. H
5. D	12. D	19. A
6. C	13. I	20. G
7. B	14. B	

Exercise 14–5

Misspelled words (correct spellings in parentheses)

1 (bronchography), 2 (bradypnea), 3 (oligopnea),
5 (pharynx), 6 (tracheotomy), 7 (diaphragm),
8 (cricoid), 9 (epiglottis), 10 (mediastinal), 11 (rhinitis),
12 (pleurisy), 13 (hyperpnea or hypercapnia),
14 (tachypnea), 15 (stridor), 16 (antrostomy),
17 (lobectomy), and 19 (antitussive)

Exercise 14–6

See Figure 14–1.

Exercise 14–7

1. difficult breathing
2. chronic obstructive pulmonary disease
3. difficult breathing brought on by exercise
4. shortness of breath
5. drugs to combat bacterial infection
6. without a fever
7. finger symptoms
8. blue color of skin
9. overinflated
10. abnormal
11. measurement of breathing capacity
12. inflammation of a lobe
13. test for Mycobacterium tuberculosis
14. pertaining to the part of the pharynx between the soft palate and the epiglottis
15. stained bacilli not decolorized by acids
16. a life-threatening respiration level
17. expansion of the bronchus
18. around the bronchus
19. depressions
20. functional
21. solidification
22. a generalized hereditary disease affecting several bodily systems
23. bronchial dilation
24. a defined part of an organ
25. the sound made by tapping
26. resonant
27. an abnormal sound when exhaling
28. an inherited respiratory disorder
29. inflammation of the lungs

Exercise 14–8

```
                1a  s   t   h   m   a       2b
                t               3p      r
            4p  n   e   u   m   o   5c  o   n   i   o   s   i   s
                l               y       e       n
                e               a       u       c
6c              c               n       m       h               7t
8r  h   i   n   i   t   i   s   o       9o  l   i   g   o   p   n   e   a
o               a               s       n       e               c
u               s               i       i       c               h
10p 11l e   u   r   i   s   y   s       a       t               y
    m           s               12a p  n   e   a               p
    p                               s                           n
    h           13b r   o   n   c   h   i   t   i   14s          e
    y           r                   s               t           a
    s           a                                   r
    e           15d y   s   p   n   e   a           i
    m           y                                   d
    a       16h y   p   e   r   p   n   e   a       o
            n                                       r
        17h y   p   e   r   c   a   p   n   i   a
            a
```

CHAPTER 15

Exercise 15–1

1. thymus
2. eating
3. pertaining to a place
4. self
5. immature; growing thing
6. affinity; love; attraction for
7. equal
8. clot
9. -immune; immun/o
10. splen/o
11. lymphangi/o
12. lymph/o
13. fluid that carries white blood cells through the body
14. lymphatic vessel that carries lymph from the left side of the body to the blood stream
15. secretion of the thymus
16. production of red blood cells
17. cell that ingests other cells
18. adenoids
19. concentration of lymphatic tissue located in the small intestine
20. lymph organs composed of lymphatic tissue located at intervals along the lymphatics
21. organ of the lymphatic system located in the abdominal cavity
22. lymph organ that secretes thymosin
23. cells of the nonspecific defense system that attack the body's own cells
24. cells of the specific defense system
25. cells that activate immune responses through chemical messages
26. part of the immune system that protects against infections in general
27. protein released by nonspecific defense system
28. secretion of phagocytes
29. protein released by nonspecific defense system
30. direct destruction of virus-infected cells and cancer cells by T-lymphocytes
31. slight increase in unequally-sized erythrocytes in the blood
32. clumping together of antigen cells
33. protein molecules that combat infectious invaders
34. cells of the immune system composed of gamma globulin
35. foreign invader that activates an immune response
36. genetically-formed site on antibody that makes it specific to a particular antigen
37. response of antibodies that travel in body fluids (humors)
38. shuffling of genes that carry the code for antigen receptors
39. an asexual copying of a cell by itself
40. resistance to disease
41. immune system that combats specific invaders
42. cloned cells
43. proteins that stimulate production of B-lymphocytes and T-lymphocytes
44. cloned B-lymphocytes and T-lymphocytes that remain in circulation for a long period
45. Kaposi's sarcoma
46. antigen
47. immunoglobulin
48. zidovudine
49. antibody
50. human immunodeficiency virus
51. hematocrit
52. mean corpuscular volume

Exercise 15–2

1. primary: red bone marrow and thymus gland; secondary: spleen, lymph nodes
2. transporting white blood cells throughout the body and transporting fat from the digestive system to the blood
3. in red bone marrow
4. skin, mucous membrane linings of the digestive, respiratory, urinary, and reproductive tracts, phagocytes, natural killer cells, interferon, complement
5. foreign invaders that activate the body's defense system (antibody generator), such as bacteria, viruses, plant pollen, or red blood cells in transplanted tissue
6. natural genetic recombination
7. secretion of lymphokines to stimulate the production of B-lymphocytes and T-lymphocytes
8. similar to plasma with fewer proteins
9. lymph nodes, thymus gland, spleen, Peyer's patches, and tonsils
10. mucous membrane lining of the tract

Exercise 15–3

1. thrombocytopenia
2. leukopenia
3. erythropenia
4. pancytopenia
5. spherocytosis
6. leukocytosis
7. erythrocytosis
8. agranulocytosis
9. anisocytosis
10. hyperbilirubinemia
11. hypercolesterolemia
12. hyperlipidemia
13. leukemia
14. hemostasis

Exercise15–4

1. E	9. D	16. N
2. H	10. I	17. S
3. F	11. S	18. S
4. A	12. N	19. S
5. J	13. S	20. N
6. G	14. N	21. S
7. C	15. N	22. S
8. B		

Exercise 15–5

1. of normal color
2. increase in unequally-sized cells
3. an erythrocyte 5 microns or less in diameter
4. small disk-shaped structures in the blood
5. immature cell
6. red cells having a nucleus
7. white blood cells that stain purple with neutral dye
8. increase in the number of leukocytes

9. structurally
10. pertaining to immature lymphocyte
11. malignant tumor of lymphatic tissue different from Hodgkin's disease
12. human immunodeficiency virus
13. organism that causes inflammation of interstitial plasma cell
14. bacteria causing disease in HIV positive patients
15. malignant tumors of lymph nodes
16. lymph node above the collarbone
17. perceptible by touch

Exercise 15–6

```
                                        ¹e
                   ²b        ³e     r    ⁴e
                ⁵a  g  r  a  n  u  l  o  c  y  t  o  s  i  ⁶s
                   n     s     l     t     s        i
                   i     o     i     h     i        d
                   s     p     p     r     n        e
                   o     h     t     e     o        r
             ⁷e    y     c     i           o  m  p  o
              r          y     l           c  i  h  p
           ⁸e  y        t     ⁹h     y     a  i     e
      ¹⁰e  r  y  t  h  r  o  c  y  t  e           t        l           n
          y  h           s           m     o              i
          t  r           i           o     s              a
          h  o           s           l     i
          r  c           y           s
          o  y                       s
          p  t                       i
          e  o       ¹¹h  e  m  o  s  t  a  s  i  s
          n  s
          i  i
          a  s
```

(Across: 5. agranulocytosis 10. erythrocyte 11. hemostasis; Down: 6. sideropenia, etc.)

CHAPTER 16

Exercise 16–1

1. glans penis
2. testicle
3. vas deferens
4. prostate
5. bladder
6. kidney
7. development; formation
8. renal pelvis
9. urine
10. ureter
11. narrowing; stricture
12. record; x-ray; writing
13. body
14. outside
15. urine
16. bursting forth; bursting forth of blood; hemorrhage
17. male; man
18. infer/o; infra-; sub-
19. -ptosis
20. -lith; lith/o
21. -tripsy
22. a cavity into which the renal pyramids drain
23. tube that carries urine out of the body from the urinary bladder
24. microscopic structures in the kidney that form urine
25. clump of glomerular capillaries in the nephron

26. Also called foot cells, these make up the third layer of tissue in the inner wall of glomerular capsule.
27. artery that carries blood away from the glomerulus
28. passage of material from the filtrate in the renal tubule to the blood in the peritubular capillaries
29. artery that carries blood into the glomerulus
30. projections on the podocytes that interlace with each other to form filtration slits in wall of the glomerular capillaries
31. fluid that circulates through the renal capsule and becomes urine
32. second or middle layer of filtration tissue in the wall of the glomerular capillaries
33. the rate at which blood moves through the glomerulus
34. passage of material from the blood in the peritubular capillaries to the filtrate in the renal tubule
35. waste material that is left in the filtrate during tubular reabsorption to be excreted in the urine
36. metabolic waste that is partially reabsorbed into the blood during tubular reabsorption
37. blood vessel that carries blood away from the kidney
38. cells in the wall of the distal convoluted tubule that are part of the juxtaglomerular apparatus
39. the collective name for two groups of specialized cells in the walls of the afferent arteriole and the distal convoluted tubule that regulate the GFR
40. cells in the wall of the afferent arteriole that are part of the juxtaglomerular apparatus
41. region of the urinary bladder in which two openings from the ureters and the opening to the urethra form three points of a triangle
42. the outer covering of the kidney
43. the cup-shaped glomerular capsule (Bowman's capsule) together with the capillaries that make up the glomerulus and sit within Bowman's capsule
44. a cavity within the kidney that opens into the ureter
45. component of the nephron made up of the glomerular capsule, the proximal convoluted tubule, the loop of Henle, and the distal convoluted tubule
46. muscle in the urinary bladder that contracts when the bladder is full
47. component of the renal tubule
48. blood vessels that surround the renal tubule
49. component of the renal tubule
50. component of the renal tubule
51. duct at the end of distal convoluted tubule to collect urine
52. cup shaped opening of each renal tubule in which the clump of glomerular capillaries (glomerulus) sits
53. filtrate fluid that carries both waste materials and excess substances out of the body
54. slits formed in the wall of the glomerular capillary by interlacing of pedicels
55. endocrine secretion of the kidney
56. endocrine secretion of the kidney
57. expandable sac in which urine collects

Exercise 16–2

1. glomerulosclerosis
2. nephritis
3. proteinuria or albuminuria
4. renal hypoplasia
5. trigonitis
6. ureterolith
7. urethrostenosis
8. nephral

Exercise 16–3

1. storage of urine for periodic excretion
2. The composition of urine is always variable, due to varying amounts of materials deposited or reabsorbed during tubular secretion and tubular reabsorption.
3. when it enters the collecting duct at the end of the distal convoluted tubule. At this point it is called urine.
4. tubular reabsorption
5. tubular secretion
6. basement cells, podocytes
7. Chemical signals sent by the macula densa can cause the afferent arteriole to dilate, increasing GFR. Chemical signals sent by the macula densa can also trigger the secretion of renin by the juxtaglomerular apparatus, leading to the secretion of angiotensin. This causes the efferent arteriole to constrict, thus increasing GFR.
8. A reflex that causes the external urethral sphincter to open so urine is excreted
9. identical to blood plasma except that proteins have been filtered out
10. efferent arteriole

Exercise 16–4

1. D	5. J	9. E
2. G	6. K	10. C
3. I	7. A	11. F
4. L	8. B	12. H

Exercise 16–5

Misspelled words (correct spelling in parentheses).
1 (calyces), 3 (urethra), 6 (loop of Henle), 7 (podocytes), 9 (macula densa)

Exercise 16–6

path of blood flow:
a. 2
b. 6
c. 5
d. 4
e. 3
f. 1

path of filtrate flow:
a. 5
b. 2
c. 6
d. 3
e. 8
f. 4
g. 1
h. 7

path of urine flow:
a. 4
b. 9
c. 2
d. 5
e. 1
f. 8
g. 3
h. 7
i. 6

Exercise 16–7

1. distention of ureter with urine
2. distention of renal pelvis and calices with urine
3. abnormal pouches in mucous membrane
4. intravenous pyelogram
5. incomplete development of kidney
6. visual inspection of bladder with endoscope
7. x-ray of kidney and ureter after introduction of contrast medium with catheter
8. abnormal position of kidney
9. abnormal narrowing of ureter
10. further from point of reference
11. surgical removal of kidney
12. inflammation of kidney and renal pelvis causing obstruction
13. pertaining to the kidneys
14. decrease in size
15. glomerular filtration rate
16. study of diseased tissue
17. excision of part of kidney
18. distension of renal pelvis and calices with urine
19. distention of ureter with urine
20. functional elements of the kidneys
21. inflammation of kidneys and renal pelvis
22. decrease in size of kidney
23. pertaining to one part or spot
24. the glomerular capillaries of the nephron
25. renal tubules of the nephron
26. persisting over a long period of time
27. an abnormal sac on the first internal tissue layer of the kidney
28. cavity that opens into the ureter
29. accumulation of fluid in intercellular spaces
30. removal of part of the prostrate through the urethra
31. a tubular instrument for inspecting the rectum
32. nonmalignant
33. pertaining to the prostate
34. a tubular instrument used to withdraw fluid

Exercise 16–8

```
[1]c  o  r  t  i  c  a  l
 a
 l
 i         [2]g [3]n                      [4]u
 c      [5]p     l  e        [6]m  [7]u  r  o  g  r  a  m
[8]e  x  t  r  a  c  o  r  p  o  r  e  a  l      e
 a      o      m  h        d                    t
 l      t      e  r        u                    e
 e      r      o           l                    r
 i      u   [9]p  y  e  l  o  g  r  a  m         o
 n      l      e           a                    l
 u      o      x        [10]t  r  i  g  o  n  i  t  i  s
 r      s      y           y                    t
 i      c              [11]d                    h
 a      l                  l
   [12]n  e  p  r  o  l  i  t  h  i  a  s  i  s
        r                  l
[13]n  e  p  h  r  o  p  t  o  s  i  s         y
        s                  s
   [14]c  h  o  l  i  n  e  r  g  i  c  s      i
        s                  s
```

CHAPTER 17

Exercise 17–1

1. cervic/o
2. vulv/o
3. hister/o; metri/o; metr/o; uter/o
4. salping/o
5. oophor/o; ovari/o
6. mamm/o; mast/o
7. woman; female
8. deficient; few; scanty
9. before
10. vagina
11. cul-de-sac (of Douglas)
12. milk
13. nipple
14. beside; near
15. surrounding; around
16. milk
17. lips
18. deoxyribonucleic acid
19. follice-stimulating hormone
20. gonadotropin-releasing hormone
21. abortion

Exercise 17–2

1. metrorrhagia
2. menorrhagia
3. menometrorrhagia
4. dysmenorrhea
5. amenorrhea
6. oligomenorrhea
7. parametrium
8. perimetrium
9. panhysterectomy
10. metroptosis
11. mastectomy
12. hysterectomy
13. intrauterine
14. colporrhaphy
15. oophoralgia

Exercise 17–3

1. All primary follicles have been used up (i.e. degenerated or expelled during ovulation).
2. mitosis
3. haploid cells have 23 chromosomes instead of 46
4. by enzymes from attacking sperm
5. the division of the cells of a fertilized ovum (zygote) by mitosis to the point at which 16 cells are present
6. chorion, amnion, yolk sac
7. cervical dilation, fetal delivery, placental delivery
8. eight days after conception
9. the pairing of chromosomes after cell division. In mitosis, all 46 chromosomes of each cell are identical to one an-

other and to the parent cell, and thus all pairs are identical. In meiosis, 23 chromosomes from the mother pair up with 23 chromosomes from the father to form pairs which are not identical to one another.
10. A lifetime supply of immature primary follicles is present at birth. At female puberty, oogenesis begins when several primary follicles begin to mature each month.
11. During cleavage, the morrula sometimes becomes separated into two groups of cells, both of which implant in the uterus. The developing infants in that case are identical twins because the blastocysts divide by mitosis. When two separate ova are fertilized by two separate sperm, the developing infants are fraternal twins, not identical, because the chromosomes of the two separate zygotes do not have identical genetic information.
12. ovaries and maturing primary follicle
13. a maximum of three days

Exercise17–4

1. E	5. C	8. B
2 H	6. D	9. G
3. A	7. F	10. I
4. J		

Exercise 17–5

Misspelled words (correct spelling in parentheses)
    3 (morula), 5 (oocyte)

Exercise 17–6

1. a woman pregnant for the fourth time
2. a woman who has delivered her third child
3. painful menstruation
4. excessive uterine bleeding during the menstrual period
5. constriction of the fallopian tube with thread-like material
6. examination of the peritoneal cavity with an endoscope
7. the development of tissue resembling the uterine mucous membrane in the pelvic cavity
8. excision of a malignant lump
9. an enclosed sac containing liquid or semisolid material
10. dilation and curettage
11. excessive uterine bleeding at the time of menstruation and at variable intervals
12. examination of the peritoneal cavity with a laser beam
13. destruction of the adhesions
14. benign tumors
15. uterus tilted backwards toward the rectum
16. uterus bent backwards toward the rectum
17. a fold of the peritoneum between the rectum and uterus
18. fibrous material; tumor
19. growth on mucous membrane lining of uterus
20. abnormality of accessory organs
21. stretched
22. instrument used for inspection of an organ interior
23. having two sets of chromosomes
24. within the cervix

Exercise 17–7

1c	e	r	v	i	c	i	t	s					2o			
o													v			
3l	a	c	t	o	g	e	n	e	s	i	s	4l	a	b	i	a	l
p												r				
5o	o	c	y	t	e							i				
p												o				
6e	n	d	o	m	e	t	r	i	u	m		r	7s			
r							8g	r	a	9g						
i	10c	11m				12p	o	l	y	t	h	e	l	i	a
n	o	e				e		n		e		p		l	
e	l	n	13p			r		e		x		i		a	
14o	o	p	h	o	r	a	l	g	i	a		c		i	n	c
p	o	p	r			m		o		s		g		t	
l	r	a	a			e		l		o		o		o	
a		u	m			t		o		p		r		r	
s	h	s	e			r		g		e		r		h	
t	a	e	t			i		i		x		h		e	
y	p	r	u			s		y		e				a	
	h		i			m		t		a					
	y		u												
			15m	e	n	a	r	c	h	e					

CHAPTER 18

Exercise 18-1

1. A	7. G	12. L
2. B	8. H	13. M
3. C	9. I	14. N
4. D	10. J	15. O
5. E	11. K	16. P
6. F		

Exercise 18-2

1. movement of a part away from the body
2. turning a part upward
3. use of electromagnetic radiation in diagnosis and treatment
4. adjective describing something that blocks x-rays
5. computer axial tomography scan
6. x-ray of the kidney and ureter
7. x-ray of the spinal cord and its nerve roots
8. examination by means of a fluoroscope
9. the frequency shift that occurs at a point with which a sound source is either opening or closing distance
10. a device for converting energy from one form to another
11. an element that emits radioactivity
12. around an axis
13. capable of producing an echo
14. front to back
15. back to front
16. x-ray technology
17. x-ray technology using a dry print process
18. x-ray of lymph vessels
19. adjective describing crystalline materials that produce an electric current when they are flexed and that flex when an electric current is passed through them
20. anterior
21. anteroposterior
22. lying down
23. computed axial tomography
24. cranial computed tomography
25. barium enema
26. computed tomography
27. intravenous pyelogram
28. intravenous urogram
29. dynamic spatial reconstructor

30. chest x-ray
31. flat plate
32. endoscopic retrograde cholangiopancreatography

Exercise 18-3

1. bronchography
2. myelography
3. mammography

4. pyelography
5. salpingography
6. lymphangiography
7. angiocardiography

Exercise 18-4

Mispelled words (correct spellings in parentheses)
   1 (radiology), 2 (salpingography),
   4 (lymphangiography), 5 (fluoroscopy), 6 (transducer),
   7 (radioisotope), 9 (myelogram), and 10 (echogenic)

Exercise 18-5

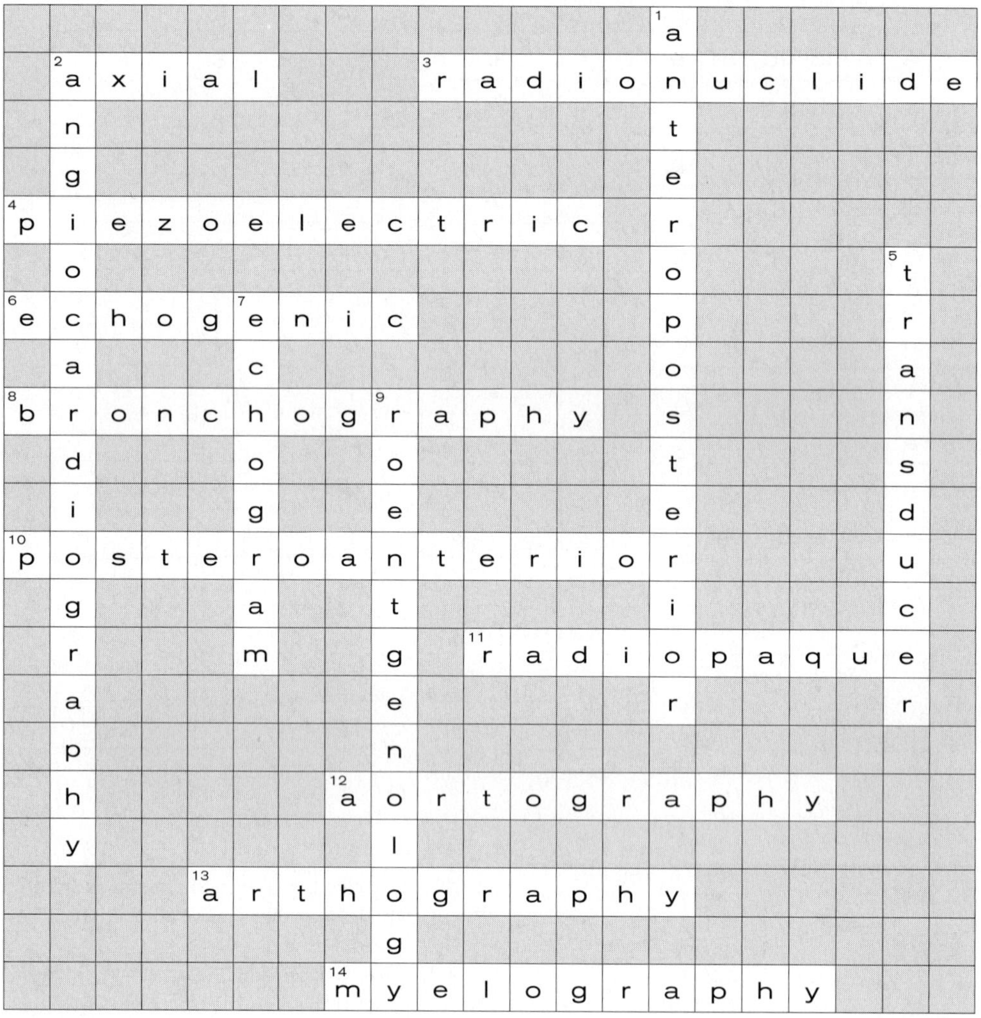

Completed crossword grid (filled letters by row):

Row 1: a
Row 2: axial — radionuclide
Row 3: n ... t
Row 4: g ... e
Row 5: piezoelectric ... r
Row 6: o ... o ... t
Row 7: echogenic ... p ... r
Row 8: a ... c ... o ... a
Row 9: bronchography ... s ... n
Row 10: d ... o ... o ... t ... s
Row 11: i ... g ... e ... e ... d
Row 12: posteroanterior ... u
Row 13: g ... a ... t ... i ... c
Row 14: r ... m ... g ... radiopaque
Row 15: a ... e ... r ... r
Row 16: h ... aortography
Row 17: y ... l
Row 18: arthography
Row 19: g
Row 20: myelography

CHAPTER 19

Exercise 19-1

1. those associated with abnormal moods or mood swings
2. bipolar and depressive
3. Major depression is marked by one or more major episodes lasting at least two weeks; dysthymia is chronic depression lasting more than two years.
4. an unreasonable fear
5. reliving a distressing experience for more than a month after its occurrence
6. hysterical neurosis
7. Both are identity-focused disorders, but psychogenic fugue includes the taking on of a new identity and travel away from familiar surroundings, while psychogenic amnesia does not.
8. an object to which one attributes magical powers
9. paraphilias and sexual dysfunctions
10. hypochondriasis

Exercise 19-2

1. an unreasonable fear of heights
2. an unreasonable fear of unfamiliar surroundings
3. an unreasonable fear of cats
4. an unreasonable fear of pain

5. an affective disorder characterized by one or more manic episodes with a history of major depressive episodes
6. an excessive concern for one's own physical appearance
7. an unreasonable fear of closed spaces
8. a physical impairment for which no physical cause can be diagnosed
9. bipolar disorder comprising many hypomanic episodes coupled with many depressive episodes
10. dissociative disorder characterized by a feeling of being only an observer of one's own mental and physical processes
11. chronic depression lasting for more than two years
12. an unreasonable fear of blushing
13. a paraphilia characterized by powerful, recurring urges to expose oneself to strangers
14. a paraphilia characterized by a disintegrative view of persons, leading to sexual arousal by reference to a body part or an item of clothing
15. a paraphilia causing one to touch unconsenting persons
16. unreasonable worry about several things, such as financial security, social acceptance, etc.
17. unreasonable concern over the state of one's health; commonly called hypochondria
18. a feeling between normal optimism and mania
19. includes at least one major depressive episode lasting two weeks or longer
20. an unreasonable fear of germs

21. fear of everything
22. commonly called sexual deviation
23. a paraphilia characterized by sexual attraction to children
24. reliving a distressing experience for more than a month after its occurrence
25. a dissociative disorder characterized by temporary assumption of a new identity, an inability to recall the original identity, and sudden and unexpected travel away from familiar surroundings
26. a paraphilia involving the desire to be humiliated or made to feel pain
27. a paraphilia involving the desire to inflict pain and humiliation
28. a somatoform disorder leading one to seek medical attention for imagined ailments
29. physical symptoms for which physical causes are unknown
30. a paraphilia characterized by intense desire to watch as people disrobe or perform the sex act
31. an unreasonable fear of foreigners

Exercise 19-3

1. D	6. I	11. M
2. H	7. F	12. J
3. A	8. B	13. O
4. G	9. E	14. K
5. C	10. N	15. L

Exercise 19-4

Across/Down crossword answers:
1. claustrophobia
2. frotteurism
3. algophobia
4. fetishism
5. hypomania
6. macrophobia
7. agoraphobia
8. xenophobia
9. depressive
10. panophobia
11. erythrophobia
12. mysophobia
13. ailuraphobia
14. somatoform
15. paraphilia

CHAPTER 20

Exercise 20-1

1. G	7. C	13. H
2. G	8. B	14. A
3. C	9. G	15. B
4. B	10. G	16. F
5. G	11. E	17. E
6. G	12. C	18. G

Exercise 20-2

1. prescription drugs
2. pharmacist
3. sublingual
4. Generic name is derived from main ingredient.
5. bacteria, yeasts, and molds
6. antihistamines
7. anticoagulant
8. ipecac
9. mydriatic cyclopegic
10. diuretics

Exercise 20-3

Misspelled words (correct spelling in parentheses)
1 (acetaminophen), 3 (erythromycin), 4 (anesthetic), 7 (ascorbic acid), 9 (ephedrine), 10 (barbiturate)

Exercise 20-4

```
 1a  2s   p  i   r  i  3n
  c   r          i
  e   o         4t  r  i  m  e  t  h  a  d 5i  o  n  e
  t   p          r                        r
  a   r          o                        o
  m   a          g        6g  u  i  n  i  d  i  n  e
  i   n  7c  a   l  c  i  u  m
  n   o           y
  o   l           c
  p   o  8p  e   n  i  c  i  l  l  i  n
  h   l           r
  e      9a  m   i  o  d  o  r  o  n 10e    11p
  n               n                  t      h
         12h  e   p  a  r  i  n       h      e
                                     o      n
13m  e  p  h  e   n  y  t  o  i 14n   t      y
                  i                  o      t
         15p  h   e  n  o  b  a  r  b  i  t  o  l
                  c                  n      i
         16e  p   h  e  d  r  i  n  e        n
                                     n
```

CHAPTER 21

Exercise 21-1

1. histopathology, clinical microbiology, immunohematology, hematology, and clinical chemistry
2. process of slicing tissue samples for examination
3. renders body cells and bacteria visible under a microscope and helps divide bacteria into two large groups
4. staphylococci
5. examination for tuberculosis
6. hemolysis
7. agglutination
8. to discover potential adverse reactions
9. hemoglobin
10. the presence of infection
11. an immune system deficiency

12. the volume percentage of red blood cells in whole blood and the test for determining it

Exercise 21-2

1. C   3. N   5. X
2. G   4. H   6. W

7. J   13. Q   19. I
8. K   14. V   20. D
9. L   15. S   21. E
10. M   16. B   22. F
11. R   17. O   23. T
12. P   18. A   24. U

Exercise 21-3

Crossword puzzle answers:
- 1 down: s
- 2 across: streptococci
- 3 down: p s s
- 4 down: c b c
- 5 across: m b c
- 6 down: b a c i l l i
- 7 down: purple / p u r p l e, phylo
- 8 across: cocci
- 9 across: diplococci
- 10 down: p c c v i d l c c
- 11 down: h e m o l y s i s
- 12 across: v l d l
- 13 down: s b e
- 14 across: agglutination
- 15 across: mic

CHAPTER 22

Exercise 22-1

1. removal of fluid from the abdomen by means of surgical puncture
2. excision of the adenoids
3. excision of the adrenal glands
4. excision of an aneurysm
5. surgical repair of vessels
6. excision of the appendix
7. surgical fusion of a joint
8. surgical repair of a joint
9. visual examination of the interior of a joint
10. surgical fixation of an eyelid
11. visual examination of the interior of bronchi
12. excision of a bursa
13. surgical fixation of the cecum
14. suturing of lips

15. excision of the gallbladder
16. incision to remove gallstones
17. excision of the colon
18. visual examination of the colon
19. a surgically created new opening in the colon
20. suturing of the vagina
21. removal of fluid from cul de sac by means of surgical puncture
22. endoscopic examination of cul de sac
23. endoscopic examination of bladder
24. surgical creation of a new opening in bladder
25. replacement of lost skin
26. suturing of the duodenum
27. surgical removal of innermost coat of an artery
28. surgical joining of small intestine and colon
29. surgical creation of a new opening in the intestine
30. suture of labia majora
31. incision of the vulva

32. excision of fascia
33. ophthalmoscopic examination
34. excision of ganglion
35. excision of the stomach
36. suturing of the tongue
37. excision of half of the colon
38. excision of half of the liver
39. excision of hemorrhoids
40. suturing of a hernia
41. excision of the hypophysis
42. excision of the uterus
43. surgical fixation of the uterus
44. excision of the ilium
45. excision of the iris
46. excision of lamina
47. endoscopic examination of the abdomen
48. incision into the abdomen
49. excision of the larynx
50. surgical fixation of a ligament
51. crushing of stones
52. excision of a lobe
53. excision of a lump
54. surgical repair of a breast
55. excision of a breast
56. incision of a maxilla
57. incision of the urinary meatus
58. excision of a meniscus
59. excision of a metacarpal
60. incision of the eardrum
61. excision of a kidney
62. incision to remove kidney stones
63. surgical fixation of a kidney
64. surgical creation of an opening into the renal pelvis
65. excision of one or both ovaries
66. surgical fixation of an ovary
67. examination of the eye with an ophthalmoscope
68. surgical fixation of an undescended testis
69. surgical repair of the ear
70. visual examination of the ear by means of an otoscope
71. surgical puncture of an ovary
72. surgical repair of the palate
73. excision of the pancreas
74. excision of a parathyroid gland
75. excision of the patella
76. suture of the perineum
77. visual examination of the peritoneal cavity by means of a peritoneoscope
78. surgical puncture of the pleural cavity to remove fluid
79. excision of all or part of a lung
80. excision of all or part of the prostate gland
81. incision to remove stones from the renal pelvis
82. incision of the pylorus muscles
83. surgical repair of the pylorus
84. surgical repair of the nose
85. excision of a uterine tube
86. excision of a uterine tube and an ovary
87. surgical fixation of a uterine tube
88. visual examination of the sigmoid colon by means of an endoscope
89. incision of a sinus
90. suture of the spleen
91. excision of the stapes

92. surgical repair of the mouth
93. excision of a tarsal bone; also excision of eyelid cartilage
94. suture of a tendon to a bone
95. suture of a tendon
96. incision of a tendon; transection of a tendon
97. surgical puncture of the chest cavity to remove fluid
98. surgical repair of the chest; removal of ribs
99. incision of the chest
100. excision of a thrombus
101. excision of the thyroid gland
102. excision of the tonsils
103. surgical creation of a new opening into the trachea
104. incision of the trachea
105. removal of fluid from the tympanic membrane
106. surgical opening of the ureter and ileum
107. surgical removal of stones from the ureter
108. surgical opening of the ureter and sigmoid colon
109. surgical opening of the ureter
110. incision of a valve
111. excision of all or part of the vas deferens
112. surgical connection of one vein to another
113. incision of a heart ventricle
114. bilateral salpingo-oophorectomy
115. cystoscopy and dilation
116. dilation and curettage
117. endoscopy
118. examination under anesthesia
119. extracapsular cataract extraction
120. general anesthesia
121. exploration of common bile duct
122. incision and drainage
123. intrauterine device
124. manipulation under anesthesia
125. operating room
126. postanesthetic recovery room
127. prepared
128. preoperative
129. postoperative
130. submucous resection
131. suture removal
132. tonsillectomy and adenoidectomy
133. therapeutic abortion
134. total abdominal hysterectomy
135. transurethral resection of prostate
136. transurethral resection

Exercise 22-2

1. perioperative patient care
2. urgent admission
3. relief of pain
4. intravenous, intramuscular, and inhalation
5. Fowler
6. McBurney (traditional; newer method now available for most appendectomies)
7. n. material used to sew up a wound or tie a blood vessel; v. to sew up a wound or tie a blood vessel
8. supine
9. approximation
10. a continuous suture around a circular wound
11. splitting open of a surgical wound after closure
12. to reduce the chance of infection

Exercise 22-3

1. D	8. J	15. B
2. F	9. C	16. A
3. H	10. G	17. C
4. E	11. C	18. E
5. B	12. A	19. B
6. I	13. D	20. A
7. A	14. A	

Exercise 22-4

Misspelled words (correct spellings in parentheses)

1 (intraoperative), 2 (scalpel), 3 (Metzenbaum), 5 (dilators), 6 (curettes), 7 (dermatome), 8 (endoscope), 9 (tourniquet), 10 (Novocain), 12 (Trendelenburg), 13 (McBurney), 14 (Pfannenstiel), 15 (monofilament), 16 (dehiscence), 18 (asepsis), 19 (dissection), and 20 (ennucleation)

Exercise 22-5

1. herniated disc
2. removal of disc
3. computed tomography scan
4. patient rendered unconscious
5. lying face down
6. preparing
7. placement of a thick sheet over the operative site
8. vertical incision into the middle region of the abdomen
9. separation of body parts
10. a process extending from the vertebral arch
11. incision of laminae
12. portion of a nerve which attaches to the spinal cord
13. a treated, absorbable suture material
14. a band of fibrous tissue
15. the layer of tissue immediately beneath the dermis
16. devices for quickly closing a surgical wound
17. free of germs
18. pain along the sciatic nerve

Exercise 22-6

Crossword puzzle solution:

Across:
- 3. retractors
- 5. sharps
- 9. endoscopes

Down:
- 1. dermatomes
- 2. gelfoam
- 3. ramous
- 4. clamps
- 6. probes
- 7. lasers
- 8. tourniquets

B ENGLISH TO MEDICAL WORD ELEMENT GLOSSARY

DEFINITION	WORD ELEMENT	DEFINITION	WORD ELEMENT
abdomen	abdomin/o celi/o lapar/o	all	pan-
		alveolus	alveol/o
abdominal wall	lapar/o	amnion	amni/o
abnormal condition	-iasis -osis	anterior	anter/o
		anus	an/o
abnormal decrease	-penia	aorta	aort/o
abnormal increase	hyper- -osis	apart	ana-
above	epi- super/o supra-	appendix	appendic/o append/o
		appetite	orex/o
accumulation of interstitial fluid	-edema	arm	brachi/o
		armpit	axill/o
acetabulum	acetabul/o	around	circum- peri-
acromion process	acromi/o		
across	trans-	artery	arteri/o
adenoids	adenoid/o	atrium	atri/o
adrenal gland	adrenal/o adren/o	attraction for	-phil
		auditory tube	salping/o
affinity	-phil	away from	ab- ex- exo-
after	post-		
again	re-		
against	anti- contra-	axis	axi/o
		back	dors/o poster/o re-
air sacs	alveol/o		

DEFINITION	WORD ELEMENT	DEFINITION	WORD ELEMENT
backbone	spin/o	body	corpor/o somato/o
backward	ana-	bone	oste/o
bad	dys- mal-	bone marrow	myel/o
base	bas/o	brain	cerebr/o encephal/o
bear (to)	-para	breakdown	-lysis
bearing	-ferous	breast	mamm/o mast/o
before	ante- pre- pro-	breath; breathing	-pnea spir/o
beginning	-arche	bronchioles (little bronchi)	bronchiol/o
behind	retro-	bronchus	bronch/i/o bronch/o
below normal	hypo-		
below; beneath	infer/o infra- sub-	bursa (fluid filled sac)	burs/o
bent	ankyl/o	bursting forth (of blood)	-rrhagia
beside	para-	calcium	calc/o
between	inter-	calculus	-lith lith/o
beyond	hyper- meta- ultra-	calyx	calic/o
bile; gall	chol/e	carbon dioxide	-capnia
bile vessel	cholangi/o	carry	-phoresis -ferent
bilirubin	bilirubin/o	cartilage	chondr/o
binary compound	-ide	cause	eti/o
binding (surgical)	-desis	cavity	sinus/o
birth	nat/i -tocin	cecum	cec/o
birth (giving birth; part with a child)	-para	cell	cellul/o -cyte cyt/o
black	melan/o		
bladder	vesic/o	cerebellum	cerebell/o
blood	hemat/o hem/o	cerebrum	cerebr/o
		cervix uteri	cervic/o
blood condition	-emia	cessation	-pause
blue	cyan/o	change	meta-

DEFINITION	WORD ELEMENT	DEFINITION	WORD ELEMENT
cheek	bucc/o	crooked	ankyl/o
cheek bone	zygomat/o	crown	coron/o
chest	pector/o steth/o thorac/o	crush (surgical)	-tripsy
		cul-de-sac (of Douglas)	culd/o
childbirth	-partum -tocin	cut (to)	cis/o sect/o tom/o -tomy
cholesterol	cholesterol/o		
choroid (middle layer of eye)	choroid/o chori/o	dark	-opaque
		death	necr/o
chorion (embryonic membrane)	chorion/o	decrease; deficient	hypo- oligo- -penia
ciliary body	cycl/o		
clavicle (collarbone)	clavicul/o	delicate	lept/o
close	proxim/o	delivery	-partum
clot	thromb/o	destruction	-lysis
coccyx (tailbone)	coccyg/o	development	-plasia -plasm -trophy
cochlea	cochle/o		
cold	cry/o	diaphragm	phren/o
colon; large intestine	col/o colon/o	different	all-
		difficult	dys-
color	chrom/o	digestion	-pepsia
common bile duct	choledoch/o	dilation (dilatation)	-ectasis mydr/o
complete	dia-		
condition	-ia -iasis -ism -sis -y	diminutive size	-ole -ule
		disc; disk	disc/o
		discharge	-rrhea
condition of no strength	-asthenia	disease	path/o
		disease process; disease	-pathy
cone-shaped	-conus		
conjunctiva	conjunctiv/o	distant	tele-
contraction	mi/o	division	-schisis
controlling	-stasis	double	dipl/o
cornea	corne/o kerat/o	down	cata-
		downward displacement	-ptosis
cortex (outer layer)	cortic/o		

DEFINITION	WORD ELEMENT	DEFINITION	WORD ELEMENT
draw	duct/o	eyelid	blephar/o palpebr/o
draw together (to)	constrict/o	falling	-ptosis
dropping	-ptosis	fallopian (uterine) tubes	salping/o
drug	pharmac/o	false	pseudo-
dry	xer/o	fascia (band of tissue surrounding the muscle)	fasci/o
dullness	ambly/o		
duodenum	duoden/o		
dura mater	dur/o	fast	tachy-
ear	auricul/o aur/o ot/o	fat	adip/o lipid/o lip/o steat/o
eat; swallowing	-phagia phag/o	fatty debris	ather/o
egg	o/o ov/o	fear (irrational)	-phobia
		female	estr/o gynec/o
electric	electr/o	femur (thighbone)	femor/o
electromagnetic radiation	radi/o	few	oligo-
ellipse	ellipt/o	fiber	fibr/o
enlarged; enlargement	-megaly	fibula (lateral bone of the lower leg)	fibul/o
epididymis	epididym/o		
epiglottis	epiglott/o	filament	filament/o
epithelium	epitheli/o	fingers	dactyl/o
equal	is/o	first	primi-
esophagus	esophag/o	fish	ichthy/o
eustachian tube	salping/o	fixation (surgical)	-desis
evaluate	-assay	flank	lapar/o
examine (to)	-scan	flesh	sarc/o
excess; excessive	hyper- ultra-	flow	-rrhea
		follicle	follicul/o
excision	-ectomy	food	aliment/o
expand	dilat/o	foot	ped/o
expert	-ician	form (shape)	morph/o
external genitalia	vulv/o	formation	-genesis -plasia -plasm -poiesis
extremity	acr/o		
eye	ocul/o ophthalm/o	formed in	-genic

DEFINITION	WORD ELEMENT	DEFINITION	WORD ELEMENT
four	tetra quadri-	hearing	audi/o audit/o -cusis
front	anter/o ventr/o	heart	cardi/o
frontal bone (forehead)	front/o	heat	-thermy
fungus	myc/o	heel	calcane/o
fusion (surgical)	-desis	hernia	-cele herni/o
fusion of parts (pathological)	ankyl/o	hidden	crypt/o
gallbladder	cholecyst/o	hip	ili/o
ganglion	gangli/o ganglion/o	hip socket	acetabul/o
gel-like	vitre/o vitr/o	hold back	isch/o
gland	aden/o	hornlike	kerat/o
glans penis	balan/o	humerus (upper arm)	humer/o
glass (glass-like)	vitr/o	hydrochloric acid	chlorhydr/o
glomerulus	glomerul/o	ileum	ile/o
glottis	glott/o	ilium	ili/o
glue	gli/o	immature	-blast
glycogen	glycogen/o	immunity (resistant to disease)	-immune -immun/o
good	eu-	in front of	pre-
granules	granul/o	in; into	in-
gray	polio-	incise; incision	cis/o -tomy
groin	inguin/o	infection	seps/o
grow (to)	-physis	inferior	infer/o
growing thing	-blast	inflammation	-itis
growth	-oma -trophy	inner ear	labyrinth/o
gums	gingiv/o	innermost	endo-
hair	cili/o pil/o	instep of foot	tars/o
half	hemi- semi-	instrument used to cut	-tome
hard; hardening	kerat/o -sclerosis	instrument used to hold something in a stable state	-stat
head	cephal/o	instrument used to measure	-meter

DEFINITION	WORD ELEMENT	DEFINITION	WORD ELEMENT
instrument used to record (instrument used to produce x-rays)	-graph	lens	phac/o phak/o
		less	mi/o
instrument used to visually examine (a body cavity or organ)	-scope	life	bi/o viv/o
insulin	insulin/o	ligament (tissue connecting bone to bone)	ligament/o
internal organs of the body	viscer/o	light	phot/o
inward	en- eso-	lips	cheil/o labi/o
iris	irid/o ir/o	liver	hepat/o
		lobe	lob/o
iron	sider/o	loosen	-lysis
irrigation	-clysis	love	-phil
ischium (posterior portion of the hip bone)	ischi/o	lower back; loins	lumb/o
		lower jaw	mandibul/o
jejunum	jejun/o	luminous	fluor/o
joined	syn-	lung	pneum/o pneumon/o pulmon/o
joint	arthr/o articul/o		
kidney	nephr/o ren/o	lymph (clear, watery fluid)	lymph/o
kill	-cidal	lymph nodes	lymphaden/o
knowledge	-gnosis	lymph tissue	lymph/o
labor	-partum -tocia -tocin	lymph vessels	lymphangi/o
		lymphatics	lymph/o
labyrinth	labyrinth/o	male	andr/o
lack of	a- an- de-	malignant tumor of connective tissue	-sarcoma
lacrimal glands	dacryoaden/o	malleolus (bony projection on the distal aspect of the fibula and tibia)	malleol/o
lacrimal sac	dacryocyst/o		
lamina (portion of the vertebra)	lamin/o	mammary gland	mamm/o
		man	andr/o
large	macro-	manufacture	-poiesis
larynx (voicebox)	laryng/o	many	multi- poly-
lead	-ducer		

DEFINITION	WORD ELEMENT	DEFINITION	WORD ELEMENT
mass	-oma	new	ne/o
			neo-
mastoid process	mastoid/o	new opening	-stomy
measurement	-meter	nipple	thel/o
medulla oblongata; medulla	medull/o	nipple-like	papill/o
meninges (membrane)	mening/o	no	a-
			an-
middle	medi/o	none	nulli-
milk	galact/o	normal	eu-
	lact/o		norm/o
month	men/o	normal measure	emmetr/o
more than the normal number	hyper-	nose	nas/o
			rhin/o
motion	-kinesia	not	a-
	kinesi/o		an-
			in-
mouth	or/o	nourishment	-trophic
	stomat/o		-trophin
movement	-kinesia	nutrition	aliment/o
	kinesi/o		-trophy
multiple	multi-	nucleus	nucle/o
muscle	muscul/o	occiput (back part of the head)	occipit/o
	my/o		
	myos/o	old age	presby-
myelin sheath	myelin/o	olecranon (elbow)	olecran/o
nail	onych/o	on	epi-
	ungu/o	one	mono-
narrowing	-stenosis		uni-
nature	physi/o	one who specializes	-er
near	juxta-		-or
	para-	opening	-tresia
	proxim/o	out of; outside; outward	ec-
neck of the body	cervic/o		ecto-
neck of the uterus	cervic/o		ex-
neoplasm	-oma		exo-
nerve	neur/o		extra-
nerve root	radicul/o	ovary	oophor/o
	rhiz/o		ovari/o
network	reticul/o	oviduct	salping/o
neutral	neutr/o	pain	-algia
			-dynia

DEFINITION	WORD ELEMENT	DEFINITION	WORD ELEMENT
painful	dys-	plastic repair	-plasty
palate	palat/o	plate	-plakia
pancreas	pancreat/o	pleura	pleur/o
paralysis	-plegia	pons (bridge)	pont/o
parathyroid gland	parathyroid/o	poor	dys-
parietal bone	pariet/o	posterior	poster/o
patch	-plakia	posterior surface of the knee	poplit/o
patella (kneecap)	patell/o		
pelvis	pelv/o	potassium	kal/i
penis	phall/o	pregnancy; pregnant	-cyesis -gravida
perineum	perine/o		
peritoneum	peritone/o	preliminary stage of growth	-blast
pertaining to	-ac -al -ar -ary -eal -ear -iac -ic -ine -ior -ory -ose -ous -tic	presence of a substance in the blood	-emia
		press	piez/o
		pressure	bar/o
		process	-iasis -ion -ism -ize -sis -y
pertaining to infection	-septic	process of cutting	-tomy
pertaining to nourishment	-trophic -trophin	process of measuring	-metry
pertaining to paralysis	-plegic	process of recording	-graphy
pertaining to a place	-stitial	process of study	-logy
phalanges (one of the bones making up the fingers or toes)	phalang/o	process of visually examining (a body cavity or organ by means of an instrument)	-scopy
pharynx (throat)	pharyng/o	produce; producing; produced by; produced from	-ferous -gen -genesis -genic gen/o -genous
physician	iatr/o		
pit	glen/o		
pituitary gland	hypophys/o pituitar/o		
place	top/o	profuse sweating	diaphor/e
plant	-phyte phyt/o	prolapse	-ptosis

DEFINITION	WORD ELEMENT
prostate gland	prostat/o
protein	protein/o
pubis	pub/o
pulse	sphygm/o
puncture to remove fluid (surgical)	-centesis
pupil	core/o pupill/o
pus	py/o
pylorus	pylor/o
pyloric sphincter	pylor/o
quick	oxy-
radius (lateral bone of the lower arm)	radi/o
rapid	oxy-
reconstruction (surgical)	-plasty
record	-gram
rectum	proct/o rect/o
red	erythemat/o erythr/o
reference to another	all/o
relaxation	-chalasis chalas/o
removal	de-
removal (surgical)	-ectomy
renal pelvis	pyel/o
repair (surgical)	-plasty
resembling	-oid
restriction	isch/o
retina	retin/o
rhythm	rhythm/o
rib	cost/o
rod-shaped	rhabd/o
rosy-red	eosin/o

DEFINITION	WORD ELEMENT
rounded	spher/o
run	-drome
rupture	-rrhexis
sac-like enlargement	alveol/o
sacrum	sacr/o
safe	immun/o; -immune
sagging	-ptosis
saliva	ptyal/o sial/o
salivary glands	sialaden/o
same	home/o
scab	eschar/o
scanty	oligo-
scapula (shoulder blade)	scapul/o
sclera	scler/o
sebum (oily secretion from the sebaceous gland)	seb/o
second	secundi-
secrete	-crine crin/o
section	tom/o
seizure	-lepsy
self	auto-
self-produced	idi/o
sensation	esthesi/o
separate	-crine -lysis
shape	-form morph/o
sharp	oxy-
shine	-lucent
shut (to)	claustr/o
side	later/o; pleur/o
sieve	ethm/o

DEFINITION	WORD ELEMENT	DEFINITION	WORD ELEMENT
sight	opt/o	spinal column	spin/o
sigmoid colon	sigmoid/o	spinal cord	myel/o
similar	home/o	spine	rach/i
sinus	sinus/o		rachi/o
skin	cutane/o		spin/o
	-derma	spiny	acanth/o
	dermat/o	spitting	-ptysis
	-dermis	spleen	splen/o
	derm/o	splitting	-schisis
skull	crani/o	stable	-stasis
sleep	narc/o	standing	-stasis
slender	lept/o	stapes	stapedi/o
slight increase in the number of cells	-cytosis	state of	-ia
			-ism
			-sis
slow	brady-	steady beat	rhythm/o
small	micro-	sternum (breastbone)	stern/o
	-ole	stiff	ankyl/o
	-ule	stimulation	-trophic
small elevation	papill/o		-trophin
small intestine	enter/o	stomach	gastr/o
smooth	lei/o	stone	-lith
socket	glen/o		lith/o
sodium	natr/o	stoppage	-pause
soft; softening	-malacia	stopping	-stasis
sound	acoust/o	straight	ortho-
	ech/o	strange	xen/o
	son/o	stretch; stretching	-ectasis
spark	scint/i		tone/o
specialist (one who specializes)	-er	striated	rhabd/o
	-ician	stricture	-stenosis
	-ist	structure	-ium
	-or	study of	-logy
specialist in the measurement of	-metrist	sudden, violent involuntary contraction or tightening of a muscle	-spasm
specialist in the study of	-logist		
spermatozoa (sperm)	spermat/o	sugar	gluc/o
	sperm/o		glyc/o
sphenoid bone	sphen/o		
spherical	spher/o		

DEFINITION	WORD ELEMENT	DEFINITION	WORD ELEMENT
surgical binding; surgical fusion	desis	thing	-us
		thirst	-dipsia
surgical crushing	-tripsy	thorax	thorac/o
surgical fixation	-pexy	thorny	acanth/o
surgical puncture to remove fluid	-centesis	thread	filament/o fil/i
surgical reconstruction; surgical repair	-plasty	three	tri-
		through	dia- per- trans-
surgical removal	-ectomy		
surrounding	peri-	throw	bol/o
suture	-rrhaphy	thymus	thym/o
sweat	hidr/o sudor/i	thyroid gland	thyr/o thyroid/o
sword	xiph/o	tibia (shin)	tibi/o
synovia (synovial fluid)	synovi/o	tissue	hist/o
synovium (synovial membrane)	synovi/o	toes	dactyl/o
		together	syn-
tarsals	tars/o	tone	ton/o
tear gland	dacryoaden/o	tongue	gloss/o lingu/o
tear sac	dacryocyst/o		
tears	dacry/o lacrim/o	tonsils	tonsill/o
		top	acr/o
teeth; tooth	dent/o odont/o	toward	ad-
temporal bone (temples)	tempor/o	toward the head	super/o
		toward the tail	caud/o
tendon	tendin/o ten/o	trachea (windpipe)	trache/o
		transmission	-phoresis
tendon sheath	synovi/o tenosynovi/o	transplant (tissue for transplant)	-graft
tension	ton/o	treatment	-therapy
testes; testicles	orchid/o orch/o testicul/o test/o	trigone	trigon/o
		tumor	-oma
		turmoil	-clonus
thalamus	thalam/o	turn	-tropion
thick	pachy-		
thin	lept/o	turning	-tropia

DEFINITION	WORD ELEMENT	DEFINITION	WORD ELEMENT
two	bi- di-	ventricles	ventricul/o
tympanic membrane (eardrum)	myring/o tympan/o	vertebra (any one of the 33 bones making up the spinal column or backbone)	spondyl/o vertebr/o
ulna (medial bone of the lower arm)	uln/o	vertebral column	spin/o
under	hypo-; sub-	vessel	angi/o vascul/o vas/o
unequal	anis/o		
union	zyg/o	vestibule (cavity or space near the entrance to a canal)	vestibul/o
up	ana-		
upon	epi-	view (to)	-opsy
upper jaw	maxill/o	vision	opt/o
upright	ortho-	vision; visual condition	-opia
urea (urea is the end product of protein metabolism and is found in urine)	ure/o	voice	-phonia
		vomiting	-emesis
ureter	ureter/o	vulva	episi/o; vulv/o
urethra	urethr/o	wall	pariet/o
urinary bladder	cyst/o	washing	-clysis
urinary tract	ur/o; urin/o	water	aque/o hydr/o
urination	-uria urin/o ur/o	wax	cerumin/o
		wedge	sphen/o
urine	-uria	white	leuc/o leuk/o
uterus	hyster/o metri/o metr/o uter/o	wide	mydr/o
		with; together	con-; syn-
uvea (includes the choroid, ciliary body and iris)	uve/o	within	en- endo- eso- intra-
uvula	staphyl/o	woman	gynec/o
vagina	colp/o vagin/o	wrist	carp/o
		writing	-gram
valve	valvul/o	x-ray film	-gram
variation	poikil/o	x-rays	radi/o roentgen/o
vas deferens	vas/o		
vein	phleb/o ven/o	yellow pigment	caroten/o

C MEDICAL WORD ELEMENT TO ENGLISH GLOSSARY

WORD ELEMENT	DEFINITION
a-; a(n)-	lack of; no; not
ab-	away from
abdomin/o	abdomen
-ac	pertaining to
acanth/o	thorny; spiny
acetabul/o	acetabulum; hip socket
acoust/o	sound
acr/o	extremity; top
acromi/o	acromion process
ad-	toward
aden/o	gland
adenoid/o	adenoids
adip/o	fat
adren/o	adrenal gland
adrenal/o	adrenal gland
-al	pertaining to
-algia	pain
aliment/o	food; nutrition
all-	different
all/o	reference to another
alveol/o	alveolus; air sacs; sac-like enlargement

WORD ELEMENT	DEFINITION
ambly/o	dullness
amni/o	amnion
anis/o	unequal
an/o	anus
ana-	apart; backward; up
andr/o	male; man
angi/o	vessel
ankyl/o	bent; crooked; fusion of parts; stiff
ante-	before
anter/o	anterior; front
anti-	against
aort/o	aorta
append/o	appendix
appendic/o	appendix
aque/o	water
-ar	pertaining to
-arche	beginning
arteri/o	artery
arthr/o	joint
articul/o	joint
-ary	pertaining to

WORD ELEMENT	DEFINITION	WORD ELEMENT	DEFINITION
-assay	to evaluate	carp/o	wrist
-asthenia	condition of no strength	cata-	down
ather/o	fatty debris	caud/o	toward the tail
atri/o	atrium	cec/o	cecum
audi/o	hearing	-cele	hernia
audit/o	hearing	celi/o	abdomen
aur/o	ear	cellul/o	cell
auricul/o	ear	-centesis	surgical puncture to remove fluid
auto-	self	cephal/o	head
axi/o	axis	cerebell/o	cerebellum
axill/o	armpit	cerebr/o	cerebrum; brain
balan/o	glans penis	cerumin/o	wax
bar/o	pressure	cervic/o	cervix uteri; neck of the body; neck of the uterus
bas/o	base		
bi/o	life	chalas/o	relaxation
bi-	two	-chalasis	relaxation
bilirubin/o	bilirubin	cheil/o	lips
-blast	immature; growing thing; preliminary stage of growth	chlorhydr/o	hydrochloric acid
		chol/e	bile; gall
blephar/o	eyelid	cholangi/o	bile vessel
bol/o	throw	cholecyst/o	gallbladder
brachi/o	arm	choledoch/o	common bile duct
brady-	slow	cholesterol/o	cholesterol
bronch/o	bronchus	chondr/o	cartilage
bronch/i/o	bronchus	chori/o	choroid (middle layer of eye)
bronchiol/o	bronchioles (little bronchi)	chorion/o	chorion (embryonic membrane)
bucc/o	cheek		
burs/o	bursa; fluid filled sac	choroid/o	choroid (middle layer of eye)
calc/o	calcium	chrom/o	color
calcane/o	heel	-cidal	to kill
calic/o	calyx	cili/o	hair
-capnia	carbon dioxide	circum-	around
card/i/o	heart	cis/o	cut; incision; incise
caroten/o	carrot	claustr/o	to shut

WORD ELEMENT	DEFINITION
clavicul/o	clavicle; collarbone
-clonus	turmoil
-clysis	irrigation; washing
coccyg/o	coccyx; tailbone
cochle/o	cochlea
col/o	colon; large intestine
colon/o	colon; large intestine
colp/o	vagina
con-	with; together
conjunctiv/o	conjunctiva
constrict/o	to draw together
contra-	against
-conus	cone-shaped
core/o	pupil
corne/o	cornea
coron/o	crown
corpor/o	body
cortic/o	cortex; outer layer
cost/o	rib
crani/o	skull
crin/o	secrete
-crine	secrete; separate
cry/o	cold
crypt/o	hidden
culd/o	cul-de-sac (of Douglas)
-cusis	hearing
cutane/o	skin
cyan/o	blue
cycl/o	ciliary body
-cyesis	pregnancy
cyst/o	urinary bladder
cyt/o	cell
-cyte	cell

WORD ELEMENT	DEFINITION
-cytosis	slight increase in the number of cells
dacry/o	tears
dacryoaden/o	tear gland; lacrimal glands
dacryocyst/o	tear sac; lacrimal sac
dactyl/o	fingers; toes
de-	lack of; removal
dent/o	tooth
derm/o	skin
-derma	skin
dermat/o	skin
-dermis	skin
-desis	surgical binding; fusion
di-	two
dia-	through; complete
diaphor/e	profuse sweating
dilat/o	to expand
dipl/o	double
-dipsia	thirst
disc/o	disc; disk
dors/o	back (often referring to the back portion of the body or of an organ)
-drome	run
-ducer	lead
duct/o	draw
duoden/o	duodenum
dur/o	dura mater
-dynia	pain
dys-	difficult; bad; painful; poor
-eal	pertaining to
-ear	pertaining to
ec-	outward
ech/o	sound

WORD ELEMENT	DEFINITION	WORD ELEMENT	DEFINITION
-ectasis	dilation (dilatation); stretching	exo-	outside; outward; away from
ecto-	outside	extra-	outside
-ectomy	excision; removal (surgical)	fasci/o	fascia (band of tissue surrounding the muscle)
-edema	accumulation of interstitial fluid	femor/o	femur; thighbone
electr/o	electric	-ferent	to carry
ellipt/o	ellipse	-ferous	bearing; producing
-emesis	vomiting	fibr/o	fiber
-emia	blood condition; presence of a substance in the blood	fibul/o	fibula (lateral bone of the lower leg)
emmetr/o	normal measure	fil/i	thread
en-	within; inward	filament/o	thread; filament
encephal/o	brain	fluor/o	luminous
endo-	within; innermost	follicul/o	follicle
enter/o	small intestine	-form	shape
eosin/o	rosy-red	front/o	frontal bone; forehead
epi-	upon; on; above	galact/o	milk
epididym/o	epididymis	gangli/o	ganglion
epiglott/o	epiglottis	ganglion/o	ganglion
episi/o	vulva	gastr/o	stomach
epitheli/o	epithelium; covering	gen/o	producing; production
-er	specialist; one who specializes	-gen	producing; produce
erythemat/o	red	-genesis	production; formation
erythr/o	red	-genic	formed in; produced by; producing
eschar/o	scab	-genous	produced by; produced from
esthesi/o	sensation	gingiv/o	gums
eso-	within; inward	glen/o	socket; pit
esophag/o	esophagus	gli/o	glue
estr/o	female	glomerul/o	glomerulus
ethm/o	sieve	gloss/o	tongue
eti/o	cause	glott/o	glottis
eu-	normal; good	gluc/o	sugar
ex-	out of; away from	glyc/o	sugar

WORD ELEMENT	DEFINITION
glycogen/o	glycogen
-gnosis	knowledge
-graft	transplant; tissue for transplant
-gram	record; x-ray film; writing
granul/o	granules
-graph	instrument used to record; instrument used to produce x-rays
-graphy	process of recording; producing images; x-ray
-gravida	pregnancy; pregnant
gynec/o	woman; female
hem/o	blood
hemat/o	blood
hemi-	half
hepat/o	liver
herni/o	hernia
hidr/o	sweat
hist/o	tissue
home/o	same; similar
humer/o	humerus; upper arm
hydr/o	water
hyper-	excessive; beyond; abnormal increase; above normal; more than the normal number
hypo-	below; under; deficient; beneath; below normal
hypophys/o	pituitary gland
hyster/o	uterus
-ia	state of; condition
-iac	pertaining to
-iasis	abnormal condition; condition; process
iatr/o	physician
-ic	pertaining to

WORD ELEMENT	DEFINITION
ichthy/o	fish
-ician	specialist; one who specializes; expert
-ide	binary compound
idi/o	self-produced
ile/o	ileum
ili/o	hip; ilium
-immun/o	safe; immunity (resistant to disease)
-immune	immunity (resistant to disease); safe
in-	in; into; not
-ine	pertaining to
infer/o	inferior; below
infra-	below; beneath
inguin/o	groin
insulin/o	insulin
inter-	between
intra-	within
-ion	process
-ior	pertaining to
ir/o	iris
irid/o	iris
is/o	equal
isch/o	hold back; restriction
ischi/o	ischium (posterior portion of the hip bone)
-ism	condition; state of; process
-ist	specialist; one who specializes
-itis	inflammation
-ium	structure
-ize	process
jejun/o	jejunum
juxta-	near
kal/i	potassium

WORD ELEMENT	DEFINITION	WORD ELEMENT	DEFINITION
kerat/o	hornlike; hard; cornea	macro-	large
kinesi/o	movement; motion	mal-	bad
-kinesia	movement; motion	-malacia	soft; softening
labi/o	lips	malleol/o	malleolus (bony projection on the distal aspect of the fibula and tibia)
labyrinth/o	labyrinth; inner ear		
lacrim/o	tears	mamm/o	mammary gland; breast
lact/o	milk	mandibul/o	lower jaw
lamin/o	lamina (portion of the vertebra)	mast/o	breast
		mastoid/o	mastoid process
lapar/o	abdomen; abdominal wall; flank	maxill/o	upper jaw
		medi/o	middle
laryng/o	larynx; voicebox	medull/o	medulla oblongata; medulla
later/o	side	-megaly	enlarged; enlargement
lei/o	smooth	melan/o	black
-lepsy	seizure	men/o	month
lept/o	slender; thin; delicate	mening/o	membrane; meninges
leuc/o	white	meta-	beyond; change
leuk/o	white	-meter	instrument used to measure; measurement
ligament/o	ligament (tissue connecting bone to bone)		
		metr/o; metri/o	uterus
lingu/o	tongue	-metrist	specialist in the measurement of
lip/o	fat		
lipid/o	fat	-metry	process of measuring
lith/o	calculus; stone	mi/o	contraction; less
-lith	calculus; stone	micro-	small
lob/o	lobe	mono-	one
-logist	specialist in the study of	morph/o	shape; form
-logy	study of; process of study	multi-	many; multiple
-lucent	shine	muscul/o	muscle
lumb/o	lower back; loins	my/o	muscle
lymph/o	lymph (clear, watery fluid); lymphatics; lymph tissue	myc/o	fungus
		mydr/o	wide; dilation (dilatation)
lymphaden/o	lymph nodes		
lymphangi/o	lymph vessels	myel/o	bone marrow; spinal cord
-lysis	breakdown; destruction; loosen; separate	myelin/o	myelin sheath

WORD ELEMENT	DEFINITION
myos/o	muscle
myring/o	tympanic membrane; eardrum
narc/o	sleep
nas/o	nose
nat/i	birth
natr/o	sodium
necr/o	death
nephr/o	kidney
neur/o	nerve
neutr/o	neutral
norm/o	normal
nucle/o	nucleus
nulli-	none
o/o	egg
occipit/o	occiput (back part of the head)
ocul/o	eye
odont/o	teeth; tooth
-oid	resembling
-ole	small; diminutive size
olecran/o	olecranon; elbow
oligo-	deficient, few; scanty
-oma	tumor; growth; neoplasm; mass
onych/o	nail
oophor/o	ovary
-opaque	dark
ophthalm/o	eye
-opia	vision; visual condition
-opsy	to view
opt/o	vision; sight
or/o	mouth
-or	specialist; one who specializes; (person or thing that does something)

WORD ELEMENT	DEFINITION
orch/o	testicles; testes
orchid/o	testicles; testes
orex/o	appetite
ortho-	straight; upright
-ory	pertaining to
-ose	pertaining to
-osis	abnormal condition; abnormal increase
oste/o	bone
ot/o	ear
-ous	pertaining to
ov/o	egg
ovari/o	ovary
oxy-	rapid; quick; sharp
pachy-	thick
palat/o	palate
palpebr/o	eyelid
pan-	all
pancreat/o	pancreas
papill/o	nipple-like; small elevation
-para	to bear; giving birth; part with a child
para-	beside; near
parathyroid/o	parathyroid gland
pariet/o	parietal bone; wall
-partum	labor; delivery; childbirth
patell/o	patella; kneecap
path/o	disease
-pathy	disease process, disease
-pause	cessation; stoppage
pector/o	chest
ped/o	foot
pelv/o	pelvis

WORD ELEMENT	DEFINITION	WORD ELEMENT	DEFINITION
-penia	deficiency; abnormal decrease; decrease	-plasm	development; formation
-pepsia	digestion	-plasty	surgical reconstruction, surgical repair; plastic repair
per-	through	-plegia	paralysis
peri-	surrounding; around	-plegic	pertaining to paralysis
perine/o	perineum	pleur/o	pleura; side
peritone/o	peritoneum	-pnea	breathing
-pexy	surgical fixation	pneum/o	lungs
phac/o	lens	pneumon/o	lung
phag/o	eating	-poiesis	formation; manufacture
-phagia	eat; swallowing	poikil/o	variation
phak/o	lens	polio-	gray
phalang/o	phalanges (one of the bones making up the fingers or toes)	poly-	many
phall/o	penis	pont/o	pons; bridge
pharmac/o	drug	poplit/o	posterior surface of the knee
pharyng/o	pharynx; throat	post-	after
-phil	affinity; love; attraction for	poster/o	back; posterior
phleb/o	vein	pre-	before; in front of
-phobia	fear (irrational)	presby-	old age
-phonia	voice	primi-	first
-phoresis	carry; transmission	pro-	before
phot/o	light	proct/o	rectum
phren/o	diaphragm	prostat/o	prostate gland
physi/o	nature	protein/o	protein
-physis	to grow	proxim/o	near; close
phyt/o	plant	pseudo-	false
-phyte	plant	-ptosis	downward displacement; dropping prolapse; sagging; falling
piez/o	press	ptyal/o	saliva
pil/o	hair	-ptysis	spitting
pituitar/o	pituitary gland	pub/o	pubis
-plakia	patch; plate	pulmon/o	lung
plasia	development; formation	pupill/o	pupil

WORD ELEMENT	DEFINITION
py/o	pus
pyel/o	renal pelvis
pylor/o	pyloric sphincter; pylorus
quadri-	four
rach/i	spine
rachi/o	spine
radi/o	x-ray; electromagnetic radiation; radius (lateral bone of the lower arm)
radicul/o	nerve root
re-	back; again
rect/o	rectum
ren/o	kidney
reticul/o	network
retin/o	retina
retro-	behind
rhabd/o	rod-shaped; striated
rhin/o	nose
rhiz/o	nerve root
rhythm/o	rhythm; steady beat
roentgen/o	x-rays (referring to the discoverer of x-rays, Wilhelm Roentgen)
-rrhagia	bursting forth; bursting forth of blood; hemorrhage
-rrhaphy	suture
-rrhea	discharge; flow
-rrhexis	rupture
sacr/o	sacrum
salping/o	fallopian tubes; uterine tubes; oviduct; auditory tube; eustachian tube
sarc/o	flesh
-sarcoma	malignant tumor of connective tissue
-scan	to examine

WORD ELEMENT	DEFINITION
scapul/o	scapula; shoulder blade
-schisis	splitting; division
scint/i	spark
scler/o	sclera
-sclerosis	hardening
-scope	instrument used to visually examine (a body cavity or organ)
-scopy	process of visually examining (a body cavity or organ by means of an instrument)
seb/o	sebum (oily secretion from the sebaceous gland)
sect/o	to cut
secundi-	second
semi-	half
seps/o	infection
-septic	pertaining to infection
sial/o	saliva
sialaden/o	salivary glands
sider/o	iron
sigmoid/o	sigmoid colon
sinus/o	sinus; cavity
-sis	state of; condition; process
somat/o	body
son/o	sound
-spasm	sudden, violent involuntary contraction or tightening of the muscle
sperm/o	spermatozoa; sperm
spermat/o	spermatozoa; sperm
sphen/o	sphenoid bone; wedge
spher/o	spherical; rounded
sphygm/o	pulse
spin/o	spine; spinal column; backbone; vertebral column

WORD ELEMENT	DEFINITION
spir/o	breath; breathing
splen/o	spleen
spondyl/o	vertebra
stapedi/o	stapes
staphyl/o	uvula
-stasis	stopping; controlling; standing; stable
-stat	instrument used to hold something in a stable state
steat/o	fat
-stenosis	narrowing; stricture
stern/o	sternum; breastbone
steth/o	chest
-stitial	pertaining to a place
stomat/o	mouth
-stomy	new opening
sub-	under; below
sudor/i	sweat
super/o	above; toward the head
supra-	above
syn-	together; with; joined
synovi/o	synovium (synovial membrane); tendon sheath; synovia (synovial fluid)
tachy-	fast
tars/o	tarsals; instep of foot
tele-	distant
tempor/o	temporal bone; temporal region; temples
ten/o	tendon
tendin/o	tendon
tenosynovi/o	tendon sheath
test/o	testicles
testicul/o	testicles
tetra-	four

WORD ELEMENT	DEFINITION
thalam/o	thalamus
thel/o	nipple
-therapy	treatment
-thermy	heat
thorac/o	chest; thorax
thromb/o	clot
thym/o	thymus
thyr/o	thyroid gland
thyroid/o	thyroid gland
tibi/o	tibia; shin
-tic	pertaining to
-tocia	labor
-tocin	childbirth; labor; birth
tom/o	cut; section
-tome	instrument used to cut
-tomy	incision; cut; incise; process of cutting
ton/o	tone; tension
tone/o	stretch
tonsill/o	tonsils
top/o	place
trache/o	trachea; windpipe
trans-	across; through
-tresia	opening
tri-	three
trigon/o	trigone
-tripsy	to crush
-trophic	nourishment; stimulation
-trophin	pertaining to nourishment; pertaining to stimulation
-trophy	development; growth; nutrition
-tropia	turning
-tropion	turn

WORD ELEMENT	DEFINITION
tympan/o	tympanic membrane; ear drum
-ule	small; diminutive size
uln/o	ulna (medial bone of the lower arm)
ultra-	excess; beyond
ungu/o	nail
uni-	one
ur/o	urinary tract; urination
ure/o	urea
ureter/o	ureter
urethr/o	urethra
-uria	urine; urination
urin/o	urinary tract; urination
-us	thing
uter/o	uterus
uve/o	uvea (includes the choroid, ciliary body and iris)
vagin/o	vagina
valvul/o	valve
vas/o	vas deferens; vessel
vascul/o	vessel

WORD ELEMENT	DEFINITION
ven/o	vein
ventr/o	front
ventricul/o	ventricles
verebr/o	vertebra (any one of the 33 bones making up the spinal column or backbone)
vesic/o	bladder
vestibul/o	vestibule (cavity or space near the entrance to a canal)
viscer/o	internal organs of the body
vitr/o	glass; glass-like
vitre/o	glass-like; gel-like
viv/o	life
vulv/o	vulva; external genitalia
xen/o	strange
xer/o	dry
xiph/o	sword
-y	process; condition
zyg/o	union
zygomat/o	cheek bone

APPENDIX

D ABBREVIATIONS GLOSSARY

ABBREVIATION	TERM
^{99}Mo	molybdenum-99
^{99m}Tc	technetium-99m
Ab	abortion; antibody
ABG	arterial blood gases
ABO	blood types: A, B, O
ABR	auditory brainstem response
AC	air conduction
ac	before meals
AC joint	acromioclavicular joint
ACh	acetylcholine
ACTH	adrenocorticotrophic hormone
AD (auris dextra)	right ear
ADH	antidiuretic hormone (vasopressin)
ADHD	attention deficit hyperactivity disorder
ad lib	as desired
AEFDV	acute encephalopathy and fatty degeneration of viscera
AFB	acid fast bacillus
AFP	alpha-fetoprotein
Ag	antigen

ABBREVIATION	TERM
AICD	automatic, implantable cardiovascular defibrillator
AIDS	acquired immunodeficiency syndrome
AIIS	anterior inferior iliac spine
ALL	acute lymphoblastic leukemia
ALS	amyotrophic lateral sclerosis
ALT	alanine transaminase
AM; am	morning
AML	acute myelogenous leukemia
amp	ampule
ANA	antinuclear antibody
ANS	autonomic nervous system
ant	anterior
AP	anteroposterior
APSGN	acute poststreptococcal glomerulonephritis
aq	water
ARDS	adult respiratory distress syndrome
ARF	acute renal failure
ARM	artificial rupture of membranes

ABBREVIATION	TERM
AS	ankylosing spondylitis
AS (auris sinistra)	left ear
ASIS	anterior iliac spine
ASHD	arteriosclerotic heart disease
AST	aspartate transaminase
AU (auris unitas)	both ears
AV	atrioventricular
AZT	azidothymidine (drug used to treat AIDS)
μg; mcg	microgram
Ba	barium
baso	basophil
BBB	blood-brain barrier
BC	bone conduction
BE	barium enema
bid	twice a day
BP	blood pressure
BPH	benign prostatic hypertrophy
BSO	bilateral salpingo-oophorectomy
BUN	blood urea nitrogen
bx	biopsy
C	cervical; Centigrade
c	with
C&D	cystoscopy and dilation
C&S	culture and sensitivity
C1, C2 . . . C7	1st cervical vertebra, 2nd cervical vertebra . . . 7th cervical vertebra
C1, C2 . . . C6-C7	intervertebral disc space between the first and second vertebrae . . . intervertebral disc space between the sixth and seventh cervical vertebrae
Ca	calcium
CA	chronological age

ABBREVIATION	TERM
CABG	coronary artery bypass graft
CAD	coronary artery disease
cap	capsule
CAPD	continuous ambulatory peritoneal dialysis
CAT	computed axial tomography
CBC	complete blood count
CBD	common bile duct
cc	cubic centimeter
CCT	cranial computed tomography
CCU	cardiac/coronary care unit
CDH	congenital dislocation of hip
CF	cystic fibrosis
CHF	congestive heart failure
CIN	cervical intraepithelial neoplasia
CIS	carcinoma in situ
CK	creatine kinase
CLL	chronic lymphocytic leukemia
CML	chronic myelogenous leukemia
CNS	central nervous system
CO	cardiac output
CO_2	carbon dioxide
COLD	chronic obstructive lung disease
COPD	chronic obstructive pulmonary disease
CP	cerebral palsy
CPAP	continuous positive airway pressure
CPK	creatine phosphokinase
CPR	cardiopulmonary resuscitation
CRF	chronic renal failure
CRH	corticotrophin releasing hormone

ABBREVIATION	TERM
CS	cesarean section
CSF	cerebrospinal fluid
CT	computed tomography
CTS	carpal tunnel syndrome
CVA	cerebrovascular accident
CVS	chorionic villus sampling
CXR	chest x-ray
D&C	dilation (dilatation) and curettage
dB	decibel
DCR	dacryocystorhinostomy
DC; disc	discontinue
DDH	developmental dysplasia of hip
decub	decubitus lying down
ddI	dideoxyinosine (drug used to treat AIDS)
DI	diabetes insipidus; diagnostic imaging
diff	differential
DIP joint	distal interphalangeal joint
DKA	diabetic ketoacidosis
DLE	discoid lupus erythematosus
DM	diabetes mellitus
DMT	dimethyltryptamine (hallucinogenic drug)
DNA	deoxyribonucleic acid
DOE	dyspnea on exertion
D/RL	dextrose with Ringer's lactate solution
DSA	digital substraction angiography
DSM-III-R	Diagnostic and Statistical Manual of Mental Disorders, Third edition, revised.
DSR	dynamic spatial reconstructor
dr	dram

ABBREVIATION	TERM
DUB	dysfunctional uterine bleeding
DW	distilled water
D_5W	dextrose, 5% in water
EBV	Epstein-Barr virus
ECBD	exploration of common bile duct
ECCE	extracapsular cataract extraction
ECG; EKG	electrocardiogram
ECM	erythema chronicum migrans
ECRP	endoscopic retrograde cholangiopancreatography
EDC	expected date of confinement
EEG	electroencephalography
EENT	eyes, ears, nose, throat
ELISA	enzyme-linked immunosorbent assay
elix	elixer
EM	erythema multiforme
EMG	electromyogram; electromyography
endo	endoscopy
ENG	electronystagmography
ENT	ear, nose, and throat
EOM	extraocular movement
eosin	eosinophil
EPS	electrophysiologic study
ERCP	endoscopic retrograde cholangiopancreatiography
ERG	electroretinography
ERS	endoscopic retrograde sphincterotomy
ERV	expiratory reserve volume
ESR	erythrocyte sedimentation rate
ESWL	extracorporeal shock wave lithotripsy

ABBREVIATION	TERM	ABBREVIATION	TERM
EUA	examination under anesthesia	GTT	glucose tolerance test
ext	extract	gtt	drops
F	Fahrenheit	Gyne; gyn	gynecology
FBS	fasting blood sugar	HAV	hepatitis A virus
FEV	forced expiratory volume	Hb, Hgb	hemoglobin
fl; fld	fluid	HBV	hepatitis B virus
FP	flat plate	HCA	heterocyclic antidepressants
FRC	functional residual capacity	hCG; HCG	human chorionic gonadotrophin
FSH	follicle-stimulating hormone		
FVC	forced vital capacity	HCL	hydrochloric acid
Fx	fracture	HCT	hematocrit
G	gravida	HCV	hepatitis C virus
GA	general anesthesia	HD	Huntington's disease
GABA	gamma-aminobutyric acid	HDL	high density lipoprotein
GAF Scale	global assessment of functioning scale (scale ranging from 1–100, where 1 refers to poor mental health and inability to function in society. 100 refers to good mental health and the ability to function well in society)	HDV	hepatitis D virus
		HHD	hypertensive heart disease
		h; hr	hour
		HIV	human immunodeficiency virus
		HLA	human leukocyte antigen
		HPV	human papilloma virus
GB	gallbladder	hs	at bedtime
GBS	gallbladder series	HSG	hysterosalpingogram
GER	gastroesophageal reflux	HSV-1	herpes simplex virus 1
GFR	glomerular filtration rate	HSV-2	herpes simplex virus 2
g; gm	gram	HVA	homovanillic acid
GGT	gamma-glytamyl transpeptidase	I&D	incision and drainage
GH	growth hormone	IABP	intra-aortic balloon pump
GHIH	growth-hormone-inhibiting hormone	IBS	irritable bowel syndrome
GHRH	growth-hormone-releasing hormone	IC	inspiratory capacity
		ICCE	intracapsular cataract extraction
GI	gastrointestinal		
GnRH	gonadotrophin-releasing hormone	IDDM	insulin dependent diabetes mellitus
gr	grains	IDU	idoxuridine

ABBREVIATION	TERM
IF	immunofluorescent
Ig	immunoglobulin
IgG, IgM, IgA, IgE, IgD	immunoglobulin: G, M, A, E, D
IM	intramuscular
IOP	intraocular pressure
IP joint	interphalangeal joint
IPPB	intermittent positive pressure breathing
IQ	intelligent quotient (measurement of intellectual functioning as obtained by a number of intelligence tests. Normal IQ is between 90–110. Subnormal IQ is below 70).
IRV	inspiratory reserve volume
IUCD	intrauterine contraceptive device
IUD	intrauterine device
IV	intravenous
IVC	inferior vena cava; intravenous cholangiogram
IVP	intravenous pyelogram
IVU	intravenous urogram
JVP	jugular venous pressure
K	potassium
KCL	potassium chloride
keV	kilo electron volt
kg	kilogram
KKUB	kidney, kidney, ureter, bladder
KS	Kaposi's sarcoma
KUB	kidney, ureter, bladder
KV	kilovolts
L	lumbar
l	liter
L1, L2 . . . L5	1st lumbar vertebra, 2nd lumbar vertebra . . . 5th lumbar vertebrae

ABBREVIATION	TERM
L1-L2 . . . L4-L5	intervertebral disc space between the first and second lumbar vertebrae . . . intervertebral disc space between the fourth and fifth lumbar vertebrae
LA	left atrium
lb	pound
LBBB	left bundle branch block
LDH	lactic dehydrogenase
LDL	low density lipoprotein
LE	lupus erythematosus
LFT	liver function test
LH	luteinizing hormone
LLL	left lower lobe
LMP	last menstrual period
LP	lumbar puncture
L/S	lecithin/sphingomyelin ratio
LSD	lysergic acid diethylamide (hallucinogenic)
LUL	left upper lobe
LV	left ventricle
MA	mental age
MAOI	monamine oxidase inhibitor (antidepressant)
MBC	minimum bactericidal concentration
MCH	mean corpuscular hemoglobin
MCHC	mean corpuscular hemoglobin concentration
MCP joint	metacarpophalangeal joint
MCV	mean corpuscular volume
MDA	methylene dioxyamphetamine (hallucinogenic drug)
meds	medication
MEN	multiple endocrine neoplasia
mEq	milliequivalent

ABBREVIATION	TERM
mg	milligram
MI	myocardial infarction
MIC	minimum inhibitory concentration
MIH	melanocyte inhibiting hormone
mono	monocyte
MRH	melanocyte-releasing hormone
MRI	magnetic resonance imaging
MS	multiple sclerosis
MSAFP	maternal serum alpha-fetoprotein
MSH	melanocyte stimulating hormone
MSS	musculoskeletal system
MTBE	methyl tert-butyl ether
MUA	manipulation under anesthesia
MV	minute volume
N&V	nausea and vomiting
Na	sodium
NaCl	sodium chloride
NB; Nb	newborn
NFP	natural family planning
NG	nasogastric
NIDDM	noninsulin dependent diabetes mellitus
NMR	nuclear magnetic resonance
noc	nocturnal; at night
non rep	do not repeat
npo	nothing by mouth; nothing per os
NS	normal saline
O_2	oxygen
OA	osteoarthritis
OB	obstetrics
OCD	obsessive compulsive disorder

ABBREVIATION	TERM
OD	once daily; overdose
OD (oculus dextra)	right eye
OR	operating room
ortho	orthopedics
os	mouth
OS (oculus sinistra)	left eye
OT	oxytocin
OU (oculus unitas)	both eyes
oz	ounce
P	phophorus; para
PA	posteroanterior
Pap smear	Papanicolaou smear
PARR	postanesthetic recovery room
pc	after meals
PCP	phencyclidine (drug affecting an individual's behavior and mind. A psychoactive drug)
PCV	packed cell volume
PD	Parkinson's disease
PDDNOS	pervasive developmental disorder not otherwise specified
PEEP	positive end-expiratory pressure
PERLA	pupils equal; react to light and accommodation
PERRLA	pupils equal; round, regular, react to light and accommodation
PET	positron emission tomography
PFT	pulmonary function test
PID	pelvic inflammatory disease
PIH	prolactin-inhibiting hormone
PIP joint	proximal interphalangeal joint
PM; pm	night

ABBREVIATION	TERM
PMN	polymorphonuclear
PMP	past menstrual period
PMS	premenstrual syndrome
PND	paroxysmal nocturnal dyspnea
PNS	peripheral nervous system
polys	polymorphonuclear leukocytes
postop; post-op	postoperative
PP	postprandial
preop; pre-op	preoperative
prep	prepared
PRH	prolactin-releasing hormone
PRK	photorefractive keratectomy
PRL	prolactin
prn	as necessary; as required; as needed
PSA	prostate specific antigen
PSP	phenolsulfonphthalein
PT	prothrombin time
pt	pint
PTC	percutaneous transhepatic cholangiography
PTCA	percutaneous transluminal coronary angioplasty
PTH	parathyroid hormone (parathormone)
PTT	partial thromboplastin time
PUVA	psoralens ultraviolet light A
PVD	peripheral vascular disease
q2h	every 2 hours
q3h	every 3 hours
qd	every day
qh	every hour
qid	four times a day
qod	every other day

ABBREVIATION	TERM
R	rectal; respiration
R	respiration
RA	rheumatoid arthritis; right atrium
RAI	radioactive iodine
RBBB	right bundle branch block
RBC	red blood cell
RDS	respiratory distress syndrome
RF	rheumatoid factor
Rh	rhesus; Rh factor in the blood
RIA	radioimmunoassay
RICE	rest, ice, compression, elevation
RL	Ringer's lactate
RLL	right lower lobe
ROM	range of motion
RUL	right upper lobe
RV	residual volume; right ventricle
R_x	take; prescription
s	without
S&D	stomach and duodenum
S_1	first heart sound
S1, S2 . . . S5	1st sacral vertebra, 2nd sacral vertebra . . . 5th sacral vertebra
S1-S2 . . . S4-S5	intervertebral disc space between the first and second sacral vertebrae . . . intervertebral disc space between the fourth and fifth sacral vertebrae
S_2	second heart sound
SA	sinoatrial
SAD	seasonal affective disorder
SAP	serum alkaline phosphatase
SBFT	small bowel follow through
SBE	subacute bacterial endocarditis

ABBREVIATION	TERM
SBS	small bowel series
SC; subcu	subcutaneous
SGOT	serum glutamic oxaloacetic transaminase
SGPT	serum glutamic pyruvic transaminase
SIDS	sudden infant death syndrome
SL	sublingual
SLE	systemic lupus erythematosus
SMR	submucous resection
SOB	shortness of breath
sol	solution
sp.gr.	specific gravity
SR	suture removal
SSSS	staphylococcal scalded skin syndrome
stat	immediately
STD	sexually transmitted disease
STS	serologic test for syphilis
supp	suppository
SVC	superior vena cava
T	temperature; thoracic
T&A	tonsillectomy and adenoidectomy
T1, T2 . . . T12	1st thoracic vertebra, 2nd thoracic vertebra . . . 12th thoracic vertebra
T1-T2 . . . T11-T12	intervertebral disc space between the first and second thoracic vertebral . . . intervertebral disc space between the eleventh and twelfth thoracic vertebrae
T_3	triiodothyronine
T_4	thyroxine
TA	therapeutic abortion
tab	tablet

ABBREVIATION	TERM
TAH	total abdominal hysterectomy
TB	tuberculosis
tbsp; T	tablespoon
Tc	technetium
TCA	tricyclic antidepressants
TGV	thoracic gas volume
THC	delta-9-tetrahydrocannabinol (major psychoactive constituent in marijuana)
TIA	transient ischemic attack
tid	three times a day
tinct	tincture
TLC	total lung capacity
TM	tympanic membrane
TPA	tissue plasminogen activator
TPN	total parenteral nutrition
TRH	thyrotrophin-releasing hormone
TSH	thyroid-stimulating hormone
TSAb	thyroid-stimulating antibodies
tsp; t	teaspoon
TUR	transurethral resection
TURP	transurethral resection of prostate
TV	tidal volume
U	unit
UGI	upper gastrointestinal
ung	ointment
up	upright
URI	upper respiratory infection
US	ultrasound
UV	ultraviolet
vag	vaginal
VC	vital capacity

ABBREVIATION	TERM
VDRL	venereal disease research laboratories
VLDL	very low density lipoprotein
VMA	vanillylmandelic acid
WBC	white blood cell
WAIS	Wechsler Adult Intelligence Scale

ABBREVIATION	TERM
WISC	Wechsler Intelligence Scale for Children
ZDV	zidovudine (drug used to treat AIDS)
ZN	Ziehl-Neelsen

A-V atrioventricular, pertaining to the atria and ventricles.

Ab antibody.

Ab abortion termination of a pregnancy, either spontaneous or by surgical means.

abdomen (ăb′-dō-měn) the portion of the trunk located between the back and front, below the diaphragm, and including the lower portion of the abdominopelvic cavity.

abdominal (ăb-dŏm′-ĭ-năl) pertaining to the abdomen.

abdominal cavity space between the diaphragm and pelvis.

abdominal paracentesis removal of abdominal fluids through a puncture made into the abdominal cavity.

abdominal quadrants four parts or divisions of the abdomen determined by drawing imaginary vertical and horizontal lines through the umbilicus. The quadrants are: right upper quadrant, RUQ; contains the liver (right lobe), gallbladder, part of the pancreas, and parts of the small and large intestines; left upper quadrant, LUQ, contains the liver (left lobe), stomach, spleen, part of the pancreas, parts of the small and large intestines; right lower quadrant, RLQ, contains parts of the small and large intestines, right ovary, right uterine (fallopian) tube, appendix, right ureter; left lower quadrant, LLQ, contains parts of the small and large intestines, left ovary, left uterine tube, and right ureter.

abdominocentesis (ăb-dŏm″-ĭ-nō-sĕn-tē′-sĭs) surgical puncture to remove fluid from the abdomen (peritoneal cavity). This procedure is done to remove fluid from a patient with ascites or for diagnostic purposes.

abdominohysterectomy (ăb-dŏm″-ĭ-nō-hĭs-tĕr-ĕk′-tō-mē) surgical incision with excision of the uterus.

abdominopelvic (ăb-dŏm″-ĭ-nō-pĕl′-vĭk) **cavity** space below the chest containing organs such as the liver, stomach, gallbladder, and intestines; also called the abdomen.

abduction (ăb-dŭk′-shŭn) movement of a limb away from the median plane of the body or, in case of digits, away from the axial line of a limb.

abductor (ăb-dŭk′-tor) muscle that draws away from the medial line of the body or to a common center.

ABG arterial blood gases.

ABO blood types: A, B, and O.

abortifacient (ă-bor-tĭ-fā′-shĕnt) anything used to cause or to induce an abortion.

abortion (ă-bor′-shŭn) termination of a pregnancy before the embryo or fetus is outside the uterus.

abruptio (ă-brŭp′-shē-ō) **placenta** premature separation of the normally implanted placenta.

absence (ăb′-sĕnz) brief temporary loss of consciousness. May occur as absentia epileptica. May also refer to the lack of structural development.

absorbable surgical clips clips made of synthetic, non-metallic material designed to maintain its strength until healing occurs. They will absorb over time and dissolve. They are sterile and do not produce tissue irritation of significance. They do not show up on x-rays or CT scans, which is advantageous in postoperative assessment.

absorbable suture sterile strand prepared from collagen or from synthetic polymer. This type of suture is absorbed and thus does not need to be removed.

absorption (ăb-sorp′-shŭn) passage of materials through the walls of the intestines into the bloodstream.

AC air conduction.

acantholysis (ă-kăn-thŏl′-ĭ-sĭs) any disease of the skin accompanied by degeneration of the cohesive elements of the cells of the outer layer of the skin.

acanthosis (ăk″-ăn-thō′-sĭs) increased thickness of prickle cell layer of skin.

accommodation (ă-kŏm″-ō-dā′-shŭn) the normal adjustment of the crystalline lens by the ciliary muscle, which makes the lens fatter or thinner to bring an object into focus on the retina.

accumulates to pile up or collect.

ACE angiotensin-converting enzyme.

ACE inhibitor a drug that lowers blood pressure and reduces the resistance in arteries, used to treat hypertension and congestive heart failure.

acetabular (ăs″-ĕ-tăb′-ū-lăr) pertaining to the acetabulum, or acetabula.

acetabular notch notch in the inferior border of acetabulum.

acetabulum (ăs″-ĕ-tăb′-ū-lŭm) **(pl. acetabula)** rounded depression or socket in the pelvic bone where the thigh bone joins with the pelvis.

acetylcholine (ăs″-ĕ-tĭl-kō′-lēn) **(ACh)** neurotransmitter chemical released at the ends of some nerve cells.

acetylsalicylic (ă-sē″-tĭl-săl′-ĭ-sĭl′-ĭk) **acid** aspirin.

achalasia (ăk″-ă-lā′-zē-ă) failure of the muscles of the lower esophagus to relax during swallowing.

acid-fast stain not decolorized easily by acids after staining. The acid-fast bacteria retain the red dye, but the surrounding tissues are decolorized.

acid-fast bacilli not readily decolorized by acids or other means when stained.

acne (ăk'-nē) skin eruptions caused by the build up of sebum and keratin in the pores of the skin.

acoustic (ă-koos'-tĭk) pertaining to sound or to the sense of hearing.

Acquired Immunodeficiency Syndrome (AIDS) disease caused by the human immunodeficiency virus (HIV) which attacks the immune system leaving the patient vulnerable to opportunistic infection.

acromegaly (ăk"-rō-mĕg'-ă-lē) enlargement of the extremities caused by hypersecretion of growth hormone from the anterior pituitary.

acromioclavicular (ă-krō"-mē-ō-klă-vĭk'-ū-lăr) pertaining to the joint of the acromion scapula and the clavicle.

acromioclavicular joint arthrodial joint between the acromion of the scapula and the clavicle.

acromion process outward extension of the scapula forming the point of the shoulder.

acromion triangular area of the scapula that articulates with the clavicle.

acrophobia an unreasonable fear of heights.

ACTH adrenocorticotrophic hormone produced by the anterior lobe of the pituitary gland; also called adrenocorticotropin. ACTH acts on the adrenal cortex, stimulating its secretion of hormones, especially cortisol.

actin (ăk'-tĭn) protein component of actomyosin in muscle.

action (ăk'-shŭn) setting into motion or causing to do something.

actomyosin (ăk"-tō-mī'-ō-sĭn) complex of actin and myosin forming the primary contractile element of muscle fiber.

acute (ă-kūt') brief, intense or severe; having rapid onset, severe symptoms, and a short course; not chronic.

acute conjunctivitis conjunctival inflammation which is not of a chronic nature.

acute lymphoblastic leukemia (ALL) form of leukemia in which immature lymphocytes (lymphoblasts) predominate, seen most often in children and adolescents.

acute myelogenous leukemia (AML) form of leukemia in which immature granulocytes (myeloblasts) predominate. Platelets and erythrocytes may be diminished because of infiltration and replacement of normal bone marrow by large numbers of myeloblasts.

acute poststreptococcal glomerulonephritis (APSGN) acute nephritis with inflammation involving glomeruli, a late complication of streptococcal infection, particularly pharyngitis.

acute renal failure acute failure of the kidney to perform its essential functions.

acyclovir (ă-sī'-klō-vĭr) a synthetic acyclic purine nucleoside with selective antiviral activity against herpes simplex virus.

AD (auris dextra) right ear.

Addison's (ăd'-ĭ-sŏnz) **disease** hypofunction of the adrenal cortex resulting in weakness, tiredness, darkened pigmentation of the skin.

adduction (ă-dŭk'-shŭn) movement of a body part toward the median plane body.

adductor (ă-dŭk'-tor) muscle that draws toward the medial line of the body or to a common center.

adductor brevis short adductor muscle.

adductor longus long adductor muscle.

adductor magnus great adductor muscle.

adenitis (ăd"-ĕ-nī'-tĭs) inflammation of lymph nodes or a gland.

adenohypophysis (ăd"-ĕ-nō-hī-pŏf'-ĭ-sĭs) anterior lobe of the pituitary gland.

adenoid (ăd'-ĕ-noyd) lymphatic tissue in the part of the throat near the nose and nasal passages, also called pharyngeal tonsils. The literal meaning is "resembling glands," since adenoids are lymphoid and are neither endocrine nor exocrine glands.

adenoidectomy (ăd"-ĕ-noyd-ĕk'-tō-mē) excision of the adenoids.

adenoma (ăd"-ĕ-nō'-mă) **(pl. adenomata, adenomas)** benign neoplasm in which tumor cells form glandlike structures.

adenopathy (ăd-ĕ-nŏp'-ă-thē) swelling and morbid change in lymph nodes.

adenovirus (ăd'-ĕ-nō-vī'-rŭs) one of a group of closely related viruses that can cause infections of the upper respiratory tract.

ADH antidiuretic hormone; vasopressin.

adhesion (ăd-hē'-zhŭn) a holding together of two surfaces or parts.

adipocele (ăd'-ĭ-pō-sēl") hernia that contains fat or fatty tissue.

adipose (ăd'-ĭ-pōz) pertaining to fat.

adipose tissue collection of fat cells.

adjuvant (ăd'-jū-vănt) **therapy** assistive treatment with curative intent. Refers in particular to treatment of neoplastic disease in which chemotherapy drugs may be given early in the course of treatment, along with surgery or radiation to attack cancer cells that may be too small to be detected by diagnostic techniques.

adnexa (ăd-nĕk'-să) any accessory part to an organ.

adolescent (ăd"-ō-lĕs'-ĕnt) young man or woman not yet fully grown.

adrenal cortex outer portion of the adrenal gland which secretes three types of steroid hormones essential to life: androgens, corticosteroids and mineralocorticoids.

adrenal (ăd-rē'-năl) **gland** endocrine glands located above each kidney.

adrenal medulla the inner portion of the adrenal gland which secretes catecholamines.

adrenal virilism excessive output of adrenal androgens.

adrenalectomy (ăd-rē"-năl-ĕk'-tō-mē) removal of the adrenal gland.

adrenaline (ă-drĕn'-ă-lēn) produced by the adrenal medulla; also called epinephrine. Adrenaline increases heart rate and blood pressure.

adrenocorticotrophic (ăd-rē"-nō-kor"-tĭ-kō-trŏp'-ĭk) **hormone (ACTH)** produced by the anterior lobe of the pituitary gland, ACTH stimulates secretion of hormones from the adrenal cortex, especially cortisol.

adventitia (ăd"-vĕn-tĭsh'-ē-ă) outermost covering of a structure or organ, such as the tunica adventitia or outer coat of an artery.

adventitious sounds sounds of external or accidental origin heard in auscultation.

AFB acid-fast bacillus (bacilli).

afebrile (ă-fĕb'-rĭl) without fever.

afferent (ăf'-ĕr-ĕnt) **arteriole** small artery, carrying blood toward the heart.

AFP (Alpha-fetoprotein) during pregnancy increases in maternal blood and amniotic fluid. May be a marker for fetal nervous system developmental abnormalities. May also be a tumor marker in hepatocellular and germ cell malignancies.

agglutination (ă-gloo″-tĭ-nā′-shŭn) clumping together.

agoraphobia (ăg″-ō-ră-fō′-bē-ă) an unreasonable fear of unfamiliar surroundings.

agranulocytosis (ă-grăn″-ū-lō-sī-tō′-sĭs) a state characterized by a deficit or absolute lack of granulocytic white blood cells.

agraphia (ă-grăf′-ē-ă) inability to express thoughts in writing. Caused by a lesion of the cerebral cortex.

AIDS acquired immunodeficiency syndrome.

ailurophobia (ă-lū″-rō-fō′-bē-ă) an unreasonable fear of cats.

air conduction (AC) conduction of sound to the inner ear via the air in the ear canal.

albinism (ăl′-bĭn-ĭzm) general term for a number of autosomal recessive inherited disorders affecting the pigment cell (melanocyte) and causing hypomelanosis or amelanosis of the skin, hair, and eyes.

albumin (ăl-bū′-mĭn) a protein that is water soluble and coagulable by heat.

albuminemia (ăl-bū″-mĭn-ē′-mē-ă) albumin in the blood.

albuminuria (ăl-bū-mĭ-nū′-rē-ă) albumin in the urine.

aldosterone (ăl-dăs′-tĕr-ōn) mineralocorticoid secreted by the adrenal cortex.

aldosteronism (ăl″-dŏ-stĕr′-ōn-ĭzm″) abnormal condition of electrolyte metabolism caused by excessive secretion of aldosterone. Also called hyperaldosteronism.

algophobia (ăl″-gō-fō′-bē-ă) unreasonable fear of pain.

alimentary (ăl″-ĭ-mĕn′-tăr-ē) pertaining to food or nutrition.

alkaline (ăl′-kă-lĭn) **phosphatase** an enzyme formed primarily in bone and liver, levels of which may be tested in the serum.

alkylating (ăl′-kĭ-lāt-ĭng) **agents** synthetic chemicals containing alkyl groups that combine easily with other substances; used in cancer treatment and are carcinogenic as well.

ALL acute lymphoblastic leukemia.

allantois (ă-lăn′-tō-ĭs) elongated bladder which contributes to development of the umbilicus and placenta.

allele (ă-lēl′) any alternative form of a gene that can occupy a particular chromosomal locus.

allergen (ăl′-ĕr-jĕn) antigenic substance capable of generating an immune response.

allergic conjunctivitis disease characterized by swelling of the eyelids and congestion, redness, and pain in the eyes.

allergic (ă-lĕr′-jĭk) **rhinitis** acute allergic congestion of the mucous membranes of the nose, marked by nasal congestion and increased mucus secretion.

allergy (ăl′-ĕr-jē) state of hypersensitivity induced by a particular antigen.

Allis forceps used to grasp or hold tissue.

allograft (ăl′-ō-grăft) tissue obtained from the same species for use in transplant procedures.

alopecia (ăl″-ō-pē′-shē-ă) absence of hair from areas where it normally grows; baldness.

alpha (ăl′-fă) **particles** radioactive particles.

ALT alanine aminotransferase, also known as serum glutamic-pyruvic transaminase (SGPT).

alveolar (ăl-vē′-ō-lăr) pertaining to the alveoli.

alveolus (ăl-vē′-ō-lŭs) **(pl. alveoli pertaining to the air sacs)** small hollow cavity.

Alzheimer's (ălts′-hī-mĕrz) **disease** organic mental disease named for Alois Alzheimer, a chronic form of dementia with onset generally between ages 40 and 60. This is a progressive disease with no known cure.

amblyopia (ăm″-blē-ō′-pē-ă) condition of dim or otherwise reduced vision.

ambulatory (ăm′-bū-lă-tō″-rĕ) able to walk or walking.

ambulatory care care provided to the patient without hospitalization.

amenorrhea (ă-mĕn″-ō-rē′-ă) absence of menstruation. Called primary amenorrhea when the patient has never menstruated and secondary amenorrhea when the patient has skipped one or more menstrual periods during life.

amitriptyline an antidepressant drug.

AML acute myelogenous leukemia.

amnesia (ăm-nē′-zē-ă) lack or loss of memory; inability to remember past experiences.

amniocentesis (ăm″-nē-ō-sĕn-tē′-sĭs) puncture of the amniotic sac through the abdominal wall to withdraw a sample of amniotic fluid. The fluid is examined to diagnose any fetal abnormality especially genetic such as Down syndrome.

ampulla (ăm-pŭl′-lă) **of Vater** hepatopancreatic ampulla; location of joining of the common bile duct and main pancreatic duct at the duodenum.

amputation (ăm″-pū-tă′-shŭn) removal of a portion or all of the extremity.

amylase (ăm′-ĭ-lās) enzyme from the pancreas which digests starch.

amyotrophic (ă-mī″-ō-trŏf′-ĭk) **lateral sclerosis (ALS)** progressive disorder characterized by degeneration of motor neurons in the spinal cord and brain stem; also called Lou Gehrig's disease.

ANA antinuclear antibodies, detection of which may aid in the diagnosis of systemic lupus erythematosus.

anabolism (ă-năb′-ō-lĭzm) process of building up complex materials (e.g., proteins) from simple materials.

anal (ā-năl) **fissure** a narrow slit in the anal canal.

anal fistula abnormal tube-like passageway near the anus, which may communicate with the rectum.

analgesia (ăn-ăl-jē′-zē-ă) loss of pain; relief of pain without loss of consciousness.

analgesic (ăn″-ăl-jē′-sĭk) type of drug, including narcotics, which reduces the patient's threshold of pain; used to alleviate mild to moderate pain or reduce fever.

anaphylaxis (ăn″-ă-fĭ-lăk′-sĭs) exaggerated or unusual hypersensitivity to an allergen.

anaplasia (ăn″-ă-plā′-zē-ă) loss of differentiation of cells; reversion to more primitive cell type.

anastomosis (ă-năs″-tō-mō′-sĭs) surgical joining of two structures that are normally separate.

anatomical (ăn″-ă-tŏm′-ĭ-kăl) **planes** three planes: frontal, sagittal, transverse.

anatomical position ten positions: anterior (front), deep, distal, inferior (caudal), lateral, medial, posterior (dorsal), prone, proximal, superficial, superior (cephalic), and supine.

androgenic (ăn″-drō-jĕn′-ĭk) producing masculinization.

androgen (ăn′-drō-jĕn) male hormone produced by the testes, and to a lesser extent, by the adrenal cortex; testosterone is an example.

anemia (ă-nē′-mē-ă) medical condition in which there is a reduction in the number of erythrocytes or amount of hemoglobin in the circulating blood.

anesthesia (ăn″-ĕs-thē′-zē-ă) absence of sense of touch or pain.

anesthesiologist (ăn″-ĕs-thē″-zē-ŏl′-ō-jĭst) physician who specializes in the study and effects of anesthesiology.

anesthetic (ăn″-ĕs-thĕt′-ĭk) drug that produces a loss of feeling or sensation which may be partial or complete; may be administered by injection or by inhalation of gaseous agents.

aneurysm (ăn′-ū-rĭzm) local widening (ballooning out of a small area) of an artery, caused by weakness in the arterial wall.

aneurysmectomy (ăn″-ū-rĭz-mĕk′-tō-mē) excision of aneurysm.

angiectasis (ăn″-jē-ĕk′-tă-sĭs) dilatation of a blood vessel; vasodilation.

angiitis (ăn″-jē-ī′-tĭs) inflammation of blood vessel or lymph vessel.

angina pectoris (ăn-jī′-nă) the pain of cardiac ischemia, usually occurring in the precordial area, which may or may not radiate. May be substernal or retrosternal. Frequently described as pressurelike or crushing.

angiocardiography (ăn″-jē-ō-kăr″-dē-ŏg′-ră-fē) x-ray of the blood vessels of the heart.

angiogram (ăn′-jē-ō-grăm) radiologic study of a blood vessel taken in rapid sequence following injection of radiopaque material into the vessel. Used to find size and shape of veins and arteries.

angiography (ăn″-jē-ŏg′-ră-fē) radiologic procedure in which contrast material is injected into the circulation and fills arteries or veins. Pictures of the fluid may be taken by x-ray. Narrowing of vessels, blood clots, cysts and tumors can be detected.

angioma (ăn″-jē-ō′-mă) blood vessels or lymph vessels forming a tumor, usually benign.

angioplasty (ăn′-jē-ō-plăs″-tē) narrowed blood vessel is opened using a balloon that is inflated after it is inserted into the blood vessel.

angiospasm (ăn′-jē-ō-spăzm) sudden, involuntary contraction of a blood vessel.

anhidrosis (ăn″-hī-drō′-sĭs) inability to sweat; may be temporary or permanent.

anisocoria (ăn-ī″-sō-kō′-rē-ă) obvious difference in pupil size from one eye to the other; may be congenital or associated with head trauma, brain lesion, or aneurysm.

anisocytosis (ăn-ī″-sō-sī-tō′-sĭs) condition of inequality in cell size.

ankyloglossia (ăng″-kĭ-lo-glŏs′-sē-ă) shortness of tongue.

ankylosing spondylitis (AS) form of chronic, progressive arthritis with stiffening of the joints of the spine.

ankylosis (ăng″-kĭ-lō′-sĭs) immobility and stiffening of the joints.

annulus (ăn′-ū-lŭs) fibrosis ring-shaped structure of fibrous tissue such as found in an intravertebral disk.

anodontia (ăn″-ŏ-dŏn′-shē-ă) condition of no teeth (a developmental condition).

anorectal (ā-nō-rĕk′-tăl) pertaining to the anus and rectum.

anoxia (ăn-ŏk′-sē-ă) without oxygen.

ant. anterior.

anteflexion (ăn-tē-flĕk′-shun) abnormal bending forward of part of an organ.

antenatal (ăn″-tē-nā′-tăl) before birth; prenatal.

anterior chamber of the eye area behind the cornea and in front of the crystalline lens and iris; contains aqueous humor.

anterior (ventral) front of the body.

anterolateral situated in front and to one side.

anteroposterior the front-to-back direction an x-ray takes through a body.

anteverted (ăn″-tē-vĕrt′-ĕd) tipped forward.

antiallergy relieving allergies.

antianginal drug drug used to reverse the effects of angina pectoris by increasing the blood supply to the heart.

antiarrhythmic (ăn″-tē-ă-rĭth′-mĭk) drug used to treat irregular heart rhythms.

antiarthritic (ăn″-tē-ăr-thrĭt′-ĭk) medicine used to help treat arthritic symptoms.

antibacterial (ăn″-tĭ-băk-tē′-rē-ăl) stopping the growth of bacteria.

antibiotics (ăn″-tĭ-bī-ŏt′-ĭks) chemical compounds that slow or arrest the growth of bacteria. They are produced by living cells such as bacteria, yeasts, or molds and can also be commercially synthesized.

antibody (ăn′-tĭ-bŏd″-ē) protein substance whose formation by lymphocytes is stimulated by the presence of antigens in the body. An antibody then helps neutralize or inactivate the antigen that stimulated its formation.

anticholinergic (ăn″-tĭ-kō″-lĭn-ĕr′-jĭk) drug which antagonizes the action of cholinergic nerve fibers.

anticholinesterase (ăn″-tĭ-kō-lĭn-ĕs′-tĕr-ās) **drug** drug used to oppose the action of cholinesterase.

anticoagulant (ăn″-tĭ-kō-ăg′-ū-lănt) type of medication used to prevent the formation of blood clots.

anticonvulsant (ăn″-tĭ-kŏn-vŭl′-sănt) drug used in the treatment of epilepsy to inhibit convulsions or seizures.

antidepressant (ăn″-tĭ-dē-prĕs′-sănt) drug used to relieve symptoms of psychological depression by altering messages between brain cells.

antidiuretic (ăn″-tĭ-dī-ū-rĕt′-ĭk) **hormone** (ADH) secreted by the posterior lobe of the pituitary gland, ADH increases reabsorption of water by the kidney; also known as vasopressin.

antiemetic (ăn″-tĭ-ē-mĕt′-ĭk) **drug** used to prevent vomiting.

antifungal (ăn″-tĭ-fŭng′-găl) drug which destroys or stops the growth of fungi.

antigen (ăn′-tĭ-jĕnz) (Ag.) a foreign material, generally a protein, which stimulates the production of an antibody. Naturally occurring antigens are the blood type factors A and B that are present at birth in some individuals.

antihistamine (ăn″-tĭ-hĭs′-tă-mēn) drug used to treat conditions in which histamines are released in response to certain allergens.

antihyperlipidemic agent used to stop or destroy an increase of lipids in the blood.

antihypertensive (ăn″-tĭ-hī″-pĕr-tĕn′-sĭv) used to control or prevent high blood pressure.

anti-infective (ăn″-tĭ-ĭn-fĕk′-tĭv) capable of destroying infectious agents or preventing them from spreading and causing infection.

antimetabolite (ăn″-tĭ-mĕ-tăb′-ō-līt) chemical that prevents cell division, used in cancer chemotherapy.

antimicrobial (ăn″-tĭ-mī-krō′-bē-ăl) agent which prevents the growth or action of microbes.

antiovulant (ăn″-tē-ŏv′-ū-lănt) used to prevent ovulation.

antipruritic (ăn″-tĭ-proo-rīt′-ĭk) used to prevent or help relieve itching.

antiseptic (ăn″-tĭ-sĕp′-tĭk) used to fight against infection.

antithrombotic (ăn″-tĭ-thrŏm-bŏt′-ĭk) **therapy** therapy of interfering with or preventing blood coagulation.

antitussive (ăn″-tĭ-tŭs′-ĭv) preventing or relieving coughing.

antiviral (ăn″-tĭ-vī′-răl) acting against a virus.

antrostomy (ăn-trŏs'-tō-mē) surgical procedure to form an opening in an antrum.

anuria (ăn-ū'-rē-ă) absence of urine production.

anus (ā'-nŭs) opening of the digestive tract to outside of the body through which waste passes.

anvil (ăn'-vĭl) second ossicle (bone) of the middle ear; also called incus.

anxiety (ăng-zī'-ĕ-tē) feeling of worry, dread, or uneasiness concerning the future.

aorta (ā-or'-tă) largest artery in the body.

aortic root replacement after excision of an aortic aneurysm a tubular graft replaces the diseased portion.

aortography (ā''-or-tog'-ră-fē) x-ray of the aorta.

aortotomy (ā''-or-tŏt'-ō-mē) incision of the aorta.

AP anteroposterior.

apex of the lung uppermost portion of the lung.

aphagia (ă-fā'-jē-ă) inability to swallow.

aphakia (ă-fā'-kē-ă) missing the crystalline lens of the eye.

aphasia (ă-fā'-zē-ă) inability to communicate using speech, writing, or signs, caused by cerebral dysfunction.

aphonia (ă-fō'-nē-ă) no voice; loss of voice.

aphthous (ăf'-thŭs) **stomatitis** inflammation of the mouth with small ulcers.

apical (ăp'-ĭ-kal) **foramen** opening at the end of a tooth which allows for blood, lymphatic, and the nerve supply to pass to the dental pulp.

aplastic (ă-plăs'-tĭk) **anemia** severe type of anemia in which the bone marrow fails to produce not only erythrocytes but leukocytes and thrombocytes as well.

apnea (ăp-nē'-ă) no breathing.

apocrine gland discharged secretions of this gland contain part of the secreting cells.

aponeurosis (ăp''-ō-nū-rō'-sĭs) **(pl. aponeuroses)** white, flat, ribbon-like fibrous sheet of connective tissue; serves to connect muscle or bone to other tissue.

appendectomy (ăp''-ĕn-dĕk'-tō-mē) removal of appendix.

appendicitis (ă-pĕn''-dĭ-sī'-tĭs) inflammation of the appendix.

appendicular (ăp''-ĕn-dĭk'-ū-lăr) **skeleton** bones of the upper and lower extremities.

appendix (ă-pĕn-dĭks) blind pouch in the right lower quadrant hanging from the first part of the colon.

approximation bringing of the edges of a wound together. This term is used in reference to the sewing up of tissues such as skin, muscle, fat, etc. The material used to approximate the edges of such tissues is called suture material.

apraxia (ă-prăk'-sē-ă) movements and behavior are not purposeful.

aqueous (ā'-kwē-ŭs) formed by water.

aqueous humor fluid produced by the ciliary body and found in the anterior chambers of the eye.

arachnoid (ă-răk'-noyd) similar to a web.

arcuate (ăr'-kū-āt) **popliteal ligament** ligament on the posterolateral side of the knee surface.

ARDS adult respiratory distress syndrome.

areola (ă-rē'-ō-lă) dark pigmented area around the breast nipple.

ARF acute renal failure.

argon (ăr'-gŏn) **laser** high-energy light.

ARM artificial rupture of membranes.

arousal state of awareness.

arrector (ă-rĕk'-tor) **pili** involuntary smooth muscle fibers, arising in the skin and extending down to the hair follicles which act to pull the hairs erect.

arrhythmia (ă-rĭth'-mē-ă) deviation from the normal heart rhythm.

arterial (ăr-tē'-rē-ăl) pertaining to arteries.

arterial blood gases (ABG) measurement of the gases present in arterial blood, i.e. oxygen and carbon dioxide.

arteriography (ăr''-tē-rē-ŏg'-ră-fē) x-ray of the arteries.

arteriole (ăr-tē'-rē-ōl) small arteries that supply capillaries.

arteriosclerosis (ăr-tē''-rē-ō-sklĕ-rō'-sĭs) hardening of an artery.

arteriostenosis (ăr-tē''-rē-ō-stĕ-nō'-sĭs) narrowing of an artery.

artery (ăr'-tĕr-ē) largest type of blood vessel; carries oxygenated blood away from the heart.

arthralgia (ăr-thrăl'-jē-ă) joint pain.

arthritis (ăr-thrī-tĭs) inflammation of joints.

arthrocentesis (ăr''-thrō-sĕn-tē'-sĭs) aspiration of synovial fluid; surgical puncture of the joint space with a needle, removing synovial fluid for analysis.

arthrodesis (ăr-thrō-dē'-sĭs) artificial ankylosis.

arthrodia (ăr-thrō'-dē-ă) synovial joint that permits only simple gliding movement.

arthrodynia (ăr''-thrō-dĭn'-ē-ă) pain in a joint.

arthrography (ăr-thrŏg'-ră-fē) process of taking x-ray pictures of a joint after injection of opaque contrast material.

arthroplasty (ăr'-thrō-plăs''-tē) replacement of one or both bone ends by a prosthesis.

arthroscope (ăr'-thrō-skōp) endoscope used to examine the interior of a joint.

arthroscopy (ăr-thrŏs'-kō-pē) visual examination of the inside of a joint with a endoscope. Surgical instruments can be passed through the arthroscope to remove tissue and repair the joint.

arthrotomy (ăr-thrŏt'-ō-mē) cutting into a joint.

articular (ăr-tĭk'-ū-lăr) relating to a joint or articulation.

articular cartilage thin layer of cartilage at the ends of bones involved in synovial joint.

articulation (connection) joint.

artificial rupture of membranes (ARM) manual rupture of the amniotic sac to assist in delivery of the fetus.

arytenoid (ăr''-ĭ-tē'-noyd) **cartilage** a laryngeal cartilage which is shaped like a jug or pitcher mouth.

AS auris sinistra; left ear.

ascending colon extends from the cecum to the under surface of the liver, where it turns left to become the transverse colon.

ascending tracts bundle of white fibers that carry impulses toward the brain.

aseptic (ā-sĕp'-tĭk) free from infectious contamination.

ASHD arteriosclerotic heart disease; heart disease secondary to arteriosclerosis.

aspermatogenesis (ă-spĕr''-mă-tō-jĕn'-ĕ-sĭs) no production of spermatozoa.

asphyxia (ăs-fĭk'-sē-ă) interference with respiration which can ultimately lead to death.

aspiration (ăs-pĭ-rā'-shŭn) fluid is withdrawn by suction from a cavity or sac with a needle.

aspirin (ăs'-pĕr-ĭn) another name for acetylsalicylic acid, an analgesic medication; an analgesic.

AST aspartate aminotransferase, also known as serum glutamicoxaloacetic transaminase (SGOT).

asthma (ăz'-mă) bronchial airway obstruction due to spasm and inflammation of bronchi.

astigmatism (ă-stĭg′-mă-tĭzm) defective curvature of the cornea or lens of the eye.

astrocyte (ăs′-trō-sīt) (astroglia) star-shaped neuroglial cell with many branching processes.

astrocytoma (ăs″-trō-sī-tō′-mă) tumor comprised of astrocytes.

asymmetry (ă-sĭm′-ĕ-trē) lacking symmetry.

asymptomatic (ā″-sĭmp-tō-măt′-ĭk) showing lack of symptoms.

ataxia (ă-tăk′-sē-ă) persistent unsteadiness on the feet, often caused by disorders of the cerebellum.

ataxic (ă-tăk′-sĭk) **gait** uncoordinated walk.

ataxic respiration irregular respiration.

atelectasis (ăt″-ĕ-lĕk′-tă-sĭs) incomplete expansion of the air sacs; collapsed, functionless, airless lung or portion of a lung.

atheroma (ăth″-ĕr-ō′-mă) occurring in atherosclerosis, fatty degeneration or thickening of larger arteries.

atherosclerosis (ăth″-ĕr-ō′-sklĕ-rō′-sĭs) accumulation of fatty debris on the tunica intima of an artery.

atlas (ăt′-lăs) first cervical vertebra; articulates above with the occipital bone and below with the axis.

atonic (ă-tŏn′-ĭk) lacking normal tension or tone.

atony (ăt′-ō-nē) without normal tone or strength.

atopic (ă-tŏp′-ĭk) **dermatitis** characterized by itching and scratching in an individual with inherently irritable skin; of unknown etiology.

atopic rhinitis non-seasonal allergic nasal inflammation.

atracurium generic name of muscle relaxant drug.

atrial (ā′-trē-ăl) pertaining to the atrium.

atrioventricular (ă″-trē-ō-vĕn-trĭk′-ū-lăr) **block** failure of proper conduction of impulses through the A-V node to the bundle of His.

atrioventricular valve (AV) specialized tissue at the base of the wall between the two upper heart chambers. Electrical impulses pass from the pacemaker (S-A node) through the A-V node to the bundle of His.

atrium (ā′-trē-ŭm) upper chamber of the heart.

atrophy (ăt′-rō-fē) wasting away.

AU (auris unitas) both ears.

audiogram (aw′-dē-ō-grăm″) recording of a hearing test.

auditory (aw′-dĭ-tō″-rē) pertaining to the sense of hearing.

auditory canal channel that leads from the flap of the ear to the eardrum.

auditory meatus auditory canal.

auditory nerve fibers nerves that carry nerve impulses from the inner ear to the brain.

auditory ossicles small bones of the ear: the malleus, incus and stapes.

auditory tube channel between the middle ear and the nasopharynx; eustachian tube.

augmentation (awg″-mĕn-tā′-shŭn) **mammoplasty** surgical enlargement of the breast.

aural (aw′-răl) pertaining to the ears.

auricle (aw′-rĭ-kl) the flap of the ear; protruding part of the external ear or pinna.

auriculotemporal (aw-rĭk″-ū-lō-tĕm′-pŏ-răl) pertaining to the ears and temporal region.

auscultation (aws″-kŭl-tā′-shun) listening with a stethoscope.

autoimmune (aw″-tō-ĭm-mūn′) self-protection from disease; pertaining to the body's ability to fight off disease.

autoimmune disease disease caused by a response of the immune system against self-antigens.

autolysis (aw-tŏl′-ĭ-sĭs) spontaneous disintegration of tissue or cells by their own autogenous enzymes.

autonomic (aw-tō-nŏm′-ĭk) **nerve** spontaneous or involuntary nerve.

autopsy (aw′-tŏp-sē) examination of a dead body to determine cause of death.

avascular (ă-văs′-kū-lăr) without a supply of blood vessels.

avascularity pertaining to the lack of supply of blood vessels.

axial (ăk′-sē-ăl) adjective meaning "around an axis."

axial skeleton bones of the cranium, vertebral column, ribs, and sternum.

axillary (ăk′-sĭ-lăr-ē) pertaining to the axilla.

axillary nodes (lymph) lymph nodes in the armpit.

axis real or imaginary straight line around which an objective rotates.

axon (ăk′-sŏn) microscopic fiber that carries the nervous impulse along a nerve cell.

axon terminal end of the microscopic fiber (axon).

azidothymidine (AZT) drug used to treat AIDS.

β blockers beta adrenergic blockers.

B-lymphocyte (B-cell) lymphocyte that transforms into plasma cell and secretes antibodies.

Ba barium.

Babcock forceps used to grasp or hold tissue.

Babinski reflex dorsiflexion of the great toe with stimulation of the sole of the foot.

bacillus (bă-sĭl′-ŭs) (pl. bacilli) rod-shaped bacteria.

bacteria (băk-tē′-rē-ă) microorganism, spherical or ovoid; may appear singly as micrococci, in pairs as diplococci, in clusters as staphylocci, or in chains as streptococci.

bacterial endocarditis inflammation of the inner lining of the heart caused by bacteria; also known as endocarditis.

bacteriuria (băk-tē″-ū′-rē-ă) accumulation of bacteria in the urine.

balanitis (băl-ă-nī′-tĭs) inflammation of the glans penis.

bandage type of dressing used to cover a wound or support an injury.

barbiturate (băr-bĭt′-ū-rāts) sedative drug used to treat nervousness and excitement.

barium sulfate radioopaque contrast medium.

barium swallow fluoroscopic x-ray examination of the pharynx and esophagus following oral intake of barium.

barotitis (băr″-ō-tī′-tĭs) media inflammation of the middle ear.

Bartholin's (băr′-tō-lĭnz) **glands** small exocrine glands at the vaginal orifice.

basal cell carcinoma malignant tumor of the basal cell layer of the epidermis.

basal ganglia four masses of gray matter at the base of the cerebral hemispheres: caudate, lentiform, amygdaloid nuclei, and claustrum.

basal layer deepest region of the epidermis; gives rise to all the epidermal cells.

basement membrane delicate non-cellular membrane serving as support and as attachment underlying a layer of epithelial cells.

basilar (băs′-ĭ-lăr) **membrane** membrane extending from crest of spiral ligament to tympanic lip of osseous spiral lamina in the cochlea of the ear.

baso basophil.

basophil (bā′-sō-fĭl) function of these cells is not clear, but they play a role in inflammation; less than 1 percent of leukocytes are this type.

BBB blood-brain barrier.

BE barium enema.

Bence Jones protein protein found in urine of patients with multiple myeloma or other diseases of the reticuloendothelial system.

benign (bē-nīn′) noncancerous; not harmful.

benign neoplasm any new or abnormal noncancerous growth.

benign prostatic hypertrophy (BPH) prostate gland enlargement, most commonly seen in males over the age of 50. The progress of this condition can interfere with urine flow by obstruction of the urethra.

beta (bā′-tă) **particles** radium-emitted particles of negative energy; penetrate more deeply than alpha rays.

beta cells insulin-secreting cells in the islets of Langerhans.

betatron (bā′-tă-trŏn) electron accelerator producing x-rays.

biceps (bī′-sĕps) muscle with two heads.

biceps brachii biceps muscle of arm.

biceps femoris biceps muscle of thigh.

biconvex (bī-kŏn′-vĕks) having two sides that are rounded, elevated, and curved evenly, like part of a sphere. The lens of the eye is a biconvex body.

bicuspid (bī-kŭs′-pĭd) **valve** valve between the left atrium and left ventricle of the heart.

bicuspid two cusps or projections, or having two cusps or projections.

bifocal (bī-fō′-kăl) **glasses** eyeglasses with each lens containing two separate or blended lens refracting powers, one for distance and one for near vision.

bilateral (bī-lăt′-ĕr-ăl) pertaining to both sides, ie., both lower extremities, both eyes, etc.

bilateral salpingo-oophorectomy (săl-pĭng″-gō-ō″-ŏf-ō-rĕk′-tō-mē) (BSO) excision of both fallopian tubes and ovaries.

bile (bīl) fluid secreted by the liver and poured into the small intestine via the bile duct.

bile duct duct formed by the union of the common hepatic and cystic ducts which empties into the duodenum at the major duodenal papilla along the pancreatic duct.

biliary (bĭl′-ē-ār-ē) pertaining to bile, bile ducts, or gallbladder.

bilirubin (bĭl-ĭ-roo′-bĭn) dark green pigment produced from hemoglobin when red blood cells are destroyed. Bilirubin is concentrated in bile by the liver and is excreted in the feces.

binocular (bĭn-ŏk′-ū-lăr) **vision** normal vision with two eyes.

biological response modifiers substances produced by normal cells that either directly block tumor growth or stimulate the immune system.

biological therapy use of the body's own defense mechanisms to fight tumor cells.

biology (bī-ŏl′-ō-jē) science that deals with the phenomena of living organisms.

biopsy (bī-ŏp-sē) removal of a piece of living tissue for microscopic examination.

bipolar (bī-pōl-ăr) pertaining to poles or processes.

bipolar (bī-pŏl′-ăr) **disorder** mood disorder characterized by the occurrence of one or more manic and depressive episodes.

bisexual (bī-sĕks′-ū-ăl) an individual who is sexually attracted to both genders. May also pertain to an individual who has imperfect genitalia of both genders.

blackhead dark-colored, oxidized sebum in a sebaceous gland.

blepharitis (blĕf″-ăr-ī′-tĭs) inflammation of the edges of the eyelids involving the hair follicles and glands. May be either ulcerative or nonulcerative.

blepharochalasis (blĕf″-ăr-ō-kăl′-ă-sĭs) upper eyelid skin hypertrophy caused by a loss of elasticity.

blepharopexy surgical fixation of the eyelid.

blepharoptosis (blĕf″-ă-rō-tō′-sĭs) drooping of the upper eyelids.

blepharospasm (blĕf′-ă-rō-spăsm) spasmodic twitching of the orbicularis oculi muscle due to spasm, eyestrain, or nervous irritability.

blind spot area 15 degrees to the outside of the visual fixation point where the optic nerve enters the eye and is without rods or cones.

blindness inability to see; without the sense of sight.

blood (blŭd) fluid that circulates through the heart, arteries, veins, and capillaries carrying oxygen and nutrients to the body cells.

blood brain barrier blood vessels (capillaries) that selectively let certain substances enter the brain tissue and keep other harmful substances out.

blood cells principal types are erythrocytes or red blood corpuscles, platelets, and leukocytes or white blood corpuscles.

blood urea nitrogen (BUN) the amount of urea nitrogen in the blood; increased amounts indicate glomerular dysfunction.

body physical makeup of the human being separate from the mind and spirit.

body dysmorphic disorder characterized by an excessive concern for one's physical appearance and by the belief that some minor defect (or even normal feature) is a disfigurement.

boil furuncle; acute circumscribed subcutaneous inflammation of the skin or hair follicle.

bolus (bō′-lŭs) rounded mass of food or pharmaceutical preparation, ready to swallow.

bone (bōn) hard form of connective tissue that constitutes the majority of the skeleton and most vertebrates, consisting of organic compounds.

bone conduction (BC) noise and vibrations felt (heard) through the bones of the ear.

bone cutters used to cut, incise, or separate tissue.

bone forceps used to grasp or hold tissue.

bone graft bone taken from the patient is used to replace a bone that has been removed or has a bony defect.

bone head rounded end of a bone separated from the body of the bone by a neck.

bone marrow inner portion of the bone consisting of blood cells.

bone marrow biopsy a needle is introduced into the bone marrow cavity, and a small amount of marrow is aspirated. The marrow is then examined under the microscope. This procedure is helpful in the diagnosis of blood disorders such as anemia, cytopenias, and leukemia.

bone marrow transplant bone marrow cells from a donor whose tissue and blood cells closely match those of the recipient are infused into a patient with leukemia or aplastic anemia.

bone scan following the intravenous injection of a radioactive phosphate substance and uptake of the substance in the bone, a scan is obtained of the bones to locate areas containing tumors, infection, inflammation, or other destructive changes.

bone shapes long, short, flat, irregular.

Book-Walter retractors retractor used for cardiovascular surgery.

borborygmus (bor″-bō-rĭg′-mŭs) gurgling, splashing, or rumbling sounds made by the intestine as gas passes through the intestine.

bowel series radiologic study of the duodenum, ileum, and jejunum, following oral intake of barium sulfate.

Bowman's (Bō′-măns) capsule cup-shaped capsule surrounding each glomerulus.

BP blood pressure.

BPH benign prostatic hypertrophy.

brachial (brā′-kē-ăl) pertaining to the arm.

brachial artery main artery of the arm located on the inside of the arm in continuation of the axillary artery.

brachial plexus lower cervical and upper dorsal spine nerve network supplying the arm, hand, and forearm with nervous impulse.

brachialis (brā″-kē-ăl′-ĭs) muscle of the arm under the biceps brachii.

brachiocephalic (brā″-kē-ō-sĕ-făl′-ĭk) pertaining to the arm and the head.

brachioradialis (brā″-kē-ō-rā″-dē-ă′-lĭs) lateral muscle in the forearm.

brachytherapy (brăk″-ē-thĕr′-ă-pē) implantation of radioactive materials in radiation therapy.

bradycardia (brăd″-ē-kăr′-dē-ă) condition of a slow heart beat.

bradykinesia (brad″-ē-kĭ-nē′-sē-ă) slow movement.

bradypnea (brăd″-ĭp-nē′-ă) slow breathing.

brain (brān) scan study of the function of the brain with radioactive isotopes.

brain stem lower portion of the brain that connects the cerebrum with the spinal cord. The pons and medulla are part of the brain stem.

brand name drug drug name assigned by the manufacturer.

Bright's disease a type of glomerulonephritis.

Broca's (Brō′-kăs) area left hemisphere of the brain at the posterior end of the inferior frontal gyrus containing speech area and responsible for control of movement of the tongue, lips, and vocal cords.

bronchi (brŏng′-kī) airway passages between the trachea and the alveoli.

bronchial (brŏng′-kē-ăl) brushings study to obtain specimens from the bronchi for diagnosis.

bronchial sounds sounds of air through the bronchi on inspiration and expiration.

bronchial tree divisions of the bronchi.

bronchial washings irrigation of the bronchi to collect cells for diagnostic study or to cleanse the bronchi.

bronchiectasis (brŏng″-kē-ĕk′-tă-sĭs) dilatation of a bronchus.

bronchiole (brŏng′-kē-ōl) smaller subdivision of the bronchi.

bronchiolectasis (brŏng″-kē-ō-lĕk′-tă-sĭs) referring to dilation of the bronchioles.

bronchiolitis (brŏng″-kē-ō-lī′-tĭs) inflammation of the bronchioles.

bronchitis (brŏng-kī′-tĭs) acute inflammation of the bronchial tree caused by a virus, often following a cold; inflammation of the bronchus.

bronchodilators drugs used to dilate the bronchi and bronchioles.

bronchography (brŏng-kŏg′-ră-fĕ) x-ray of the lung after instillation of a radioactive substance.

bronchopneumonia (brŏng″-kō-nū-mō′-nē-ă) consolidation along the bronchus.

bronchoscope (brŏng′-kō-skōp) lighted, flexible fiberoptic scope used to examine the lumen of the bronchial tree.

bronchoscopy (brŏng-kŏs′-kō-pē) examination of the bronchial tubes by passing a lighted, flexible fiberoptic tube through the nose, throat, larynx, and trachea into the bronchi.

bronchospasm (brŏng′-kō-spăzm) spasm of the parabronchial smooth muscle accompanied by coughing and wheezing. Present in asthmatic and bronchitic conditions.

bronchovesicular (brŏng″-kō-vĕ-sĭk′-ū-lăr) pertaining to sounds made in the bronchial tubes and alveoli.

bronchus (brŏng′-kŭs) branch of the trachea (windpipe) that acts as a passageway into the air spaces (alveoli) of the lung; bronchial tube.

Brudzinski sign pain on hip flexion when the neck is flexed from a supine position. Commonly seen with meningitis.

bruit (brwē) adventitious sounds of a venous or arterial nature.

Brunner's (brŭn′-ĕrz) glands glands of the duodenum and upper jejunum embedded in submucous tissue and lined with columnar epithelium.

BSO (bilateral salpingo-oophorectomy) surgical excision of both fallopian tubes and both ovaries.

buccal cavity (bŭk′-ăl) mouth.

buccal mucosa pertaining to the mucous membrane of the cheek inside the mouth.

buccinator (bŭk′-sĭn-ā-tor) cheek muscle.

Bucket handle tear tear of the cruciate ligament resembling the handle of a bucket with tissue remaining attached on either side of the tear.

bulbourethral (bŭl″-bō-ū-rē′-thrăl) Cowpers glands, two exocrine glands near the male urethra.

bulbous (bŭl′-bŭs) bulb-shaped.

bulla (bŭl′-lă) blister or skin vesicle filled with fluid.

BUN blood urea nitrogen.

bundle of His specialized muscle fibers in the wall between the ventricles that carry the electric impulses to the ventricles.

bunion (bŭn′-yŭn) abnormal valgus deviation of the joint between the big toe and the first metatarsal bone.

bunionectomy excision and removal of a bunion.

burn (bĕrn) injury to tissues caused by heat. First-degree burn: superficial epidermal lesions, erythema, hyperesthesia and no blisters. Second-degree burn: epidermal and dermal lesions, erythema, blisters, and hyperesthesia. Third-degree burn: epidermis and dermis are destroyed (necrosis of skin), and subcutaneous layer is damaged leaving charred, white tissue.

bursa (bŭr′-să) sac of fluid near a joint.

bursectomy (bŭr-sĕk′-tō-mē) excision of a bursa.

bursitis (bŭr-sī′-tĭs) inflammation of a bursa.

butterfly self-adhesive bandage used in place of sutures to keep wound edges in close approximation so that healing can occur.

butterfly rash rash on the skin of both cheeks joined across the nose; commonly seen in systemic lupus erythematosus.

buttocks (bŭt′-ŭks) formed by the gluteal muscles in the lower posterior hip region.

C&D cystoscopy and dilation.

C&S culture and sensitivity.

C1, C2 . . . C7 first cervical vertebra, second cervical vertebra, etc.

Ca calcium.

CABG coronary artery bypass graft.

CAD coronary artery disease.

cafe au lait spots (cafe au lait macules) small, pale brown areas on the skin with irregular borders caused by increased melanin deposition in the skin, appearing in infancy and usually disappearing with age. May increase in number in certain pathologic conditions such as neurofibromatosis.

calcaneal (kăl-kā'-nē-ăl) pertaining to the calcaneous (heel bone).

calcaneal (Achilles) tendon tendon of the gastrocnemius and soleus muscles of the leg.

calcaneus (kăl-kā'-nē-ŭs) os calcis or heel bone.

calcify (kăl'-sē-fī) to harden, as in the formation of bone.

calcitonin (kăl''-sĭ-tō'-nĭn) hormone produced by the parathyroid glands which lowers calcium levels in the blood; also called thyrocalcitonin.

calcium (kăl'-sē-ŭm) one of the mineral constituents of bone; generic name for a mineral supplement.

calcium carbonate white, tasteless, odorless powder used as an antacid.

calcium channel blockers drugs used to treat angina and hypertension. They dilate blood vessels.

calcium phosphate powder used as an antacid for treatment of hyperacidity.

calculus (kăl'-kū-lŭs) a stone. May occur in the gallbladder, kidneys, ureters, bladder, or urethra.

Caldwell-Luc surgical procedure involving opening of the maxillary sinus through the supradental fossa to remove dental roots or abnormal sinus tissue.

caliceal (kăl''-ĭ-sē'-ăl) pertaining to the calices.

canal of Schlemm sinus through which aqueous humor is drained from the anterior chamber of the eye.

cancellous (kăn'-sĕl-ŭs) bone spongy, porous, trabecular bone tissue.

canines (kā'-nīn) upper and lower eye teeth, between incisors and molars.

canker (kăng'-kĕr) sore ulcer of the mouth or lips.

canthus (kăn'-thŭs) corners of the eyelids where upper and lower lids meet on either side of the eye.

CAPD continuous ambulatory peritoneal dialysis.

capillary (kăp'-ĭ-lā''-rē) small blood vessel connecting arterioles and venules, serves as the delivery and collection vessel between the blood stream and the body's cells.

capitate (kăp'-ĭ-tāt) rounded extremity, shaped like the head; one of the bones of the wrist.

capitulum (kă-pit'-ū-lŭm) articulation at the lower end of the humerus where it meets the radial head.

carbohydrate (kăr''-bō-hī'-drāt) chemical substance including glycogen, starches, sugar, dextrins, and celluloses.

carbon (kăr'-bŭn) dioxide (CO_2) waste gas released by body cells and transported via veins to the heart and then to the lungs to be expelled.

carbuncle (kăr'-bŭng''-k'l) common pyogenic skin eruption on the neck, upper back and buttocks, characterized by a painful nodule covered by tight erythematous skin that eventually perforates and drains pus.

carbunculosis (kăr-bŭng''-kū-lō'-sĭs) presence of several carbuncles at one time or in succession.

carcinogenic (kăr''-sĭ-nō-jĕn'-ĭk) cancer producing.

carcinogens (kăr-sĭn'-ō-jĕn) agents that cause cancer; may include chemicals, drugs, and radiation.

carcinoma malignant neoplasm of epithelial origin.

carcinoma (kăr''-sĭ-nō-mă) in-situ referring to localized tumor cells that have not invaded adjacent structures.

carcinomata alternative plural of carcinoma.

cardia (kăr'-dē-ă) origin of stomach at the esophagus.

cardiac (kăr'-dē-ăk) pertaining to the heart.

cardiac arrest sudden stoppage of the heart.

cardiac catheterization a thin, flexible tube (catheter) is introduced into a vein or artery and is guided into the heart for purposes of detecting pressures and patterns of blood flow. Dye can also be injected and x-rays taken (angiocardiography).

cardiac cycle systole and diastole. The process of blood entering and exiting the heart.

cardiac disease pertaining to any disease of the heart.

cardiac monitor used to check the heart's rhythm.

cardiac muscle myocardium or heart muscle in which branched fibers anastomose to form a contractile network.

cardiac notch accomodation along anterior margin of the left lung where the heart lies.

cardiac output (CO) measurement of blood discharged from the right or left ventricle each minute.

cardiogram (kăr'-dē-ō-grăm'') (electrocardiogram) recording of the electrical impulses of the heart.

cardiograph (kăr'-dē-ō-grăf'') (electrocardiograph) recording device used to monitor the electrical impulses of the heart.

cardiography (kăr''-dē-ŏg'-ră-fē) (electrocardiography) study of recordings of electrical impulses of the heart.

cardiology (kăr-dē-ŏl'-ō-jē) study of the heart.

cardiomegaly (kăr''-dē-ō-mĕg'-ă-lē) enlarged heart, particularly left ventricular hypertrophy.

cardiomyopathy (kăr'-dē-ō-mī-ŏp'-ă-thē) disease of the heart muscle or myocardium.

cardiopathy (kăr''-dē-ŏp'-ă-thē) disease of the heart.

cardioplegia (kăr''-dē-ō-plē'-jē-ă) paralysis of the heart. The temporary and deliberate interruption of the heart's impulses.

cardiopulmonary (kăr''-dē-ō-pŭl'-mō-nĕr-ē) bypass use of a pump-oxygenator to take over the function of the heart and lungs during heart surgery.

cardiovascular (kăr''-dē-ō-văs'-kū-lăr) pertaining to the heart and blood vessels.

cardiovascular surgery surgery of the heart and supporting vessels.

carditis (kăr-dī'-tĭs) inflammation of the heart.

carotene (kăr'-ō-tēn) yellowish pigment present in plant and animal tissues. It is stored in the liver and converted to vitamin A.

carotenemia (kăr''-ō-tĕ-nē'-mē-ă) yellow skin caused by carotene in the blood. The conjunctivae are not affected as in jaundice.

carotenoderma yellow-colored skin caused by excess carotene.

carpal (kăr'-păl) pertaining to the carpus; the eight bones of the wrist joint.

carpal tunnel syndrome (CTS) compression of the median nerve as it passes beneath the transverse carpal ligament and the bones and tendons of the wrist (the carpal tunnel).

cartilage (kăr'-tĭ-lĭj) flexible connective tissue attached to bones at joints, surrounding the trachea, and part of the external ear and nose.

cartilaginous (kăr''-tĭ-lăj'-ĭ-nŭs) pertaining to or made up of cartilage.

CT scan method of three dimensional imaging using x-rays; computed axial tomography.

catabolism (kă-tăb'-ō-lĭzm) destructive phase of metabolism with breaking down of complex substances into simpler substances causing energy release.

cataract (kăt'-ă-răkt) clouding of the lens, causing decreased vision.

cataract extraction surgical excision of a cataract from the eye. May include intraocular lens replacement.

catecholamine (kăt″-ĕ-kōl′-ă-mēn) hormone derived from an amino acid and secreted by the adrenal medulla.

catgut natural absorbable suture material made from the collagen of mammals. Strength varies with the amount of collagen used. Catgut can be treated with chromium salts to increase its strength and prolong the absorption rate. Treated catgut is called chromic catgut while untreated is called plain catgut.

cathether (kăth′-ĕ-tĕr) tube for injecting or removing fluids.

catheterization (kăth″-ĕ-tĕr-ĭ-zā′-shŭn) insertion of a tubular instrument for injecting or removing fluids into a body cavity. In particular, insertion into the bladder of a flexible tube for withdrawal of urine.

cathode (kăth′-ōd) **ray tube** vacuum tube which generates cathode rays, or x-rays.

cauda (kaw′-dă) **equina** ("horse tail") a collection of spinal nerves below the end of the spinal cord at the level of the second lumbar vertebra.

caudal (kawd′-ăl) pertaining to a tail-like structure.

caudate (kaw′-dāt) having a tail.

caudate nucleus portion of the basal ganglia resembling a tail, or comma, composed of gray matter.

cautery (kaw′-tĕr-ē) destruction of tissue by means of freezing, electrocution, or corrosive chemicals.

CBC complete blood count.

CBD common bile duct.

CCT cranial computed tomography.

CCU cardiac/coronary care unit.

CDH congenital dislocation of hip.

cecopexy (sē′-kō-pĕk″-sē) surgical fixation of the cecum.

cecum (sē′-kŭm) first part of the large intestine.

cell (sĕl) basic component of the tissues of the body.

cell-mediated immune response immune response involving T cell lymphocytes; antigens are destroyed by direct action of cells.

cellulitis (sĕl-ū-lī′-tĭs) inflammation of skin or connective tissue.

cellular (sĕl′-ū-lăr) **oncogenes** pieces of DNA that, when broken or dislocated, can cause a normal cell to become malignant.

cementoblast a cell of dental sac of developing teeth which deposits cementum on the dentin of the root of the tooth.

cementum (sē-mĕn′-tŭm) calcified dental tissue formed by cementoblasts.

centesis (sĕn-tē′-sĭs) puncture into a body cavity.

central nervous system (CNS) the brain and the spinal cord.

central sulcus fissure dividing the frontal and parietal lobes of each cerebral hemisphere.

cephalgia (sĕf-făl′-jē-ă) headache.

cephalodynia (sĕf″-ă-lō-dĭn′-ē-ă) headache.

cephalopelvic (sĕf″-ă-lō-fĕl′-vĭk) **disproportion** pelvic outlet is smaller than the size of the fetus.

cerebellum (sĕr-ĕ-bĕl′-ŭm) posterior part of the brain responsible for coordinating voluntary muscle movements and maintaining balance.

cerebral (sĕr′-ĕ-brăl; sĕ-rē′-brăl) pertaining to the cerebrum.

cerebral cortex outer region of the cerebrum.

cerebrospinal (sĕr″-ĕ-brō-spī′-năl) pertaining to the brain and spinal cord.

cerebrospinal fluid (CSF) fluid surrounding the brain and spinal cord which cushions these structures from physical impact.

cerebrovascular (sĕr″-ĕ-brō-văs′-kū-lăr) **accident (CVA)** interruption of the blood supply to nerve cells of a part of the brain, also called a stroke.

cerebrovascular disease disease of the blood vessels of the brain.

cerebrum (sĕr′-ĕ-brŭm) two hemispheres that make up the largest portion of the brain.

cerumen (sĕ-roo′-mĕn) a waxy substance secreted by the external ear; also called ear wax.

ceruminous (sĕ-roo′-mĭ-nŭs) pertaining to cerumen.

ceruminous glands glands in the skin lining the external auditory canal which are actually modified sweat glands that secrete cerumen.

cervical (sĕr′-vĭ-kăl) **(C1-C7)** pertaining to the first seven cervical vertebra of the spinal column, or to the uterine cervix.

cervical conization surgical procedure in which sharp instrument is used to remove a piece of uterine of cervix shaped like a cone.

cervical intraepithelial neoplasia (CIN) dysplastic changes of the uterine cervix which may range from mild dysplasia to carcinoma-in-situ.

cervical mucus mucosal secretions of the cervix.

cervical (lymph) nodes lymph nodes in the neck region.

cervical plexus nerve complex in the neck region.

cervical polyp benign tumor (papilloma) of the cervix. Polyps are usually pedunculated and extend into the cervical cavity where they can be surgically removed.

cervical punch biopsy and cautery sharp circular instrument is used to remove a piece of cervix for microscopic study. Hemostasis may be maintained by cautery, the application of heat of electric current to the bleeding vessel.

cervicitis (sĕr-vĭ-sī′-tĭs) inflammation of the cervix uteri.

cervix (sĕr′-vĭks) lower, neck-like portion of the uterus.

cervix uteri lower, neck-like portion of the uterus.

cesarean (sē-sār′-ē-ăn) **section** removal of the fetus by incision into the uterus through the abdominal wall.

chalazion (kă-lā′-zē-ŏn) small, hard, cystic mass on the eyelid; formed from chronic inflammation of a meibomian gland.

characteristics traits that make up an organism.

CHD congenital heart disease.

cheilitis (kī-lī′-tĭs) inflammation of the lip.

cheiloplasty (kī′-lō-plăs″-tē) surgical repair of the lip.

cheilorrhaphy (kī-lor′-ă-fē) suturing or repair of the lip, as in cleft lip repair.

chemotherapy (kē″-mō-thĕr′-ă-pē) treatment with drugs.

chest fluoroscopy use of a fluoroscope to examine the chest cavity radiographically.

chest pain pain in the chest, may have many etiologies of cardiac, pulmonary, gastric or musculoskeletal origin.

Cheyne-Stokes (chān′-stōks′) breathing pattern characterized by a brief period of apnea followed by increased depth and frequency of respiration.

CHF (congestive heart failure) failure of the heart to pump adequately (more blood enters the heart from the veins than leaves through the arteries).

childbirth act of giving birth to an infant through a series of uterine contractions up to and including vaginal expulsion.

chisel (chĭs′l) used to cut, incise, or separate tissue.

chlamydia (klă-mĭd′-ē-ă) group of organisms causing a variety of human diseases, including sexually transmitted disease. May be treated with antibiotics.

chloride (klō′-rīd) component of blood serum consisting of a salt.

cholangiogram (kō-lăn′-jē-ō-grăm″) x-ray of a bile duct.

cholangiography (kō-lăn″-jē-ŏg′-ră-fe) x-ray of the biliary ducts.

cholangiopancreatography x-ray of the biliary and pancreatic ducts.

cholecystectomy (kō″-lē-sĭs-těk′-tō-mē) excision of the gallbladder.

cholecystitis (kō″-lē-sĭs-tī′-sĭs) inflammation of the gallbladder.

cholecystogram (kō″-lē-sĭs-′tō-grăm) oral (OCG) x-ray of the gallbladder following oral contrast administration.

cholecystographic agent drug that makes the gallbladder visible on x-rays after having become absorbed into the blood and concentrated in the gallbladder.

cholecystography (kō″-lē-sĭs-tŏg′-ră-fē) x-ray of the gallbladder.

cholecystolithiasis (kō″-lē-sĭs″-tō-lĭ-thī′-ă-sĭs) condition of stones in the gallbladder.

choledochectomy (kō-lěd′-ō-kěk′-tō-mē) excision of common bile duct.

choledocholithiasis (kō-lěd″-ō-kō-lĭ-thī′-ă-sĭs) condition of stones in the gallbladder and common bile duct.

choledocholithotomy (kō-lěd″-ō-kō-lĭth-ŏt′-ō-mē) removal of gallstones from the gallbladder and bile ducts through an incision.

choledochotomy (kō″-lěd-ō-kŏt′-ō-mē) incision into the bile duct.

cholelith (kō′-lē-lĭth) gallstone.

cholelithiasis (kō″-lē-lĭ-thī′-ă-sĭs) condition of gallstones that form in the gallbladder.

cholelithotomy (kō″-lē-lĭ-thŏt′-ō-mē) removal of stones from the gallbladder through an incision.

cholestasia (kō″-lē-stā′-zē-ă) stoppage of the flow of bile through the biliary system.

cholesteatoma (kō″-lē-stě″-ă-tō′-mă) collection of skin cells and cholesterol in a sac within the middle ear.

cholesterol (kō-lěs′-těr-ŏl) a widely distributed sterol in animal tissues. A major constituent of bile and of gallstones.

cholinergic (kō″-lĭn-ěr′-jĭk) drug which stimulates certain parasympathetic nerves, such as those found in the bladder.

chondroma (kŏn-drō′-mă) slow-growing cartilaginous tumor.

chondromalacia (kŏn-drō-măl-ā′-shē-ă) softening of the cartilage, most commonly seen in the patella.

chondrosarcoma (kŏn-drō-săr-kō′-mă) malignant tumor of cartilage.

chordae tendineae (kor′-dē těn-dĭn′-ē-ē) fibrous cords connecting the free edges of atrioventricular valves and papillary muscles.

chordotomy (kor-dŏt′-ō-mē) incision of the spinal cord with division to eliminate pain in a region.

chorionic (kō-rē-ŏn′-ĭk) **villus sampling** (CVS) samples of fetal tissue are taken from the chorionic villi (finger-like projections from the chorion), for the purpose of diagnosing fetal abnormalities.

chorioretinitis (kō″-rē-ō-rět″-ĭn-ī′-tĭs) inflammation of the choroid and retina.

choroid (kō′-royd) portion of the eye consisting of the vascular coating between the sclera and the retina.

choroid layer the middle, vascular layer of the eye between the retina and the sclera.

chorion outermost, multilayered fetal membrane.

chromaffin (krō-măf′-ĭn) pigmented cells found in the adrenal medulla.

chromatin (krō-mă-tĭn) substance present in the nucleus of cells that contains genetic material. This deeply staining substance is a deoxyribonucleic acid attached to a protein base.

chromic (krō′-mĭc) **catgut** natural absorbable suture material made for the collagen of mammals with increased strength and prolonged absorption from treatment with chromium salts.

chromosomal pairs DNA in form of a linear thread found in the nucleus of a cell. There are 23 pairs in all somatic cells constituting the dipoloid number. 22 pairs of these are considered autosomes and one pair are the sex chromosomes. These are the make up of the cell structure of every human being.

chromosome (krō′-mō-sōm) DNA in form of a linear thread in the nucleus of a cell.

chronic (krŏn′-ĭk) ongoing disease showing little change or progressing very slowly.

chronic bronchitis cough productive of mucus signifying inflammation of the bronchi, persisting for more than three months each year.

chronic obstructive pulmonary disease (COPD) chronic condition of persistent obstruction of air flow through the bronchial tubes and lungs. Chronic bronchitis and emphysema are the two conditions usually causing COPD.

chyle (kīl) content of the lacteal and lymphatic vessels of the intestines. This is a product of digestion of fats which is carried by the lymphatic vessels into the bloodstream.

chylomicron small fat particles in the blood following digestion and absorption of fats in foods.

chyme nearly liquid mass of partially digested food and digestive secretions found in the small intestine and stomach while a meal is being digested.

cicatrix (sĭk′-ă-trĭks) contracted-appearing, non-elastic scar without pigmentation.

cilia (sĭl′-ē-ă) eyelashes.

ciliary body structure on each side of the crystalline lens that connects the choroid and the iris. It contains the ciliary muscles, which control the shape of the lens, and secretes aqueous humor.

ciliary muscle (sĭl′-ē-ěr′-ē) smooth muscle of the eye which causes the lens to accomodate or change shape.

ciliary process circular structure in the eye which serves as an attachment for the suspensory ligament and the lens.

CIN cervical intraepithelial neoplasia.

cinefluorography (sĭn″-ě-floo″-or-ŏg′-ră-fē) fluoroscopic examination with the use of motion pictures to document findings.

circulating nurse a registered nurse working in the operating suite. With the medical doctor, a circulating nurse is responsible for patient safety and for ensuring that supplies and equipment are ready perioperatively.

circulation regular movement in a circular course.

circulatory system cardiovascular system.

circumcision (sěr″-kŭm-sĭ′-zhŭn) removal of the prepuce or foreskin.

circumduction (sěr″-kŭm-dŭk′-shŭn) swinging of the limbs; movement of the eye in a circular pattern.

circumvallate (sĕr″-kŭm-văl′-āt) completely enclosed by a wall or raised structure, as in the circumvallate papillae of the tongue.

cirrhosis (sĭ-rō′-sĭs) chronic disease of the liver with degeneration of liver cells.

CIS carcinoma "in situ."

CK creatine kinase.

clamps used to control bleeding and to grasp tissue.

claustrophobia (klaws-trō-fō′-bē-ă) an unreasonable fear of closed spaces.

clavicle (klăv′-ĭ-k'l) (collarbone) bone in the chest region that articulates with the sternum and scapula.

clavicular (klă-vĭk′-ū-lăr) pertaining to the collarbone.

clavicular notch point of articulation between the clavical and the sternum.

claw toe dorsal flexion of the first phalanx with plantar flexion of the second and third phalanx causing the toe to curl under somewhat. Also referred to as hammer toe.

cleft (klĕft) lip separation of the upper lip, may be associated with cleft palate.

cleft palate fissure in the roof of the mouth causing a passageway between the mouth and nasal cavities. This is a common birth defect.

clinical actual observation of a patient to form conclusions rather than basing conclusions on data or facts obtained from pathology.

clinical microbiology microscopic examination of disease-causing micro-organisms including bacteria, viruses, yeasts, and fungi.

clitoris (klĭ′-tō-rĭs) organ of sensitive erectile tissue anterior to the urinary meatus in female genitalia.

CLL chronic lymphocytic leukemia.

clone (klōn) artificially reproduced cells or plants; structures with the identical character of the original cell, plant or structure. A group of cells descended from a single cell, not produced from seed.

clonic (klŏn′-ĭk) alternate contraction and relaxation of muscle.

cloning reproduction of a cell, plant or structure from a single cell.

CML chronic granulocytic leukemia.

CNS central nervous system.

CO cardiac output.

CO₂ carbon dioxide.

coagulant (kō-ăg′-ū-lănt) an agent which causes blood to clot.

coagulation therapy administration of medication to aid in regulation of blood clotting.

cobalt-57 (kō′-bălt) radioactive isotope with half-life of 272 days.

cobalt-60 radioactive isotope with half-life of 5.27 years.

cocci (kŏk′-sī) round-shaped bacteria.

coccidioidomycosis (kŏk-sĭd″-ĭ-oyd-ō-mī-kō′-sĭs) a type of fungal infection of the lungs. May rarely spread to the visceral organs, bones and skin.

coccygeal (kŏk-sĭj′-ē-ăl) pertaining to the tailbone; caudal-most four vertebral bodies.

coccyx (kŏk′-sĭks) tailbone; caudal-most four vertebral bodies.

cochlea (kŏk′-lē-ă) snail-shaped, spirally wound tube in the inner ear; contains sensitive hearing receptor cells.

cochlear (kŏk′-lē-ăr) pertaining to the cochlea.

cochlear nerve eighth cranial nerve.

coitus (kō′-ĭ-tŭs) sexual intercourse; copulation.

colchicine (kŏl′-chĭ-sĭn) medication used to treat acute gout.

colectomy (kō-lĕk′-tō-mē) surgical excision of all or part of the colon.

colic (kŏl′-ĭk) painful, spasmodic contractions of any hollow organ such as the bile ducts, intestines, abdomen, or kidneys. May also involve the uterus when associated with menstruation.

colitis (kō-lī′-tĭs) inflammation of the colon.

collagen (kŏl′-ă-jĕn) nonsoluble fibrous structural protein in connective tissue such as bones, skin, ligaments, and cartilage.

collateral (kō-lăt′-ĕr-ăl) accessory branch of a blood vessel or nerve.

colocolostomy (kō″-lō-kō-lŏs′-tō-mē) creation of a new opening or connection between two portions of the colon.

colon (kō′-lŏn) large intestine; ascending, transverse, and descending parts.

colonoscope (kō-lŏn′-ō-skōp) instrument or scope used to view the internal aspect of the colon.

colonoscopy (kō″-lŏn-ŏs′-kō-pē) process of viewing the colon with the aid of an instrument or scope.

color blindness inability to distinguish colors.

colostomy (kō-lŏs′-tō-mē) creation of a new opening from the colon through the abdominal wall allowing feces to pass through the colon and into a bag or pouch.

colpoperineoplasty (kŏl″-pō-pĕr″-ĭn-ē′-ō-plăs″-tē) surgical reconstruction of the vagina and perineum.

colporrhaphy (kŏl-por′-ă-fē) suturing the vagina.

colposcopy process of visually examining the vagina and cervix, usually under magnification.

colpotomy (kŏl-pŏt′-ō-mē) vaginotomy. Incision of the vagina.

coma (kō′-mă) deep unconscious state without arousal from external or painful stimuli.

comatose (kō′-mă-tōs) condition of being in a coma.

combination chemotherapy use of several chemotherapeutic agents together in the treatment of tumors.

compact bone hard, dense bone tissue.

complete blood count (CBC) series of tests including a hemoglobin, a hematocrit, white cell count and differential, and calculations of the volume of red blood cells.

computed axial tomography (CAT scan) two-dimensional radiographic study in transverse planes of tissues. The computerized analysis of absorption variances reconstructs an image of the studied area.

computed tomography (CT scan) CAT scan.

concave (kŏn′-kāv) depressed or hollow surface.

conception (kŏn-sĕp′-shŭn) to form an idea; the joining of the male sperm with the female ovum resulting in fertilization and pregnancy.

conduction (kŏn-dŭk′-shŭn) system Purkinje fibers and atrioventricular bundle (AV bundle or bundle of His), right and left bundle branches.

condyle (kŏn′-dĭl) rounded, knuckle-like process at a joint.

condyloma (kŏn″-dĭ-lō′-mă) acuminatum viral wart in the genital or perianal area, usually sexually transmitted.

cone biopsy removal of a cone-shaped piece of tissue; often used to remove a piece of uterine cervical tissue for biopsy.

cones photosensitive receptor cells in the retina that change light energy into a nerve impulse. Cones make the perception of color possible.

congenital (kŏn-jĕn′-ĭ-tăl) present at birth.

congenital heart disease (CHD) disease of the heart, present at birth.

congenital megacolon extremely dilated colon, present at birth.

congested (kŏn-jĕs′-tĕd) containing an abnormally high volume of blood.

congestive heart failure (CHF) failure of the heart due to an abnormally high volume of blood. Related to inability to process and evacuate blood with regularity thus the blood volume backs up in the heart.

conization (kŏn″-ĭ-zā′-shŭn) removal of a cone-shaped piece of tissue; often used to remove a piece of uterine tissue for biopsy.

conjunctiva (kŏn″-jŭnk-tī′-vă) delicate membrane lining the inner eyelids and covering the exposed surfaces of the sclera.

conjunctival membrane delicate membrane lining the inner eyelids and covering the exposed surfaces of the sclera.

conjunctivitis (kŏ-jŭnk″-tĭ-vī′-tĭs) inflammation of the conjunctival membrane, also known as pinkeye.

connective bound together.

connective tissue tissue that binds together with other tissue to support parts of the body.

consciousness state of awareness.

consolidation (kŏn-sŏl-ĭ-dā′-shŭn) accumulation of a substance to form a solid structure.

constrict to bind or squeeze.

contact dermatitis skin irritation and inflammation following contact with an irritating chemical or substance.

contact lens a refractive correctional device that is worn on the cornea of the eye to correct defective vision.

contagious (kŏn-tā′-jŭs) transmitted easily from one person to another. Communicable organism that causes disease.

continuous (kŏn-tĭn′-ū-ŭs) suture a single thread is used to close the entire wound. There is a knot at the beginning and end of the suture. The suture line is uninterrupted.

contraction (kŏn-trăk′-shŭn) shortening or tightening of a muscle.

contralateral (kŏn″-tră-lăt′-ĕr-ăl) affecting the opposite side of the body.

contrast (kŏn′-trăst) media used in radiologic studies, a radio-opaque substance that provides contrast density between the tissue or organ being studied and the medium.

contusion (kŏn-too′-zhŭn) a bruise. The skin is not broken.

conus (kō′-nŭs) medullaris conical portion of the lower spinal cord.

convergence (kŏn-vĕr′-jĕns) moving of objects or rays of light toward a common point.

convergent (kŏn-vĕr′-jĕnt) movement toward a common point.

conversion (kŏn-vĕr′-zhŭn) change from one state to another.

conversion disorder psychological distress which manifests itself as physical illness, such as paralysis, blindness, inability to speak, etc. A diagnosis for this disorder is accurate only if an actual organic reason for the impairment cannot be found.

convex (kŏn′-vĕks) arched or curved surface.

convulsion (kŏn-vŭl′-shŭn) involuntary muscular contraction and relaxation.

COPD see chronic obstructive pulmonary disease.

coracoid (kor′-ă-koyd) process process on anterior surface of the scapula at its upper portion.

corium (kō′-rē-ŭm) middle layer of skin; dermis.

cornea (kor′-nē-ă) fibrous layer of clear tissue that extends over the anterior portion of the eyeball.

corneal abrasion scratch or abraded area on the corneal surface.

corneal transplant involves replacement of a section of an opaque cornea with normal, transparent cornea in an effort to restore vision.

corneum (kor′-nē-ŭm) horny layer of the skin.

coronal (kō-rō′-năl) suture junction of the parietal and frontal bones of the cranium

coronary pertaining to the crown or encircling blood vessels that supply blood to the heart.

coronary (kor′-ō-nă-rē) arteries blood vessels that branch from the aorta and carry oxygen-rich blood to the heart muscle.

coronary artery bypass graft (CABG) a shunt placed surgically to permit blood to travel from the aorta or other artery to a branch of a coronary artery at a point past an obstruction.

coronary artery disease (CAD) loss of oxygen and nutrients to the heart muscle caused by diminished coronary blood flow through the coronary blood vessels.

coronary bypass surgery surgical treatment procedure used to improve the blood supply to the heart muscle when narrowed coronary arteries reduce the flow of blood. Vessel grafts are connected to existing coronary arteries to detour around blockages in the coronary arteries and keep the myocardium supplied with oxygenated blood.

coronoid (kor′-ō-noyd) fossa oval depression on the anterior surface of the distal humerus.

coronoid process process on the proximal end of the ulna.

coronoid process of mandible process on anterior ramus at the upper end for attachment of temporalis muscle.

corpus callosum portion of the brain between the cerebral hemispheres.

corpus luteum (kor′-pŭs lū′-tē-ŭm) empty follicle that secretes estrogen and progestogen after release of the egg cell.

corpuscle (kor′-pŭs-ĕl) red blood cell. Erythrocyte.

corrosive (kŏ-rō′-sĭv) pertaining to destruction or wearing away by a destructive substance.

corrugator (kor′-ū-gā″-tor) muscle superior to the eye orbit arising from the frontal bone functioning to draw the eyebrow medially and interiorly.

cortex (kor′-tĕks) outer region; the renal cortex is the outer region of the kidney.

cortical (kor′-tĭ-kăl) pertaining to the outer layer or cortex of the kidney.

corticosteroid (kor″-tĭ-kō-stēr′-oyd) steroid hormone produced by the adrenal cortex.

cortisol (kor′-tĭ-sŏl) (hydrocortisone) produced by the adrenal cortex, regulates the use of sugars, fats, and proteins in cells.

costal (kŏs′-tăl) pertaining to the rib.

costal angle pertaining to the angle of a rib.

costal groove pertaining to a groove in a rib.

costal surface pertaining to the surface of a rib.

costovertebral (kŏs″-tō-vĕr′-tĕ-brăl) pertaining to the rib and vertebra.

Cowper's glands bulbourethral glands.

coxa (kŏk′-să) valga inward rotation of the hips.

coxa vara outward rotation of the hips.

coxa pertaining to hip bones.

CPAP continuous positive airway pressure.

CPK creatine phosphokinase.

CPR cardiopulmonary resuscitation.

crackles abnormal crackling sound heard during inspiration (rales).

cradle cap scaly seborrheic dermatitis of the newborn appearing on the scalp.

cranial (krā'-nē-ăl) pertaining to the skull.

cranial bone hard, dense bone tissue of the skull.

cranial cavity space in the head containing the brain and surrounded by the skull.

craniotome (krā'-nē-ō-tōm) instrument used to forcibly perforate the skull.

craniotomy (krā-nē-ŏt'-ō-mē) incision into the skull.

cranium (krā'-nē-ŭm) portion of the skull that contains the brain.

creatine (krē'-ă-tĭn) colorless, crystalline substance which serves as a source of high energy phosphate released in anaerobic phase of muscle contraction.

creatine kinase enzyme present in cardiac muscle, brain and skeleton.

creatine phosphokinase an improper term for creatine kinase.

creatinine (krē-ăt'-ĭn-ĭn) waste product of muscle metabolism; nitrogenous waste excreted in urine.

creatinine clearance test measures the ability of the kidney to remove creatinine from the blood.

crepitation (krĕp-ĭ-tā'-shŭn) crackling or grating sound.

crest prominent ridge or elongation.

cretinism (krē'-tĭn-ĭzm) extreme hypothyroidism during infancy and childhood which leads to a lack of normal physical and mental growth.

CRF chronic renal failure.

CRH corticotrophin-releasing hormone.

crib death sudden infant death syndrome. Unexpected and unexplained death in an apparently healthy infant during sleep.

cribriform (krĭb'-rĭ-form) plate perforated, sieve-like part of the ethmoid bone through which the olfactory nerves pass.

cricoid (krī'-koyd) cartilage lowermost of the laryngeal cartilages, resembling a circular shape.

crista (krĭs'-tă) galli ridge on ethmoid bone that serves as attachment to the falx cerebri.

Crohn's (Krōnz) disease chronic inflammation of the intestinal tract, most commonly the last part of the ileum.

crossmatch testing of blood for compatibility prior to transfusion.

croup (kroop) viral disease of childhood, characterized by inflammation and obstruction of the upper and lower respiratory tracts; also called laryngotracheobronchitis.

cruciate (kroo'-shē-āt) (crossing) ligaments cross-shaped ligaments supporting the knee.

crust lesions seen in eczema, seborrhea, syphilis, impetigo, and ringworm with a dry scab-like coating. May drain brown, yellow, green or red colored exudate.

cryosurgery (krī-"ō-sĕr'-jĕr-ē) use of cold temperatures to destroy tissue. The freezing temperature is produced by a probe using liquid nitrogen.

cryotherapy (krī-ō-thĕr'-ă-pē) therapeutic exposure to cold or freezing temperatures.

cryptorchidism (krĭpt-or'-kĭd-ĭzm) undescended testicles.

crypts of Lieberkuhn (krĭptz lē'-bĕr-kē) glands of the intestine, appearing in a tubular form, which secrete intestinal juices.

crystalline (krĭs'-tă-lĭn) lens a transparent, biconvex body behind the pupil of the eye. It bends light rays to bring them into focus on the retina.

CSF cerebrospinal fluid.

CSF culture microscopic study of the cerebrospinal fluid used to diagnose meningitis.

CTS carpal tunnel syndrome.

cubic millimeter unit of measurement.

cuboid (kū'-boyd) shaped like a cube.

cul-de-sac (kŭl'-dĭ-săk') region of the abdomen midway between the rectum and the uterus.

culdocentesis (kŭl"-dō-sĕn-tē'-sĭs) removal of fluid by surgical puncture of the cul-de-sac of Douglas for diagnostic purposes.

culdoscope (kŭl'-dō-skōp) instrument used to examine the cul-de-sac (of Douglas).

culdoscopy (kŭl-dŏs'-kō-pē) process of visually examining a cul-de-sac.

culture (kŭl'-tūr) growing out microorganisms in a speical medium to help in the diagnosis of disease and treatment of disease.

culture and sensitivity (C&S) the growing of microorganisms in a special medium then exposing the organisms to antibiotics to determine which antibiotic is most effective in the treatment of the disease.

cuneiform (kū-nē'-ĭ-form) cartilage elastic cartilage lying in the aryepiglottic fold immediately anterior to the arytenoid cartilage.

curet, curette (kū-rĕt') instrument used to cut, incise, separate, or scrape out foreign matter from a cavity.

curvature bending or sloping; a curve.

Cushing's (koosh'-ĭng) disease hyperfunctioning of the adrenal cortex with increased glucocorticoid secretion.

cuspid (kŭs'-pĭd) canine teeth.

cutaneous (kū-tā'-nē-ŭs) pertaining to the skin.

cuticle (kū'-tĭ-k'l) band of epidermis extending from the nail wall onto the nail surface.

CVA cerebrovascular accident.

CVP central venous pressure.

CVS chorionic villus sampling.

CXR chest x-ray.

cyanosis (sī-ă-nō'-sĭs) bluish skin coloration due to inadequate oxygen delivery to the tissues.

cycloplegia (sī"-klō-plē'-jē-ă) term used for paralysis of the ciliary muscle of the eye.

cycloplegic (sī"-klō-plē'jĭk) producing cycloplegia.

cyclothymia (sī"-klō-thī'-mē-ă) mild fluctuations of manic depressive nature.

cyclotron (sī'klō-trŏn) particles are rotated between magnets with increasing speed on each rotation.

cyst (sĭst) closed sac or pouch. May contain fluid or solid material. Usually results from developmental anomalies as from obstruction of ducts.

cystectomy (sĭs-tĕk'-tō-mē) surgical excision of a cyst.

cystic (sĭs'-tĭk) pertaining to a cyst.

cystic duct duct of the gallbladder, uniting with the hepatic duct from the liver to form the common bile duct.

cystic fibrosis (CF) inherited disease of exocrine glands (pancreas, sweat glands, and membranes of the respiratory tract) leading to airway obstruction.

cystitis (sĭs-tī'-tĭs) inflammation of the bladder.

cystocele (sĭs'-tō-sēl) hernia of the bladder that protrudes into the vagina.

cystojejunostomy (sĭs"-tō-jē-jū-nŏs'-tō-mē) new opening between the bladder and jejunum.

cystoplegia (sĭs"-tō-plē'-jē-ă) paralysis of the bladder.

cystoscope (sĭst'-ō-skōp) instrument usd to visually examine the inside of the bladder.

cystoscopy (sĭs-tŏs'-kō-pē) process of visually examining the bladder.

cystotomy (sĭs-tŏt'-ō-mē) incision of the bladder.

cystourethrography (sĭs"-tō-ū-rē-thrŏg'-ră-fē) x-ray of the bladder and urethra following injection of a contrast medium into the bladder through a cathether; x-ray of the bladder and urethra.

cytology (sī-tŏl'-ō-jē) study of formation, structure and function of cells.

cytomegalovirus (sī"-tō-mĕg"-ă-lō-vī'-rŭs) herpes virus strain.

cytoplasm (sī'-tō-plăzm) protoplasm of a cell, outside of the nucleus.

cytosol (sī'-tō-sŏl) clear fluid portion of a cell.

cytotoxic (sī'-tō-tŏks'ĭk) destruction of cells.

cytotoxic T-lymphocytes T-cells (killer cells) that directly kill foreign cells; also called CD8 cells.

D&C (dilation of the cervix and curettage of the uterus) dilation (widening) of the cervical opening is accomplished by inserting a series of probes of increasing size. Curettage (scraping) is then performed using a curette (metal loop at the end of a long, thin handle) to remove the lining of the uterus.

dacryoadenitis (dăk"-rē-ō-ăd"-ĕn-ī'-tĭs) inflammation of the lacrimal gland.

dacryocystorhinostomy (dăk"-rē-ō-sĭs"-tō-rī-nŏs'-tō-mē) (DCR) surgical procedure in which the lumen of the tear sac is connected with the nasal cavity.

day surgery scheduled procedure on an outpatient basis. The patient is discharged on the same calendar day as admitted.

dB (decibels) unit of measure of sound.

DCR dacryocystorhinostomy surgical procedure in which the lumen of the tear sac is connected with the nasal cavity.

DDH developmental dysplasia of hip.

deafness inability to hear.

Deaver retractors retractor used for inside the abdomen.

debris (dě-brē') remains of damaged or broken-down tissues or cells.

deciduous (dē-sĭd'-ū-ŭs) teeth first teeth, baby teeth. Primary teeth.

decompression release of pressure from a specific body area such as the brain or abdomen.

decongestants release of congestion or reduction of swelling.

decub lying down; decubitus.

decubitus (dē-kū'-bĭ-tŭs) lying down.

decubitus ulcers bed sores. Ulcerative skin lesions caused by constant pressure from lying or sitting in one position for extended periods of time.

dedifferentiation loss of differentiation of cells; reversion to a more primitive, embryonic cell type; anaplasia.

deep away from the surface.

deep tendon reflexes involuntary response of tissues deep to the surface of the skin.

deep vein thrombosis (DVT) formation of blood clots in deep veins.

defecation (dĕf-ĕ-kā'-shŭn) evacuation of feces from the bowel.

defibrillation (dē-fĭb"-rĭ-lā'-shŭn) stopping fibrillation by use of drugs or electrical countershocks to the heart; cardioversion.

deficiency (dē-fĭsh'-ĕn-sē) below the normal amount.

deformity (dē-form'-ĭ-tē) acquired or congenital deviation from normal appearance.

deglutition (dē"-gloo-tĭsh'-ŭn) swallowing.

dehiscence (dē-hĭs'-ĕns) splitting open of the operative incision suture line.

deltoid (dĕl'-toyd) refers to the shoulder anteriorly, posteriorly, and laterally.

dendrite (dĕn'-drīt) microscopic branching fiber of a nerve cell that is the first part to receive the nervous impulse.

dens (dĕnz) tooth.

dental caries tooth decay (caries means decay).

dentin major tissue composing teeth, covered by the enamel in the crown and a protective layer of cementum in the root.

deoxygenated (dē-ŏk'-sĭ-jĕn"-āt-ĕd) blood blood that is oxygen-poor.

deoxyribonucleic (dē-ŏk"-sē-rī"-bō-nū-klē'-ĭk) acid (DNA) genetic material within the nucleus of a cell; controls cell division and protein synthesis.

depersonalization disorder condition in which a patient has become socially or occupationally impaired because of a feeling of detachment, a mere observer of his own mental or bodily process.

depersonalization neurosis characterized by feeling of robotic or dream state.

depigmentation (dē"-pĭg-mĕn-tā'-shŭn) removal of pigmentation from the skin by chemical or physical process.

depression (dē-prĕsh'-ŭn) indentation or hollow region.

derm, derma cutis vera or skin.

dermal pertaining to the skin.

dermatitis (dĕr"-mă-tī'-tĭs) inflammation of the skin.

dermatology (dĕr"-mă-tŏl'-ō-jē) study of diseases of the skin.

dermatome (dĕr'-mă-tōm) instrument used to remove slices of skin for skin grafting; variations in the thickness of the donor skin can be obtained by adjusting the dermatomes; area of skin supplied by a single spinal nerve root.

dermatomycosis (dĕr"-mă-tō-mī-kō'-sĭs) skin infection caused by a fungus.

dermatophyte (dĕr'-mă-tō-fīt) fungal parasite growing in or on the skin.

dermatophytosis (dĕr'-mă-tō-fī-tō'-sĭs) fungal infection of the hair, skin or nails.

dermatoplasty (dĕr'-mă-tō-plăs"-tē) instrument used to cut into the skin or small skin lesions.

dermis (dĕr'-mĭs) corium; true skin.

descending colon portion of the colon through which products of digestion travel in a downward direction.

desquamation (dĕs"-kwă-mā-shŭn) shedding the epidermis.

deterioration retrogression.

deviated nasal septum nasal passage irregularity in which the nasal septum or center line is away from its normal location.

deviation (dē-vē-ā'-shŭn) departure from normal.

diabetes (dī"-ă-bē'-tēz) disease characterized by excess urination.

diabetes insipidus (DI) inadequate secretion of vasopressin, or resistance of the kidney to the action of antidiuretic hormone.

diabetes mellitus inadequate secretion or improper utilization of insulin.

diabetic nephropathy kidney abnormality associated with diabetes.

diabetic retinopathy retinal effects of diabetes mellitus include microaneurysms, hemorrhages, dilation of retinal veins, and neovascularization.

diagnosis (dī"-ăg-nō'-sĭs) name given to denote the disease or syndrome affecting an individual.

diagnostic pertaining to disease.

diagnostic aid drug any of the multitude of agents used to dye, highlight, enhance, or label for benefit of study and reaching a diagnosis.

dialysis (dī-ăl'-ĭ-sĭs) waste materials such as urea are separated from the bloodstream by artificial means when the kidneys can no longer function.

diapedesis (dī"-ă-pĕd-ē'-sĭs) passage of blood cells through the intact wall of a capillary.

diaphoresis (dī"-ă-fō-rē'-sĭs) profuse sweating; feeling cool or clammy.

diaphoretic (dī"-ă-fō-rĕt'-ĭk) agent used to induce sweating; the state of diaphoresis.

diaphragm (dī'-ă-frăm) muscle separating the abdominal and thoracic cavities.

diaphysis (dī-ăf'-ĭ-sĭs) shaft, or midportion, of a long bone.

diarthrosis (dī"-ăr-thrō'-sĭs) articulation in which opposing bones move freely.

diastole (dī-ăs'-tō-lē) relaxation phase of the heartbeat.

diathermy (dī'-ă-thĕr"-mē) use of an electric current to coagulate blood vessels and thus stop bleeding. It will also destroy or cut tissue. Also known as cautery.

diencephalon (dī"-ĕn-sĕf'-ă-lŏn) portion of the brain situated between the telencephalon and mesencephalon.

dietary (dī'-ĕ-tā"-rē) **iodine** regulated allowance of iodine in the diet.

diff. differential.

differentiation specialization of cells.

diffuse (dĭ-fūs) spreading evenly throughout the affected tissue.

digestion breakdown of complex foods to simpler forms.

digestive (dī-jĕs'-tĭv) **system** consisting of all organs and glands necessary to digest food from the mouth to the anus.

digit (dĭj'-ĭt) finger or toe.

digital (dĭj'-ĭ-tăl) **subtraction angiography (DSA)** an x-ray of contrast-injected blood vessels is produced by taking two x-rays (the first without contrast) and using a computer to subtract obscuring shadows from the image.

digitalis (dĭj"-ĭ-tăl'-ĭs) drug that increases the strength and regularity of the heartbeat.

dilated expanded organ, orifice or vessel.

dilation to expand an organ, orifice or vessel.

dilation and curettage (D&C) widening the cervical opening with an instrument called a dilator and insertion of a second instrument called a curet (curette) for the scraping out of the endometrial lining.

dilator (dī-lā'-tor) instrument used to widen an organ, orifice or vessel.

diminished reduced.

DIP joint distal interphalangeal joint.

diplegia (dī-plē'-jē-ă) paralysis of like organs on both sides of the body.

diplococci (dĭp"-lō-kŏk'-sē, dĭp"-lō-kŏk'-ī) bacteria appearing in pairs.

diploid (dĭp'-loyd) two sets of chromosomes.

diplopia (dĭp-lō'-pē-ă) double vision.

disarticulation amputation through a joint.

discectomy surgical excision of a disc.

discharge (dĭs-chărj') release of a secretion or excretion of pus, feces or urine or the release of accumulated energy; to release a patient from the physician's care as in release from the hospital.

discoloration change in the usual color.

disease (dĭ-zez') pathological condition of the body in which a group of clinical signs and symptoms correlate with laboratory findings to differentiate and substantiate a diagnostic finding separating the condition from others with dissimilar findings.

disk (disc) pad of cartilage between each vertebra.

dislocation displacement of a bone from its joint.

disopyramide (dī-sō-pĕr'-ă-mīd) generic antiarrhythmic drug.

disorder abnormal pathological condition of the body or mind.

dissection (dī-sĕk'-shŭn) separation of body parts.

dissectors used to cut, incise, or separate tissue.

dissociative disorder affects the patient's identity, consciousness, or memory.

distal (dĭs'-tăl) far from the point of attachment to the trunk or far from the beginning of a structure.

diuretic (dī"-ū-rĕt'-ĭk) drug used to reduce fluid retention in body tissues by enhancing water excretion by the kidneys.

diverticulitis (dē"-vĕr-tĭk'-ū-lī'-tĭs) inflammation of diverticulum in the intestinal tract.

diverticulosis (dī"-vĕr-tĭk'-ū-lō'-sĭs) condition of diverticula in the colon without inflammation or symptomatology.

diverticulum (dī"-vĕr-tĭk'-ū-lŭm) **(pl. diverticula)** small sacs or pouches in the walls of an organ such as the intestines.

DKA diabetic ketoacidosis.

DLE discoid lupus erythematosus.

DNA deoxyribonucleic acid.

DOE dyspnea on exertion.

dominant genetic trait or characteristic that is passed from one generation to the next.

donor person who donates blood, tissues or organs to another person.

dopamine (dō'-pă-mēn) drug used to treat hypotension.

Christian Johann Doppler (Dŏp'-lĕr) Austrian scientist who pioneered studies regarding how sound waves travel through the body.

doppler (dŏp'-lĕr) **effect** frequency shift that occurs at a reference point moving, in relative terms, either toward or away from a sound source.

doppler ultrasound an instrument is used to focus sound waves on a blood vessel, and blood flow is measured as echoes bounce off of red blood cells. Arteries or veins in the arms, neck, or legs may be examined to detect vascular occlusion (blockage due to clots or atherosclerosis).

dorsal pertaining to the back; posterior.

dorsal recumbent lying face up, head straight. Most common surgical position.

dorsiflexion decreasing the angle of the ankle joint so that the foot bends backward (upward).

Down syndrome condition caused by three # 21 chromosomes instead of two. Symptoms may include heart malformations and mental retardation. Some cases are fatal in infancy but most people with this condition live to adulthood.

doxylamine (dŏk-sĭl'-ă-mēn) a generic antihistamine drug.

drain (drān) used during or following an operation to remove air or fluids (serum, blood, lymph, pus, bile, intestinal secretions) from the operative site and to prevent the development of a deep wound infection. The drain is inserted directly into the incision or into a separate wound, called a stab wound, near the incision site.

drainage (drān'-ĭj) removal of air or fluid in a free flowing fashion from a wound or body cavity.

draping placement of a thick sheet (drape) over the operative site, with an opening over the incision for accessibility. The purpose of the draping is to reduce the chance of infection.

dressing a covering for a wound, may be sterile or nonsterile. The simplest type of dressing is a gauze pad held in place by tape. Other examples include: Elastoplast, plaster of Paris, stockinette, Teflon strips, skin tapes, flannel and pads.

drills used to cut, incise, or separate tissue.

droperidol (drō-pĕr′-ĭ-dŏl) generic name for a general anesthetic drug which is administered intravenously.

DSR dynamic spatial reconstructor.

DUB dysfunctional uterine bleeding.

Duchenne (dū-shĕn′) **muscular dystrophy** condition characterized by weakness and pseudohypertrophy of affected muscles beginning in childhood and progressing with age. This condition affects the shoulder and pelvic girdle muscles predominantly in males.

duct narrow vessel or channel.

ductus (dŭk′-tŭs) **deferens** better known as the vas deferens, this is a duct that carries sperm from the epididymis to the ejaculatory duct.

dullness without normal resonance or percussion.

duodenojejunostomy (dū′-ō-dē′-nō-jĕ-joo-nŏs′-tō-mē) creation of a new passage between the duodenum and the jejunum.

duodenorrhaphy (dū″-ō-dĕ-nor′-ă-fē) suturing of the duodenum.

duodenum (dū″-ō-dē′-nŭm) first part of the small intestine, the duodenum measures approximately 12 inches in length.

Dupuytren's contracture inability to extend the ring and little fingers from a bent position due to contracture of the palmar fascia.

dura (dū′-ră) **mater** outermost layer of the meninges surrounding the brain and spinal cord.

DVT deep vein thrombosis.

dwarfism congenital hyposecretion of growth hormone; hypopituitary dwarfism.

dyschromia discoloration of the nails of the fingers and toes and the skin.

dyscrasia (dĭs-krā′-zē-ă) general term for pathologic condition, usually applied to diseases of the blood.

dysesthesia (dĭs″-ĕs-thē′-zē-ă) sense or feeling of burning, prickling, tingling, numbness, or cutting pain on the skin in the absence of clinical findings.

dysfunction (dĭs-fŭnk′-shŭn) impaired or abnormal function of a part or organ.

dyskinesia (dĭs″-kĭ-nē′-sē-ă) impairment of muscle movement.

dysmenorrhea (dĭs″-mĕn-ō-rē′-ă) painful menstruation due to strong uterine contractions.

dysmorphophobia (dĭs″-mor-fō-fō′-bē-ă) characterized by an excessive concern for one's physical appearance and by the belief that some minor defect (or even normal feature) is a disfigurement.

dyspareunia (dĭs″-pă-rū′-nē-ă) pain on coitus (intercourse).

dyspepsia (dĭs-pĕp′-sē-ă) indigestion.

dysphagia (dĭs-fā′-jē-ă) difficult, painful swallowing.

dysphonia (dĭs-fō′-nē-ă) difficulty in speaking.

dysplastic displaying a highly abnormal but not clearly cancerous appearance.

dyspnea (dĭsp-nē′-ă) difficulty in breathing.

dysrhythmia (dĭs-rĭth′-mē-ă) abnormal rhythm.

dysthymia (dĭs-thī′-mē-ă) depression, chronic and mild in nature, that has been present for two or more years. Occurs most frequently in females.

dystocia (dĭs-tō′-sē-ă) difficult labor.

dystonia (dĭs-tō′-nē-ă) abnormal tone or tension of muscle.

dystrophy (dĭs′-trō-fē) defective development due to insufficient metabolism or nutrition.

dysuria painful urination.

earwax (ēr′-wăks) waxy substance secreted by the external ear, also called cerumen.

eardrum (ēr′-drŭm) membrane between the outer and the middle ear; also called tympanic membrane.

ECBD exploration of common bile duct.

ECCE extracapsular cataract extraction.

ecchymosis (ĕk-ĭ-mō′-sĭs) **(pl. ecchymoses)** bluish-black hemorrhagic mark of the skin that eventually fades to a yellowish color before disappearing.

eccrine (ĕk′-rĭn) sweat gland.

ECG; EKG electrocardiogram.

echocardiogram (ĕk″-ō-kăr′-dē-ō-grăm) recording of the heart made by an echocardiograph.

echocardiography (ĕk″-ō-kăr′-dē-ŏg′-ră-fē) pulses of high-frequency sound waves (ultrasound) are transmitted into the chest, and echoes returning from the valves, chambers, and surfaces of the heart are electronically plotted and recorded. This procedure can show the structure and movement of the heart.

echoencephalography (ĕk″-ō-ĕn-sĕf′-ă-lŏg′-ră-fē) recording of the brain with the use of ultrasonography.

echogenic refers to the body structures that reflect sound.

echogram (ĕk′-ō-grăm) image produced by ultrasound imaging.

eclampsia (ĕ-klămp′-sē-ă) condition during pregnancy or shortly after, marked by high temperature, hypertension, edema of face, legs and feet, albuminuria, severe headaches, dizziness, epigastric pain, nausea and convulsions. The etiology is unknown.

ectogenous (ĕk-tŏj′-ĕ-nŭs) ability to grow or having an origin outside of the body.

ectopic (ĕk-tŏp′-ĭk) **pregnancy** implantation of the embryo in a site outside the uterus. The most common site of implantation is the fallopian tube. In some cases the tube ruptures after implantation and the bleeding can be life-threatening to the mother.

ectropion (ĕk-trō′-pē-ŏn) outward turning of a margin or edge, such as of the eyelid.

EDC expected date of confinement. Estimated date of delivery of fetus.

edema (ĕ-dē′-mă) localized or generalized swelling secondary to fluid retention.

edematous (ĕ-dĕm′-ăt-ŭs) pertaining to swelling secondary to fluid retention.

EEG electroencephalogram.

effector cells active cells of the immune system responsible for destruction of foreign antigens.

efferent arteriole small artery that carries blood away from a structure, in particular, the vessel that carries blood away from the glomerular capillaries.

efferent nerves nerves that carry impulses away from the brain and spinal cord to the muscle, glands, and organs.

effusion (ĕ-fū′-zhŭn) leakage or escape of fluid into a body part.

ejaculation (ē-jăk′-ū-lā′-shŭn) ejection of sperm and fluid from the male urethra.

ejaculatory ducts extension of the vas deferens as it joins the urethra.

electrocardiogram (ē-lĕk″-trō-kăr′-dē-ō-grăm″) (ECG, EKG) a recording of the electrical activity of the heart.

electrocardiograph (ē-lĕk″-trō-kăr′-dē-ō-grăf) an instrument for recording the electrical activity of the heart.

electrocardiography the process, study, or interpretation of the recording of the electrical activity of the heart.

electrocautery (ē-lĕk″-trō-kaw′-tĕr-ē) the destruction of tissue by high frequency current.

electrocochleography (ē-lĕk″-trō-kŏk-lē-ŏg′-ră-fē) recording of the electrical activity of the cochlea.

electrodesiccation (ē-lĕk″-trō-dĕs″-ĭ-kā′-shŭn) method of surgery using high frequency electricity to destroy tissue by dehydration or drying.

electroencephalograph (ē-lĕk-trō-ĕn-sĕf′-ă-lō-grăf) an instrument for recording the brain's electrical activity.

electroencephalography (EEG) the recording and study of the electrical activity of the brain.

electrolysis (ē″-lĕk-trŏl′-ĭ-sĭs) decomposition of body tissues by application of a directed electrical current.

electrolyte (ē-lĕk′-trō-līt) mineral salt found in the blood and tissues and necessary for proper functioning of cells; potassium, sodium, and calcium are examples.

electromagnetic pertaining to an electromagnet consisting of a length of wire wound around a soft iron core.

electromyelogram (ē-lĕk″-trō-mī′-ō-gram) (EMG) a graphic recording of the strength of muscle contraction in response to electrical stimulation.

electromyography (ē-lĕk″-trō-mī-ŏg′-ră-fē) process, study, or interpretation of electromyograms.

electroretinograph a recording of the electrical activity of the retina in response to stimuli.

electron a minute particle with a negative electrical charge which revolves around the central core or nucleus of an atom.

electrophysiologic (ē-lĕk″-trō-fĭz-ē-ŏl′-ō-gē) study the study of the effects of electrical stimulation upon tissues; commonly refers to a procedure permitting the diagnosis of cardiac arrythmia or cardiac conduction system abnormality by electrical stimulation of the conduction pathways of the heart.

electrosurgical unit a device which use an electric current to destroy tissue, to incise tissue, and to maintain hemostasis of cut blood vessels; common term is cautery.

eleidin (ĕ-lē′-ĭ-dĭn) acidophil substance present in the stratum lucidum of the epidermis.

elevation (ĕl′-ĕ-vā′-shŭn) raising above. A raised area protruding above the surrounding area.

elevator curved retractor for holding eyelid away from eye, also used to raise depressed bones.

elliptocyte (ē-lĭp′-tō-sīt) oval-shaped red blood cell.

elliptocytosis (ē-lĭp″-tō-sī-tō′-sĭs) increase in the number of oval shaped red blood cells as seen in some forms of anemia.

emaciation (ē-mā″-sē-ā′-shŭn) the state of being excessively thin.

embolectomy (ĕm″-bō-lĕk′-tō-mē) removal of an embolus by surgical means or the destruction of an embolus with the use of clot-dissolving enzymes.

embolism (ĕm′-bō-lĭzm) obstruction of a blood vessel by an embolus.

embolus (ĕm′-bō-lŭs) (pl. emboli) blood clot that has detached from the vessel wall and moves through the blood stream. Air, amniotic fluid, bacteria and fat may also cause emboli.

embryo (ĕm′-brē-ō) stage in development from fertilization of the ovum through the second month of pregnancy.

emergency department area in the hospital for treating patients who need immediate care.

emesis (ĕm′-ĕ-sĭs) expulsion of gastric contents through the mouth.

emetic (ĕ-mĕt′-ĭk) agent which induces vomiting. May be used to treat medication overdoses or the ingestion of some poisons.

EMG electromyography.

emmetropia (ĕm″-ĕ-trō′-pē-ă) condition of having normal vision with light rays focused exactly upon the retina.

emollient (ē-mŏl′-yĕnt) soothing agent that softens and moisturizes the skin.

emphysema (ĕm″-fĭ-sē′-mă) overinflation of the air sacs of the lung with associated destruction of alveolar walls. Pulmonary emphysema; air within the connective tissue.

empyema pus within a body cavity, particularly used in reference to pus in the pleural cavity.

en bloc (ĕn-blŏk) resection surgical procedure in which an entire tumor is removed along with a large area of surrounding tissue containing affected lymph nodes.

encapsulated surrounded by a capsule.

encephalitis (ĕn-sĕf′-ă-lī′-tĭs) inflammation of the brain.

encephalocele (ĕn-sĕf′-ă-lō-sēl) extension and protrusion of brain tissue and meninges through a fissure in the cranium.

encephalomeningitis (ĕn-sĕf′-ă-lō-mĕn″-ĭn-jī′-tĭs) condition of inflammation of the brain and its surrounding membranes.

encephalomyelitis (ĕn-sĕf′-ă-lō-mī-ĕl-ī′-tĭs) condition of inflammation of the brain and spinal cord.

encephalomyelopathy (ĕn-sĕf′-ă-lō-mī″-ĕl-ŏp′-ă-thē) disease of the brain and spinal cord.

encephalopathy (ĕn-sĕf′-ă-lŏp′-ă-thē) disease of the brain.

encephalotome (ĕn-sĕf′-ă-lō-tŏm) instrument used to cut into the brain tissue.

endarterectomy (ĕnd″-ăr-tĕr-ĕk′-tō-mē) removal of the inner layer of the arterial wall.

endocardiomyopathy any disease of the innermost layer of the heart.

endocarditis (ĕn″-dō-kăr-dī′-tĭs) inflammation of the inner lining of the heart, often but not always caused by bacteria.

endocardium inner lining of the heart.

endocrine (ĕn′-dō-krĭn) pertaining to ductless glands that secrete hormones into the bloodstream and lymph.

endocrine system pertaining to the hormonal secretion of a ductless gland.

endodontist specialist concerned with the treatment and prevention of diseases of the dental pulp and surrounding tissues.

endogenous (ĕn-dŏj′-ĕ-nŭs) originating within (an organism, organ, tissue or cell).

endolymph (ĕn′-dō-lĭmf) fluid contained in the inner ear.

endometrial (ĕn″-dō-mē′-trē-ăl) ablation permanent destruction of the endometrium by cautery or other means. Used as a treatment for menometrorrhagia.

endometriosis (ĕn″-dō-mē″-trē-ō′-sĭs) endometrium (uterine lining) that adheres to the pelvis or abdominal wall causing pelvic pain, adnexal masses, and infertility.

endometritis inflammation of the endometrium.

endometrium (ĕn-dō-mē′-trē-ŭm) refers to the innermost structure (layer) of the uterus.

endoplasmic reticulum microscopic canals or tubes crossing through the nucleus of cells and cytoplasm.

endorphin (ĕn-dor′-fĭn) naturally occurring chemical substance produced in nerve tissue which has analgesic properties.

endoscopic retrograde cholangiopancreatography (ERCP) x-ray of biliary and pancreatic ducts performed by the injection of contrast medium through the hepatopancreatic ampulla into the biliary tree through an endoscope.

endoscopic surgery surgery which utilizes an endoscope to allow visual examination of the internal cavities of the body. The endoscope is often equipped with a videocamera which provides a clear picture of the internal structures. Common accessories include light, knife, biopsy forceps, suction and electrosurgery devices.

endoscopy (ĕn-dŏs′-kō-pĕ) visual inspection of internal body organs with an endoscope.

endosteum (ĕn-dŏs′-tē-ŭm) lining of the medullary cavity of bone.

endothelium (ĕn″-dŏ-thē′-lē-ŭm) layer of flat cells lining the heart, blood vessels, lymph vessels, and serous cavities.

endotracheal intubation procedure in which a flexible tube is placed through the nose or mouth, through the pharynx and larynx, and into the trachea to establish an airway.

ENT ear, nose, and throat.

enteritis (ĕn″-tĕr-ī′-tĭs) inflammation of the small intestine.

enterocele (ĕn′-tĕr-ō-sēl) herniation containing a portion of the intestine.

enterocolectomy (ĕn″-tĕr-ō-kō-lĕk′-tō-mē) surgical excision of the ascending colon, terminal ileum, and cecum.

enterolith (ĕn′-tĕr-ō-lĭth) stone in the intestine.

enterostomy (ĕn″-tĕr-ŏs′-tō-mē) creation of a new opening from the intestine through the wall of the abdomen.

entropion (ĕn-trō′-pē-ŏn) inward turning of a margin or edge, such as of the eyelid.

enucleation (ē-nū″-klē-ă′-shŭn) removal of the eyeball from its socket.

enuresis (ĕn″-ū-rē′-sĭs) involuntary bedwetting.

enzyme (ĕn′-zīm) chemical that speeds up a reaction between substances. Digestive enzymes help in the breakdown of food from complex molecules to simpler molecules.

enzyme-linked immunosorbent assay (ELISA) laboratory test used to screen for the presence of a specific antigen. A type of ELISA can be used to detect antibodies to HIV.

EOM extraocular muscles. Extraocular movement.

eosin (ē′-ō-sĭn) red acid dye.

eosinophil (ē″-ō-sĭn′-ō-fĭl) white blood cell with dense, reddish granules having an affinity for the red acid dye eosin; may be active and elevated in allergic conditions. About 3 percent of leukocytes are of this type.

ependymal (ĕp-ĕn′-dĭ-măl) **cell** cell making up the lining of the cerebral ventricles and internal spinal cord.

ephedrine (ĕ-fĕd′-rĭn) generic name for a sympathomimetic drug.

epicardial (ĕp″-ĭ-kărd′-ē-ăl) pertaining to the epicardium.

epicardium visceral layer of pericardium. Outer surface layer of the heart.

epicranius (ĕp″-ĭ-krā′-nē-ŭs) musculature and scalp covering the skull.

epidermis (ĕp″-ĭ-dĕr′-mĭs) outermost portion of the skin.

epidermoid (ĕp″-ĭ-dĕr′-moyd) resembling epithelial cells. Often used to describe tumors arising from epithelial cells.

epididymis (ĕp″-ĭ-dĭd′-ĭ-mĭs) (**pl. epididymides**) tube located on top of each testis which carries and stores sperm cells before they enter the vas deferens.

epididymitis (ĕp″-ĭ-dĭd″-ĭ-mī′-tĭs) inflammation of the epididymis.

epidural anesthesia local anesthetic injected into the extradural space of the lumbar spine blocking pain sensation leading to the lower abdomen and pelvis. Often used in obstetrical surgery.

epigastric pertaining to the epigastrium.

epigastric incision also referred to as midline incision. A surgical cut in the midline above the umbilicus, adjacent to the stomach. Used to reach the stomach, duodenum, and pancreas.

epigastric region epigastrium.

epigastrium (ĕp″-ĭ-găs′-trē-ŭm) the upper central area of the abdomen.

epiglottis (ĕp″-ĭ-glŏt′-ĭs) lid-like piece of cartilage that covers the opening of the larynx.

epiglottitis (ĕp″-ĭ-glŏt-ī′-tĭs) inflammation of the epiglottis.

epilepsy (ĕp′-ĭ-lĕp″-sē) disorder characterized by sudden, transient (passing) disturbances of brain function secondary to seizures.

epimysium (ĕp″-ĭ-mĭz′-ē-ŭm) connective tissue enclosing skeletal muscle.

epinephrine (ĕp″-ĭ-nĕf′-rĭn) catecholamine produced by the adrenal medulla which increases heart rate and blood pressure; also called adrenaline.

epiphyseal (ĕp″-ĭ-fĭz′-ē-ăl) **plate** cartilaginous area at the ends of long bones where lengthwise growth takes place.

epiphysis (ĕ-pĭf′-ĭ-sĭs) a secondary center of bone growth, distinct from the shaft and separated from it by a layer of cartilage.

episcleritis (ĕp″-ĭ-sklē-rī′-tĭs) inflammation of the sclera in the subconjunctival layers.

episiorrhaphy (ĕ-pĭs″-ē-or′-ă-fē) suturing of the vulva.

episiotomy (ĕ-pĭs″-ē-ŏt′-ō-mē) surgical incision of the vulva generally done just prior to childbirth to facilitate delivery.

epispadias (ĕp″-ĭ-spā′-dē-ăs) congenital abnormality in which the meatal opening is on the dorsum (top side) of the penis.

epistaxis nosebleed.

epithelial (ĕp″-ĭ-thē′-lē-ăl) pertaining to epithelium.

epithelial cell skin cell that lines the external body surface and the internal surface of organs.

epithelium (ĕp″-ĭ-thē′-lē-ŭm) layer of skin cells forming the outer and inner surfaces of the body.

eponychium (ĕp″-ō-nĭk′-ē-ŭm) cuticle of the nail.

Epstein-Barr virus (EBV) virus that causes infectious mononucleosis.

equilibrium balance.

ERCP endoscopic retrograde cholangiopancreatography.

erect standing or sitting in an upright position.

erection engorgement of the penis with blood to a swollen, hardened, stiffened state upon sexual arousal.

ERG electroretinogram.

erosion (ē-rō′-shŭn) destruction of a surface by wearing away or eating away.

error of refraction a defect in the shape of the eyeball causing light rays to fall on the retina out of focus. Includes astigmatism, myopia and presbyopia.

ERS endoscopic retrograde sphincterotomy

eructation (ĕ-rŭk-tā′-shŭn) belching of gas from the stomach.

ERV expiratory reserve volume.

erysipelas (ĕr″-ĭ-sĭp′-ĕ-lăs) localized inflammation and redness of skin and subcutaneous tissue generally caused by group A streptococci.

erythema (ĕr″-ĭ-thē′-mă) redness of skin.

erythema multiforme reddened skin areas, consisting of erythematous spots or macules which may be surrounded by a concentric ring, giving a target-like appearance.

erythematous (ĕr″-ĭ-thĕm′-ă-tŭs) characterized by red coloration of the skin.

erythremia (ĕr″-ĭ-thrē′-mē-ă) increase in red blood cell mass and total blood volume. Polycythemia rubra vera.

erythroblast (ĕ-rĭth′-rō-blăst) nucleated red blood cell precursor.

erythroblastosis (ĕ-rĭth″-rō-blăs-tō′-sĭs) fetalis hemolytic disease of the newborn, caused by a blood group (Rh factor) incompatibility between the mother and the fetus.

erythrocyte (ē-rĭth′-rō-sīt) red blood cell. Red corpuscle.

erythrocyte count red blood cell count.

erythrocyte sedimentation rate (ESR) test which measures the speed at which erythrocytes settle out of plasma. Venous blood is collected, anticoagulant is added, and the blood is placed in a tube in a vertical position. The distance that the erythrocytes fall in a given period of time is the sedimentation rate. The rate is altered in conditions that increase the immunoglobulin content of the blood, such as infections, inflammation, and malignancy.

erythrocytosis (ĕ-rĭth″-rō-sī-tō′-sĭs) increase in total red blood cell mass in response to a known external stimulus.

Erythromycin (ĕ-rĭth″-rō-mī′-sĭn) generic antibiotic drug.

erythropoiesis (ĕ-rĭth″-rō-poy-ē′-sĭs) erythrocyte production.

erythropoietin (ĕ-rĭth″-rō-poy′-ē-tĭn) hormone secreted by the kidney which stimulates the production of red blood cells.

eschar (ĕs′-kăr) sloughing scar tissue produced by a burn.

escharotomy (ĕs-kăr-ŏt′-ō-mē) surgical release of constricted burned tissue.

esophageal (ē-sŏf′-ă-jē′-ăl) pertaining to the esophagus.

esophageal atresia congenital failure of the esophageal lumen to develop fully.

esophageal hiatus opening in the diaphragm through which the esophagus passes.

esophageal regurgitation backward flow of gastric contents into the esophagus.

esophageal sphincter muscular ring at the end of the esophagus.

esophageal varices swollen, dilated, engorged veins at the distal end of the esophagus.

esophagus (ē-sŏf′-ă-gūs) tube connecting the throat to the stomach.

esophagotomy (ē-sŏf-ă-gŏt′-ō-mē) surgical opening into the esophagus.

esotropia (ĕs-ō-trō′-pē-ă) condition in which one eye is turned inwardly toward the other, which may cause diplopia in certain fields of vision.

ESR erythrocyte sedimentation rate.

estradiol (ĕs-tră-dī′-ŏl) estrogen (female hormone) produced by the ovaries.

estrogen (ĕs′-trō-jĕn) hormone produced by the ovaries; responsible for female secondary sex characteristics and buildup of the uterine lining during the menstrual cycle.

ESWL extracorporeal shock wave lithotripsy.

ether generic anesthetic drug.

ethmoid (ĕth′-moyd) sieve-like structure.

ethmoid bone irregularly shaped bone forming a portion of the nasal cavity.

ethmoidal sinuses pertaining to the airspaces of the paranasal sinuses located within the ethmoid bone.

etiology (ē″-tē-ŏl′-ō-jē) cause or origin, particularly of disease.

EUA examination under anesthesia.

eupnea (ūp-nē′-ă) normal breathing.

eustachian (ū-stā′-kē-ăn) tube auditory tube.

euthyroid (ū-thī′-royd) goiter condition of swelling or enlargement in a normally functioning thyroid gland.

eversion (ē-vĕr′-zhŭn) a turning outward of a body part.

evisceration (ē-vĭs″-ĕr-ā′-shŭn) protrusion of viscera outside of the abdominal cavity.

evoked response reaction brought about by a particular stimulus.

Ewing's (ū′-ĭngz) tumor malignant bone tumor.

exacerbation (ĕks-ăs″-ĕr-bā′-shŭn) increase in the severity of a condition or disease.

examination under anesthesia (EUA) examination of a body part, organ or cavity under anesthesia, particularly as refers to a pelvic exam while anesthetized.

excision (ĕk-sĭ′-zhŭn) surgical removal of a part or organ.

excisional biopsy removal of tumor and a margin of normal tissue. This procedure provides a specimen for diagnosis and may be curative for small tumors.

excoriation (ĕks-kō-rē-ă′-shŭn) scratch or abrasion of the skin.

excretion (ĕks-krē′-shŭn) waste material that is eliminated by the body or process of such elimination, such as the passage of feces from the bowel or urine from the bladder.

excretory urogram (ĕks′-krē-tō-rē ū′-rō-grăm) radiologic examination of the urinary tract to observe size, shape, and location of kidneys, ureters, and bladder following intravenous injection of a contrast medium. Also referred to as an intravenous excretory urogram or IVU.

exenteration (ĕks-ĕn″-tĕr-ā′-shŭn) wide surgical resection involving removal of a tumor, its organ of origin, and all surrounding tissue in a body space, such as in the pelvis.

exercise test exercise on a treadmill or other device under controlled conditions with monitoring of the electrocardiogram, pulse and blood pressure for the purpose of detecting cardiac disease.

exfoliation (ĕks″-fō-lē-ā′-shŭn) shedding, scaling or desquamation of epidermal cells.

exfoliative cytology microscopic examination of exfoliated cells.

exhibitionism psychosexual disorder in which the patient is overcome by the need to expose the genitalia to unsuspecting or involuntary subjects.

exocrine (ĕks′-ō-krĭn) pertaining to the outward secretion of a gland from a duct.

exocrine glands glands that secrete through a duct.

exogenous (ĕks-ŏj′-ĕ-nŭs) originating outside of an organism, organ, tissue or cell.

exophthalmia (ĕks″-ŏf-thăl′-mē-ă) condition in which the eyeballs protrude.

exophthalmometry a test measuring the extent of eyeball protrusion.

exophthalmos (ĕks″-ŏf-thăl′-mōs) protrusion of the eyeballs.

exotropia (ĕks″-ō-trō′-pē-ă) condition in which one eyeball turns away from the other which may cause diplopia in certain fields of vision.

expected date of confinement (EDC) the expected date an infant will be born.

expectorant (ĕk-spĕk′-tō-rănt) agent that brings about the expulsion of mucus or fluids from the lungs or nasal passages.

expiration (ĕks″-pĭ-rā′-shŭn) to exhale air from the lungs; to die, cease to live.

expiratory reserve volume (ERV) the amount of air remaining in the lungs after exhalation.

exploration of common bile duct (ECBD) examination of the contents of the common bile duct surgically, endoscopically, or fluoroscopically.

extension (ĕks-tĕn′-shŭn) return from flexion to an unflexed position; increasing the angle between two bones; straightening out a limb.

extensor digitorum longus muscle allowing extension of the four lateral toes.

extensor digitorum muscle allowing extension of the fingers.

external acoustic meatus the outer opening of the ear.

external auditory meatus external acoustic meatus.

external canthus outer or lateral junction of the upper and lower eyelids.

external ear outer, visible portion of the ear.

external genitalia portion of the reproductive anatomy at the outermost portion of the body; the penis and scrotum in males, the clitoris, labia minora, and labia majora in females.

external nares nostrils.

external respiration the exchange of gases in the lungs, as distinguished from the exchange at the tissues.

external urethral sphincter ring-like muscular structure which constricts the urethra.

extracapsular (ĕks″-tră-kăp′-sū-lăr) **cataract extraction (ECCE)** surgical removal of the anterior capsule of the lens and the lens contents, leaving the posterior capsule of the lens in place.

extracellular (ĕks″-tră-sĕl′-ū-lăr) pertaining to the outside of a cell.

extracellular fluid fluid or liquid outside a cell, including the interstitial fluid and the plasma.

extracorporeal (ĕks″-tră-kor-por′-ē-ăl) outside of, or unrelated to, the body.

extraction the process of pulling out or drawing away.

extradural (ĕks-tră-dū′-răl) **hemorrhage** hemorrhage into epidural space of the cranium.

extraocular (ĕks″-tră-ŏk′-ū-lăr) adjacent to but outside of the eyeball.

extravasation (ĕks-trăv″-ă-sā′-shŭn) escape of fluid, such as blood, from a blood vessel.

extremities the arms and legs.

extrinsic (ĕks-trĭn′-sĭk) **ocular (extraocular) muscles** muscles responsible for movement of the eye.

exudate (ĕks′-ū-dāt) fluid composed of cells, protein, and solid materials that has leaked from blood vessels into or onto a body tissue.

facet (făs′-ĕt) plane surface on a bone where it articulates with another structure.

facial bones bones of the face: lacrimal, mandible, maxillae, nasal, vomer and zygomatic.

fallopian (fă-lō′-pē-ăn) pertaining to the uterine tubes.

fallopian tubes uterine tubes.

false vocal cords folds of mucous membrane within the larynx which do not function in voice production.

fascia (făsh′-ē-ă) fibrous membrane separating and enveloping muscles, deep to the skin surface.

fascial (făsh′-ē-ăl) pertaining to the fascia.

fasciculation (fă-sĭk″-ū-lā′-shŭn) muscle contraction visible through skin.

fasciculus (fă-sĭk′-ū-lŭs) pertaining to a fascicle; a small bundle of nerves, muscles or tendon fibers.

fasciectomy (făsh″-ē-ĕk′-tō-mē) excision of the fascia.

fasciitis (fă-sī′-tĭs) inflammation of the fascia.

fasciorrhaphy (făsh-ē-or′-ă-fē) suturing of the fascia.

fasting blood sugar (FBS) test which measures blood glucose when the patient is fasting (has refrained from eating for 12 to 24 hours beforehand).

fat white or yellowish adipose tissue forming a cushioning layer between organs.

fatal (fāt′-l) bringing about death.

fatigue (fă-tēg) exhaustion of energy due to prolonged exertion.

FBS fasting blood sugar.

febrile (fē′-brĭl) having an increased body temperature.

feces (fē′-sēz) waste matter composed of digested food, bacteria, cells, and intestinal secretions.

femoral (fĕm′-or-ăl) pertaining to the thighbone.

femur (fē′-mŭr) the long bone extending from the pelvis to the knee in the leg. This is the largest bone in the body.

fertile (fĕr′-tĭl) **days** days of ovulation when egg is available for fertilization by sperm.

fertilization fusion of the sperm and ovum.

fetal (fē′-tăl) pertaining to the fetus.

fetish (fĕt′-ĭsh) an inanimate object which is regarded as having magical or erotic qualities.

fetoscope optical device used to view the fetus in the womb.

fetoscopy examination of the fetus using a fetoscope. Used to diagnose normal and abnormal fetal development.

fetus (fē′-tŭs) embryo from the third month (after 8 weeks) to birth.

FEV$_1$ forced expiratory volume in one second, a measure of the volume of air which can be expelled from the lungs in the first second of a forced expiration.

fibrinogen (fī-brĭn′-ō-jĕn) protein threads that form the basis of a blood clot.

fibroadenoma (fī″-brō-ăd″-ĕ-nō′-mă) benign rubbery tumor of the breast composed of glandular elements and connective tissue.

fibroblast (fī′-brō-blăst) fiber-producing cell from which connective tissue develops.

fibroid (fī′-broyd) uterine leiomyoma, a benign tumor of the uterus.

fibroma (fī-brō′-mă) (pl. fibromas, fibromata) benign tumor composed of fibrous connective tissue.

fibromyoma (fī″-brō-mī-ō′-mă) leiomyoma containing substantial fibrous connective tissue.

fibrous (fī′-brŭs) containing or composed of fibers.

fibula (fĭb′-ū-lă) lateral and smaller of the two lower leg bones.

fibular pertaining to the fibula.

filiform (fĭl′-ĭ-form) threadlike. In microbiology, a bacterial growth that is uniform along the inoculation line in stab or streak cultures.

filtrate (fĭl′-trāt) fluid that a filter allows to pass through.

filum (fī′-lŭm) **terminale** long, slender connective tissue filament at the end of the spinal cord.

fimbria (fĭm′-brē-ă) (pl. **fimbriae**) finger-like end of the fallopian tubes.

fissure (fĭsh′-ūr) narrow, deep, slit-like opening.

fixation act of immobilizing, making rigid.

flaccid (flăk′-sĭd) absent of muscular form; flabby, or relaxed.

flagellum (flă-jĕl′-ŭm) hair-like process which propels a sperm cell.

flat in percussion, without resonance.

flatplate radiographic term used to describe examination requiring a frontal projection of the abdomen or other body part with the patient in a supine position.

flat plate of abdomen x-ray of abdominal organs without use of a contrast medium. Sometimes called kidneys, ureters and bladder (KUB), as these organs are highlighted.

flatulence (flăt′-ū-lĕns) presence of an increased amount of intestinal gas.

flatus (flā′-tŭs) gas expelled from the stomach or intestine.

flexion (flĕk′-shŭn) decrease of the angle at a joint.

floating kidney kidney which is moveable from its normal bed of fat and connective tissue.

fluorescein (floo″-ō-rĕs′-ē-ĭn) dye.

fluorescein angiography diagnostic procedure in which fluorescein is injected intravenously allowing the movement of blood through the retina to be photographed; allows detection of vascular lesions of the retina.

fluoroscopy x-ray examination which permits visualization of a moving image, such as movement of substances or contrast through the digestive tract.

Foley catheter drain used to remove contents of the urinary bladder.

folic (fō′-lĭk) **acid** member of the vitamin B complex used in the treatment of sprue.

follicle small, gland-like sac.

follicle-stimulating hormone (FSH) gonadotrophin produced by the anterior lobe of the pituitary gland. FSH stimulates hormone secretion and egg production by the ovaries and sperm production by the testes.

fontanel (fŏn″-tă-nĕl′) soft spot in the skull of a fetus or neonate present between the cranial bones before they have fused.

foramen (for-ā′-mĕn) opening in bone or membrane.

foramen magnum opening in the occipital bone through which the spinal cord passes to the brain.

foramen ovale in the fetus, an opening between the atria of the heart.

foramen rotundum opening in the great wing of the sphenoid bone through which the maxillary branch of the trigeminal nerve passes.

forceps (for′-sĕps) also known as fingers, tissues, or pickups, are used to grasp or hold tissue. Non-toothed forceps handle delicate tissue, while toothed forceps handle thick or difficult to manage tissue. Common forceps are tenaculum, Babcock, Kocher, Allis and obstetrical.

forceps delivery use of a tong-shaped instrument to grasp the fetus by the head and aid its passage through the birth canal.

forebrain anterior portion of the brain of the embryo.

foreign bodies slivers, dirt, cinders, or small objects that may lodge in the eyes, skin, or nose, or internally.

foreskin skin covering the tip of the penis.

fornix (pl. **fornices**) the arch-shaped roof of an anatomical space. Fornices are present in the brain, conjunctivae, pharynx and vagina.

fossa (fŏs′-ă) shallow cavity.

fovea (fō′-vē-ă) **capitis** depression of the head of the femur for attachment of the ligamentum teres.

fovea centralis tiny pit or depression in the retina that is the region of clearest vision.

Fowler position posture in which patient is seated in a position with the back angle half way between vertical and horizontal at 45 degree angle. Used for some shoulder procedures and in the recovery room.

fractionation method of administering radiation therapy in small, repeated doses rather than a few large doses. Fractionation allows a larger total dose to be given with less damage to normal tissue.

fracture breaking of a bone.

fragment (frăg′-mĕnt) broken-off part from a larger entity.

fraternal (dizygotic) twins twins resulting from the fertilization of two separate eggs concurrently.

free radical molecule containing an odd number of electrons.

free tie ligation a solitary strand of suture material placed around a blood vessel which is held by a hemostat; the free tie is then tightened and knotted, occluding the vessel.

fremitus (frĕm′-ĭ-tŭs) vibratory tremors, most commonly felt through the chest wall by palpation.

frequency the increased urge to micturate or void, often with a reduced volume of urine.

frontal pertaining to the forehead bone; anterior.

frontal bone cranial bone which forms the forehead and the superior portion of the orbits.

frontal (coronal) plane vertical plane dividing the body into an anterior and a posterior portion.

frontal sinuses hollow pair of spaces in the frontal bone located above the orbits.

frotteurism fetish involving sexual excitement derived from rubbing or touching another individual without consent.

FSH follicle-stimulating hormone.

fulguration (fŭl-gū-rā′-shŭn) electrical destruction of tissue.

fundoscopy (fŭn-dŏs′-kō-pē) visual examination of the fundus of the eye.

fundus (fŭn′-dŭs) larger part, base of body of a hollow organ.

fungal (fŭn′-găl) caused by or pertaining to a fungus.

fungating (fŭn′-gāt-ĭng) mushrooming pattern of growth in which cells pile one on top of another and project from a tissue surface.

fungiform (fŭn′-jĭ-form) fungus-shaped.

fungiform papillae small rounded eminences on middle and anterior parts of the tongue, many of which contain taste buds.

fungus (fŭn′-gŭs) (pl. **fungi**) plant-like organism that subsists on organic matter.

furosemide generic diuretic drug.

furuncle (fū′-rŭng-k′l) boil.

furunculosis (fū-rŭng″-kū-lō′-sĭs) condition marked by the presence of boils.

fusion (fū′-shŭn) uniting, meeting or joining together, particularly through heat.

Fx fracture.

G gravida.

GA general anesthesia.

gait (gāt) manner of walking.

galactorrhea (gă-lăk″-tō-rē′-ă) excessive discharge of milk from the breast. May be seen with pituitary gland tumors.

galea (gā′-lē-ă) **aponeurotica** flat fibrous sheet of connective tissue of the scalp which connecting the frontal and occipital bellies of the occipitofrontalis muscle.

gallbladder (GB) a small sac under the liver which stores bile.

gallbladder series (GBS) series of x-ray films studing the gallbladder.

gamete (găm′-ēt) sex cell; sperm or ovum.

gamma emitter substance that emits gamma radiation.

gamma globulin fraction of serum globulin with which most of the immune antibodies are associated.

gamma rays electromagnetic radiation emitted by a radioactive substance.

gammopathy a disturbance of immunoglobulin production.

ganglion (găng′-lē-ŏn) **(pl. ganglia, ganglions)** knot-like collection of nerve cell bodies outside of the brain and spinal cord; cystic mass arising from a tendon sheath, frequently in the wrist.

ganglionectomy (găng″-lē-ō-něk′-tō-mē) excision of a ganglion.

gastralgia (găs-trăl′-jē-ă) pain in the stomach.

gastrectomy (găs-trĕk′-tō-mē) surgical removal all or part of the stomach.

gastric (găs′-trĭk) pertaining to the stomach.

gastric analysis study of gastric contents for levels of hydrochloric acid and pH.

gastritis (găs-trī′-tĭs) inflammation of the stomach mucosa.

gastrocnemius (găs″-trŏk-nē′-mē-ŭs) large muscle of the posterior lower leg.

gastroenterology (găs″-trō-ĕn″-tĕr-ŏl′-ō-jē) study of the pathology and physiology of the gastrointestinal tract.

gastroenterostomy (găs″-trō-ĕn-tĕr-ŏs′-tō-mē) surgical creation of an artificial opening between the stomach and small bowel.

gastroesophageal reflux (GER) the involuntary backwash of stomach contents from the stomach into the esophagus; may be a cause of dyspepsia or "heartburn".

gastrointestinal pertaining to the stomach and intestine.

gastrojejunostomy (găs-trō-jĕ-jū-nŏs′-trō-mē) surgical creation of an artificial opening between the stomch and jejunum.

gastrology (găs-trŏl′-ō-jē) study of function and diseases of the stomach.

gastropathy (găs-trŏp′-ă-thē) any disorder of the stomach.

gastropexy (găs′-trō-pĕk″-sē) the suturing of the stomach to the abdominal wall to prevent displacement.

gastrorrhexis (găs-trō-rĕk′-sĭs) rupture of the stomach.

gastroscope (găs′-trō-skōp) endoscope for visually inspecting the interior of the stomach.

gastroscopy (găs-trŏs′-kō-pē) the precedure of visually inspecting the interior of the stomach with an endoscope.

gastrospasm (găs′-trō-spăzm) sudden, involuntary contractions of the stomach.

gastrotomy (găs-trŏt′-ō-mē) incision into the stomach.

gavage (gă-văzh′) feeding via a nasogastric tube.

GB gallbladder.

GBS gallbladder series.

general anesthesia (GA) the state of complete loss of feeling or sensation produced by a gneeral anesthetic agent.

general anesthetic drug which produces complete loss of consciousness, blocks pain sensation, and induces muscle relaxation.

generalized anxiety disorder psychiatric disorder characterized by unreasonable apprehension which is not caused by any clearly identifiable stimulus.

generator (gĕn′-ĕr-ā″-tor) in nuclear medicine, a device for manufacturing a radionuclide from another radionuclide by radioactive decay.

generic (jĕn-ĕr′-ĭk) **drug** a drug named according to its main chemical ingredient, regardless of manufacturer.

gene (gēn) basic unit of heredity.

geneticist (jĕn-ĕt′-i-sĭst) one who specializes in genetics.

genetics (jĕn-ĕt-ĭkz) study of heredity and its variations.

genital (jĕn′-ĭ-tăl) **herpes** sexually transmitted disease causing painful vescular lesions on the external genitalia.

genitalia (jĕn-ĭ-tāl′-ē-ă) reproductive organs, also called genitals.

genitals (jĕn′-ĭ-tăls) reproductive organs.

genitourinary (jĕn″-ĭ-tō-ūr′-ĭ-nār-ē) pertaining to the genitals and urinary organs.

genu (jē′-nū) **valgum** knock-kneed.

genu varum bowlegged.

GER gastroesphageal reflux.

gestation (jĕs-tā′-shŭn) pregnancy.

GFR glomerular filtration rate.

GGT gamma-glutamyl transpeptidase.

GH growth hormone.

GHIH growth-hormone-inhibiting hormone.

GHRH growth-hormone-releasing hormone.

GI gastrointestinal.

GI series gastrointestinal series.

giant cell tumor tumor of bone, usually benign, seen most commonly in the long bones of young adults.

gigantism (jī′-găn-tĭzm) condition of abnormal size of the body or any of its parts, may be caused by oversecretion of growth hormone from the pituitary gland.

gingiva (jĭn′-jĭ-vă) gums, the tissue that surrounds the necks of the teeth.

gingivitis (jĭn-jĭ-vī′-tĭs) inflammation of the gums.

gingivolabial (jĭn″-jĭ-vō-lā′-bē-ăl) pertaining to the gums and cheek.

glans penis sensitive tip of the penis.

glaucoma (glaw-kō′-mă) increased intraocular pressure, resulting in damage to the retina and optic nerve.

glenohumeral (glē″-nō-hū′-mĕr-ăl) pertaining to the humerus and the glenoid cavity.

glenoid (glē′-noyd) giving the appearance of a socket.

glenoid cavity socket in the scapula that receives the head of the humerus.

glioblastoma (glī″-ō-blăs-tō′-mă) **multiforme** neoplasm of the central nervous system.

globulin (glŏb′-ū-lĭn) plasma protein; separates into alpha, beta, and gamma types by electrophoresis.

globus globe or sphere.

globus pallidus pale-appearing section within the lenticular nucleus of the brain.

glomerular filtration rate (GRF) the volume of fluid filtered by the glomerulus in a given time, usually expressed in milliliters per minute.

glomerulonephritis (glō-mĕr″-ū-lō-nĕ-frī′-tĭs) inflammation of the kidney glomerulus.

glomerulosclerosis (glō-mĕr″-ū-lō-sklē-rō′-sĭs) scarring of the renal glomeruli, frequently in association with arteriosclerosis.

glomerulus (glō-mĕr′-ū-lŭs) **(pl. glomeruli)** tiny ball of capillaries (microscopic blood vessels) in cortex of the kidney.

glossorrhaphy (glō-sor′-ă-fē) suture of wound of the tongue.

glottis (glŏt′-ĭs) the true vocal cords and the opening between.

glucagon (gloo′-kă-gŏn) peptide hormone produced by the islet cells of the pancreas. Glucagon stimulates the conversion of glycogen (starch) to glucose and antagonizes the action of insulin.

glucocorticoid (gloo″-kō-kort′-ĭ-koyd) a class of steroid hormone naturally secreted by the adrenal cortex; necessary for the metabolism of sugars, fats, and proteins and for the body's normal response to stress.

gluconeogenesis (gloo″-kō-nē″-ō-jĕn′-ĕ-sĭs) formation of sugar from proteins and fats.

glucose (gloo′-kōs) a simple sugar which is the main source of cellular energy.

glucose (gloo′-kōs) **tolerance test** (GTT) the measurement of blood glucose levels at timed intervals following an oral glucose load. Abnormally elevated glucose levels during the test may be indicative of diabetes mellitus.

glycogen (glī′-kō-jĕn) animal starch; glucose is stored as glycogen in liver cells.

glycogenolysis (glī″-kō-jĕn-ŏl′-ĭ-sĭs) breakdown of glycogen to form glucose.

glycolysis (glī-kŏl′-ĭ-sĭs) anaerobic breakdown of glucose to lactic acid.

GnRH gonadotrophin-releasing hormone.

goblet cell mucus-secreting cell found in the epithelium of the intestinal and respiratory tracts.

goiter (goy′-tĕr) enlargement of the thyroid gland.

gonads (gō′-nădz) organs in the male and female that produce gametes; ovaries and testes.

gonioscopy (gō″-nē-ŏs′-kō-pē) inspection of the anterior chamber of the eye.

gonococcal (gŏn″-ō-kŏk′-ăl) related to or caused by gonococci.

gonococcus (gŏn″-ō-kŏk′-ŭs) (pl. **gonococci**) bacterium that causes gonorrhea.

gonorrhea (gŏn″-ō-rē′-ă) sexually transmitted disease causing inflammation in either the male or female reproductive tract. May be treated with antibiotics.

gout (gowt) a metabolic disease in which deposition of uric acid crystals in the joints may cause a form of acute arthritis.

gracilis (grăs′-ĭ-lĭs) long slender muscle on the medial aspect of the thigh.

grading of tumors evaluating the microscopic appearance of tumor cells to determine the degree of anaplasia.

grafting (grăft′-ĭng) transfer of tissue taken from elsewhere to another location.

gram (grăm) **stain** a stain added to material such as body fluid to be microscopically examined for the presence of bacteria. The stain performs two functions: it renders the bacteria visible under the microscope and it helps to divide bacteria into two large groups. Gram-positive bacteria will turn purple and Gram-negative bacteria will appear pink. Each of these groups can then be further divided according to their shape. The shapes include cocci which are round, and bacilli which are rod-shaped.

granulocyte (grăn′-ū-lō-sīt″) white blood cells with granules; eosinophils, neutrophils, and basophils.

granulocytic pertaining to the granulocyte.

grasper an instrument to grasp and hold tissue.

Graves' disease a form of hyperthyroidism named for Robert J. Graves, an Irish physician (1796–1853), characterized by weight loss, tremulousness and tachycardia, and commonly but not invariably, exophthalmos.

gray matter nervous tissue of grayish color in which myelinated nerve fibers do not predominate.

gross (grōs) **anatomy** anatomy which can be studied without the use of a microscope.

gross description of tumors the visual appearance of tumors: may be described as cystic, fungating, inflammatory, medullary, necrotic, polypoid, ulcerating, or verrucous.

growth hormone (GH) peptide hormone produced by the anterior pituitary which stimulates the growth of bones and tissues; also called somatotropin.

growth hormone inhibiting hormone (GHIH) peptide hormone produced by the hypothalamus which inhibits the pituitary's production of growth hormone.

GTT glucose tolerance test.

guarding body defense mechanism to prevent further injury to an already injured body part.

Guillain-Barre syndrome an inflammatory polyneuritis of unknown etiology, thought to have an autoimmune basis.

gynecology (gī″-nĕ-kŏl′-ō-jē) study of diseases of the female reproductive organs.

gynecological (gī″-nĕ-kō-lŏj′-ĭ-kăl) pertaining to gynecology or the study of diseases peculiar to women.

gynecologist (gī″-nĕ-kŏl′-ō-jĭst) specialist in the study of the diseases and treatment of the female genital tract.

gynecomastia (gī″-nĕ-kō-măs′-tē-ă) overdevelopment of the male mammary glands.

gyrus (jī′-rŭs) (pl. **gyri**) elevation in the surface of the cerebral cortex.

hair cell a sensory epithelial cell present in the ear and in the taste buds, possessing threadlike nonmotile cilia.

hair follicle sac or pit in which a hair grows.

half-life the time required for a radioactive substance to lose half of its original radioactivity by radioactive decay.

hallucination (hă-loo-sĭ-nā′-shŭn) a strongly experienced false perception which seems real but which has no basis in fact.

hallux (hăl′-ŭks) great toe.

hallux valgus displacement of the tip of the great toe towards the other toes. Commonly referred to as a bunion.

hallux varus displacement of the tip of the great toe away from the other toes.

halothane (hăl′-ō-thăn) generic name for a general anesthetic gas which is administered through inhalation.

hamate (hăm′-ăt) "hooked"; one of the bones of the wrist.

hammer first ossicle of the middle ear; also called malleus.

hammer toe any toe with dorsal flexion of the first phalanx and plantar flexion of second and third phalanges.

hamstring one of the tendons that form both the medial and lateral boundaries of the popliteal space.

Hanks dilators used to widen the cervix uteri.

haploid (hăp′-loyd) possessing a single set of chromosomes.

haustra (haws′-tră) sacculated pouches of the colon.

HAV hepatitis A virus.

Hawkins dilators used to widen the cervix uteri.

Hb, Hgb hemoglobin.

HBV hepatitis B virus.

hCG human chorionic gonadotropin.

HCl hydrochloric acid.

HCT hemoglobin.

HCV hepatitis C virus.

HDL high-density lipoprotein.

HDV hepatitis D (or delta) virus.

head anterior, proximal, or upper extremity of a structure or body.

hearing aid device which amplifies sound, used by those with hearing impairments.

heart (hărt) muscular hollow contractile organ which is the center of the circulatory system.

heart block (atrioventricular block) condition in which there is improper conduction of impulses through the A-V node to the bundle of His. May result in an irregular rhythm or slowed heart rate.

heart transplant surgical transplantation of the heart from a donor, frequently a victim of trauma, to a recipient.

Hegar (hā′-găr) **dilators** used to widen the cervic uteri.

helper T-lymphocytes T cells that aid B cells in recognizing antigens; also called CD4 cells.

hemangioma (hē-măn″-jē-ō′-mă) common, benign tumor consisting of dilated blood vessels.

hematemesis (hĕm-ăt-ĕm′-ĕ-sĭs) the vomiting of blood.

hematocele (hē′-mă-tō-sēl) the accumulation of blood into the tunica vaginalis of the testis.

hematocrit (hē-măt′-ō-krĭt) test to measure the percentage of cells in a given volume of blood. A sample of blood is spun in a centrifuge so that the erythrocytes fall to the bottom of the sample.

hematology (hē″-mă-tŏl′-ō-jē) study of the anatomy, physiology and pathology of the blood and blood-forming organs.

hematoma (hē″-mă-tō′-mă) mass of blood, normally clotted, confined to a tissue, organ or space, caused by a break in a blood vessel.

hematopoiesis (hē″-mă-tō-poy-ē′-sĭs) the process of formation and development of blood cells.

hematosalpinx (hē″-mă-tō-săl′-pĭnks) accumulation of blood in the fallopian tube.

hematuria (hē″-mă-tū′-rē-ă) blood in the urine.

hemianopia (hĕm″-ē-ă-nŏ′-pē-ă) hemianopsia.

hemianopsia (hĕm″-ē-ă-nŏp′-sē-ă) reduced vision or blindness in half of the visual field of one or both eyes.

hemicolectomy (hĕm″-ē-kō-lĕk′-tō-mē) excision of a portion of the colon.

hemihepatectomy (hĕm″-ē-hĕp″-ă-tĕk′-tō-mē) surgical excision of a portion of the liver.

hemiplegia (hĕm-ē-plē′-jē-ă) paralysis of one side of the body.

hemisphere (hĕm′-ĭ-sfĕr) half of the cerebrum or cerebellum.

hemocytoblast (hē″-mō-sī′-tō-blăst) stem cell found in bone marrow from which all cells normally present in blood are thought to arise.

hemoglobin (hē″-mō-glō′-bĭn) a blood protein found in red blood cells which enables the red blood cell to carry oxygen; laboratory test to measure hemoglobin concentration in the blood.

hemolysis (hē-mŏl′-ĭ-sĭs) the rupture of blood cells.

hemolytic anemia anemia resulting from the rupture of red blood cells.

hemolytic (hē″-mō-lĭt′-ĭk) **disease of the newborn** erythroblastosis fetalis, caused by a blood group (Rh factor) incompatibility between the mother and the fetus.

hemopericardium (hē″-mō-pĕr″-ĭ-kăr′-dē-ŭm) blood in the pericardial sac.

hemophilia (hē″-mō-fĭl′-ē-ă) an inherited clotting disorder caused by a deficiency in one of the protein substances necessary for coagulation.

hemoptysis (hē-mŏp′-tĭ-sĭs) the coughing of blood arising from the lungs or bronchial tree.

hemorrhage (hĕm′-ē-rĭj) bleeding, particularly if severe or profuse.

hemorrhagic (hĕm-ō-răj′-ĭk) characterized by or pertaining to hemorrhage.

hemorrhoidectomy (hĕm″-ō-royd-ĕk′-tō-mē) surgical excision of hemorrhoidal tissue.

hemorrhoid (hĕm′-ō-royd) a dilated, varicose vein in the anal region.

hemostasis (hē-mŏs′-tă-sĭs) stoppage of bleeding or circulation.

hemostat (hē′-mō-stăt) **clamp** an instrument used to control bleeding and to grasp tissue.

hemothorax (hē″-mō-thō′-răks) blood in the pleural cavity.

Hemovac surgical drain used to drain blood.

heparin (hĕp′-ă-rĭn) anticoagulant drug.

hepatic (hĕ-păt′-ĭk) **duct** canal that receives bile from the liver.

hepatic flexure bend of the colon under the liver.

hepatitis (hĕp″-ă-tī′-tĭs) inflammation of the liver. May be caused by a variety of conditions, infections, inflammatory and toxic. Hepatitis A is transmitted via feces and contaminated water. Hepatitis B is transmitted by contaminated blood and body fluids. May be transmitted sexually. Hepatitis C is transmitted similarly to hepatitis B.

hepatitis B surface antigen antigen to a portion of the hepatitis B virus, presence of which in the blood indicates hepatitis B infection.

hepatocyte (hĕp″-ă-tō-sīt) parenchymal liver cell.

hepatology (hĕp″-ă-tŏl′-ō-jē) study of the liver.

hepatoma (hĕp″-ă-tō′-mă) tumor of the liver.

hepatopathy (hĕp-ĕ-tŏp′-ă-thē) pertaining to any disease of the liver.

hepatosplenomegaly (hĕp″-ă-tō-splē″-nō-mĕg′-ă-lē) enlargement of the liver and spleen.

heredity (hĕ-rĕd′-ĭ-tē) transmission of characteristics from parent to child.

hernia (hĕr′-nē-ă) protrusion of an organ or part through the muscle normally containing it.

herniated disk abnormal protrusion of an intervertebral pad into the neural canal or onto a spinal nerve.

herniorrhaphy (hĕr-nē-or′-ă-fē) the suturing and repair of a hernia.

herpes simplex (hĕr′-pēz-sĭm′-plĕx) infectious disease caused by herpes simples virus types I or II.

herpes zoster (hĕr′-pēz zŏs′-tĕr) shingles. The reactivation of latent varicella (chicken pox) virus within a peripheral nerve causing a blistering rash and pain along the path of that nerve.

heterograft (hĕt′-ĕ-rō-grăft) a tissue graft taken from an animal of a different species from the recipient.

heterosexual (hĕt′-ĕr-ō-sĕk′-shū-ăl) pertaining to the opposite gender.

HHD hypertensive heart disease.

hidradenitis (hī-drăd-ĕ-nī′-tĭs) inflammation of the sweat glands.

hillock (hĭl′-ŏk) small eminence or projection.

hilum (hī′-lŭm) depression in or that part of an organ where blood vessels and nerves enter and leave. Also called a hilus.

hindbrain (hīnd′-brān) most caudal of the three divisions of the embryonic brain.

Hirschsprung (hĭrsh′-sprŭngz) **disease** a congenital dilatation of a portion of the colon because of the absence of nerve ganglion cells in the portion of bowel distal to it. A cause of chronic constipation.

hirsutism (hŭr′-sūt-ĭzm) the presence of excessive body or facial hair, particularly in women.

histamine (hĭs′-tă-mĭn) substance released by mast cells during an allergic reaction.

histiocyte (hĭs′-tē-ō-sīt) large phagocyte present in connective tissue of the skin.

histology (hĭs-tŏl′-ō-jē) the study of tissue.

histopathology (hĭs″-tō-pă-thŏl′-ō-jē) the laboratory study of surgically removed and chemically fixed tissue. The size, shape, color, and texture of the tissue are appraised and samples are then studied under the microscope.

histoplasma (hĭs″-tō-plăz′-mă) **capsulatum** fungus which is the etiologic agent of histoplasmosis.

histoplasmosis (hĭs″-tō-plăz-mō′-sĭs) an infection resulting from inhalation of spores of histoplasma capsulatum. May cause disease of the lungs or reticuloendothelial system.

HIV human immunodeficiency virus.

HNP History and Physical.

Hodgkin (hŏj′-kĭn) **disease** solid tumor of the lymphorecticular system, named for Thomas Hodgkin (1798–1866).

holders instruments which grasp and hold tissue.

Holter monitor portable electrocardiograph worn by a patient during normal activity.

homeostasis (hō″-mē-ō-stā′-sĭs) tendency in an organism to maintain an equilibrium or constant, stable state.

homosexual (hō″-mō-sĕks′-ū-ăl) one sexually attracted to another of the same gender.

hordeolum (hor-dē′-ō-lŭm) (**stye**) localized, purulent, inflammatory staphylococcal infection of the eyelid.

horizontal parallel to or in the plane of the horizon.

horizontal mattress sutures stitches which run parallel to the wound, passing under the surface to be tied off on the other side.

hormone (hor′-mōn) substance produced by an endocrine gland which travels through the blood to modify the structure or function of a distant organ or gland.

horny cell keratin-filled cell in the epidermis.

HSG hysterosalpingogram.

Hubbard tank tank used for active or passive underwater exercises.

human chorionic gonadotropin (hCG) hormone produced by the placenta to stimulate the mother's ovaries to produce estrogen and progesterone.

human immunodeficiency virus (HIV) virus that causes human AIDS.

humeral (hū′-mĕr-ăl) pertaining to the upper arm.

humerus (hū′-mĕr-ŭs) upper bone of the arm proximal to the elbow.

humoral (hū′-mor-ăl) **immune response** the portion of the immune response in which B cells transform into plasma cells and secrete antibodies.

hyaline (hī′-ă-lĭn) **membrane disease** a respiratory problem of the premature neonate caused by lack of protein surfactant in the alveoli, resulting in collapse of the lungs. Also known as respiratory distress syndrome of the newborn.

hydrocele (hī′-drō-sēl) an accumulation of water within the tunica vaginalis of the testis.

hydrocephalus (hī-drō-sĕf′-ă-lŭs) the accumulation of excessive fluid in the spaces of the brain.

hydrochloric (hī″-drō-klōr′-ĭk) **acid** a substance produced by the stomach; necessary for the digestion of food.

hydrogen (hī′-drō-jĕn) colorless, odorless, and tasteless gas.

hydrogen peroxide (H_2O_2) an oxidizing agent used as a mild antiseptic.

hydronephrosis (hī″-drō-nĕf-rō′-sĭs) dilation of the renal collecting system caused by the obstructed outflow of urine.

hydrosalpinx (hī″-drō-săl′-pĭnks) the accumulation of fluid in the fallopian tube.

hydrothorax (hī″-drō-thō′-răks) a collection of watery fluid in the pleural cavity.

hyoid (hī′-oyd) **bone** bone shaped like a horseshoe, lying at the base of the tongue.

hyperaldosteronism (hī″-pĕr-ăl″-dō-stĕr′-ōn-ĭzm) abnormal condition of electrolyte balance caused by excessive secretion of aldosterone.

hyperbilirubinemia (hī″-pĕr-bĭl″-ĭ-roo-bĭn-ē′-mē-ă) excessive amounts of bilirubin in the blood.

hypercapnia (hī″-pĕr-kăp′-nē-ă) excessive carbon dioxide levels in the blood.

hypercholesterolemia (hī″-pĕr-kō-lĕs″-tĕr-ŏl-ē′-mē-ă) excessive amount of cholesterol in the blood.

hyperchromia (hī″-pĕr-krō′-mē-ă) excessive pigmentation.

hyperemesis (hī″-pĕr-ĕm′-ĕ-sĭs) **gravidarium** excessive and persistent vomiting during pregnancy which may be accompanied by exhaustion and weight loss.

hyperesthesia (hī″-pĕr-ĕs-thē′-zē-ă) increased sensitivity to touch.

hyperextension (hī″-pĕr-ĕks-tĕn′-shŭn) extension beyond the normal position.

hyperglycemia high blood sugar.

hyperhidrosis (hī″-pĕr-hī-drō′-sĭs) abnormal or increased sweating.

hyperinsulinism (hī″-pĕr-ĭn′-sū-lĭn-ĭzm) excess secretion of insulin, causing hypoglycemia.

hyperkeratosis (hī″-pĕr-kĕr′-ă-tō-sĭs) a condition of hypertrophy of the horny layer of the epidermis.

hyperkinesia (hī″-pĕr-kī-nē′-zē-ă) excessive movement, fast movement.

hyperlipidemia (hī″-pĕr-lĭp-ē′-mē-ă) an excess of blood lipids.

hypermetropia (hī″-pĕr-mē-trō′-pē-ă) farsightedness.

hyperopia (hī″-pĕr-ō′-pē-ă) farsightedness.

hyperparathyroidism (hī″-pĕr-păr″-ă-thī′-roy-dĭzm) a condition resulting from excessive production of parathyroid hormone, causing an elevated serum calcium.

hyperpituitarism (hī″-pĕr-pĭ-tū′-ĭ-tăr-ĭsm) a condition of overactivity of the anterior lobe of the pituitary gland.

hyperplasia (hī″-pĕr-plā′-zē-ă) abnormal increase or multiplication in the number of normal cells within a tissue.

hyperpnea (hī″-pĕrp-nē′-ă) abnormal increase in the rate and depth of respirations.

hyperresonance (hī″-pĕr-rĕz′-ō-năns) increased resonance.

hypersensitivity (hī″-pĕr-sĕn″-sĭ-tĭv′-ĭ-tē) condition in which the body reacts with an exaggerated immune response; the immune system produces tissue damage and disordered function rather than immunity.

hypertension (hī″-pĕr-tĕn′-shŭn) blood pressure higher than 140/90.

hypertensive heart disease (HHD) high blood pressure affecting the heart.

hyperthyroidism (hī″-pĕr-thī′-royd-ĭzm) overactivity of the thyroid gland.

hypertrophy (hī-pěr′-trŏ-fē) enlargement of an organ due to an increase in its own bulk.

hypertropia (hī″-pěr-trō′-pē-ă) a type of vertical strabismus in which one eye is permanently deviated upward.

hyperventilation (hī″-pěr-věn″-tĭ-lā′-shŭn) abnormal rapid, deep breathing.

hyphema (hī-fē′-mă) bleeding within the anterior chamber of the eye.

hypnotic (hĭp-nŏt′-ĭk) **sedative** sedative drug used to induce sleep.

hypoadrenalism (hī″-pō-ăd-rē′-năl-ĭzm) reduced activity of the adrenal gland.

hypocalcemia (hī″-pō-kăl-sē′-mē-ă) abnormally low blood calcium.

hypochrondriac (hī″-pō-kŏn′-drē-ăk) an individual possessing an abnormal or excessive fear of disease, especially when appearing healthy.

hypochrondriac region the upper right and left regions of the abdomen beneath the ribs.

hypochrondriasis (hī″-pō-kŏn-drī′-ă-sĭs) a psychiatric condition, also known as hypochondriacal neurosis, in which the individual believes he has a serious disease, medical assurances to the contrary notwithstanding.

hypochromia (hī″-pō-krō′-mē-ă) condition where the red blood cells have a reduced hemoglobin content.

hypodermic (hī″-pō-děr′-mĭk) inserted or used under the skin; hypodermic needle.

hypoesthesia (hī″-pō-ěs-thē′-zē-ă) reduced sensitivity to touch.

hypogastric (hī″-pō-găs′-trĭk) pertaining to the region of the abdomen inferior to the umbilicus.

hypogastric region the lower middle region of the abdomen inferior to the umbilical region.

hypoglossal (hī″-pō-glŏs′-ăl) located under the tongue.

hypoglycemia (hī″-pō-glī-sē-mē-ă) deficient amounts of sugar in the blood.

hypoglycemic (hī″-pō-glī-sē′-mĭk) **agent** a drug which reduces the level of glucose in the blood.

hypomania (hī″-pō-mā′-nē-ă) excitement and mild degree of mania.

hypomaniac (hī″-pō-mā′-nĭk) the condition or state of hypomania; someone who is afflicted with hypomania.

hypoparathyroidism (hī″-pō-păr-ă-thī′-royd-ĭzm) deficient production of parathyroid hormone, resulting in a low serum calcium level.

hypophysectomy (hī-pŏf″-ĭ-sĕk′-tō-mē) the removal of the hypophysis (anterior pituitary gland) by surgical or other means.

hypophysis (hī-pŏf′-ĭ-sĭs) the pituitary gland.

hypopituitarism (hī″-pō-pĭ-tū′-ĭ-tă-rĭzm) the lack or diminished secretion of pituitary hormones.

hypospadias (hī″-pō-spā′-dē-ăs) a congenital abnormality in which the meatal opening is on the ventral (underside) of the penis.

hypothalamus (hī″-pō-thăl′-ă-mŭs) the portion of the brain beneath the thalamus; controls sleep, appetite, body temperature, and the secretions from the pituitary gland.

hypothyroidism (hī″-pō-thī′-royd-ĭzm) underactivity of the thyroid gland.

hypotropia (hī″-pō-trō′-pē-ă) a type of vertical strabismus in which one eye is permanently deviated downward.

hypoxia (hī″-pŏks′-ē-ă) lack of oxygen.

hypoxyphilia a form of sexual masochism characterized by the desire to be deprived of oxygen.

hysterectomy (hĭs-tĕr-ĕk′-tō-mē) the surgical excision of the uterus.

hysteria (hĭs-tē′-rē-ă) obsolete, broad term which refers to a wide variety of symptoms of psychogenic orgin

hysterosalpingography (hĭs″-tĕr-ō-săl″-pĭn-gŏg′-ră-fē) (HSG) x-ray of the uterus and fallopian tubes following injection of contrast medium into the uterus.

hysteroscopy (hĭs″-tĕr-ŏs′-kō-pē) examination of the uterus using a special endoscope.

hysterotomy incision into the uterus.

Hz (Hertz) unit of frequency; one hertz equals one cycle per second.

I&D incision and drainage.

IABP intra-aortic balloon pump.

iatrogenic (ī″-ăt-rō-jĕn′-ĭk) **disorder** an adverse condition which is an effect of the treatment process itself.

IBS irritable bowel syndrome.

ichthyosis (ĭk″-thē-ō′-sĭs) condition where the skin becomes dry and scaly, appearing fish-like.

icterus (ĭk′-tĕr-ŭs) the yellow staining of the tissues, secretions, and membranes with bile pigments as in hyperbilirubinemia.

identical (monozygotic) twins twins resulting from the separation of one fertilized egg into two distinct embryos.

idiopathic (ĭd″-ē-ō-păth′-ĭk) pertaining to spontaneous origin, conditions without clear pathogenesis, or disease without recognizable cause.

idoxuridine (ī-dŏks-ūr′-ĭ-dēn) (IDU) drug used for the treatment of herpesvirus infections of the eye.

IEP immunoelectrophoresis.

ileectomy (ĭl″-ē-ĕk′-tō-mē) removal of the ileum.

ileocecal (ĭl″-ē-ō-sē′-kăl) **valve** the point where the small intestine opens into the ascending colon.

ileostomy (ĭl′-ē-ŏs′-tō-mē) the surgical creation of an artificial passage from the ileum through the abdominal wall.

ileum (ĭl′-ē-ŭm) the third part of the small intestine, from the Greek *eilos* meaning twisted; so named because when the abdomen was viewed at necropsy (autopsy), the intestine appeared twisted.

iliac (ĭl′-ĭ-ăk) pertaining to the ilium or hip bone.

iliac crest long curved upper border of the ilium.

iliac region the lower right and left regions of the abdomen near the groin.

iliosacral (ĭl″-ē-ō-sā′-krăl) pertaining to the ilium and sacral regions.

iliotibial (ĭl″-ē-ō-tib′-ē-ăl) pertaining to or extending between the ilium and tibia.

ilium (ĭl′-ē-ŭm) one of the bones the pelvis; hip bone.

IM intramuscular.

imbalance out of balance.

imipramine (ĭ-mĭp′-ră-mēn) an antidepressant drug.

immature (ĭm″-mă-tūr′) not yet fully developed.

immobilization making an extremity or part immobile.

immune (ĭm-ūn′) protected against disease.

immunity process where one is protected or immune to disease.

immunoelectrophoresis (ĭ-mū″-nō-ē-lĕk″-trō-fō-rē′-sĭs) process by which the amount and character of proteins and antibodies in body fluids is determined by the use of electrophoresis.

immunofluorescence (ĭm″-ū-nō-floo″-rĕ′-sĕnce) the use of fluorescein-stained or fluorescein labeled antibodies to locate antigens in tissues.

immunoglobulin (ĭm″-ū-nō-glŏb′-ū-lĭn) protein (globulin) with antibody activity; examples are IgG, IgM, IgA, IgE, IgD.

immunohematology (ĭ-mū-nō-hēm″-ă-tŏl′-ō-jē) the cross-matching of donated blood with a sample of the patient's blood by determination of the ABO and Rh antigens present on red blood cells before a transfusion.

immunology (ĭm″-ū-nŏl′-ō-jē) study of the immune system.

impetigo (ĭm-pĕ-tī′-gō) an inflammatory skin disease of bacterial origin characterized by vesicles, pustules, and crusted lesions.

implantation (ĭm″-plăn-tā′-shŭn) the grafting of tissues or the insertion of an organ such as skin, tooth, or tendon into a new location.

impotence (ĭm′-pō-tĕnz) sexual dysfunction characterized by the inability to maintain a sufficient erection for intercourse.

impulse (ĭm′-pŭls) a spontaneous act performed without thought.

in vitro (ĭn vē′-trō) within a test tube or other artificial environment.

in vivo (ĭn vē′-vō) within the living body.

incision (ĭn-sĭzh′-ŭn) a surgical cut. Several layers of tissue must often be incised in order to reach an intended organ or cavity. For example, to reach the abdominal organs, the surgeon must incise the skin, subcutaneous tissue, fascia, muscle and peritoneum.

incisional biopsy procedure in which only a piece of tissue is removed for examination to establish a diagnosis.

incisor (ĭn-sī′-zor) one of four front teeth in the dental arch.

incontinence a loss of sphincter control causing the inability to retain urine or feces.

incus (ĭng′-kŭs) second ossicle (bone) of the middle ear; also called anvil.

indapamide a diuretic drug.

index (ĭn′-dĕks) (pl. indices) forefinger.

indigestible (ĭn″-dĭ-jĕs′-tĭ-bl) food which cannot be broken down to be utilized by the body.

indurated (ĭn′-dū-rāt-ĕd) firm or hardened.

infancy the earliest part of life during which a child is unable to walk or to feed itself.

infant child in the first year of life, from birth to the first birthday.

infantilism (ĭn-făn′-tĭl-ĭzm) state of slow development of mind and body.

infarct an area of tissue death resulting from local loss of blood supply.

infarction formation of an infarct.

infectious arthritis inflammation in a joint caused by infection.

inferior (ĭn-fē′-rē-or) below, lower, smaller.

inferior (caudal) referring to the lower anatomical plane.

inferior palpebra lower eyelid.

infertile days the days during the menstrual cycle when the egg is not available for fertilization.

infertility the inability to impregnate or to become pregnant.

infiltrate (ĭn-fĭl′-trāt) to pass through into another space, cavity.

infiltrative that which extends beyond normal tissue boundaries.

inflammation a complex of reactions which occurs in tissues in response to injury, infection or other stimulation including, but not limited to, erythema and edema.

inflammatory characterized by inflammation.

influenza (ĭn″-flū-ĕn′-ză) an acute viral respiratory infection.

infracostal (ĭn″-fră-kŏs′-tăl) below the rib.

infundibulum (ĭn″-fŭn-dĭb′-ū-lŭm) funnel-shaped structure or passage.

infusion (ĭn-fū′-zhŭn) introduction of a liquid substance into the body via a vein for therapeutic purposes.

inguinal (ĭng′-gwĭ-năl) pertaining to the region of the groin.

inguinal nodes lymph nodes in the inguinal region.

inguinal region lower right and left regions near the groin. Also called the iliac region.

inhalation (ĭn″-hă-lā′-shŭn) breathing in (inspiration).

inhalation therapy the administration of medicines, vapors, gases, or anesthetics by inhalation.

inhibit (ĭn-hĭb′-ĭt) to restrain.

innervate (ĭn-nĕr′-vāt) to supply nervous stimulation to a part of the body.

innominate (ĭ-nŏm′-ĭ-nāt) **bones** pelvic bones, which include the ilium, ischium, and pubis.

inotropic (ĭn″-ō-trŏp′-ĭk) that which influences the force of muscular contractility.

insertion movable attachment of the distal end of a muscle; placing of something into something else.

inspiration (ĭn″-spĭr-ā′-shŭn) inhalation; the act of drawing air into the lungs.

insufflation the process of blowing a gas into a cavity.

insufflation of fallopian tubes test for the patency of the fallopian tubes. Carbon dioxide is instilled into the fallopian tubes via the uterus. If the fallopian tubes are open, the gas will enter the abdominal cavity and will show up on x-ray.

insula (ĭn′-sū-lă) central lobe of the cerebral hemisphere.

insulin (ĭn′-sū-lĭn) a peptide hormone produced by the endocrine cells of the pancreas. It permits the entry of glucose into cells from the blood and stimulates glycogen formation by the liver.

integumentary (ĭn-tĕg-ū-mĕn′-tă-rē) **system** the skin and its accessory structures such as hair and nails.

interatrial (ĭn″-tĕr-ā′-trē-ăl) situated between the atria of the heart.

interatrial septum walls between the atria.

intercellular (ĭn″-tĕr-sĕl′-ū-lăr) between the cells of a structure.

intercondylar eminence an elevation on the tibia between its two condyles.

intercourse introduction of the male penis into the female vagina.

interferon (ĭn-tĕr-fēr′-ŏn) antiviral protein secreted by T-lymphocytes.

interleukin protein that stimulates the growth of T-lymphocytes and activate immune responses.

intermittent (ĭn″-tĕr-mĭt′-ĕnt) **claudication** sporadic blood clotting.

internal (ĭn-tĕrn′-ăl) innermost portion of a part, organ, or surface.

internal respiration the exchange of gases at the tissue level.

internal acoustic meatus internal auditory canal.

interphalangeal (ĭn″-tĕr-fă-lăn′-jē-ăl) pertaining to the area between the phalanges.

interrupted suture suture which is individual and isolated by a knot.

interstitial (ĭn″-tĕr-stĭsh′-ăl) **fluid** fluid in the spaces between cells. This fluid becomes lymph when it enters the lymph capillaries.

interstitial pneumonia an inflammation of the lungs in which fluid builds up in the tissue between the alveoli.

intertrochanteric (ĭn″-tĕr-trō″-kăn-tĕr′-ĭk) **crest** the ridge between the greater and lesser trochanters of the femur.

interventricular between the ventricles.

intestinal obstruction blockage of the lumen of the intestine.

intestine (ĭn-tĕs′-tĭn) portion of the alimentary canal extending from the pylorus to the anus.

intolerance an inability to withstand.

intracapsular cataract extraction surgical procedure in which the entire lens, including its capsule, is removed.

intracellular (ĭn″-tră-sĕl′-ū-lăr) within a cell.

intracoronary within the arterial supply of the heart.

intracranial within the skull.

intracranial abscess abscess within the skull cavity, usually within the brain.

intraocular within the eyeball.

intraocular lens manufactured lens for refraction of light which is placed within the eye itself to replace the clouded native lens removed during a cataract extraction.

intraocular lens implant implantation of a manufactured or transplanted lens in the intraocular space of the eye.

intraocular pressure the pressure of fluid within the eye.

intraoperative (ĭn″-tră-ŏp′-ĕr-ă″-tĭv) during surgery.

intrauterine (ĭn″-tră-ū′-tĕr-ĭn) within the uterine cavity.

intravenous within or into a vein.

intravenous pyelogram (IVP) a radiographic procedure in which contrast material is injected into a vein and travels to the kidney where it is filtered into the urine. X-rays are then taken showing the dye filling the kidneys, ureters, bladder, and urethra. These x-rays provide an index of renal function as well as show cysts, tumors, infections, hydronephrosis and calculi.

intravenous urography (IVU) an x-ray of the urinary system using contrast medium.

intussusception (ĭn″-tŭ-sŭ-sĕp′-shŭn) telescoping of one segment of intestine within another.

invasive that which enters the body.

inversion (ĭn-vĕr′-zhŭn) reversal of a normal relationship; a turning inward of a body part.

involuntary muscle a muscle which moves independently of conscious will.

ion a charge-carrying particle.

ionizing radiation energy given off by radioactive atoms and x-rays which produces small particles called ions.

IP interphalangeal joint.

ipecac (ĭp′-ĕ-kăk) an emetic drug.

ipodate (ĭ′-pō-dāt) a radiopaque contrast medium.

IPPB intermittent positive pressure breathing.

iridectomy (ĭr″-ĭd-ĕk′-tō-mē) surgical removal of the iris or a portion thereof.

iridocyclitis (ĭr″-id-ō-sī-klī′-tĭs) inflammation of the iris and ciliary body.

iridotomy (ĭr-ĭ-dŏt′-ō-mē) incision of the iris.

iris (ĭ′-rĭs) colored portion of the eye.

iris forceps a type of small forceps used to grasp or hold tissue.

iritis (ī-rīt′-ĭs) inflammation of the iris.

iron (ī′-ĕrn) a mineral supplement.

irradiation (ĭ-rā′-dē-ā-shŭn) exposure to protons, electrons, neutrons, or other ionizing radiation.

irreducible (ĭr″-rē-dū′-sĭ-bl) not capable of being reduced or made smaller.

ischemia (ĭs-kē′-mē-ă) inadequate circulation of blood to a body part.

ischial (ĭs′-kē-ăl) pertaining to the ischium.

ischium (ĭs′-kē-ŭm) lower portion of the hip bone.

islets (ī-lĕtz) **of Langerhans** (after Paul Langerhans, pathologist, 1847–1888) clusters of hormone-producing cells in the pancreas.

isoenzyme (ī″-sō-ĕn′-zīm) one of a group of enzymes which have similar catalytic properties but which have differing electrophoretic mobility.

isoflurane general anesthetic gas.

isolate remove from others, separate.

isoniazid (ī″-sō-nī′-ă-zĭd) (INH) antituberculous drug.

isotope (ī′-sō-tōp) chemical element having the same atomic number as another.

isthmus (ĭs′-mŭs) narrow passage that connects two spaces or cavities.

IUCD intrauterine contraceptive device.

IUD intrauterine device.

IVC intravenous cholangiogram.

IVC inferior vena cava.

IVP intravenous pyelogram.

IVU intravenous urography.

jaundice (jawn′-dĭs) yellow pigmentation of the skin caused hyperbilirubinemia.

jejunum (jē-jū′-nŭm) second part of the small intestine. The Latin *jejunus* means empty as this part of the intestine was always empty when a body was examined after death.

Jobst garment elastic garment, fabricated to apply various amounts of pressure to an area of the body healing after a burn.

joint an articulation.

jugular (jŭg′-ū-lăr) **foramen** opening between the occipital and temporal bones through which passes the jugular vein as well as nerves and arteries.

juxtaglomerular (jŭks″-tă-glō-mĕr′-ū-lăr) **apparatus** a collection of cells surrounding the arteriole leading to the glomerulus of the kidney, consists of specialized cells which secrete renin and monitor blood pressure.

juxtaglomerular cells specialized cells present in the juxtaglomerular apparatus resembling those of the carotid body.

JVP jugular venous pressure.

K potassium.

Kaposi's (kăp′-ō-sē″) **sarcoma** malignant tumor arising from the lining of capillaries and appearing as bluish-red skin nodules.

karyotype (kăr′-ē-ō-tīp) the full chromosome set of a given individual.

Kelly clamp surgical instrument used to control bleeding and to grasp tissue.

keloid (kē′-lŏyd) enlarged, thickened scar.

keratin (kĕr′-ă-tĭn) hard, protein material found in the epidermis, hair, and nails.

keratinization development of or conversion into keratin.

keratinocyte (kĕ-răt′-ĭ-nō-sīt) epidermal cell that synthesizes keratin.

keratitis inflammation of the cornea.

keratoconjunctivitis (kĕr″-ă-tō-kŏn-jŭnk″-tĭ-vī′-tĭs) inflammation of the cornea and the conjunctiva.

keratoconus (kĕr-ă-tō-kō′-nŭs) a conical protrusion in the center of the cornea which is without inflammation.

keratolytic (kĕr″-ă-tō-lĭt′-ĭk) characterized by, or producing, or pertaining to desquamation or loosening of the horny layer of the skin.

keratomycosis (kĕr″-ă-tō-mī-kō′-sĭs) a fungal infection of the cornea.

keratoplasty (kĕr′-ă-tō-plăs″-tē) procedure involving replacement of a section of an opaque cornea with normal, transparent cornea in a effort to restore vision; also called corneal transplant

keratosis (kĕr-ă-tō′-sĭs) thickened area of the epidermis.

Kernig's (kĕr′-nĭgz) **sign** (after Vladimir Kernig, physician, 1840–1917) pain and reflex contraction in the hamstring muscles when attempting to extend the leg after flexing the thigh upon the body, a sign of meningitis.

ketamine hydrochloride a general anesthetic drug which is administered intramuscularly.

ketosteroid a steroid molecule with ketone groups attached, generally produced in the adrenal cortex.

keV kilo electron volt.

kidney an organ, situated alongside the spinal column, purple-brown in color, that filters blood and excretes the end-products of body metabolism in the form of urine.

kidney transplant removal of a kidney from a donor and its placement into a recipient.

kidneys, ureters, and bladder (KUB) term to denote a supine x-ray of the abdomen which demonstrates the size and location of the kidneys in relationship to other organs in the abdominopelvic region.

Kimmelstiel-Wilson syndrome degeneration of the glomerular function following long-term diabetes mellitus.

kinesiometer an instrument used to measure movement.

Klebsiella (klĕb″-sē-ĕl′-ă) **pneumoniae** an encapsulated species of bacterium that can cause pneumonia.

knee joint the articulation of the femur and tibia.

knee replacement the replacement of a knee joint with a manufactured joint.

Kocher forceps surgical instrument used to grasp or hold tissue.

kraurosis (krō-rō′-sĭs) a dry and wrinkled appearance of the external genitalia, especially the vulva. Most frequently seen in post-menopausal women.

KS Kaposi's sarcoma.

KUB kidneys, ureter, and bladder.

kyphosis (kī-fō′-sĭs) excessive angulation of the normal posterior curve of the spine.

L lumbar.

L/S ratio lecithin/sphingomyelin ratio.

LA left atrium.

label radioactive part of a radiopharmaceutical.

labia (lā′-bē-ă) lips of the vulva.

labia minora smaller innermost lips of the vulva.

labia majora larger outermost lips of the vulva.

labial (lā′-bē-ăl) pertaining to the lips.

labioglossopharyngeal (lā″-bē-ō-glŏs″-ō-făr-ĭn′-jē-ăl) pertaining to the lips, tongue and throat.

labor process by which the fetus is expelled from the uterus and vagina to the outside of the body.

labyrinth (lăb′-ĭ-rĭnth) maze-like series of canals in the inner ear; includes the cochlea, semicircular canals, saccule, and utricle.

labyrinthitis (lăb″-ĭ-rĭn-thī′-tĭs) inflammation of the labyrinth.

laceration (lăs″-ĕr-ā′-shŭn) open wound with jagged edges.

lacrimal (lăk′-rĭm-ăl) pertaining to tears.

lacrimal apparatus a group of structures which form and secrete tears.

lacrimal bones two paired bones which are located at the corner of each eye. These thin, small bones contain fossae for the lacrimal gland (tear gland) and canals for the passage of the lacrimal duct.

lacrimal duct one of two ducts that convey tears.

lacrimal duct probe a surgical instrument used to treat stenosis of the lacrimal duct.

lacrimal gland a tear gland located near the eye.

lacteal (lăk′-tē-ăl) a lymphatic vessel which carries chyle from the intestine.

lactate dehydrogenase (LDH) cardiac profile.

lactiferous (lăk-tĭf′-ĕr-ŭs) **duct** tube that carries milk within the breast.

lamina (lăm′-ĭ-nă) (pl. laminae) thin flat layer or plate.

laminectomy (lăm″-ĭ-nĕk′-tō-mē) the excision of a posterior vertebral arch or lamina.

LAO left anterior oblique.

laparoscope (lăp′-ă-rō-skōp″) endoscope used for visual examination of the abdominal cavity.

laparoscope-assisted vaginal hysterectomy surgical procedure in which the uterus is removed through the vaginal opening while being viewed through the laparoscope.

laparoscopic hysterectomy surgical removal of the uterus utilizing laparoscopic guidance.

laparascopic laser endometriosis vaporization laparoscope equipped with laser capabilities is inserted through a small incision into the pelvic cavity. The laser beam is used to destroy the ectopic endometrium.

laparoscopic surgery any surgery using a laparoscope.

laparoscopy (lăp-ăr-ŏs′-kō-pē) procedure in which an endoscope is inserted into the abdomen through a small incision in the abdominal wall. Through the laparoscope, the abdominopelvic organs can be visualized.

laparotomy (lăp-ăr-ŏt′-ō-mē) surgical procedure in which the abdomen is opened.

large intestine portion of the colon extending from the ileum to the anus.

laryngectomy (lăr″-ĭn-jĕk′-tō-mē) surgical excision of the larynx.

laryngitis (lăr-ĭn-jī′-tĭs) inflammation of the larynx.

laryngopharynx (lăr-ĭn″-gō-făr′-ĭnks) the lower portion of the pharynx.

laryngotracheobronchitis (lă-rĭng″-gō-trē″-kē-ō-brŏng-kī′-tĭs) inflammation of the larynx, trachea and bronchi; also known as croup.

larynx (lăr′-ĭnks) (pl. larynges) voice box; a box-like structure located at the upper part of the trachea which is made of cartilage.

laser (lā′-zĕr) an instrument used for cutting, hemostasis, and destruction of tissue with light rays. Laser is an acronym that has been accepted as a word. It refers to light amplification by stimulated emission of radiation.

laser iridectomy use of a laser to surgically remove a portion of the iris.

laser photocoagulation procedure in which an argon laser beam is used to coagulate tissue in the interior of the eye.

laser surgery a narrow beam of light energy is absorbed by tissue, generating heat which is used to coagulate, destroy and dissect. It is employed in abdominal, ophthalmic, orthopedic, gynecological and urinary surgery.

laser therapy any therapeutic use of a laser.

lateral (lăt′-ĕr-ăl) pertaining to the side. Farther from the median.

lateral condyle rounded knuckle at the side of a bone.

lateral decubitus the position of lying on the side with the arms stretched out.

lateral malleolus outside prominence of the ankle composed of the lower end of the fibula.

lateral rectus the muscle responsible for lateral movement of the eye.

lateral sulcus the lateral groove which is the deepest of the fissures of the brain; Sylvian fissure.

lavage (lă-văzh′) to irrigate or wash out a hollow organ such as the intestine.

LBBB left bundle branch block.

LDH lactate dehydrogenase.

LDL low-density lipoprotein.

left subcostal incision surgical cut below the ribs used to reach the spleen.

Legionella pneumophila rod-shaped bacterium that causes Legionnaires' disease.

leiomyoma (lī″-ō-mī-ō′-mă) benign smooth muscle tumor which frequently occurs in the uterus. Also known as fibroids, myomas and fibromyomas.

leiomyosarcoma (lī″-ō-mī″-ō-săr-kō′-mă) a malignant tumor of smooth muscle.

lens (lĕnz) manufactured transparent refracting medium, usually made of glass; the natural refracting medium of the eye, located behind the pupil.

lentiform (lĕnt′-ĭ-form) shaped like a lens.

lesion (lē′-zhŭn) a wound, injury or circumscribed pathologic change of the tissues.

lesser omentum portion of the omentum that passes from the lesser curvature of the stomach to the transverse fissure of the liver.

lesser trochanter minor of the two bony processes below the neck of the femur.

lethargic (lĕ-thăr′-jĭk) sluggish.

leukemia (loo-kē′-mē-ă) an excessive proliferation of abnormal white blood cells.

leukocyte (loo′-kō-sĭt) white blood cell.

leukocytosis (loo″-kō-sī-tō′-sĭs) an increase in the number of leukocytes in the circulating blood.

leukoderma (loo-kō-dĕr′-mă) the lack of pigmentation in the skin.

leukopenia (loo″-kō-pē′-nē-ă) a decrease in the number of leukocytes in the circulating blood.

leukoplakia (loo″-kō-plā′-kē-ă) white, thickened patches on the mucous membranes of the tongue, cheek or genitalia.

leukorrhea (loo″-kō-rē′-ă) a whitish discharge from the vaginal canal.

levator ani (lē-vā′-tor ăn′-ĭ) wide muscle that helps form the floor of the pelvis.

levator palpebrae superioris the muscle that lifts the upper eyelid.

lever (lĕv′-ĕr) action of one structure moving against another to lift and enable movement.

leverage action or mechanical power of a lever.

Levin's (lĕ-vĭnz′) **tube** type of surgical drain inserted into the stomach through the nose to drain stomach contents.

levodopa a drug used in the treatment of Parkinson's disease.

LH luteinizing hormone.

licensed proof of qualification to perform a professional function.

lichenification (lī-kĕn″-ĭ-fĭ-kā′-shŭn) thickening of the skin with exaggeration of the normal skin markings, giving the skin a leathery, barklike appearance.

lidocaine (lī′-dō-kān) **hydrochloride** a local, epidural, regional spinal anesthetic drug. Also used as an antiarrythmic.

ligament (lĭg′-ă-mĕnt) connective tissue binding bones to other bones; supports and strengthens the joint.

ligamentopexis (lĭg″-ă-mĕn″-tō-pĕks′-ĭs) a surgical procedure to shorten the round ligaments.

ligamentous (lĭg″-ă-mĕn′-tŭs) pertaining to ligaments.

ligate (lī′-gāt) to tie or suture a blood vessel.

ligation (lī-gā′-shŭn) **and stripping** method of removing varicose veins in the legs by which the veins are cut, tied, and removed.

ligature (lĭg′-ă-chūr) suture material used to tie blood vessels.

linea alba (lĭn′-ē-ă ăl′-bă) white line of connective tissue in the center of the abdomen that runs from the sternum to pubis.

linea aspera a rough ridge located on the posterior surface of the middle third of the femur.

linear (lĭn′-ē-ăr) **accelerator** an electronic device that produces high-energy x-ray beams for the radiation therapy of tumors.

lipoma (lī-pō′-mă) fatty tumor.

lithoid (lĭth′-oyd) stone-like.

lithotomy (lĭth-ŏt′-ō-mē) **position** lying face up with the lower body in a sitting position; knees supported or suspended in stirrups. Used for hemorrhoidectomies and gynecological procedures.

lithotripsy (lĭth′-ō-trĭp″-sē) a procedure for crushing urinary tract stones.

liver (lĭv′-ĕr) large organ predominantly in the RUQ of the abdomen. It secretes bile, stores sugar, iron, and vitamins, produces blood proteins, and destroys worn out red blood cells, among other functions.

liver function tests enzymes found in liver tissue which are detected in small quantities in the blood. These enzymes are as follows: alanine transaminase (ALT), aspartate transaminase (AST), lactic dehydrogenase (LDH), alkaline phosphatase and gamma-glytamyl transpeptidase (GGT).

LMP last menstrual period.

lobar (lō′-băr) **pneumonia** partial or complete consolidation of a lobe of lung.

lobectomy (lō-bĕk′-tō-mē) removal of a lobe of the lung.

local anesthetic drugs that produce anesthesia of a localized area of tissue. The patient remains conscious.

locus (lō′-kŭs) a place or specific site. May refer to a location on a gene.

loop of Henle (Hĕn′-lē) ascending and descending limbs of the nephron.

lordosis (lor-dō′-sĭs) condition of abnormal curvature of the spine.

Lou Gehrig's disease amyotrophic lateral sclerosis (ALS). A progressive disorder characterized by degeneration of motor neurons in the spinal cord and brain stem.

lower gastrointestinal series x-ray of the lower digestive tract, including the small and large intestines, using contrast material.

lower clamp surgical instrument used to control bleeding and to grasp tissue.

LP lumbar puncture.

lubricate to make smooth or slippery.

lumbar (L1–L5) refers to lumbar spine of which there are five vertebrae; L1, L2, L3, L4 and L5.

lumbar plexus a nerve plexus formed by the second to fifth lumbar vertebral nerves.

lumbar puncture (LP) placement of a needle into the subarachnoid space of the spinal column at the level of the fourth intervertebral space.

lumbar region the middle right and left flank regions near the waist.

lumen area within a tube, such as that within a vein, artery, intestine or injection needle.

lumpectomy (lŭm-pĕk′-tō-mē) surgical excision of a breast lump only, leaving the remaining breast tissue in place.

lunate (lū′-nāt) crescent- or moon-shaped bone of the proximal row of the carpus.

lung (lŭng) spongy cone-shaped organ of the respiratory system located within the pleural cavity.

lunula (lū′-nū-lă) half-moon-shaped, white area at the base of the nail.

lupus (lū′-pŭs) **erythematosus** a multi-organ system autoimmune disease which may be characterized by exacerbations and remission. Also called systemic lupus erythematosus (SLE).

luteinizing (loo″-tē-nī′-zĭng) **hormone (LH)** hormone produced by the pituitary gland; promotes ovulation in females and stimulates hormone secretions by the testes in males.

LV left ventricle.

lymph (lĭmf) a clear colorless or milky fluid found in the lymphatic vessels.

lymph duct a tube or passage through which lymph passes.

lymph node a round body of lymphatic tissue located along the course of the lymphatic vessels.

lymphadenitis (lĭm-făd″-ĕn-ī′-tĭs) inflammation of the lymph glands.

lymphadenopathy (lĭm-făd″-ĕ-nŏp′-ă-thē) disease of the lymph nodes.

lymphangitis (lĭm″-făn-jī′-tĭs) inflammation of the lymphatic vessels.

lymphangiogram (lĭm-făn′-jē-ō-grăm) a specialized x-ray procedure in which contrast material is injected into the lymph vessels of the foot, and x-rays are taken to visualize the flow of lymph upwards toward the chest.

lymphangiography (lĭm-făn″-jē-ŏg′-ră-fē) the performance of a lymphangiogram.

lymphatic capillary the smallest lymph vessel.

lymphatic (lĭm-făt′-ĭk) pertaining to the lymph nodes and vessels.

lymphedema (lĭmf-ĕ-dē′-mă) swelling of the lymph vessels, usually a result of lymphatic obstruction.

lymphoblast (lĭm′-fō-blăst) an immature lymphocyte.

lymphocytes (lĭm′-fō-sīt) **(pl. lymphocyte)** a white blood cell which fights disease by the production of antibodies and lymphokines.

lymphokines (lĭm′-fō-kīnz) substances with immune modulating functions which are released by lymphocytes as they contact antigens.

lymphoma (lĭm-fō′-mă) malignant tumor of lymph nodes and lymph tissue.

lymphopenia (lĭm-fō-pē′-nē-ă) deficiency of lymphocytes in the blood.

lysis (lī′-sĭs) **of adhesions** the division of bands of fibrous tissue within the abdominopelvic cavity by surgical or other means.

lysosome (lī′-sō-sōm) a particle within a cell which contains hydrolytic enzymes.

lysozyme (lī′-sō-zīm) an enzyme with bactericidal properties. Now called muramidase.

macrocyte (măk′-rō-sīt) erythrocyte of abnormally large (extending 10 microns) diameter.

macrocytosis (măk″-rō-sī-tō′-sĭs) condition of abnormally large macrocytes.

macrophage (măk′-rō-fāj) large phagocytes that destroy worn-out red blood cells and engulf foreign material in body tissues.

macula densa a group of closely packed cells, close to the juxtaglomerular apparatus of the kidney.

macula lutea (măk′-ū-lă lū′-tē-ă) yellowish region on the retina; contains the fovea centralis.

macular (măk′-ū-lăr) **degeneration** deterioration of the macula lutea of the retina.

macule (măk′-ūl) a discolored (often reddened) flat lesion of the skin.

maculopapular (măk″-ū-lō-păp′-ū-lăr) pertaining to macules and papules, i.e., a rash which is both raised and discolored.

malaise (mă-lāz′) feeling of general bodily discomfort.

malignant (mă-lĭg′-nănt) tending to become worse and resulting in death; tumors having the characteristics of invasiveness, anaplasia, and metastasis.

malignant melanoma (mă-lĭg′-nănt mĕl″-ă-nō′-mă) cancerous growth of the skin composed of melanocytes.

malleable (măl′-ē-ă-b′l) **retractor** a retractor that a surgeon is able to bend into the desired shape. Used in surgery of the abdomen and skull.

malleolar (măl-ē′-ō-lăr) pertaining to the malleolus.

malleolus (măl-ē′-ō-lŭs) **(pl. malleoli)** a rounded process on either side of the ankle joint.

mallet toe fixed flexion of the midphalangeal joint of the toe.

malleus (măl′-ē-ŭs) first ossicle of the middle ear; also called the hammer.

malposition (măl-pō-zĭ′-shŭn) **of uterus** an abnormal position of the uterus.

malrotation (măl″-rō-tā′-shŭn) failure during embryonic development of the intestinal tract to rotate to its proper position.

mammary (măm′-ă-rē) pertaining to the breast.

mammary glands glands that secrete milk in the female.

mammography (măm-ŏg′-ră-fē) the x-ray examination of the breast.

mammoplasty (măm′-ō-plăs″-tē) surgical reconstruction of the breast following mastectomy; surgical reduction or augmentation of the breast.

mandible (măn′-dĭ-bl) a horseshoe-shaped bone which forms the lower jaw.

mandibular (măn-dĭb′-ū-lăr) pertaining to the lower jaw.

mandibular bone the mandible or lower jaw bone. Both the maxilla and the mandible contain the sockets called alveoli in which the teeth are embedded. The mandible joins the skull at the region of the temporal bone, forming the temporomandibular joints (TMJ) on either side of the skull.

manic (măn'-ĭk) a frenzied emotional state characterized by excessive energy, poor impulse control and psychosis.

Mantoux (măn-tū') **skin test** (after Charles Mantoux, physician 1877–1947) the intracutaneous injection of PPD (purified protein derivative); a skin test for the detection of tuberculosis.

manubrium (mă-nū'-brē-ŭm) any handle-shaped structure or bone.

mass number total amount of neutrons and protons in the nucleus of an atom.

mast cell cell found in connective tissue and in the corium layer of the skin which secretes histamine and heparin.

mastectomy (măs-tĕk'-tŏ-mē) surgical excision of the breast.

mastication (măs-tĭ-kā'-shŭn) the process of chewing.

mastitis (măs-tī'-tĭs) inflammation of the breast.

mastoid (măs'-toyd) breast-shaped.

mastoid process a round projection of the temporal bone behind the ear.

mastoiditis (măs-toyd-ī'-tĭs) inflammation of the mastoid antrum and air cells.

mastopexy (măs'-tō-pĕks-ē) surgical fixation of the breasts to correct sagging.

matrix (mā'-trĭks) the basic structure from which a thing is made or develops.

maxilla (măk-sĭ'-lă) irregularly-shaped bone with several processes that forms the skeletal base of the upper face, roof of the mouth, sides of the nasal cavity, and floor of the orbit.

maxillary (măk'-sĭ-lĕr'-ē) **bones** two large bones which compose the upper jaw bones (maxillae). They are joined by a suture in the median plane. If the two bones do not come together normally before birth, the condition known as cleft plate exists.

maxillary sinus air cavity in the maxilla which opens into the meatus of the nose.

maxillotomy (măk″-sĭ-lŏt'-ō-mē) surgical incision of the maxilla.

MBC minimum bactericidal concentration.

McBurney incision surgical cut above the McBurney point used to reach the appendix during appendectomy.

MCH mean corpuscular hemoglobin.

MCHC mean corpuscular hemoglobin concentration.

MCP joint metacarpophalangeal joint.

MCV mean corpuscular volume.

meatotomy (mē″-ă-tŏt'-ō-mē) incision of the urinary meatus.

meatus (mē-ā'-tŭs) an opening to a canal.

medial (mē'-dē-ăl) pertaining to the middle or near the middle plane of the body.

mediastinal (mē″-dē-ăs-tī'-năl) pertaining to the mediastinum.

mediastinum the middle partition of the thoracic cavity.

medical (mĕd'-ĭ-kăl) pertaining to medicine; the study of the art and science of caring for those who are ill.

medulla (mĕ-dŭl'-lă) inner region; the renal medulla is the inner region of the kidney.

medulla oblongata a part of the brain just above the spinal cord; controls breathing, heartbeat, and the tone of blood vessels.

medullary (mĕd'-ū-lār-ē) pertaining to the medulla.

medullary cavity the central, hollowed-out area in the shaft of a long bone.

meibomian gland mucus secreting glands along the margin of the eyelid.

meibomian (mī-bō'-mē-ăn) **cyst** cystic degeneration of a meibomian gland, also called a chalazion.

meiosis (mī-ō'-sĭs) a special method of cell division, occurring in the maturation of sex cells.

Meissner's (mīs'-nĕrz) **corpuscle** (after Georg Meissner, histologist, 1829–1905) a medium-sized encapsulated nerve ending found in the skin, most commonly in the palms and soles.

Meissner's plexus small aggregations of ganglion cells localed in the submucosa of the intestine.

melanemesis (măl-ăn-ē'-mē-sĭs) black vomit caused by blood in the upper gastrointestinal tract.

melanin (mĕl'-ăn-ĭn) black pigment formed by melanocytes in the epidermis.

melanocyte-stimulating (mĕl'-ăn-ō-sīt) **hormone** (MSH) a peptide hormone produced by the anterior lobe of the pituitary gland which increases the pigmentation of the skin.

melanocyte (mĕl'-ăn-ō-sīt) the pigment-forming cell of the skin.

melanoma (mĕl″-ă-nō'-mă) a tumor arising from the melanocytes of the skin.

melatonin a hormone produced by the pineal gland in mammals which inhibits gonadal development.

melena (măl'-ĕ-nă) black, dark brown, tarry stools; feces containing blood.

membrane (mĕm'-brān) thin layer of tissue that lines a cavity, covers a structure or organ, or separates one part from another.

MEN multiple endocrine neoplasia.

menarche (mĕn-ăr'-kē) the beginning of the regular menstrual cycle, usually at approximately the age of 12.

Menetrier's disease giant hypertrophic gastritis, a form of inflammation of the stomach mucosa.

Meniere's (mān″-ē-ārz') **disease** condition of the inner ear causing vertigo, tinnitus and progressive hearing loss.

meninges (mĕn-ĭn'-jēz) three protective membranes that surround the brain and spinal cord.

meningioma (mĕn-ĭn″-jē-ō'-mă) a slow-growing tumor arising from the arachnoidal tissue of the meninges.

meningitis (mĕn-ĭn-jī'-tĭs) inflammation of the meninges.

meningocele (mĕn-ĭn'-gō-sēl) herniation of the meninges through an opening in the skull or spinal column.

meningomyelocele (mĕn-in″-gō-mī-ĕl'-ō-sēl) myelomeningocele. Protrusion of the meninges and spinal cord through a defect in the spinal column.

meniscectomy (mĕn″-ĭ-sĕk'-tō-mē) excision of an intra-articular meniscus, as in the knee joint.

meniscus (mĕn-ĭs'-kŭs) (pl. menisci) crescent-shaped structure; frequently refers to the knee cartilage shaped like a crescent.

menometrorrhagia (mĕn″-ō-mĕt-rō-rā'-jē-ă) irregular and excessive menstrual bleeding.

menopause (mĕn'-ō-pawz) the permanent cessation of menstruation.

menorrhagia (mĕn″-ō-rā'-jē-ă) excessive or profuse menstrual bleeding.

menstruation (mĕn-stroo-ā'-shŭn) monthly shedding of the uterine lining.

mental foramen (mĕn'-tăl fō-rā'-mĕn) opening on the lateral part of the body of the mandible, opposite the second biscupid tooth, for passage of the mental nerve and vessels.

meperidine (mĕ-pĕr'-ĭ-dēn) a narcotic analgesic drug.

mesentery (mĕn'-ĕn-tĕr"-ē) the membranous folds of peritoneum attaching the small intestine to the posterior body wall, also called the mesenterium.

mesocolon (mĕs"-ō-kō'-lŏn) the fold of peritoneum attaching the colon to the posterior abdominal wall.

mesovarium (mĕs"-ō-vā'-rē-ŭm) a portion of the broad ligament of the uterus holding the ovary in place.

metabolic (mĕt"-ă-bŏl'-ĭk) pertaining to metabolism.

metabolism (mĕ-tăb'-ō-lĭzm) sum of all physical and chemical changes that take place within an organism.

metacarpal (mĕt"-ă-kăr'-păl) pertaining to the bones of the hand between the wrist and fingers.

metacarpectomy (mĕt"-ă-kăr-pĕk'-tō-mē) surgical excision or resection of a metacarpal.

metacarpophalangeal (mĕt"-ă-kăr"-pō-fă-lăn'-jē-ăl) **joint (MCP joint)** the joint between the head of the metacarpal bone and the proximal phalanx.

metaplasia (mĕt"-ă-plā'-zē-ă) changing of one kind of tissue into a form that is not normal for that tissue.

metastasis (mĕ-tăs'-tă-sĭs) the spread of a malignant tumor to a secondary site.

metatarsal (mĕt"-ă-tăr'-săl) pertaining to one of the bones of the arch of the foot.

metroptosis (mē-trō-tō'-sĭs) the downward displacement of the uterus.

metrorrhagia (mĕt"-rō-rā'-jē-ă) irregular uterine bleeding especially at a time other than the menstrual period.

Metzenbaum dissecting scissors a type of surgical scissors.

MI myocardial infarction.

MIC minimum inhibitory concentration.

microaneurysm (mī"-krō-ăn'-ū-rĭzm) small aneurysm, such as that occurring in the retinal blood vessels of diabetics.

microbiology (mī"-krō-bī-ŏl'-ō-jē) the study of microorganisms.

microcytosis (mī"-krō-sī-to'-sĭs) the presence of many abnormally small red blood cells in the blood.

microencephaly (mī"-krō-ĕn-sĕf'-ă-lē) micrencephaly. Possessing a small brain.

microfilament (mī"-krō-fĭl'-ă-mĕnt) one of the submicroscopic elements of a cell.

microglial (mī-krŏg'-lē-ăl) **cell** a type of neuroglial cell.

microorganism (mī-krō-or'-găn-ĭzm) small living organism not able to be seen with the human eye.

microscopic (mī-krō-skŏp'-ĭk) pertaining to the microscope.

microtomy (mī-krŏt'-ō-mē) the cutting of thin sections of tissue for examination under a microscope. In the process, water is removed and replaced with wax to produce a solid tissue sample that can be sliced. The slices may be less than one cell thick and are placed on a slide and stained for microscopic examination. The entire process takes approximately 48 hours. A faster method, in which the tissue sample is frozen, is used when quick answers are needed during a surgical procedure already in progress.

microtubule (mī"-krō-tū'-būl) hollow tubular structure present in the cell.

microvilli (mī"-krō-vĭl'-ī) microscopic projections from the free surface of cell membranes.

micturition (mĭk-tū-rĭ'-shŭn) urination; the act of voiding.

micturition reflex relaxation of the urinary sphincter and contraction of the walls of the bladder in response to a full bladder.

midbrain portion of the brain consisting of the crura cerebri, the aqueduct of Sylvius and the corpora quadrigemina, connecting the hemispheres of the cerebrum with the pons and the cerebellum.

middle ear portion of the ear consisting of the malleus, incus, stapes and oval window.

midline (mĭd'-līn) **incision** also referred to as an epigastric incision. A surgical cut in the midline above the umbilicus, adjacent to the stomach. Used to reach the stomach, duodenum and pancreas.

mimic (mĭm'-ĭk) to duplicate the mannerisms of something or someone else.

mineral supplement an aid in maintenance of health in cases where diets are deficient or in cases where absorption of nutrients is inhibited by disease.

mineralocorticoid (mĭn"-ĕr-ăl-ō-kor'-tĭ-koyd) steroid hormone produced by the adrenal cortex to regulate the mineral salts (electrolytes) and water balance in the body.

minimally invasive surgery an alternative to the traditional open cavity surgery, in which a procedure such as a hysterectomy, tubal ligation, cholecystectomy, or nephrectomy can be performed by insertion of a laparoscope through a single incision.

miosis (mī-ō'-sĭs) contraction of the pupil.

miotic drug that causes the pupil to contract.

miscarriage discharge of the fetus before it is viable outside the uterus. Approximately 50 percent of miscarriages are caused by chromosomal abnormalities.

mitochondrion (mīt"-ō-kŏn'-drē-ă) a structure in the cell cytoplasm where the release of energy takes place.

mitosis (mī-tō'-sĭs) replication of cells; a stage in the cell life cycle involving the production of two identical cells from a parent cell.

mitral (mī'-trăl) **valve** the valve found between the left atrium and the left ventricle of the heart.

mitral valve prolapse (MVP) an improper bowing of the mitral valve into the left atrium during contraction of the left ventricle. May or may not be associated with mitral valve regurgitation.

mitral valve regurgitation the backflow of blood from the left ventricle into the left atrium during systole caused by failure of the mitral valve to close fully.

mitral valve stenosis obstruction or narrowing of the mitral valve. Results in decreased blood flow from the atrium to the ventricle.

mittelschmerz (mĭt'-ĕl-shmărts) abdominal pain at time of ovulation.

mobility being able to move.

Mohs surgery surgical technique for removal of skin cancer in which thin layers of a growth are removed, and each is examined successively under a microscope.

molar back, grinding tooth; three are present on each side of each jaw.

Molybdenum hard, heavy metallic element.

Molybdenum-99 a radioactive tracer.

monocyte (mŏn'-ō-sīt) a type of leukocyte which engulfs debris after neutrophils have attacked foreign cells.

monofilament suture a suture material consisting of a single strand.

monoplegia (mŏn-ō-plē'-jē-ă) paralysis of a single limb.

mons pubis (mŏns pū'-bĭs) the elevated fleshy prominence overlying the symphysis pubis.

morphine (mor'-fēn) a narcotic analgesic.

morphology (mor-fŏl′-ō-jē) the science of structure or form without regard to function.

mosquito another name for a small hemostat.

motor pertaining to movement.

motile (mō′-tĭl) able to move.

MRH melanocyte-releasing hormone.

MRI magnetic resonance imaging.

MS multiple sclerosis.

MSAFP maternal serum alpha-feto protein.

MSH melanocyte-stimulating hormone.

MSS musculoskeletal system.

MUA manipulation under anesthesia.

MVP mitral valve prolapse.

mucosa (mū-kō′-să) mucous membrane.

mucous (mū′-kŭs) **membrane** a thin layer of tissue serving as a covering, lining, partition or connection.

multifilament suture a suture material consisting of several strands braided together.

multiform (mŭl′-tĭ-form) having many forms or shapes.

multigravida (mŭl″-tĭ-grăv′-ĭ-dă) a woman who has been pregnant two or more times, written gravida II, gravida IV, gradiva V etc., G II, G III, G IV.

multipara (mŭl-tĭp′-ă-ră) a woman who has given birth two or more times. Written para II, III, IV, etc.

multiple myeloma a malignant tumor of bone marrow. Also called plasma cell myeloma.

multiple sclerosis (MS) a neurologic disease characterized by the destruction of the myelin sheath on neurons in the central nervous system and its replacement by plaques of sclerotic (hard) tissue. Symptoms may include paralysis, weakness, numbness and tremor.

multiple personality disorder dissociative psychiatric disorder affecting the patient's identity. The patient may assume multiple different personalities of various ages, races and social backgrounds.

murmur a blowing sound indicative of turbulent blood flow.

muscle (mŭs′-ĕl) **relaxant** a drug which interferes with the transmission of nerve impulses at the myoneuonal junction.

muscular pertaining to muscle.

muscular dystrophy group of inherited diseases characterized by progressive weakness and degeneration of muscle fibers without involvement of the nervous system.

multiple endocrine neoplasia (MEN) a group of genetically based disorders causing tumors in several endocrine tissues simultaneously.

myalgia (mī-ăl′-jē-ă) muscle pain.

myasthenia (mī-ăs-thē′-nē-ă) abnormal fatigue associated with muscle weakness.

myasthenia gravis a neuromuscular disorder characterized by relapsing weakness of skeletal muscles.

mycobacterium (mī″-kō-băk-tē′-rĭ-ŭm) a slender, nonmotile, acid-fast organism which is the cause of tuberculosis and leprosy.

Mycobacterium avium a cause of opportunistic infection.

Mycobacterium tuberculosis bacterium which is the cause of tuberculosis.

mydriasis (mĭd-rī′-ă-sĭs) abnormal dilation of the pupil.

mydriatic (mĭd-rē-ăt′-ĭk) **cyclopegic** an agent used to dilate the pupil of the eye and block the response of the ciliary muscles during eye examinations.

mydriatic (mĭd-rē-ăt′-ĭk) any drug that dilates the pupil.

myelin (mī′-ĕ-lĭn) **sheath** the lipid-protein complex which surrounds the axon of some nerve fibers.

myelination (mī″-ĕl-ĭn-ā′-shŭn) the formation of a myelin sheath.

myelitis (mī-ĕ-lī′-tĭs) inflammation of the bone marrow or spinal cord.

myelocele (mī′-ĕ-lō-sēl) the protrusion of the spinal cord in spina bifida.

myelogenous (mī-ĕ-lŏj′-ĕn-ŭs) originating in the bone marrow.

myelogram (mī′-ĕ-lō-grăm) an x-ray taken after dye is injected into the membranes around the spinal cord.

myelography (mī-ĕ-lŏg′-ră-fē) the performance of a myelogram.

myeloid (mī′-ĕ-loyd) dervied from bone marrow cells.

myeloma (mī-ĕ-lō′-mă) a tumor of bone marrow.

myocardial (mī-ō-kăr′-dē-ăl) **infarction (MI)** necrosis of cardiac muscle tissue caused by ischemia of the heart muscle.

myocardiorrhaphy suture of the muscular layer of the heart.

myocarditis (mī″-ō-kăr-dī′-tĭs) inflammation of the myocardium.

myocardium (mī-ō-kăr′-dē-ŭm) the muscle layer of the heart.

myoclonus (mī-ŏk′-lō-nŭs) the twitching of a muscle or group of muscles.

myofibrosis (mī″-ō-fī-brō′-sĭs) degeneration of a muscle with formation of increased connective or fibrous tissue.

myoma (mī-ō′-mă) a tumor which contains muscle tissue.

myometrium (mī″-ō-mē′-trē-ŭm) the muscular wall of the uterus.

myopathy (mī-ŏp′-ă-thē) any muscular disease.

myopia (mī-ō′-pē-ă) nearsightedness.

myosarcoma (mī″-ō-sar-kō′-mă) malignant tumor derived from muscular tissue.

myosin (mī′-ō-sĭn) a protein present in muscle fibrils.

myositis (mī-ō-sī′-tĭs) inflammation of a muscle.

myotonia (mī″-ō-tō′-nē-ă) failure of a muscle to relax following muscle contraction.

myringotomy (mĭr-ĭn-gŏt′-ō-mē) incision of the tympanic membrane.

mysophobia (mī″-sō-fō′-bē-ă) unreasonable fear of germs or dirt.

myxedema (mĭks-ĕ-dē′-mă) advanced hypothyroidism in adulthood.

N&V nausea and vomiting.

Na sodium.

nail bed portion of the finger or toe covered by the nail.

nail matrix portion of the nail bed on which the root of the nail rests.

narcotic analgesic drug used to alleviate moderate to severe pain. Narcotic analgesics are habit-forming. They are sometimes prescribed as analgesics in combination with aspirin or acetaminophen.

naris (nā′-rĭs) **(pl. nares)** nostril.

nasal (nā′-zl) pertaining to the nose.

nasal bone two slender bones supporting the bridge of the nose. They join with the frontal bone superiorly to form part of the nasal septum.

nasal cavity the area between the floor of the cranium and the roof of the mouth.

nasal septum wall dividing the two nasal cavities.

nasal speculum an instrument used to hold back tissue within the nasal cavity.

nasogastric intubation procedure of inserting a nasogastric tube through the nose and into the stomach.

nasogastric (nā″-zō-găs′-trĭk) **tube** tube placed through the nose into the stomach.

nasolacrimal (nā″-zo-lăk′-rĭm-ăl) **duct** duct which drains tears from the lacrimal sac into the nasal cavity.

nasopharynx (nā″-zō-făr′-ĭnks) the part of the pharynx situated above the soft palate.

nausea (naw′-sē-ă) the feeling of discomfort associated with the urge to vomit.

navicular (nă-vĭk′-ū-lăr) "boat-shaped"; one of the bones of the wrist.

necrosis (nĕ-krō′-sĭs) irreversible damage to tissue causing cell death.

necrotic that which pertains to or contains dead tissue.

needle biopsy the recovery of tissue for pathologic examination through a needle.

needle driver forceps a surgical instrument used to grasp or hold tissue.

Neisseria (nī-sē′-rē-ă) **meningitidis** the species of bacteria causing a type of cerebrospinal meningitis.

neonatal (nē″-ō-nā′-tăl) pertaining to the first four weeks after birth.

neoplasm (nē′-ō-plăzm) new growth; an abnormal tissue that grows by rapid cell division, often used as a synonym for tumor.

neostigmine (nē-ō-stĭg′-mĭn) a cholinergic drug.

nephrectasis (nĕf-rĕk′-tă-sĭs) distention of the kidney.

nephrectomy (nĕ-frĕk′-tō-mē) the removal of a kidney.

nephritis (nĕf-rī′-tĭs) inflammation of a kidney.

nephroblastoma (nĕf″-rō-blăs-tō′-mă) Wilm's tumor. A malignant neoplasm of the kidney containing embryonic tissue which occurs in children.

nephrolithiasis (nĕf″-rō-lĭth-ī′-ă-sĭs) stones in the kidney.

nephrolithotomy (nĕf″-rō-lĭth-ŏt′-ō-mē) an invasive procedure for the removal of renal calculi through an incision into the kidney.

nephron (nĕf′-rŏn) the structural and functional unit of the kidney.

nephropathy (nĕ-frŏp′-ă-thē) any disease of the kidney.

nephropexy (nĕf′-rō-pĕks-ē) surgical fixation of the kidney.

nephroptosis (nĕf″-rŏp-tō′-sĭs) a downward displacement of the kidney.

nephrostomy (nĕ-frŏs′-tō-mē) development of an artificial fistula into the renal pelvis.

nerve a macroscopic ropelike structure consisting of axons and dendrites in bundles.

neural (nū′-răl) pertaining to nerves or connected with the nervous system.

neurilemma (nū′-rĭ-lĕm″-mă) a cell which covers the axon of a peripheral nerve.

neuroanastomosis (nū″-rō-ă-năs″-tō-mō′-sĭs) surgical procedure that attaches from one end of a severed nerve to the other end.

neurofibril (nū-rō-fī′-brĭl) numerous tiny filaments extending in many directions within the cytoplasm of the body of a nerve cell.

neurofibroma (nū″-rō-fī-brō′-mă) a benign tumor of the neurilemma.

neuroglia (nū-rŏg′-lē-ă) cells in the nervous system that do not carry impulses but are supportive and connective in function.

neurohypophysis (nū″-rō-hī-pŏf′-ĭs-ĭs) the posterior pituitary gland.

neurolysis (nū-rŏl′-ĭs-ĭs) the destruction of nerve tissue or freeing of adhesions from around a nerve.

neuron (nū′-rŏn) nerve cell.

neuropathy (nū-rŏp′-ă-thē) any disease of the nerves.

neurosis (nū-rō′-sĭs) **(pl. neuroses)** a psychological disorder manifested by anxiety.

neurosurgery (nū″-rō-sŭr′-jĕ-rē) surgery of the nervous system.

neutron (nū′-trŏn) subatomic particle without an electrical charge.

neutrophil (nū′-trō-fĭl) a type of granulocyte (white blood cell).

nevus (nē′-vŭs) **(pl. nevi)** mole. A colored lesion of the skin.

NFP natural family planning.

NG nasogastric.

niacin (nī′-ă-sĭn) nicotinic acid.

nicotinic acid (nĭk″-ō-tĭn′-ĭk) niacin. Part of the vitamin B complex.

nipple (nĭp′-l) the conical protrusion of the breast from which the lactiferous ducts discharge.

nitroglycerin a vasodilator drug used to treat angina pectoris.

nitrous oxide an anesthetic drug sometimes referred to as "laughing gas".

NMR nuclear magnetic resonance.

nocturia (nŏk-tū′-rē-ă) urination at night.

node (nōd) a small circumscribed mass of tissue.

nodes of Ranvier constrictions of the myelin sheath of a myelinated nerve fiber.

nodule (nŏd′-ūl) a small aggregation of cells; a small node.

nodular (nŏd′-ū-lăr) having the characteristics of a nodule.

non-toothed forceps a surgical instrument used to handle delicate tissue.

nonabsorbable surgical clip surgical clip used for hemostasis or tissue approximation which is removed at a later time (if superficial) or which is left permanently in place (if deep). They are made of steel, titanium or tantalum and thus appear on radiopaque x-rays.

nonabsorbable suture any suture material that cannot be absorbed by the body over a period of time. The material resists being broken down by the action of living tissue. They may be made of either natural or synthetic material. Natural nonabsorbable sutures include silk, cotton, linen, and stainless steel wires. Synthetic nonabsorbable sutures include nylon, polyester, and polypropylene.

nonviral hepatitis exposure to toxic chemicals.

norepinephrine (nor-ĕp″-ĭ-nĕf′-rĭn) a catecholamine hormone produced by the adrenal medulla; also called noradrenalin. Norepinephrine causes increases in heart rate and blood pressure.

normochromia (nor″-mō-krō′-mē-ă) the state of normal color of red blood cells seen when the hemoglobin content of blood is normal.

NSAIDs nonsteroidal anti-inflammatory drugs.

nucleolus (nū-klē′-ō-lŭs) spherical body made up of granules and dense fibers within the cell nucleus.

nucleus (nū′-klē-ŭs) the central portion of a cell, substance or structure.

nucleus pulposus the gelatinous central portion of the intervertebral disk.

nuclide (nū′-klīd) a species of an element characterized by the quantum state of its atom's nucleus.

nulligravida (nŭl-lĭ-grăv'-ĭd-ă) woman who has never been pregnant.

nullipara (nŭl-ĭp'-ă-ră) woman who has never given birth.

nutrient (nū'-trē-ĕnt) any substance or food that provides the body with the necessary elements for metabolism.

nystagmus (nĭs-tăg'-mŭs) oscillatory movement of the eyeball.

OA osteoarthritis.

obesity (ō-bē'-sĭ-tē) the state of having an abnormal amount of body fat.

oblique (ō-blēk') diagonal.

obstetrical forceps an instrument used for delivering babies.

obstetrics (ŏb-stĕt'-rĭks) the branch of medicine dealing with the management of women during pregnancy and childbirth.

obturator (ŏb'-tū-rā"-tor) **foramen** a large opening in the anterior part of the hip bone between the pubis and ischium.

occipital (ŏk-sĭp'-ĭ-tăl) **bone** a bone located at the back of the skull above the neck.

occipital lobe a portion of the cerebral hemisphere located posteriorly that is shaped like a three-sided pyramid.

occlude (ŏ-klūd') to close up, obstruct, or join together.

occupational therapy therapeutic use of self-care, work and play activities to increase independent function and enhance development while preventing disability.

OCG oral cholecystogram.

odontalgia (ō-dŏn-tăl'-jē-ă) a toothache.

odontorrhagia (ō-dŏn"-tō-rā'-jē-ă) hemorrhaging from the tooth.

olecranon (ō-lĕk'-răn-ŏn) a large process of the humerus forming the tip of the elbow.

olfactory (ŏl-făk'-tō-rē) pertaining to the sense of smell.

oligodendrocyte (ŏl"-ĭ-gō-dĕn'-drō-sīt) type of neuroglial cell having few and delicate processes.

oligomenorrhea (ŏl"-ĭ-gō-mĕn"-ō-rē'-ă) scanty uterine bleeding at the time of menstruation.

oligopnea (ŏl-ĭ-gŏp'-nē-ă) infrequent respiration.

oligospermia (ŏl"-ĭ-gō-spĕr'-mē-ă) deficient amounts of spermatozoa in the semen.

oliguria (ŏl-ĭg-ū'-rē-ă) diminished urine output.

onychomalacia (ŏn"-ĭ-kō-mă-lā'-sē-ă) an abnormal softening of the nails.

onychomycosis (ŏn"-ĭ-kō-mī-kō'-sĭs) a fungal infection of the nails.

oocyte (ō'-ō-sīt) an immature egg cell which develops into an ovum.

oogenesis (ō"-ō-jĕn'-ĕ-sĭs) the development of the ovum.

oophoralgia (ō"-ŏf-ō-răl'-jē-ă) pain in the ovary.

oophorectomy (ō"-ŏf-ō-rĕk'-tō-mē) surgical excision of an ovary.

opaque (ō-pāk') not transparent.

open not closed.

operating room the area of the hospital in which surgery is performed. The term includes the operating theater, ancillary rooms for storage and supply, and the recovery room.

operating room suite the surgical area of the hospital. The term includes the operating theater, ancillary rooms for storage and supply, and the recovery room.

operating room theater room within the operating room suite where the surgery is actually carried out; also known as operating room (OR) or theater.

ophthalmia (ŏf-thăl'-mē-ă) **neonatorum** severe purulent conjunctivitis in a newborn.

ophthalmologist (ŏf-thăl-mŏl'-ō-jĭst) physician that specializes in the treatment of disorders of the eye.

ophthalmoplegia (ŏf-thăl"-mō-plē'-jē-ă) paralysis of the ocular muscles.

ophthalmorrhagia (ŏf-thăl"-mō-rā'-jē-ă) hemorrhage from the eye.

ophthalmorrhea (ŏf-thăl"-mō-rē'-ă) a purulent discharge from the eye.

ophthalmoscope (ŏf-thăl'-mō-skōp) an instrument for examining the retina and the interior of the eye.

ophthalmoscopy (ŏf-thăl-mŏs'-kō-pē) the process of visually examining the interior of the eye.

opium (ō'-pē-ŭm) a narcotic analgesic.

optic (ŏp'-tĭk) **chiasm** point at which fibers of the optic nerves cross in the brain.

optic disc region at the back of the eye where the optic nerve meets the retina; the blind spot of the eye.

optic nerve cranial nerve that carries impulses from the retina to the brain.

optic tract the continuation of the optic nerve behind the optic chiasm.

optician (ŏp-tĭsh'-ăn) one who specializes in the making of optical lenses or eyeglasses.

optometrist (ŏp-tŏm'-ĕ-trĭst) a professional who treats diseases of the eye and prescribes eyeglasses.

OR operating room.

oral (or'-ăl) pertaining to the mouth.

oral cavity (mouth) body cavity formed by the cheeks, lips and dental arches.

orbit (or'-bĭt) the bony cavity of the skull that protects and contains the eyeball.

orbital (or'-bĭ-tăl) pertaining to the orbits.

orchiectomy (or"-kē-ĕk'-tō-mē) surgical excision of a testicle; castration.

orchiopexy the surgical fixation of the testicle to the scrotum used as treatment for an undescended testicle.

orchitis (or-kī'-tĭs) inflammation of the testicle.

organ (or'-găn) any part of the body having a specific function.

organelle (or"-găn-ĕl') a part of a cell that performs a specific function.

organism (or'-găn-ĭzm) any living plant or animal.

organomegaly (or"-gă-nō-mĕg'-ă-lē) the enlargement of a visceral organ.

origin (or'-ĭ-jĭn) a starting point; a fixed or unmovable point of attachment of a muscle.

oropharyngeal (or"-ō-făr-ĭn-jē'-ăl) **airway** tube which is inserted into the mouth of an unconscious person to prevent the tongue from obstructing the airway.

oropharynx (or"-ō-făr'-ĭnks) that portion of the pharynx located below the nasopharynx and behind the oral cavity.

ortho straight, normal, or correct.

orthodontia a branch of dentistry dealing with the correction of misaligned teeth.

orthodontist (or"-thō-dŏn'-tĭst) dentist who specializes in orthodontia.

orthopedic (or"-thō-pē'-dĭk) pertaining to the correction or prevention of musculoskeletal abnormalities.

orthopedic surgery a branch of surgery involved with the correction of musculoskeletal abnormalities.

orthopnea (or″-thŏp′-nĕ-ă) difficulty breathing except in the upright position.

orthoptic (or-thŏp-tĭk) training eye muscle exercises for the purpose of correcting strabismus and restoring normal coordination of the eyes.

os a bone

os coxa (ŏs kŏx′-ă) (os coxae) hip bone.

ossicle (ŏs′-ĭ-kl) a small bone, such as those found in the ear.

osseous (ŏs′-ē-ŭs) tissue bone tissue.

ossification (ŏs″-ĭ-fĭ-kā′-shŭn) the process of bone formation.

osteitis (ŏs-tē-ī′-tĭs) inflammation of a bone.

osteoarthritis (ŏs″-tē-ō-ăr-thrī′-tĭs) (OA) a progressive, degenerative joint disease characterized by the loss of articular cartilage and hypertrophy of the bone at the articular surfaces.

osteoblast (ŏs′-tē-ō-blăst) a bone-forming cell.

osteoclast (ŏs′-tē-ō-klăst) a bone cell that absorbs and removes unwanted bone tissue.

osteocyte (ŏs′-tē-ō-sīt′) a bone cell.

osteogenesis (ŏs″-tē-ō-jĕn′-ĕ-sĭs) the regeneration of bone.

osteogenic sarcoma a malignant tumor of bone.

osteoma (ŏs-tē-ō′-mă) benign tumor of bone-forming tissue.

osteomalacia (ŏs″-tē-ō-măl-ā′-shē-ă) a condition characterized by softening of the bones.

osteomyelitis (ŏs″-tē-ō-mī″-ĕl-ī′-tĭs) a bacterial infection of bone.

osteoporosis (ŏs″-tē-ō-por-ō′-sĭs) a decrease in bone density; thinning and weakening of bone.

osteosarcoma (ŏs″-tē-ō-săr-kō′-mă) osteogenic sarcoma, a malignant sarcoma of bone.

osteotome (ŏs′-tē-ō-tōm) a surgical instrument used to cut, incise, or separate bone.

TO oxytocin.

otalgia (ō-tăl′-jē-ă) pain in the ear, earache.

otitis (ō-tī′-tĭs) inflammation of the ear.

otitis media inflammation of the middle ear.

otoconium (ō″-tō-kō′-nē-ŭm) a small particle, containing calcium carbonate, found in the inner ear.

otolaryngology (ō″-tō-lar″-ĭn-gŏl′-ō-jē) the medical specialty involved with the study and treatment of diseases of the ears, nose, and throat.

otolith (ō′-tō-lĭth) otoconium.

otomycosis (ō″-tō-mī-kō′-sĭs) fungal infection of the external auditory canal of the ear.

otoplasty (ō′-tō-plăs″-tē) plastic surgery to correct defects and deformities of the ear.

otorrhea (ō″-tō-rē′-ă) a discharge from the ear.

otosclerosis (ō″-tō-sklē-rō′-sĭs) the hardening of the tissue of the labyrinth of the ear.

otoscope (ō′-tō-skŏp) a device used to examine the ear.

otoscopy (ō-tŏs′-kō-pē) the visual examination of the ear with an otoscope.

oval (ō′-văl) window membrane between the middle and the inner ear.

ovarian (ō-vā′-rē-ăn) pertaining to or resembling an ovary.

ovarian cyst a closed sac or cavity on the surface of ovary containing fluid, semi-solid or solid material. These cysts can be described as follicular cysts involving the graafian follicle or lutein cysts involving the corpus luteum.

ovariocentesis (ō-vā″-rē-ō-sĕn-tē′-sĭs) surgical procedure in which an ovarian cyst is punctured and drained.

ovariorrhexis (ō-vā″-rē-ō-rĕk′-sĭs) rupture of an ovary.

ovary (ō′-vă-rē) one of two female gonads which produce ova and hormones.

over and over sutures technique of surgical suturing in which edges of a wound are approximated by piercing the skin an equal distance on either side of the wound. The needle is placed into the skin on one side and pulled out on the other. Can be continuous or interrupted.

over-the-counter (OTC) drug drug that can legally be dispensed without a prescription.

oviduct (ō′-vĭ-dŭkt) a uterine or fallopian tube.

ovulation (ŏv″-ū-lā′-shŭn) cyclic ripening and rupture of the mature graafian follicle followed by the discharge of the ovum.

ovum (ō′-vŭm) (pl. ova) the female reproductive cell; egg.

oxygen (ŏk′-sĭ-jĕn) a gas that is essential to animal and plant life.

oxygen monitor instrument which monitors oxygen concentration in the blood.

oxygenation (ŏk″-sĭ-jĕn-ā′-shŭn) the addition of oxygen to the blood or tissues.

oxyntic (ŏk-sĭn′-tĭk) that which manufactures or secretes acid.

oxytocia (ŏk″-sē-tō′-sē-ă) rapid birth.

oxytocin (ŏk″-sē-tō′-sĭn) (TO) a peptide hormone secreted by the posterior lobe of the pituitary gland which stimulates contraction of the uterus during labor and childbirth.

P waves first deflection on the electrocardiogram, representing atrial depolarization.

P para.

P-R interval the interval between P and R waves on the electrocardiogram, a measurement of the period of time that impulses from the SA node take to reach the Purkinje fibers in the AV node.

PA posteroanterior.

pacemaker (pās′-māk-ĕr) the rhythmic tissue in the sinoatrial (SA) node of the right atrium that initiates the heartbeat.

palatine (păl′-ă-tīn) pertaining to the palate.

palatine tonsils the rounded masses of lymph tissue in the oropharynx.

palatopharyngeal (păl′-ă-tō-fă-rĭn′-jē-ăl) pertaining to the palate and pharynx.

palatoplasty (păl′-ăt-ō-plăs″-tē) surgical repair of the palate.

pallor (păl′-or) lack of color.

palmar (păl′-măr) pertaining to the palm of the hand.

palpation (păl-pā′-shŭn) the applying of hands to the external surface of the body to detect deformities or abnormities.

palpebra (păl′-pĕ-bră) eyelid.

palpebral (păl′-pĕ-brăl) pertaining to the eyelid.

palpitation (păl-pĭ-tā′-shŭn) forcible, rapid or unusual heart beat of which the patient is consciously aware.

pancarditis (păn-kăr-dī′-tĭs) inflammation of all the heart layers. Included are the epicardium, myocardium, and endocardium.

pancreas (păn′-krē-ăs) an organ located under the stomach which produces insulin (for transport of sugar into cells) and enzymes (for the digestion of foods).

pancreatectomy (păn″-krē-ăt-ĕk′-tō-mē) the surgical removal of all or part of the pancreas.

pancreatic (păn″-krē-ăt′-ĭk) duct one or more ducts which carry pancreatic juice to the duodenum.

pancreatic juice the exocrine secretion of the pancreas.

pancreatogenic (păn″-krē-ă-tō-jĕn′-ĭk) produced by or formed in the pancreas.

pancytopenia (păn″-sī-tō-pē′-nē-ă) decrease in all cellular elements of the blood.

panhypopituitarism (păn-hī″-pō-pĭ-tū′-ĭ-tăr-ĭzm) a condition in which all pituitary hormones are deficient.

panhysterectomy (păn″-hĭs-tĕr-ĕk′-tō-mē) complete removal of the uterus.

panophobia (păn-ō-fō′-bē-ă) state of generalized anxiety marked by fear of everything.

pansinusitis (păn″-sī-nŭs-ī′-tĭs) inflammation of all of the paranasal sinuses.

Pap (păp) **smear** (**Papanicolaou smear**) the microscopic study of cells scraped from the uterine cervix for the early detection of cancer cells.

papilla (pă-pĭl′-ă) (**pl. papillae**) any small nipple-like projection.

papillary (păp′-ĭ-lăr-ē) forming small, finger-like or nipple-like projections of cells.

papillary muscle one of several muscular eminences in ventricles of the heart which attach to the chordae tendineae.

papilledema (păp″-ĭl-ĕ-dē′-mă) edema of the optic disk, generally caused by elevated intracranial pressure.

papilloma (păp′-ĭ-lō′-mă) any benign epithelial tumor.

papule (păp′-ūl) a small (less than 1 cm. in diameter), solid elevation of the skin.

papulopustular (păp″-ū-lō-pŭs′-tū-lăr) characterized by the presence of both pustules and papules.

papulosquamous (păp″-ū-lō-skwā′-mŭs) characterized by the presence of both pustules and scales.

para (**P**) a woman who has given birth; the state of parity.

parainfluenza virus a virus that may cause acute respiratory infections, especially in children.

paralysis (pă-răl′-ĭ-sĭs) the loss of voluntary movement of a muscle caused by an abnormal disruption of the connection between nerve and muscle.

paralytic (păr″-ă-lĭt′-ĭk) **ileus** nonmechanical obstruction of the bowel caused by paralysis of the intestines.

paramedian (păr″-ă-mē′-dē-ăn) **incision** surgical cut beside the midline used to reach pelvic structures and the colon.

parametrium (păr-ă-mē′-trē-ŭm) structures which are adjacent to or beside the uterus.

paranasal structures beside the nasal cavity.

paraphilia (păr″-ă-fĭl′-ĭ-ă) psychosexual mental disorder characterized by intense, unnatural sexual urges.

paraplegia (păr-ă-plē′-jē-ă) paralysis of lower portion of the body and of both legs.

parathyroid (păr-ă-thī′-royd) **gland** one of four endocrine glands embedded within the connective tissue of the thyroid gland which secretes parathyroid hormone (PTH).

parathyroid hormone or **parathormone** (**PTH**) a peptide hormone produced by the parathyroid gland, regulates calcium metabolism.

parathyroidectomy (păr″-ă-thī-royd-ĕk′-tō-mē) the surgical excision of the parathyroid gland.

parenchyma (păr-ĕn′-kĭ-mă) the essential or distinguishing cells of an organ.

paresthesia (păr″-ĕs-thē′-zē-ă) an abnormal sensation of burning or tingling.

parietal (pă-rī′-ĕ-tăl) forming or pertaining to the wall of a cavity.

parietal bone one of two flat bones of irregular shape that forms the roof and upper part of the cranium.

parietal lobe division of the brain lying beneath each parietal bone.

Parker retractors a type of surgical retractor used for minor surgery.

Parkinson's disease the degeneration of nerves in the basal ganglia brain, leading to tremors, weakness of muscles, and slowness of movement.

paronychia (păr-ō-nĭk′-ē-ă) inflammation and swelling of the soft tissue around the nail.

parotid (pă-rŏt′-ĭd) describing any structure located near the ear.

parotid duct a duct which transports secretions from the parotid gland to the oral cavity.

parotid gland the largest of the salivary glands, located in front of each ear.

paroxysmal (păr″-ŏk-sĭz′-măl) the sudden onset of symptoms of a disease.

PARR postanesthetic recovery room.

Louis Pasteur 19th century French scientist who demonstrated that germs cause disease.

partial thromboplastin time (**PTT**) a laboratory test for measuring the integrity of the coagulation pathways.

patch (păch) area differing from the rest of the surface in either color or texture.

patch test a test for allergies, performed by applying to the skin a small piece of gauze or filter paper on which has been placed a suspected allergen.

patella (pă-tĕl′-ă) the kneecap, a small flat bone that lies in front of the articulation between the femur and the lower leg.

patella ligament a broad ligament which is the continuation of the quadriceps muscle of the thigh. It runs from the patella to attach to the tuberosity of the tibia.

patellapexy (pă-tĕl′-ă-pĕk″-sē) the surgical fixation of the patella to the lower end of the femur.

patellar (pă-tĕl′-ăr) pertaining to the kneecap.

patellectomy (păt′-ĕ-lĕk′-tō-mē) the surgical excision or removal of the patella.

pathogenic (păth″-ō-jĕn′-ĭk) pertaining to the production of disease.

pathologist (pă-thŏl′-ō-jĭst) a physician who examines biopsy samples, performs post-mortem examinations, and practices laboratory medicine.

pathology (pă-thŏl′-ō-jē) the study of the nature and cause of disease.

patient (pā′-shĕnt) individual under treatment.

patient's bracelet an identification band worn by the patient while hospitalized.

PCV packed cell volume.

pectoral (pĕk′-tō-răl) pertaining to the chest.

pectoralis major the large triangular muscle that extends from the anterior chest wall to the humerus.

pediatrician (pē-dē-ă-trĭsh′-ăn) specialist in the treatment of children's diseases.

pedicel (pĕd′-ĭ-sĕl) a footlike part.

pedicle (pĕd′-ĭ-k'l) a stalklike attachment.

pediculosis (pē-dĭk″-ū-lō′-sĭs) infestation with lice.

pedophilia (pē″-dō-fĭl′-ē-ă) a psychosexual disorder of sexual attraction to children.

peduncle (pĕ-dŭn′-kl) a stemlike connecting part. Pedicle.

PEEP positive end-expiratory pressure.

pelvic (pĕl′-vĭk) pertaining to the pelvis.

pelvic cavity space below the abdomen containing the urinary bladder and reproductive organs.

pelvic girdle the hip bones and the sacrum which support the trunk and to which the lower extremities are attached.

pelvic inflammatory disease (PID) bacterial infection of the uterus, cervix uteri, fallopian tubes, ovaries or parametrium. Causative microorganisms include streptococci, staphylococci, gonococci and Chlamydia. Responds well to antibiotic therapy, but if left untreated may cause sterility.

pelvimeter (pĕl-vĭm′-ĕ-tĕr) an apparatus used to measure the pelvis.

pelvis (pĕl′-vĭs) (pl. pelves) the ring of bone at the lower portion of the trunk formed by the hip bones, sacrum and coccyx.

pemphigus a blistering skin disorder.

penetrating (pĕn′-ĕ-trāt-ĭng) entering, piercing deeply.

penicillin (pĕn-ĭ-sĭl′-ĭn) an antibiotic drug.

penis (pē′-nĭs) the male organ of copulation through which the urethra passes.

Penrose drain surgical drain used to drain fluid or blood.

pepsinogen (pĕp-sĭn′-ō-jĕn) a proenzyme secreted by the chief cells of the gastric mucosa from which pepsin, a digestive enzyme, is made.

peptide two or more amino acids linked together in sequence.

percussion (pĕr-kŭsh′-ŭn) a procedure for determining the density of an underlying structure by tapping over its surface.

percutaneous (pĕr′-kū-tā′-nē-ŭs) **transhepatic cholangiography (PTC)** fluoroscopic examination of the biliary system following injection of contrast medium through a catheter placed through the skin into the liver's duct system.

perforation (pĕr″-fō-rā′-shŭn) an abnormal opening into a hollow organ.

perfusion (pĕr-fū′zhŭn) passing of fluids through blood vessels.

perianal (pĕr″-ē-ā′-năl) pertaining to the area around the anus.

periarthritis (pĕr″-ē-ăr-thrī′-tĭs) inflammation of the structures around a joint.

peribronchial (pĕr″-ĭ-brŏng′-kē-ăl) surrounding or enclosing a bronchus.

pericardial (pĕr″-ĭ-kăr′-dē-ăl) pertaining to the pericardium.

pericardial cavity the membranous sac surrounding the heart.

pericardial fluid the fluid within the pericardial cavity.

pericardial tamponade compression of the heart as a result of accumulation of excessive fluid within the pericardial cavity.

pericarditis (pĕr-ĭ-kăr-dī′-tĭs) inflammation of the pericardium.

perilymph (pĕr′-ĭ-lĭmf) the fluid contained in the labyrinth of the inner ear.

perimetrium (pĕr-ĭ-mē′-trē-ŭm) the outermost layer of the uterus.

perimysium (pĕr″-ĭ-mĭs′-ē-ŭm) a fibrous sheath enclosing a primary bundle of skeletal muscle fibers.

perineorrhaphy (pĕr″-ĭ-nē-or′-ă-fē) suturing of the perineum.

perineum (pĕr″-ĭ-nē′-ŭm) the area between the anus and the scrotum in the male and the anus and vulva in the female.

perineuritis (pĕr″-ĭ-nū-rī′-tĭs) inflammation of the connective tissue surrounding a peripheral nerve.

periodic (pēr-ē-ŏd′-ĭk) **table** identifies the over 100 known elements and assigns each one a position based upon the number of protons found in its nucleus.

periodontal (pĕr″-ē-ō-dŏn′-tăl) around a tooth.

periodontitis (pĕr″-ē-ō-dŏn-tī′-tĭs) inflammation of the periodontium, which surrounds a tooth.

perioperative the period before and after surgery.

periosteum (pĕr-ē-ŏs′-tē-ŭm) the membrane surrounding a bone.

peripheral (pĕr-ĭf′-ĕr-ăl) located away from the center.

peripheral nervous system (PNS) nerves located outside of the brain and spinal cord.

peripheral vascular disease impairment of circulation in the extremities, caused by obstruction of the arterial lumen.

peripheral vision that part of the field of vision found at either side when the eye is motionless.

periphery (pĕr-ĭf′-ĕ-rē) the part located away from center.

perirenal (pĕr″-ĭ-rē′-năl) **fat** the fatty tissue surrounding the kidney.

peristalsis (pĕr-ĭ-stăl′-sĭs) the rhythmic contractions of tubular structures, such as the intestinal tract.

peristaltic (pĕr″-ĭ-stăl′-tĭk) pertaining to peristalsis.

peritonitis (pĕr″-ĭ-tō-nī′-tĭs) inflammation of the peritoneum.

peritoneal (pĕr″-ĭ-tō-nĕ′-ăl) concerning the peritoneum.

peritoneal cavity thin potential space between the parietal and the visceral peritoneum, normally empty except for a small amount of serous fluid that keeps the surfaces moist.

peritoneoscopy (pĕr″-ĭ-tō″-nē-ŏs′-kō-pē) laparoscopy. A procedure to inspect the abdominal cavity. A laparoscope is inserted into the peritoneal cavity through a small incision in the abdominal wall.

peritoneum (pĕr″-ĭ-tō-nē′-ŭm) the membrane that lines the abdominal cavity.

peritonitis (pĕr″-ĭ-tō-nī′-tĭs) inflammation of the peritoneum.

periumbilical (pĕr″-ē-ŭm-bĭl′-ĭ-kăl) around the navel.

periungual (pĕr″-ē-ŭng′-gwăl) around the nail.

permanent teeth teeth that develop at the second dentition.

pernicious (pĕr-nĭsh′-ŭs) **anemia** a form of anemia resulting from inability to absorb vitamin B12 from the intestinal tract; characterized by abnormally large blood corpuscles (macrocytes).

peroneus (pĕr″-ō-nē′-ŭs) one of the several muscles in the leg that act to move the foot.

PET scan positron emission tomography scan.

petechia (pē-tē′-kē-ă) (pl. petechiae) small, pinpoint hemorrhages visible in the skin.

Pfannenstiel curved abdominal surgical incision just above the symphysis pubis. Used in gynecological surgery to reach the uterus, fallopian tubes and ovaries.

phacoemulsification (făk″-ō-ē-mŭl′-sĭ-fĭ-kā″-shŭn) method of breaking up and removing a cataract of the eye.

phacomalacia (făk″-ō-mă-lā′-shē-ă) softening of the lens of the eye.

phagocyte (făg′-ō-sīt) a cell which possesses the ability to engulf and ingest bacteria or other foreign material.

phagocytosis (făg″-ō-sī-tō′-sĭs) the ingestion and digestion of particles and bacteria by phagocytes.

phalangeal (fă-lăn′-jē-ăl) pertaining to a phalanx.

phalanx (făl′-ănks) (pl. phalanges) any of the bones of the fingers or toes.

pharmacist (făr′-mă-sĭst) one who dispenses drugs.

pharmacologist (făr″-mă-kŏl′-ō-jĭst) a professional involved in the research and development of new drugs.

pharmacology (făr″-mă-kŏl′-ō-jē) the study of drugs.

pharyngeal (făr-ĭn′-jē-ăl) pertaining to the pharynx.

pharyngeal tonsil a collection of lymphoid tissue at the posterior wall of the naso pharynx.

pharyngitis (făr″-ĭn-jī′-tĭs) inflammation of the pharynx.

pharynx (făr′-ĭnks) throat. Passageway for food to travel from the mouth to the esophagus and air to pass from the nose to the trachea.

phenobarbital (fē″-nō-băr′-bĭ-tăl) sedative hypnotic drug.

phenylpropanolamine (fĕn″-ĭl-prō″-pă-nŏl′-ă-mĕn) a sympathomimetic drug.

phenytoin (fĕn′-ĭ-tō-ĭn) an anticonvulsant drug.

phimosis (fĭ-mō′-sĭs) a tightened foreskin which cannot be pulled back.

phlebitis (flĕ-bī′-tĭs) inflammation of a vein.

phlebothrombosis (flĕb″-ō-thrŏm-bō′-sĭs) an abnormal condition of clots in a vein.

phobia (fō′-bē-ă) irrational fear of an object or situation.

phosphatase (fŏs′-fă-tās) group of enzymes that catalyze the hydrolysis of phosphoric acid esters.

phospholipid (fŏs″-fō-lĭp′-ĭd) lipoid substance containing phosphorus.

phosphorus (fŏs′-for-ŭs) a mineral substance found in bones, muscles and nerves.

photodermatitis (fō″-tō-dĕr-mă-tī′-tĭs) inflammation of the skin caused by exposure to ultraviolet light.

photoelectricity (fō″-tō-ē-lĕk trī′-sĭ-tē) electricity produced by the action of light.

photoreceptor (fō″-tō-rē-sĕp′-tor) a sensory nerve ending which is stimulated by light.

phrenic (frĕn′-ĭk) pertaining to the diaphragm.

phrenic nerve nerve arising in the cervical plexus which is the main motor nerve for the diaphragm.

phrenoplegia (frĕn-ō-plē′-jē-ă) paralysis of the diaphragm.

phrenotomy incision into the diaphragm.

physical therapy the use of natural forces (massage, hydrotherapy, exercise, etc.) in the treatment of disease.

physician (fĭ-zĭsh′-ŭn) a practitioner of medicine, licensed in the care of the sick.

physiology (fĭz″-ē-ŏl′-ō-jē) study of the chemical and physical processes of living organisms.

physiotherapy (fĭz″-ē-ō-thĕr′-ă-pē) physical therapy.

pia mater (pē′-ă mā′-tĕr) thin, delicate, inner membrane of the meninges.

pickups generic term for any forceps used to hold or grasp tissue.

PID pelvic inflammatory disease.

piezoelectricity (pī-ē″-zō-ē-lĕk-trī′-sĭ-tē) production of electricity by applying pressure to crystals such as mica or quartz.

pigmentation (pĭg″-mĕn-tā′-shŭn) coloration because of the deposition of pigments.

pigmented (pĭg′-mĕnt-ĕd) colored by pigment.

PIH prolactin-inhibiting hormone.

piles (pīls) persistent dilation of the veins in the anal region caused by increased venous pressure; also known as hemorrhoids.

pilonidal (pī″-lō-nī′-dăl) relating to dermoid cyst containing hairs in a nest formation.

pilonidal cyst congenital pit containing hair found over the midline sacral area of the back.

pilosebaceous (pī″-lō-sē-bā′-shŭs) pertaining to the hair and sebaceous glands.

pineal (pĭn′-ē-ăl) gland a structure located in the central portion of the brain which secretes melatonin.

pinealectomy (pĭn″-ē-ăl-ĕk′-tō-mē) removal of the pineal gland.

pink eye conjunctivitis. Inflammation of the conjunctivae membrane.

pinna (pĭn′-ă) auricle or flap of the ear.

pisiform (pī′-sĭ-form) pea-shaped.

pituitary (pĭ-tū′-ĭ-tār″-ē) relating to or concerning the pituitary gland.

pituitary gland an endocrine gland at the base of the brain.

pityriasis (pĭt″-ĭ-rī′-ă-sĭs) a skin disease characterized by fine scales.

pityriasis rosea an acute self-limited eruption of scaly macules on the trunk and extermities.

placenta (plă-sĕn′-tă) a vascular organ attached to the uterine wall that develops during pregnancy and serves as a communication between the maternal and the fetal bloodstreams.

placenta previa a displaced placenta implanted in the lower region of the uterine wall.

plain chest radiograph x-ray of the chest in the AP position.

plantar (plăn′-tăr) concerning the sole of the foot.

plantar flexion motion that extends the foot downward toward the ground as when pointing the toes.

plantar wart a wart found on the sole of the foot.

plaque (plăk) patch found on the skin or a mucous membrane.

plasma (plăz′-mă) liquid portion of blood; contains water, proteins, salts, nutrients, hormones, and vitamins.

plasma cell cell that secretes antibodies and originates from B cell lymphocytes.

platelet (plāt′-lĕt) smallest formed element in the blood, a thrombocyte.

platelet count number of platelets per cubic millimeter of blood. Platelets normally average between 200,000 to 500,000 per mm^3.

pleomorphic (plē-ō-mor′-fĭk) composed of a variety of types of cells.

pleura (ploo′-ră) (pl. pleurae) double-layered membrane surrounding each lung.

pleural cavity the potential space between the pleurae.

pleural effusion the escape of fluid into the pleural cavity.

pleurisy (ploo-rĭs′-ē) inflammation of the pleura.

pleuritis (ploo-rī′-tĭs) pleurisy. Inflammation of the pleura.

pleurocentesis (ploo″-rō-sĕn-tē′-sĭs) thoracentesis. Puncture of the pleural cavity.

plexus (plĕks′-ŭs) (pl. plexuses) large, interlacing network of nerves or blood vessels.

plicae (plī′-kē) circulares one of the many transverse folds of the small intestine.

PMN polymorphonuclear leukocyte.

PMP past menstrual period.

pneumoconiosis (nū″-mō-kō″-nē-ō′-sĭs) black lung. Abnormal condition caused by the inhalation of mineral dust into the lungs, with resultant chronic inflammation and bronchitis.

Pneumocystis (nū″-mō-sĭs′-tĭs) carinii organism that causes pneumonia in immunocompromised individuals.

pneumonectomy (nū″-mŏn-ĕk′-tō-mē) the surgical removal of a lung.

pneumonia (nū-mō′-nē-ă) inflammation of the lung, specifically when secondary to an acute infectious process.

pneumonitis (nū″-mō-nī′-tĭs) inflammation of the lung.

pneumothorax (nū-mō-thō′-răks) the presence of air or gas in the pleural cavity.

PNS peripheral nervous system.

podocyte (pŏd′-ō-sīt) an epithelial cell within the glomerulus of the kidney.

poikilocytosis (poy″-kĭl-ō-sī-tō′-sĭs) irregularity in the shape of red blood cells. Occurs in certain types of anemia.

poliomyelitis (pōl′-ē-ō-mī″-ĕl-ī′-tĭs) viral disease causing inflammation of the gray matter of the spinal cord, leading to paralysis of the muscles that rely on the damaged neurons.

polychromasia (pŏl″-ē-krō-mā′-zē-ă) polychromatophilia. A

property of staining of certain red blood cells with several different types of dye.

polycystic (pŏl″-ē-sĭs′-tĭk) **ovary syndrome** a condition associated with multiple ovarian cysts and primary anovulation.

polycythemia (pŏl″-ē-sī-thē′-mē-ă) excess of blood cells.

polycythemia rubra vera increase in red blood cells.

polymorphonuclear (pŏl″-ē-mor″-fō-nū′-klē-ăr) having nuclei of various forms; refers to a type of leukocyte.

polymorphonuclear (pŏl″-ē-mor″-fō-nū′-klē-ăr) **leukocyte** neutrophil. An important disease fighting white blood cell which is phagocytic and possesses a multilobed nucleus. Almost 60 percent of leukocytes are neutrophils.

polymyositis (pŏl″-ē-mī″-ō-sī′-tĭs) a chronic inflammatory myopathy of uncertain etiology.

polyneuritis (pŏl″-ē-nū-rī′-tĭs) the simultaneous inflammation of two or more nerves.

polyp (pŏl′-ĭp) mushroom-like growth extending on a stalk from the surface of a mucous membrane.

polypoid (pŏl′-ē-polyd) resembling a polyp.

polythelia (pŏl″-ē-thē′-lē-ă) the condition of having more than two nipples.

polyuria (pŏl″-ē-ū′-rē-ă) the excretion of large amounts of urine.

pons (pŏnz) the bridge-like part of the brainstem between the medulla and the midbrain.

popliteal (pŏp″-lĭt-ē′-al) pertaining to the posterior region of the knee.

pore (por) a minute opening.

positron (pŏz′-ĭ-trŏn) an atomic particle having a positive charge.

posterior (pŏs-tē′-rē-or) behind or after.

posterior chamber area behind the iris containing aqueous humor.

posteroanterior (pŏs″-tĕr-ō-ăn-tĕr′-ē-or) back-to-front direction an x-ray beam takes through a body (posterior to anterior).

posterolateral (pŏs″-tĕr-ō-lă′-tĕr-ăl) located behind and to the side.

postmenopausal (pōst″-mĕn-ō-paw′-zăl) after the cessation of menopause.

postnatal (pōst-nā′-tăl) occurring after birth.

postoperative after surgery.

post partum (pōst-păr′-tŭm) with reference to the mother, the period after delivery.

postprandial (pōst-prăn′-dē-ăl) following a meal.

postural (pŏs′-tū-răl) pertaining to or affected by posture.

posture (pŏs′-tŭr) the attitude or position of the body.

potassium (pō-tăs′-ē-ŭm) an electrolyte found throughout the body.

PTT partial thromboplastin time.

practitioner (prăk-tĭsh′-ŭn-ĕr) one who is licensed to provide health care service, i.e., physician, nurse, dentist, physical therapist, etc.

pre-eclampsia (prē″-ē-klămp′-sē-ă) hypertension with proteinuria and/or edema during pregnancy.

pregnancy (prĕg′-năn-sē) the gravid state of a female from the time of conception to birth.

premenstrual (prē-mĕn′-stroo-ăl) **syndrome** (PMS) physical and emotional distress occurring in a cyclical pattern related to the menstrual cycle. May include symptoms such as edema, fatigue, irritability and depression.

premolar (prē-mō′-lĕr) a bicuspid tooth.

prenatal (prē-nā′-tl) with reference to the fetus, pertaining to the time before birth.

pre-op (prē-ŏp) preoperative.

preoperative (prē-ŏp′-ĕr-ă-tĭv) before surgery.

prep (prĕp) prepared.

prepuce (prē′-pūs) foreskin.

presbycusis (prĕz-bĭ-kū′-sĭs) the loss of hearing with age.

presbyopia (prĕz-bē-ō′-pē-ă) farsightedness. Loss of the ability of the eye to accomodate with age.

prescription written orders from the physician to the pharmacist on the dispensing of medication.

prescription (prē-skrĭp′-shŭn) **drug** drug that must be dispensed and taken with medical supervision only. Cannot be legally dispensed without orders from a physician.

presenile (prē-sē′-nĭl) displaying characteristics of premature old age.

PRH prolactin-releasing hormone.

primary suture line sutures that hold the edges of an incision in approximation.

primigravida (prī-mĭ-grăv′-ĭ-dă) woman who is pregnant for the first time.

primipara (prī-mĭp′-ă-ră) woman who has given birth for the first time.

probe (prōb) a surgical instrument used to explore cavities, wounds, ducts or fistulae.

procainamide an antiarrhythmic drug.

procaine (prō′-kān) **hydrochloride** a local anesthetic drug.

proctoclysis (prŏk-tŏk′-lĭ-sĭs) irrigation of the rectum.

progesterone (prō-jĕs′-tĕr-ōn) the hormone produced by the corpus luteum of the ovary and by the placenta.

prognosis (prŏg-nō′-sĭs) prediction about the outcome of an illness.

progressive (prō-grĕs′-ĭv) advancing.

projection (prō″-jĕk′-shŭn) physical act of pushing out or throwing forward.

prolactin (prō-lăk′-tĭn) (PRL) a peptide hormone produced by the anterior lobe of the pituitary gland which promotes milk secretion.

pronation (prō-nā′-shŭn) rotation of the forearm so as to turn the palm backward.

prone (prōn) the condition of lying on the stomach.

prone position lying face down. Used for back surgery and heel surgery.

prophylactic (prō-fĭ-lăk′-tĭk) that which prevents disease.

propranolol an antianginal and antihypertensive medication.

prostate (prŏs′-tāt) **gland** a structure lying at the base of the male bladder surrounding the urethra which secretes fluid to support the viability of sperm.

prostatectomy (prŏs″-tă-tĕk′-tō-mē) surgical excision of all or part of the prostate gland.

prostatitis (prŏs″-tă-tī′-tĭs) inflammation of the prostate.

prosthesis (prŏs-thē′-sis) an artificial device to temporarily or permanently replace a missing or defective body part.

prosthetics (prŏs-thĕt′-ĭks) the science of manufacturing and adjusting artificial body parts.

proteinuria (prō″-tē-ĭn-ū′-rē-ă) the excretion of increased amounts of protein in the urine.

proton (prō′-tŏn) positively charged atomic particle.

protoplasm (prō′-tō-plăzm) the substance of which cells are formed.

protraction (prō-trăk′-shŭn) an extension forward, particularly in reference to tooth position.

protrusion (prō-troo'-zhŭn) the state of being thrust forward.

proximal (prŏk'-sĭm-ăl) nearest the trunk or near the point of origin of a structure.

pruritus (proo-rī'-tĭs) itching.

pruritus ani (proo-rī'-tĭs ā'-nī) itching of the anus.

pruritus vulvae (proo-rī'-tĭs vŭl'-vē) severe itching of the vagina.

pseudocyesis (soo"-dō-sī-ē'-sĭs) false pregnancy.

psoas (sō'-ăs) a large retroperitoneal muscle which flexes the thigh.

psoriasis (sō-rī'-ă-sĭs) a chronic, recurrent dermatosis marked by itchy, scaly, red patches covered by silvery gray scales.

psychosis (sī-kō'-sĭs) (pl. psychoses) a severe mental disorder in which the patient withdraws from reality into an inner world of disorganized thinking.

PTC percutaneous transhepatic cholangiography.

PTCA percutaneous transluminal coronary angioplasty.

PTH parathormone or parathyroid hormone.

ptosis (tō'-sĭs) the sagging of an organ or body part.

ptyalism (tī'-ă-lĭzm) the excessive secretion of saliva.

puberty (pū'-bĕr-tē) the beginning of the fertile period when gametes are first produced and secondary sex characteristics appear.

pubes the hair on and around the external genitalia.

pubic (pū'-bĭk) pertaining to the pubes.

pubic symphysis the area of fusion of the two pubic bones. They are joined together by a piece of fibrocartilage.

pubis (pū'-bĭs) the pubic bone.

pubofemoral (pū"-bō-fĕm'-or-ăl) ligament the ligament between the pubis and femur.

pulmonary (pŭl'-mō-nĕ-rē) pertaining to the lung.

pulmonary angiography radiographic procedure in which dye is injected into a blood vessel, and x-rays are taken of the arteries in the lung.

pulmonary artery artery carrying oxygen-poor blood from the right ventricle of the heart to the lungs.

pulmonary function tests (PFT) group of tests measuring ventilation including the quantity of air moved into and out of the lungs under normal conditions.

pulmonary tuberculosis (TB) Mycobacterium tuberculosis infection of the lungs.

pulp (pŭlp) the soft tissue within a tooth containing nerves and blood vessels.

punch biopsy a procedure utilizing a sharp circular instrument to remove a piece of tissue for microscopic examination.

pupil (pū'-pĭl) dark opening of the eye, surrounded by the iris, through which light rays pass.

purpura (pŭr'-pū-ră) hemorrhage into the skin.

purse-string suture a type of continuous suture around a circular wound which acts as a drawstring.

purulent (pūr'-ū-lĕnt) containing or pertaining to pus.

pustule (pŭs'-tūl) small elevation of the skin containing pus.

putamen (pū-tā'-mĕn) darker outer layer of the lenticular nucleus of the brain.

PUVA Psoralen-ultraviolet A.

PVD peripheral vascular disease.

pyelogram (pī'-ĕ-lō-grăm) see intravenous pyelogram (IVP).

pyelography (pī"-ĕ-lŏg'-ră-fē) the process of taking x-ray images of the kidney, urethra, bladder and ureters with the use of radiopaque contrast (dye).

pyelolithotomy (pī"-ĕ-lō-lĭth-ŏt'-ō-mē) removal of calculus from the pelvis of a kidney through an incision.

pyelonephritis (pī"-ĕ-lō-nĕ-frī'-tĭs) inflammation of the renal parenchyma and pelvis due to a bacterial infection.

pylorectomy (pī"-lō-rĕk'-tō-mē) surgical removal of the pylorus.

pyloric (pī-lor-ĭk) pertaining to the opening between the stomach and the duodenum.

pyloric stenosis narrowing of the opening of the stomach between the stomach and the duodenum.

pyloromyotomy (pī-lor"-ō-mī-ŏt'-tō-mē) incision of the pyloric sphincter.

pyloroplasty (pī-lor'-ō-plăs"-tē) surgical procedure to repair the pylorus.

pylorospasm (pī-lor'-ō-spăzm) sudden, involuntary contraction of the pylorus.

pylorostenosis (pī-lor"-ō-stĕn-ō'-sĭs) pyloric stenosis.

pylorus (pī-lor'-ŭs) lower muscular tissue surrounding lower opening of the stomach into the duodenum.

pyogenic (pī-ō-jĕn'-ĭk) that which produces pus.

pyosalpinx (pī"-ō-săl'-pĭnks) the accumulation of pus in the fallopian tube.

pyothorax (pī"-ō-thō'-răks) a collection of pus (empyema) in the chest.

pyuria (pī-ū'-rē-ă) the presence of pus in the urine.

QRS complex the group of waves on the electrocardiogram representing ventricular depolarization.

quadriceps a four-headed muscle.

quadriplegia (kwŏd"-rĭ-plē'-jē-ă) paralysis of all four extremities.

quinidine (kwĭn'-ĭ-dēn) an antiarrhythmic drug.

RA right atrium.

rachischisis (ră-kĭs'-kĭ-sĭs) congenital condition in which one or more of the vertebral arches fail to develop or fail to fuse dorsally. Occurs most commonly in the lumbar region and is a cause of spina bifida.

rachitis (ră-kī'-tĭs) rickets. A condition of a deficiency of calcium and vitamin D, causing the bones to become soft, bend easily, and become deformed.

radial (rā'-dē-ăl) pertaining to the radius.

radiation (rā-dē-ā'-shŭn) the emission of radiant energy carried by a stream of particles.

radiation therapy the treatment of cancer with high energy radiation, usually x-rays.

radical (răd'-ĭ-kăl) hysterectomy the surgical removal of the entire uterus, including the cervix and upper vagina in one procedure.

radical mastectomy the surgical removal of the breast, lymph nodes, and adjacent chest wall muscles in a single procedure.

radioactive (rā"-dē-ō-ăk'-tĭv) substance a material possessing radioactivity.

radioactivity (rā"-dē-ō-ăk"-tĭv'-ĭ-tē) the property of certain materials of spontaneously emitting rays of subatomic particles.

radiocurable (rā"-dē-ō-kūr'-ă-bl) tumor tumor that can be completely eradicated by radiation therapy. These are usually localized tumors with no evidence of metastasis.

radiography (rā-dē-ŏg'-ră-fē) the process of recording x-rays.

radioimmunoassay (rā"-dē-ō-ĭm"-ū-nō-ăs'-ā) (RIA) measurement of an antigen-antibody interaction using a radiopharmaceutical.

radioisotope (rā"-dē-ō-ī'-sō-tōp) form of a radioactive element having an atomic weight different from that of the element itself; radionuclide.

radiologist (rā-dē-ŏl′-ō-jĭst) physician who specializes in the practice of diagnostic radiology.

radiology (rā-dē-ŏl′-ō-jē) use of electromagnetic radiation in the diagnosis and treatment of disease.

radiolucent (rā″-dē-ō-lū′-sĕnt) refers to structures through which x-rays can pass. Such structures appear black on an x-ray film.

radionuclide (rā″-dē-ō-nū′-klīd) element that emits radioactivity.

radionuclide (rā″-dē-ō-nū′-klīd) **scan** a diagnostic procedure in which a radiopharmaceutical is injected intravenously allowing visualization of an organ in question with a special camera.

radiopaque (rā-dē-ō-pāk′) refers to structures through which x-rays cannot pass. Such structures appear white on an x-ray film.

radiopharmaceutical (rā″-dē-ō-fărm″-ă-sū′-tĭ-kăl) a chemical carrying a radioactive substance used in nuclear medical diagnostic studies.

radioresistant tumor a tumor that requires large doses of radiation to produce the death of cells. These high doses of radiation may have a damaging effect on surrounding normal tissues.

radiosensitive tumor a tumor in which irradiation easily causes the death of cells, avoiding serious damage to surrounding normal tissue.

radiotherapy (rā″-dē-ō-thĕr′-ă-pē) the use of x-rays and radiation from radioactive substances to treat cancer.

radius (rā′-dē-ŭs) lateral lower arm bone (in line with the thumb).

RAI radioactive iodine.

rake retractor a type of surgical retractor used for both minor and major surgery.

rales (rălz) (**crackles**) abnormal crackling sounds heard during inspiration produced in the alveoli.

raspatory (rasp) an instrument used to scrape bone.

Raynaud's (rā-nōz′) **disease** a disease of the peripheral vascular system characterized by spasmodic contraction of the arterioles of the fingers and toes cutting off circulation to these areas.

RBBB right bundle branch block.

RBC red blood cells.

RDS respiratory distress syndrome.

receptor (rē-sĕp′-tor) a sensory nerve ending that receives a nervous stimulus.

recessive (rē-sĕs′-ĭv) that which recedes or falls back; not dominant.

recovery (rĭ-kŭv′-ĕr-ē) **room** an area where patients are monitored closely immediately after surgery and anesthesia.

rectal (rĕk′-tăl) pertaining to the rectum.

rectocele (rĕk′-tō-sēl) a herniation of the rectum toward the vagina.

rectum (rĕk′-tŭm) the terminal portion of the colon.

rectus (rĕk′-tŭs) straight, not bent.

recumbent general term meaning lying down in any of a number of positions.

recurrent (rĭ-kŭr′-ĕnt) symptoms or disease which returns after an interval of remission.

red blood cell count (RBC) a laboratory which measures the number of erythrocytes per cubic millimeter of blood. The normal number is 4.5–6 million per cu mm^3.

red blood cell morphology the form or shape of stained red blood cells under the microscope. The presence of anisocytosis, poikilocytosis, sickle cells, and hypochromia is noted.

red bone marrow found in cancellous bone; the site of hemopoiesis.

red blood cells (RBC) erythrocytes.

reduction (rĭ-dŭk′-shŭn) **division** the reduction in chromosomes which occurs during gamete function.

reduction mammoplasty the surgical reduction of the size and diameter of the breast.

reflex (rē′-flĕks) any involuntary response to stimulus.

reflux (rē′-flŭks) backwards flow.

refract (rĭ-frăkt′) to bend a light ray.

refraction (rĭ-frăk′-shŭn) the bending of light rays by the cornea, lens, and fluids of the eye to bring light rays into focus on the retina.

regional (rē′-jŭn-ăl) **nerve block** a local anesthetic injected into a nerve plexus. Such anesthesia covers a greater area than a localized injection.

renal (rē′-năl) pertaining to the kidney.

renal angiography an x-ray of the renal blood vessels following injection of a contrast medium into the renal vasculature.

renal artery vessel which carries blood to the kidney.

renal biopsy excision of a piece of tissue from the kidney for microscopic examination.

renal calculi kidney stones; may be composed of uric acid or of calcium salts.

renal hypoplasia an underdeveloped kidney.

renal pelvis the central collecting region in the kidney which is continuous with the ureter.

renal tubules microscopic tubes in the kidney where urine is formed and water, sugar, and salts are reabsorbed into the bloodstream.

renal vein the vessel which carries blood away from the kidney.

renin (rĕn′-ĭn) a substance, made in the kidney, that increases blood pressure by causing the formation of angiotensin II.

reproduction (rē-prō-dŭk′-shŭn) act of duplicating; procreation.

resection (rē-sĕk′-shŭn) excision of all or part of an organ or structure.

resectoscope (rē-sĕk′-tō-skōp) a surgical instrument used to visualize and remove tissue, especially the prostate.

resonance (rĕz′-ō-nănce) a vibrating sound produced by the percussion of a hollow structure.

respiration (rĕs-pĭr-ā′-shŭn) mechanical process of breathing; the repetitive unconscious exchange of air between the lungs and the external environment.

respiratory (rĕs-pĭr′-ă-tō-rē) **failure** condition in which the respiratory system is unable to function, causing hypoxia and a buildup of carbon dioxide in the body.

respiratory insufficiency the failure to adequately provide oxygen to and remove carbon dioxide from the cells of the body.

retention sutures secondary line of sutures, typically one to two inches to either side of the primary line. It eases the tension on the primary suture line thus resisting the splitting open of the operative incision site.

reticulocyte (rĕ-tĭk′-ū-lō-sīt) a developing red blood cell with a network of granules in its cytoplasm.

reticulocyte count laboratory measurement of maturing red blood cells.

reticuloendothelial relating to macrophages and phagocytes or structures containing these, such as the spleen, liver, lymph nodes and bone marrow.

retina (rĕt'-ĭ-nă) sensitive nerve cell layer of the eye that contains receptor cells called rods and cones.

retinal (rĕt'-ĭ-năl) **tear** a tear in the retina of the eye.

retinal detachment a condition in which the retina separates from the choroid.

retinopathy (rĕt"-ĭn-ŏp'-ă-thē) any disorder of the retina.

retinopexy (rĕt"-ĭn-ŏ-pĕk'-sē) a surgical procedure to repair the retina.

retinoschisis (rĕt"-ĭ-nŏs'-kĭ-sĭs) splitting of the retina into two layers with cyst formation between the layers.

retraction (rĭ-trăk'-shŭn) act of drawing back or shrinking.

retractor a surgical instrument to hold back tissue from the operative site to provide a clear surgical field.

retroflexed (rĕt'-rō-flĕkst") bent backward.

retrograde (rĕt'-rō-grād) **pyelogram** a procedure in which contrast material is introduced directly into the bladder and ureters through a cystoscope, allowing x-rays to be taken to determine the presence of an obstruction.

retrograde urography x-ray of the urinary system by injection of contrast material into the ureters.

retroperitoneal (rĕt"-rō-pĕr"-ĭ-tō-nē'-ăl) located behind the peritoneum.

Reye's (Rīz) **syndrome** a multisystem disorder characterized by vomiting, increased intracranial pressure, and dysfunction of the liver.

RF rheumatoid factor.

Rh factor antigen normally found on red blood cells of certain individuals said to be Rh-positive.

Rh Rh factor.

rhabdomyolysis (răb"-dō-mī-ŏl'-ĭ-sĭs) the destruction of striated muscle tissue.

rhabdomyoma (răb"-dō-mī-ō'-mă) a benign tumor of striated muscle.

rhabdomyosarcoma (răb"-dō-săr-kō'-mă) malignant tumor of striated muscle.

rheumatoid arthritis chronic disease in which joints become inflamed and painful, caused by an immune reaction against joint tissues.

rheumatoid factor an immunoglobulin found in the serum of patients with rheumatoid arthritis.

rhinitis (rī-nī'-tĭs) inflammation of the nasal mucosa.

rhinoplasty (rī'-nō-plăs"-tē) the surgical reconstruction of the nose.

rhinorrhea (rī"-nō-rē'-ă) a discharge from the nose.

rhizolysis (rī-zŏl-ĭ-sĭs) a radiofrequency neurotomy.

rhizotomy (rī-zŏt'-ō-mē) the division of a spinal nerve root for the relief of pain or spasticity.

rhodopsin (rō-dŏp'-sĭn) visual purple; a protein found in the retinal rods.

rhomboideus (rŏm-bō-ĭd'-ē-ŭs) **major** a muscle of the upper back attching to the scapula.

rhonchus (rŏng'-kus) (**pl. rhonchi**) abnormal, musical sounds heard during inspiration produced in the bronchi.

RIA radioimmunoassay.

rib (rĭb) one of 24 curved bones forming the bony wall of the chest. There are 12 pairs of ribs, the first seven join the sternum anteriorly through cartilaginous attachments called costal cartilages. These are called true ribs. Ribs eight to ten are called false ribs as they join with the vertebral column in the back but join the seventh rib anteriorly instead of attaching to the sternum. Ribs 11 and 12 are floating ribs because they are completely free at their anterior border.

ribonucleic (rī"-bō-nū"-klē-ĭk) **acid** (RNA) a cellular substance (located within and outside the nucleus) that, along with DNA, plays an important role in the synthesis of proteins in a cell.

ribosome (rī-bō-sōm) location of protein synthesis (manufacture) within a cell.

Richardson retractor a type of retractor used for abdominal surgery.

right subcostal incision surgical cut below the ribs used to reach the gallbladder and biliary tract.

rigid (rĭ-jĭd') straight, unbending, fixed.

Ringer (rĭng'-ĕr) **lactate** a type of intravenous solution used for rehydration.

ringworm (rĭng'-wŭrm) a fungal infection of the skin.

Rinne (rĭn'-nē) **test** vibration source (tuning fork) is placed on the mastoid process and then in front of the external auditory meatus to test bone and air conduction.

RNA ribonucleic acid.

rod (rŏd) photosensitive receptor cell of the retina that transforms light waves into nerve impulses. Rods contain rhodopsin.

roentgenography (rĕnt"-gĕn-ŏg'-ră-fē) radiography.

roentgenology (rĕnt"-gĕn-ŏl'-ō-jē) an alternate term for x-ray technology.

ROM rupture of membranes.

Romberg (rŏm'-bĕrg) **sign** (after Moritz Heinrich Romberg, physician, 1795–1873) a test of proprioception which is positive if the individual is unable to maintain equilibrium with the eyes closed and the feet close together.

rongeur (rŏn-zhŭr') a forceps used for gouging away bone.

rotation (rō-tā'-shŭn) circular movement around an axis.

rubella (roo-bĕl'-lă) **titer** a serologic study to diagnose rubella or the presence of antibodies to rubella.

Rubin (roo-bĭn) **test** act of filling the fallopian tubes with carbon dioxide to test for their patency.

ruga (roo'-gē) (**pl. rugae**) a ridge on the hard palate and on the wall of the stomach.

rupture (rŭp'-chūr) to burst, open.

RV right ventricle.

S-A sinoatrial.

S&D stomach and duodenum.

S1 first heart sound.

S2 second heart sound.

SBE subacute bacterial endocarditis.

saccule organ in the inner ear that is associated with maintaining equilibrium.

sacral pertaining to the sacrum.

sacral plexus part of the lumbosacral plexus formed by the fourth and fifth lumbar and the first through third sacral nerves.

sacroiliac pertaining to the sacrum and ilium.

sacrum (sā'-krŭm) (S1–S5) a bone of the vertebral column consisting of S1–S5 which are fused together.

SAD (**seasonal affective disorder**) a psychiatric condition marked by mental depression during the winter months, believed related to reduced exposure to sunlight.

sagittal (săj'-ĭ-tăl) arrowlike or in the anteriposterior direction.

sagittal plane a vertical plane dividing the body into right and left sides.

saliva (să-lī′-vă) the digestive juice produced by the salivary glands.

salivary (săl′-ĭ-vĕr-ē) pertaining to saliva.

salivary glands structures for the production of saliva. Major salivary glands include the parotid, sublingual, and submandibular.

salpingectomy (săl″-pĭn-jĕk′-tō-me) the surgical removal of the fallopian tubes.

salpingitis (săl″-pĭn-jī′-tĭs) inflammation of the fallopian tubes.

salpingo-oophorectomy (săl-pìng″-gō-ō″-ŏf-ōrĕk′-tō-mē) surgical excision of the fallopian tubes and ovaries.

salpingopexy (săl-pĭng′-ō-pĕk″-sē) the surgical fixation of the fallopian tubes.

Saratoga sump type of surgical drain.

sarcoma (săr-kō′-mă) a cancerous tumor derived from connective tissue.

sarcomere (săr′-kō-mēr) a unit of muscle; the striated muscle fibril lying between adjacent dark lines.

saw a surgical instrument for cutting bone.

SBFT small bowel follow through.

SBS small bowel series.

scabicide (skă′-bĭ-sīd) substance that kills mites.

scabies (skā′-bē-ēz) infestation with a contagious mite which causes skin rash and intense pruritus.

scala (skā′-lă) **tympani** a division of the spiral canal of the cochlea.

scale (skāl) small, thin, dry exfoliation of the skin.

scalpel (skăl′-pĕl) a surgical instrument used to cut tissue.

scaphoid (skăf′-oyd) boat-shaped or hollow.

scapula (skăp′-ū-lă) shoulder bone; one of two flat, triangular bones, one on each dorsal side of the dorsal thorax.

Schiller's (shĭl′-ĕrz) **test** (after Walter Schiller, pathologist, 1887–1960) test for superficial cancer of the cervix.

schizophrenia (skĭz″-ō-frē′-nē-ă) a psychiatric condition marked by psychosis, delusions and hallucinations. A frequent delusion includes the belief that one's thoughts are controlled by an outside force, or that one's thoughts are being broadcast to the world at large.

Schwann (shvŏnz) **cells** (after Theodore Schwann, anatomist, 1810–1882) cells which form a nerve axon's myelin sheath.

sciatic nerve (sī-ăt′-ĭk) a large nerve arising from the sacral plexus which passes down the posterior thigh.

sciatica (sī-ăt′-ĭ-kă) neuralgia of the sciatic nerve.

scintiscan (sĭn′-tĭ-skăn) image created by the gamma radiation emitted from a radiopharmaceutical.

scirrhous (skĭr′-rŭs) hard or densely packed; especially as relates to a tumor overgrown with fibrous tissue commonly found in the breast.

scissors (sĭz′-ors) an instrument used to cut, incise, or separate tissue.

sclera (sklĕr′-ă) **(pl. sclerae)** tough, white, outer coat of the eyeball.

scleral buckle the suturing of a silicone band to the sclera directly over a detached portion of the retina. The band brings together the two layers of a detached retina.

sclerectomy (sklĕ-rĕk′-tō-mē) the surgical excision of a portion of the sclera.

scleroderma (sklĕr″-ĕ-dĕr′-mă) chronic disease of the skin and other organs with hardening and shrinking of the connective tissue.

sclerosis (sklĕ-rō′-sĭs) a hardening due to chronic inflammation, especially within the nervous system.

sclerotherapy (sklĕr″-ō-thĕr′-ă-pē) using hormones as treating agents.

scoliosis (skō″-lē-ō′-sĭs) lateral curvature of the spinal column.

scotoma (skō-tō′-mă) area of blindness or reduced vision within the visual field.

scrotum (skrō′-tŭm) the external sac that contains the testes.

scrub hand wash prior to surgery lasting a prescribed length of time. Antibacterial soaps are used to scrub the skin from the finger tips to the elbows.

sebaceous (sē-bā′-shŭs) pertaining to sebum.

sebaceous gland oil-secreting gland in the corium of the skin that is associated with the hair follicles.

seborrhea (sĕb-or-ē′-ă) overactivity of the sebaceous glands.

seborrheic (sĕb″-ō-rē′-ĭk) relating to seborrhea.

seborrheic dermatitis a scaly erythematous oily eruption of the skin.

seborrheic keratosis a superficial yellow-brown warty lesion of the skin occurring in older individuals.

sebum (sē′-bŭm) oily substance secreted by the sebaceous glands.

secondary suture line secondary line of sutures, typically one to two inches on either side of the primary suture line. Used to lend support to the primary line. It eases the tension on the primary suture line.

secretion substance which is the product of cellular or glandular activity.

secundigravida (sē-kŭn″-dĭ-grăv′-ĭd-ă) woman pregnant for the second time.

secundipara (sē″-kŭn-dĭp′-ă-ră) woman who has given birth to two viable offspring.

sedative (sĕd′-ă-tĭv) drug used to depress the central nervous system and reduce nervousness or excitement or induce sleep.

sella turcica (sĕl′-ă tŭr′-sĭ-kă) cavity in the skull that contains the pituitary gland.

semen (sē-mĕn) spermatozoa and fluid.

semicircular (sĕm″-ē-sŭr′-kū-lăr) **canal** one of three bony tubes in the labyrinth of the inner ear that are associated with the maintenance of equilibrium.

semifowler position body position in which patient is seated in a position with back at a 30 degree angle from the horizontal. Used for shoulder procedures and in the recovery room.

semimembranosus (sĕm″-ē-mĕn″-brăn-ō′-sŭs) a muscle of the inner and back part of the thigh.

seminiferous (sĕm-ĭn-ĭf′-ĕr-ŭs) **tubules** the narrow, coiled tubules in the testes which are the location of sperm production.

seminoma (sĕm″-ĭ-nō′-mă) a malignant tumor of the testis.

seminal (sĕm′-ĭ-năl) **vesicle** gland that secretes fluid which is a component of semen.

semipermeable (sĕm″-ē-per′-mē-ă-bl) that which will allow passage of some substances, but not others.

semitendinosus (sĕm″-ē-tĕn″-dĭn-ō′-sŭs) a muscle of the posterior and inner part of the thigh.

Senn retractor a type of retractor used for superficial surgical procedures.

sensorineural (sĕn″-sō-rē-nū′-răl) pertaining to a sensory nerve.

sensory (sĕn′-sō-rē) pertaining to sensation, feeling.

septum (sĕp′-tŭm) **(pl. septa)** partition; in the cardiovascular system, a partition between the right and the left sides of the heart.

serological (sē-rō-lŏj′-ĭk-ăl) **test for syphilis** a laboratory study for the diagnosis of syphilis.

serology (sē-rŏl′-ō-jē) the study of blood serum.

serosa (sē-rō′-să) serous membrane; the outermost coat of a visceral structure.

serous (sēr′-ŭs) pertaining to a thin, watery fluid (serum).

serous otitis media a noninfectious inflammation of the middle ear with the accumulation of serum.

serum (sē′-rŭm) **acid phosphatase** an enzyme found in the prostate which can be measured in small quantities in the blood.

serum calcium measurement of the amount of calcium in blood.

serum glutamic oxalaxetic transaminase (SGOT) an enzyme found in serum and body tissue, particularly in heart and liver.

serum phosphorus measurement of the amount of phosphorus in blood.

sesamoid (sĕs′-ă-moyd) having the size or shape of a grain of sesame; a bone located over a joint.

sessile (sĕs′-l) having a broad base of attachment with no stem.

seventh cranial nerve the facial nerve.

sex chromosome the chromosome which determines sex.

sexual dysfunction difficulty in completing the sexual response cycle.

sexually transmitted disease (STD) a disease acquired during sexual relations with an infected person.

SGOT serum glutamic oxaloacetic transaminase.

sheath (shēth) any covering or enveloping structure.

shingles (shĭng′-lz) herpes zoster.

SIADH syndrome of inappropriate antidiuretic hormone secretion.

sialoadenitis (sī″-ă-lō-ăd″-ĕ-nī′-tĭs) inflammation of a salivary gland.

sickle (sĭk′-l) **cell anemia** hereditary condition characterized by abnormally shaped erythrocytes and by hemolysis.

sideropenia (sĭd″-ĕr-ō-pē′-nē-ă) iron deficiency.

SIDS sudden infant death syndrome.

sigmoid (sĭg′-moyd) **colon** the "S" shaped part of the colon just proximal to the rectum.

sigmoidoscopy (sĭg″-moy-dŏs′-kō-pē) the procedure of visually examining the sigmoid colon.

sign (sīn) any objective indication of illness on physical examination.

sinoatrial (sīn″-ō-ā′-trē-ăl) **node** (S-A node) group of cells located in the right atrial wall which can initiate an electrical impulse spontaneously at a rate of 75 to 100 times per minute. Called the pacemaker, as it sets the heart's basic rhythm.

sinus (sī′-nŭs) channel, cavity or passage.

sinusotomy (sī-nŭs-ŏt′-ō-mē) an incision into a sinus.

skeletal (skĕl′-ē-tăl) pertaining to the skeleton.

skeletal muscle tissue muscle connected to bones; also called voluntary or striated muscle.

skin outermost covering of the body.

skin grafting using skin from a healthy part of the body or from a donor individual to repair a defect or wound.

skin preparation a procedure preceding surgery to reduce the chance of postoperative infection. The body hair near the surgical site is shaved or clipped and the surgical site is washed with an antibacterial solution.

slit lamp an instrument for examination of the eye under magnification.

slit lamp biomicroscopy test using a slit lamp for the micro-scopic study of the cornea, conjunctiva, iris, lens, and vitreous humor.

small bowel follow through upper GI series in combination with small bowel series.

small bowel series x-ray and fluoroscopic examination of the small duodenum, jejunum, and ileum following oral intake of barium sulfate.

SMR submucous resection.

snaps slang for hemostat.

SOB shortness of breath; dyspnea.

soleus (sō′-lē-ŭs) flat, broad muscle located in the calf of the leg.

somatotropin (sō″-măt-ō-trō′-pĭn) a peptide hormone produced by the anterior lobe of the pituitary gland; also known as growth hormone (GH).

sonogram (sō′-nō-grăm) examination by ultrasonography.

sonolucent (sō″-nō-loo′-sĕnt) permitting the passage of ultra-sound; the opposite of sonogenic.

sp. gr. specific gravity.

spasm any sudden involuntary movement.

spastic (spăs′-tĭk) hypertonic; pertaining to spasms.

speculum an instrument for examining the interior of a canal.

speculum (spĕk′-ū-lŭm) **retractor** special type of retractor which is inserted into a body cavity.

speech therapy the study, diagnosis and treatment of defects and disorders of speech.

sperm (spĕrm) spermatozoon; a male sex cell.

spermatic (spĕr-măt′-ĭk) **cord** the cord formed by the vas def-erens and associated structures as they pass into the scrotum.

spermatocele (spĕr-măt′-ō-sēl) a cyst of the epididymis contain-ing spermatozoa.

spermatocidal (spĕr″-mă-tō-sī′-dăl) pertaining to an agent used to kill spermatozoa.

spermatogenesis (spĕr″-măt-ō-jĕn′-ĕ-sĭs) formation of mature functional spermatozoa.

spermatozoon (sper″-măt-ō-zō′-ŏn) (pl. **spermatozoa**) sperm cell.

sphenoid (sfē′-noyd) wedge-shaped.

sphenoid bone bat-shaped bone extending behind the eye and forming part of the base of the skull.

spherocytosis (sfē″-rō-sī-tō′-sĭs) an increased number of fragile, rounded erythrocytes in the blood.

sphincter (sfĭngk′-tĕr) a ring of muscles within a tube.

sphincter ani sphincter that closes the anus.

sphincter of Oddi sphincter within the ampulla of the hepato-pancreatic duct.

sphincterotomy (sfĭngk″-tĕr-ŏt′-ō-mē) incision of a sphincter.

sphygmomanometer (sfĭg″-mō-măn-ŏm′-ĕt-ĕr) blood pressure cuff.

spina bifida (spī′-nă) a congenital defect in the spinal column due to imperfect union of vertebral parts.

spina bifida cystica spina bifida associated with a meningocele.

spina bifida occulta spina bifida without herniation of the spi-nal cord or its membranes. In its most minor form, there is no defect in the skin, and the only evidence of its presence may be a small dimple with a tuft of hair.

spinal (spī′-năl) pertaining to the spine or spinal cord.

spinal anesthesia drugs injected into the subarachnoid or epi-dural space of the spinal cord resulting in blockage of nerve impulses at the nerve roots.

spinal cavity the space within the spinal column (backbone) containing the spinal cord.

spinal cord the nervous tissue within the spinal cavity.

spinal column the bone tissue surrounding the spinal cavity; vertebral column.

spinous (spī'-nŭs) process the prominence at posterior part of each vertebra.

spirometry (spī-rŏm'-ĕ-trē) the measurement of breathing capacity and lung volume.

spleen (splēn) the large lymphatic organ located in the left upper quadrant of the abdomen, adjacent to the stomach.

splenectomy (splē-nĕk'-to'-mē) surgical removal of the spleen.

splenomegaly (splē''-nō-mĕg'-ă-lē) enlargement of the spleen.

splenorrhagia (splē''-nō-rā'-jē-ă) hemorrhage from a ruptured spleen.

splenorrhaphy (splē-nor'-ă-fē) the suturing of a wound of the spleen.

spondylitis (spŏn-dĭl-ī-tĭs) inflammation of one or more vertebrae.

spondylolisthesis (spŏn''-dĭ-lō-lĭs''-thē'-sis) a forward slipping of one vertebrae on the one below it.

spondylolysis (spŏn''-dĭ-lŏl'-ĭ-sĭs) a breaking down of the vertebral structure.

spondylomalacia (spŏn''-dĭ-lō-mă-lā'-shē-ă) softening of the vertebrae.

spondylosis (spŏn''-dĭ-lō'-sĭs) vertebral ankylosis.

sponge forceps used to grasp or hold a gauze sponge during surgery.

spontaneous (spŏn-tā'-nē-ŭs) without apparent cause.

spontaneous abortion discharge of the fetus before it is viable outside the uterus. Approximately 50 percent of miscarriages are caused by chromosomal abnormalities.

sprain (sprān) trauma to a joint with pain, swelling, and injury to ligaments.

squamosal (skwā-mō'-săl) suture the line uniting the temporal and parietal bones of the skull.

squamous (skā'-mŭs) scale-like.

squamous epithelium composed of a layer of flat, scale-like cells.

squamous cell carcinoma malignant tumor of the squamous epithelium.

squint (skwĭnt) abnormal deviation of the eye. Slang term for strabismus.

stab (stăb) wound wound inflicted by a sharp instrument; a separate incision made at the time of a surgical procedure into which a surgical drain is placed to remove fluids from the operative site.

stapedectomy (stā''-pē-dĕk'-tō-mē) the surgical removal of the stapes of the ear. After its removal, a prosthetic device is used to connect the incus and the oval window.

stapedius (stā-pē'-dē-ŭs) a small muscle of the inner ear.

stapes (stā'-pēz) third ossicle of the middle ear.

staphylococci (stăf''-ĭl-ō-kŏk'-sē) common gram-positive bacteria appearing in clusters under the microscope.

Staphylococcus (stăf''-ĭl-ō-kŏk'-ŭs) aureus a species of gram-positive bacteria commonly present on skin and mucous membranes.

staphylorrhaphy repair of a cleft palate.

staple extractor a device for removing staples from the skin after a surgical procedure.

stay sutures secondary line of sutures, typically one to two inches to either side of the primary suture line which eases the tension on the primary suture line.

STD sexually transmitted disease.

steatoma (stē''-ă-to'-mă) lipoma; a fatty tumor.

steatorrhea (stē''-ă-tō-rē'-ă) discharge of fat in the feces.

stereotaxic (stĕr''-ē-ō-tăk'-sĭk) neurosurgery use of an instrument that, when fixed onto a skull, can locate a neurosurgical target by three dimensional measurement.

sterilization (stĕr''-ĭl-ĭ-zā'-shŭn) rendering incapable of reproduction; the destruction of all microorganisms in or around an object.

sternal (stĕr'-năl) pertaining to the sternum or breastbone.

sternoclavicular (stĕr''-nō-klă-vĭk'-ū-lăr) concerning the sternum and clavicle.

sternocleidomastoid (stĕr''-nō-klī''-dō-măs-toyd) one of two muscles in the neck arising from the sternum and inner part of the clavicle.

sternohyoid (stĕr''-nō-hī'-oyd) a muscle extending from the medial end of the clavicle and sternum to the hyoid bone.

sternum (stĕr'-nŭm) narrow, flat bone in the middle of the chest.

steroid (stĕr'-oyd) a group of complex chemicals of which many hormones are made.

stethoscope (stĕth'-ō-skōp) instrument used to listen to body sounds.

stick tie ligation needle attached to suture material is used to secure the suture material to the tissue before occlusion of the blood vessel.

stimulus (stĭm'-ū-lŭs) (pl. stimuli) change in the internal or external environment that can evoke a response.

stomach (stŭm'-ăk) muscular organ that receives food from the esophagus. Food is digested in the stomach and sent to the duodenum.

stomatitis (stō-mă-tī'-tĭs) inflammation of the mouth.

stomatoplasty (stō'-mă-tō-plăs''-tē) plastic surgery to repair the mouth.

stool analysis feces are placed in a growth medium to test for the presence of microorganisms; guaiac is added to a stool sample to reveal the presence of blood in the feces.

strabismus (stră-bĭz'-mŭs) abnormal deviation of the eye.

strabismus repair surgical repair of the eye muscles.

stratified (străt'-ĭ-fīd) epithelium epithelium in superimposed layers with differently shaped cells in various layers.

stratum (strā'-tŭm) (pl. strata) layer of cells.

stratum basale the outermost layer of the endometrium; the deepest layer of the epidermis.

stratum corneum outermost layer of the epidermis, which consists of flattened, keratinized (horny) cells.

stratum germinativum the stratum basale and stratum spinosum.

stratum granulosum the granular layer of the epidermis.

stratum lucidum the translucent layer of the epidermis.

stratum spinosum the prickle cell layer of the epidermis.

streptococci (strĕp''-tō-kŏk'-sī) common gram-positive bacteria appearing in long chains under the microscope; responsible for strep throat, tonsillitis, rheumatic fever and certain kidney ailments.

streptococcus pneumoniae species of bacteria, appearing as paired ovals under the microscope, responsible for many cases of pneumonia.

streptococcus pyogenes a species of group A hemolytic streptococcus.

streptococcus viridans group of streptococci that are normally present in the upper respiratory tract.

streptokinase (strĕp″-tō-kī′-nās) drug that dissolves clots.

stress (strĕs) **incontinence** involuntary micturition due to increased intra-abdominal pressure from coughing, laughing, or bending.

stress test diagnostic procedure to determine the heart's response to physical exertion.

striated (strī′-ā-tĕd) **muscle** skeletal muscle.

stricture (strĭk′-chŭr) abnormal narrowing of an opening or passageway.

stridor (strī′-dor) strained, high-pitched, noisy breathing associated with obstruction of the larynx or a bronchus.

stroke (strōk) also called a cerebrovascular accident; nerve cells of the brain become injured when deprived of blood because of vascular injury.

STS serological test for syphilis.

sty (stī) hordeolum; localized, purulent, inflammatory staphylococcal infection of a marginal gland of the eyelid.

styloid (stī′-loyd) **process** a pole-like process on the temporal bone.

subarachnoid (sŭb″-ă-răk′-noyd) below or under the arachnoid membrane and pia mater of the covering of the brain.

subarachnoid hemorrhage bleeding below or under the arachnoid membrane of the brain.

subcutaneous (sŭb″-kū-tā′-nē-ŭs) below or introduced beneath the skin.

subcutaneous tissue (superficial fascia) the fatty connective tissue underlying the dermis.

subcuticular (sŭb″-kū-tĭk′-ū-lăr) **suture** skin suture placed just under the skin. Can be continuous or interrupted.

subdeltoid (sŭb-dĕl′-toyd) beneath the deltoid muscle.

subdural (sŭb-dū′-răl) **hemorrhage** bleeding below the dura of the meninges of the brain.

subinvolution (sŭb″-ĭn-vō-lū′-shŭn) failure of the uterus to return to its normal size following pregnancy.

sublingual (sŭb-lĭng′-gwăl) under the tongue; a route of administering medication.

sublingual gland one of two major salivary glands found under the tongue.

subluxation (sŭb″-lŭks-ā-shŭn) partial or complete dislocation of any joint.

submammary (sŭb-măm′-ă-rē) below the mammary gland.

submandibular below the lower jaw or mandible.

submandibular gland one of two major salivary glands located just under the mandible.

submucous (sŭb-mū′-kŭs) **resection (SMR)** excision of the tissues below the mucosa.

suborbital (sŭb-or′-bĭ-tăl) below the orbit.

subscapular (sub-skăp′-ū-lăr) below the scapula.

subtotal (sŭb-tō′-tăl) **hysterectomy** an incomplete hysterectomy leaving a portion of the uterus intact.

suction aspiration; the act of sucking.

sudoriferous (sū-dor-ĭf′-ĕr-ŭs) **glands** sweat-secreting glands of the skin.

sulcus (sŭl′-kŭs) **(pl. sulci)** a depression in the surface of the cerebral cortex; fissure.

superficial (soo″-pĕr-fĭsh′-ăl) on the surface.

superior (soo-pē′-rē-or) **(cephalic)** above another structure.

supination (sū″-pĭn-ā′-shŭn) rotation of the forearm so as to turn the palm upward.

supine (sū-pīn′) lying on the back.

supine position lying face up, head straight. Most common surgical position.

suprapubic (soo″-pră-pū′-bĭk) **prostatectomy** removal of the prostate through a suprapubic abdominal incision.

suprapubic incision surgical cut above the symphysis pubis.

surgery (sŭr′-jĕr-ē) correction of deformities and defects, or repair of injuries by operation.

surgical (sŭr′-jĭ-kăl) pertaining to surgery.

surgical clips small clips used to ligate small structures such as veins, arteries and nerves. Clips offer significant advantages over sutures in terms of speed and ease of use. Thus, when bleeding must be controlled quickly, or when the structure to be ligated is deep or difficult to reach, clips may be the method of choice.

surgical staples staples applied with a stapler when closing skin incisions or wound closures. Staples are advantageous because they can be used to close a wound quickly, thus reducing the time the patient is anesthetized. Their use can also minimize tissue damage because less handling of the tissue is required. Staples can result in less scarring of certain wounds. They may also be used for anastomosis (joining parts of organs not normally joined).

surgical neck shaft of the humerus below the tuberosities which is constricted.

suspensory (sŭs-pĕn′-sō-rē) **ligaments** any ligaments that support a specific organ or structure.

suture (sū′-chŭr) suture material used to sew up a wound or tie a blood vessel (noun); the act of sewing up a wound or tying of a blood vessel (verb); a fibrous joint of two flat bones (sagittal, coronal, lambdoidal and squamosal).

suturing technique ways of sewing together two edges of a wound with different stitches depending upon the need. Common suturing techniques include the continuous, interrupted, mattress, purse-string, subcuticular, and retention stitches. Each describes the method in which two edges of the wound are approximated.

SVC superior vena cava.

sweat (swĕt) **glands** simple, coiled, tubular glands found on all body surfaces except the margin of lips, glans penis, and inner surface of the prepuce.

symblepharon (sĭm-blĕf′-ă-rŏn) adhesion, due to previous injury, of the conjunctiva of the lid to that of the eyeball.

symmetry (sĭm′-ĕt-rē) the same shape, size and relative position on opposite sides of a body.

sympathectomy (sĭm″-pă-thĕk′-tō-mē) excision of a portion of a sympathetic nerve.

sympathomimetic (sĭm″-pă-thō-mĭm-ĕt′-ĭk) agent whose effect mimics the impulses of the sympathetic nervous system. May be used in the treatment of asthma and allergic reactions.

symphysis (sĭm′-fĭ-sĭs) type of joint in which the bony structures are firmly united by a plate of cartilage.

symphysis pubis junction of the pubic bones at the midline in the front.

symptom (sĭm′-tŭm) any change from normal as experienced by the patient which is indicative of disease.

symptomatology (sĭmp″-tō-mă-tŏl′-ō-jē) the science of symptoms of disease and the indications they furnish.

synapse (sĭn′-ăps) space between one neuron and another or between a neuron and a muscle cell through which a nervous impulse is transmitted.

syncope (sĭn′-kō-pē) fainting, loss of consciousness caused by inadequate flow of blood to the brain.

syndactylism (sĭn-dăk′-tĭl-ĭzm) the condition of two or more fingers or toes being fused together.

syndrome (sĭn′-drōm) group of signs or symptoms that commonly occur together and indicate a particular disease or abnormal condition.

syndrome of inappropriate ADH (SIADH) the excessive secretion of antidiuretic hormone.

synechia (sĭn-ĕk′-ē-ă) adhesions of the iris to the cornea or lens.

synovia (sĭn-ō′-vē-ă) the transparent alkaline fluid in joint cavities, bursae and tendon sheaths.

synovial (sĭn-ō′-vē-ăl) pertaining to synovia.

synovial cavity space between bones in a synovial joint.

synovial fluid the viscous fluid within the synovial cavity. Synovial fluid is similar in viscosity to egg white; this accounts for the origin of the term.

synovial joint freely movable joint.

synovial membrane membrane lining the synovial cavity.

synovitis (sĭn″-ō-vī′-tĭs) pain and inflammation of the synovial membrane.

synovium (sĭn-ō′-vē-ŭm) synovial membrane.

synthetic (sĭn-thĕt′-ĭk) **absorbable suture** suture material made from non-animal materials.

syphilis (sĭf′-ĭ-lĭs) sexually transmitted disease initially causing lesions on the external genitalia, later causing multiorgan involvement; may be cured with antibiotics.

syringe (sĭr-ĭng′) an instrument for injecting fluid.

systemic (sĭs-tĕm′-ĭk) affecting the body as a whole.

systemic circulation flow of blood from the body cells to the heart and back again.

systemic lupus erythematosus (SLE) chronic inflammatory disease involving the joints, skin, kidneys, nervous system, heart and lungs.

system organized grouping of related structures.

systole (sĭs′-tō-lē) contraction phase of the heart beat.

T wave portion of the electrocardiogram denoting ventricular repolarization.

T and B lymphocyte subset enumeration a test for B and T cell deficiency.

T-tube surgical drain for removal of bile following exploration of the common bile duct.

T&A tonsillectomy and adenoidectomy.

T3 triiodothyronine.

T4 thyroxine.

tachycardia (tăk″-ē-kăr′-dē-ă) a fast heart beat of greater than 100 beats per minute.

tachypnea (tăk″-ĭp-nē′-ă) fast breathing.

tactile (tăk′-tĭl) pertaining to touch.

TAH total abdominal hysterectomy.

talus most superior of the tarsal bones; articulates with the tibia and fibula forming the ankle joint.

tarsal pertaining to the ankle bones, the seven short bones that correspond to the carpal bones of the wrist.

tarsectomy excision of a tarsal bone.

TB tuberculosis.

Tc technetium.

tears (tērs) liquid excreted into the eyes by the lacrimal glands.

technetium-99m (tĕk-nē′-shē-ŭm) commonly used gamma emitter used as the radionuclide in liver and spleen scans.

telemetry transmission of information electronically, used especially in reference to a type of electrocardiographic monitoring.

temporal (tĕm′-por-ăl) pertaining to the temples.

temporal bone one of two bones forming the lower sides and base of the cranium. Each bone encloses an ear and contains a fossa for joining with the mandible (lower jaw bone).

temporalis (tĕm″-pō-rā′-lĭs) the muscle of lateral region of the head above the zygomatic arch and the mandible.

temporomandibular (tĕm″-pō-rō-măn-dĭb′-ū-lăr) **joint (TMJ)** articulation between the temporal and mandibular bones.

tenaculum (tĕn-ăk′-ū-lŭm) a forceps used to grasp or hold tissue.

tendinitis (tĕn″-dĭn-ī-tĭs) inflammation of a tendon.

tendinous (tĕn′-dĭ-nŭs) pertaining to a tendon.

tendon (tĕn′-dŭn) connective tissue that binds muscles to bones.

tenodesis (tĕn-ŏd′-ĕ-sĭs) the surgical transferring of a tendon to a new point of attachment.

tenorrhaphy (tĕn-or′-ă-fē) suturing of a tendon.

tenosynovitis (tĕn″-ō-sĭn″-ō-vī′-tĭs) inflammation of the tendon sheath.

tenotomy (tĕ-nŏt′-ō-mē) the cutting of a tendon.

tension (tĕn′-shŭn) **sutures** secondary line of sutures, typically one to two inches to either side of the primary suture line, easing the tension on the primary suture line.

teratoma (tĕr-ă-tō′-mă) tumor composed of several tissues not normally found in the organ of origin.

testis (tĕs′-tĭs) **(pl. testes)** the male gonad that produces spermatozoa and the hormone testosterone.

testicles (tĕs′-tĭ-klz) testis; the male gonad.

testicular (tĕs-tĭk′-ū-lăr) pertaining to the testicles.

testicular torsion the twisting of the spermatic cord causing ischemia to the testis.

testosterone (tĕs-tŏs′-tĕr-ōn) a steroid hormone secreted by the interstitial tissue of the testes; responsible for male sex characteristics.

tetanus (tĕt′-ă-nŭs) an often fatal infectious disease caused by a bacterial toxin.

tetracaine hydrochloride a local anesthetic drug.

thalamus (thăl′-ă-mŭs) the main relay center of the brain; incoming sensory messages are relayed through the thalamus to appropriate centers in the cerebrum.

thalassemia (thăl-ă-sē′-mē-ă) inherited defect in the ability to produce hemoglobin.

Thallium-201 (thăl′-ē-ŭm) a radionuclide used in cardiac imaging.

thelitis (thē-lī′-tĭs) inflammation of the nipple.

therapy (thĕr′-ă-pē) any treatment of disease.

thoracentesis (thō″-ră-sĕn-tē′-sĭs) surgical puncture of the thorax to remove fluid from the pleural cavity.

thoracic (thō-răs′-ĭk) pertaining to the chest or thorax.

thoracic cage bony structure surrounding the thorax, consisting of ribs.

thoracic cavity space in the chest containing the heart, lungs, bronchial tubes, trachea, esophagus, and other organs.

thoracic duct the largest lymph vessel in the body.

thoracoplasty (thō′-ră-kō-plăs″-tē) surgical reconstruction of the thorax.

thoracostomy (thō″-răk-ŏs′-tō-mē) the placement of a tube into the pleural cavity for drainage of air or fluid.

thoracotomy (thō″-răk-ŏt′-ō-mē) a surgical procedure involving the cutting of the chest wall.

thorax (thō′-răks) **(pl. thoraces)** that portion of the anatomy that is situated between the base of the neck superiorly and the diaphragm inferiorly.

thrombectomy (thrŏm-bĕk′-tō-mē) excision of a thrombus.

thrombocyte (thrŏm′-bō-sīt) platelets; the tiny blood elements formed in the bone marrow which are necessary for blood clotting.

thrombocytopenia (thrŏm″-bō-sī″-tō-pē′-nē-ă) a decrease in the number of platelets.

thrombocytosis (thrŏm″-bō-sī-tō′-sĭs) increase in the number of platelets.

thrombolysis (thrŏm-bōl′-ĭ-sĭs) the breaking up of a thrombus.

thrombolytic (thrŏm-bō-lĭt′-ĭk) pertaining to or causing the breaking up of a thrombus.

thrombophlebitis (thrŏm″-bō-flē-bī′-tĭs) inflammation of a vein with associated clot formation.

thrombosis (thrŏm-bō′-sĭs) formation or presence of a blood clot.

thrombotic (thrŏm-bŏt′-ĭk) occlusion the blocking of the artery by a clot.

thrombus (thrŏm′-bŭs) blood clot in the heart or blood vessels.

thrush (thrŭsh) a fungal (yeast) infection of the mouth and throat.

thymectomy (thī-mĕk′-tō-mē) surgical removal of the thymus gland.

thymosin hormone that is important in the development of the immune response in newborns.

thymus (thī′-mŭs) an unpaired lymphatic organ located in the mediastinal cavity anterior to and above the heart; involutes with advancing age.

thyrocalcitonin (thī″-rō-kăl″-sĭ-tō′-nin) calcitonin. A hormone produced by the thyroid gland. Calcitonin lowers calcium levels in the blood.

thyroid (thī′-royd) pertaining to a ductless secretory gland located in the neck.

thyroid carcinoma cancer of the thyroid gland.

thyroid cartilage the largest of the cartilages of the larynx; produces the prominence on the neck known as the Adam's apple.

thyroid function tests measure the levels of T4, T3, and TSH in the bloodstream.

thyroid gland endocrine gland that surrounds the trachea in the neck.

thyroid scan a nuclear medicine procedure for visualization of the thyroid gland.

thyroid sonogram an ultrasound examination of the thyroid.

thyroid-stimulating hormone (TSH) a peptide hormone produced by the anterior lobe of the pituitary gland; TSH acts on the thyroid gland to promote its secretion of T4 and T3; also called thyrotropin.

thyroidectomy (thī″-royd-ĕk′-tō-mē) surgical excision of the thyroid gland.

thyrotropin (thī″-rō-trōp′-ĭn) thyroid stimulating hormone.

thyroxine (thī-rŏks′-ĭn) (T4) produced by the thyroid gland; also called tetraiodothyronine. T4 regulates metabolism in cells.

TIA transient ischemic attack.

tibia (tĭb′-ē-ă) the larger and more medial of the bones of the leg between the knee and ankle.

tibial (tĭb′-ē-ăl) pertaining to the tibia.

tibialis (tĭb″-ē-ā′-lĭs) pertaining to the tibia.

tic (tĭk) a spasmodic muscular contraction.

tinea (tĭn′-ē-ă) infection of the skin caused by a fungus.

tinea barbae a fungal infection of the skin in the beard area.

tinea capitis a fungal infection of the scalp.

tinea corporis tinea of the body.

tinea cruris a fungal infection of the skin of the scrotal, crural, anal, and genital areas.

tinea pedis athlete's foot; a fungal infection of the foot.

tinea unguium onychomycosis; a fungal infection of the nail.

Tinel's (tĭn-ĕlz′) sign (after Jules Tinel, neurologist, 1879–1952) a tingling sensation produced by percussion over a damaged peripheral nerve, particularly the median nerve in the wrist.

tinnitus (tĭn-ī′-tŭs) noise (ringing, buzzing, roaring) in the ears.

TLC total lung capacity.

TLE temporal lobe epilepsy.

tomogram (tō′-mō-grăm) x-ray examination using slices taken at different depths of focus through the patient.

tomography (tō-mŏg′-ră-fē) method of x-ray examination in which the x-ray device is moved to generate sections or slices at different depths of focus.

tongue (tŭng) a muscle which extends across the floor of the oral cavity and is attached to the lower jaw bone.

tonic (tŏn′-ĭk) pertaining to tone or tension.

tonoclonic (tŏn″-ō-klŏn′-ĭk) denoting rhythmic muscular contractions such as those present during a generalized seizure.

tonometry (tōn-ŏm′-ĕ-trē) measurement of the tension or pressure within the eye.

tonsillar (tŏn′-sĭ-lăr) pertaining to the tonsils.

tonsillectomy (tŏn-sĭl-ĕk′-tō-mē) surgical removal of the tonsils.

tonsillitis (tŏn-sĭl-ī′-tĭs) inflammation of the tonsils.

tonsils (tŏn′-sĭlz) masses of lymphatic tissue.

toothed forceps surgical instrument used to handle thick or difficult to manage tissue.

topical pertaining to a definite area; local.

topical anesthesia the administration of anesthetic drugs to the skin surface.

torticollis (tor″-tĭ-kŏl′-ĭs) the spasmodic contraction of the muscles of the neck causing the head to be drawn to one side.

tourniquet (toor′-nĭ-kĕtz) a device used to compress an extremity thereby temporarily stopping blood flow to it.

toxemia (tŏks-ē′-mē-ă) an obsolete term for eclampsia and preeclampsia.

toxic (tŏks′-ĭk) pertaining to a poison.

toxin (tŏks′-ĭn) a poisonous substance of animal or plant origin.

tPA (tissue plasminogen activator) drug that dissolves clots, useful in treating coronary thrombosis.

TPN total parenteral nutrition.

trabecula (tră-bĕk′-ū-lă) the spongy latticework found in the epiphyses of long bones and in the middle portion of most other bones of the body.

trabeculoplasty a surgical procedure involving the trabecular network of the eye.

trachea (trā′-kē-ă) windpipe; the tube leading from the throat to the bronchial tubes.

tracheostomy (trā″-kē-ŏs′-tō-mē) the creation of a new opening into the trachea.

tracheotomy (trā″-kē-ŏt′-ō-mē) the process of cutting into the trachea.

tracheorrhagia (trā″-kē-ō-rā′-jē-ă) hemorrhage from the trachea.

trachoma (trā-kō′-mă) a chronic infectious conjunctivitis caused by Chlamydia trachomatis.

tract (trăkt) a passageway or path.

tranquilizer (trăn″-kwĭ-līz′-ĕr) a drug used to control anxiety.

transducer (trăns-dū′-sĕr) device for converting energy from one form to another.

transection (trăn-sĕk′-shŭn) cutting across.

translucent (trăns-lū′-sĕnt) able to be seen through.

transurethral (trăns″-ū-rē′-thrăl) pertaining to anything that extends through the urethra.

transurethral resection of the prostate (TURP) special endoscope (resectoscope) is inserted through a catheter into the urethra, and pieces of the prostate gland are removed by electrocautery (burning) or cryogenic (freezing) techniques.

transverse crosswise.

transverse colon (trăns-vĕrs′) that portion of the large bowel which passes horizontally toward the spleen, and turns downward into the descending colon.

transverse incision surgical cut across the abdomen.

transverse plane the horizontal plane dividing the body into upper and lower portions (cross section).

transverse process portion of the vertebral arch.

trapezium (tră-pē′-zē-ŭm) geometric figure having four sides, none of which are parallel; one of the bones of the wrist having this shape.

trapezius (tră-pē′-zē-ŭs) the triangular muscle covering the shoulders and neck.

trauma (traw′-mă) wounds caused by a physical injury.

treatment (trēt′-mĕnt) any medical, surgical, dental or psychiatric care for a patient.

tremor (trĕm′-or) uncontrolled muscle quivering.

Trendelenburg (trĕn-dĕl′-ĕn-bŭrg) body position in which the patient is lying face up, knees slightly flexed, with the head and feet below height of knees.

TRH thyrotrophin-releasing hormone.

triceps (trī′-sĕps) possessing three heads; the large muscle which extends the elbow.

tricuspid (trī-kŭs′-pĭd) valve the valve located between the right atrium and the right ventricle of the heart; it has three leaflets, or cusps.

trigeminal (trī-jĕm′-ĭn-ăl) neuralgia severe pain in one or more branches of the facial nerve.

triglyceride (trī-glĭs′-ĕr-īdz) a product of fat digestion.

trigone (trī′-gōn) triangular area in the bladder where the ureters enter and the urethra exits.

trigonitis (trĭg″-ō-nī′-tĭs) inflammation of the trigone of the bladder.

triiodothyronine (trī″-ī-ō″-dō-thī′-rō-nēn) (T3) produced by the thyroid gland; T3 regulates metabolism in cells.

triquetrum (trī-kwē′-trŭm) a three sided bone within the wrist.

trocar (trō′-kăr) a surgical instrument used for puncturing a cavity.

trochanter (trō-kăn′-tĕr) one of two large processes on the femur for the attachment of muscle.

trochlea (trŏk′-lē-ă) apparatus having a function of a pulley; refers especially to the fibrous loop in the orbit through which the tendon of the superior oblique muscle passes.

troponin (trō′-pō-nĭn) a muscle protein concerned with the binding and inhibition of cross-bridge formation.

true vocal cords structures in the larynx which produce sound by vibrating as air moves over them.

TSH thyroid stimulating hormone.

TSS toxic shock syndrome.

tubal (tū′-băl) ligation a sterilization procedure in which the fallopian tube is cut and tied.

tubercle (tū′-bĕr-kl) a small, rounded process on many bones for attachment of tendons or muscles.

tuberculin (tū-bĕr′-kū-lĭn) skin test skin test to determine the presence of an immune response to tuberculosis.

tuberculosis (tū-bĕr″-kū-lō′-sĭs) (TB) an infectious disease caused by Mycobacterium tuberculosis; most commonly affects the lungs but any organ in the body may be involved.

tuberosity (tū-bĕr-ŏs′-ĭ-tē) a large, rounded process on many bones for attachment of muscles of tendons.

tumor (tū′-mor) a neoplastic growth.

tunica (tū′-nĭ-kă) adventitia outermost fibroelastic layer of a blood vessel of other tubular structure.

tunica intima the innermost fibroelastic layer of a blood vessel or tubular structure.

tunica media middle layer in the wall of a blood vessel or tubular structure.

tunica vaginalis a serous membrane surrounding the front and sides of the testicle.

turbinate (tŭr′-bĭ-nāt) shaped like an inverted cone; the bony plates within the nasal cavity.

turgor (tŭr′-gor) fullness.

TURP transurethral resection of the prostate.

tympanic (tĭm-păn′-ĭk) membrane membrane between the outer and the middle ear; also called eardrum.

tympanoplasty (tĭm″-păn-ō-plăs′-tē) surgical reconstruction of the middle ear.

UA urinalysis.

UGI upper gastrointestinal.

ulcer (ŭl′-sĕr) open sore caused by the superficial loss of tissue.

ulcerating characterized by an open, exposed surface resulting from death of overlying tissue.

ulna (ŭl′-nă) the more medial of the two lower arm bones.

ultrasonography (ŭl-tră-sŏn-ŏg′-ră-fē) use of high frequency sound waves to produce an image of a body part.

ultrasound use of inaudible sound waves to produce an image or photograph of an organ or tissue.

ultraviolet (ŭl″-tră-vī′-ō-lĕt) rays beyond the visual spectrum at its violet end.

umbilical (ŭm-bĭl′-ĭ-kăl) region the central region of the abdomen near the navel.

undifferentiated (ŭn-dĭf″-ĕr-ĕn-shē-ā′-tĕd) lacking structures typical of normal, fully mature cells.

unilateral (ū″-nĭ-lăt′-ĕr-ăl) pertaining to only one side.

unmyelinated (ŭn-mī′-ĕ-lĭ-nāt″-ĕd) nerve without a myelin sheath.

unremarkable no significant abnormality, within normal limits.

up upright.

upper respiratory tract infection (URI) an infection of the nose, nasal cavity pharynx, and larynx. The common cold is the most common upper respiratory infection.

upper gastrointestinal (UGI) series x-ray of the upper digestive tract, including the esophagus, stomach, and duodenum following oral intake of barium sulfate.

urea (ū-rē′-ă) the major nitrogenous waste product excreted in urine.

uremia (ū-rē′-mē-ă) the accumulation of waste products in the blood due to loss of renal function.

ureter (ū′-rĕ-tĕr) the tube which conveys urine from the kidney to the urinary bladder.

ureteral stricture a narrowing of the ureters, resulting in a complete or partial blockage.

ureterolith (ū-rē′-tĕr-ō-lĭth) a stone or calculus in the ureter.

ureterolithotomy (ū-rē″-tĕr-ō-lĭth-ŏt′-ō-mē) surgical procedure for the removal of a stone or calculus from the ureter.

ureterostomy (ū-rē″-tĕr-ŏs′-tō-mē) the creation of a permanent external fistula for the drainage of a ureter.

urethra (ū-rē′-thră) canal from the bladder to the outside for the discharge of urine.

urethral (ū-rē′-thrăl) pertaining to the urethra.

urethrorrhagia (ū-rē″-thror-ā′-jē-ă) hemorrhage from the urethra.

urethral stenosis (ū-rē″-thrăl-stĕn-ō′-sĭs) a narrowing of the urethra.

urgency the sudden need to micturate or void.

uric (ū′-rĭk) **acid** nitrogenous waste which is a breakdown product of protein metablism and is excreted in the urine.

urinalysis (ū″-rĭ-năl′-ĭ-sĭs) examination of the urine.

urinary (ū′-rĭ-năr″-ē) pertaining to urine or the urinary tract.

urinary bladder the sac that holds urine.

urine (ū′-rĭn) the fluid excreted by the kidneys consisting of water, salts, and acids.

urobilinogen (ū″-rō-bī-lĭn′-ō-jĕn) colorless byproduct of the intestinal bacteria, a derivative of bilirubin.

urogenital (ū″-rō-jĕn′-ĭ-tăl) pertaining to the reproductive and urinary organs.

urogram (ū′-rō-grăm) an x-ray record of the urinary tract.

urologic (ū-rō-lŏj′-ĭk) pertaining to urology.

urologist (ū-rŏl′-ō-jist) one who specializes in the study of urology.

urology (ū-rŏl′-ō-jē) study of the urinary tract of both sexes and the genital tract in males.

URI upper respiratory tract infection.

urticaria (ŭr-tĭ-kā′-rē-ă) immunologic reaction in which red, round wheals develop on the skin.

US ultrasound.

uterine (ū′-tĕr-ĭn) **fibroid** a benign smooth muscle tumor of the uterus.

uterine prolapse the falling of the uterus into the vagina.

uterine tube duct through which the egg travels from the ovary into the uterus; also called fallopian tube or oviduct.

uteropexy (ū′-tĕr-ō-pĕks″-ē) surgical fixation of the uterus.

uterovesical (ū″-tĕr-ō-vĕs′-ĭ-kăl) pertaining to the uterus and bladder.

uterus (ū′-tĕr-ŭs) the womb; the organ that holds the embryo and fetus as it develops. Comprised of a body, fundus, and a cervix.

UTI urinary tract infection.

utricle (ū′-trĭk′l) tiny, sac-like structure in the inner ear that, along with the saccule and semicircular canals, is associated with maintaining equilibrium.

uvea (ū′-vē-ă) that portion of eye lying beneath the sclera including the iris, ciliary body and choroid.

uveitis (ū-vē-ī′-tĭs) inflammation of the uvea.

uvula (ū′-vū-lă) the soft tissue suspended from the soft palate in the mouth.

vacuole (văk′-ū-ōl) a clear space within the cell protoplasm.

vagina (vă-jī′-nă) a sheathlike tube extending from the uterus to the exterior of the body.

vaginal (văj′-ĭn-ăl) pertaining to the vagina.

vaginal speculum an instrument inserted into the vagina for the examination of its interior.

vaginal hysterectomy a surgical procedure in which the uterus is removed through the vaginal opening.

vaginitis (văj-ĭn-ī′-tĭs) inflammation of the vagina.

valve (vălv) structure in veins or in the heart, permits the flow of blood in only one direction.

valve replacement surgical replacement of a deteriorated heart valve with a prosthesis made of man-made material or animal tissue.

valvuloplasty (văl′-vū-lō-plăs″-tē) the surgical repair of a valve.

valvulotomy (văl″-vū-lŏt′-ō-mē) act of cutting through a valve.

varicella-zoster (văr″-ĭ-sĕl′-ă) **immune globulin** immune globulin with a high antibody titer to varicella-zoster virus used to convey passive immunity.

varicocele (văr′-ĭ-kō-sēl) the dilation of testicular veins inside the scrotum.

varicose (văr′-ĭ-kōs) **veins** abnormally swollen and dilated veins, usually occurring in the legs.

varix (vā′-rĭks) (pl. varices) dilated and twisted vein.

vas deferens (văs dĕf′-ĕr-ĕns) the narrow tube that carries sperm from the epididymis into the urethra.

vascular (văs′-kū-lar) pertaining to a vessel.

vasectomy (văs-ĕk′-tō-mē) bilateral excision of a portion of the vas deferens for the purpose of sterilization.

vasoconstriction (văs″-ō-kŏn-strĭk′-shŭn) the process of drawing together the walls of a vessel; narrowing of the lumen of a vessel.

vasoconstrictor (văs″-ō-kŏn-strĭk′-tor) a drug which narrows blood vessels.

vasodilation (văs″-ō-dī-lā′-shŭn) process of vessel expansion; widening of the vessel lumen.

vasodilator (văs″-ō-dī-lā′-tor) a drug used for the treatment of angina or hypertension which relaxes blood vessels.

vasopressin (văs″-ō-prĕs′-ĭn) a peptide hormone secreted by the posterior lobe of the pituitary gland; also called antidiuretic hormone.

vasospasm (văs′-ō-spăzm) the sudden, involuntary contraction of the walls of a vessel.

VC vital capacity.

VCUG voiding cystourethrogram.

VDRL venereal disease research laboratories.

vein (vān) a thin-walled blood vessel that carries oxygen-poor blood from the body tissues to the heart.

vena cava (vē′-nă cā′-vă) (pl. venae cavae) largest vein in the body. The superior and inferior venae cavae bring blood into the right atrium of the heart.

venereal (vē-nē′-rē-ăl) **disease** a disease transmitted by sexual contact.

venereal warts a reddish elevation on the anus and genitals transmitted by sexual contact.

venography (vē-nŏg′-ră-fē) an x-ray image of veins is taken after introducing contrast medium intravenously.

venostasis (vē″-nō-stā′-sĭs) abnormally sluggish movement of blood through the veins.

venous (vē′-nŭs) pertaining to a vein.

venovenostomy (vē″-nō-vē-nŏs′-tō-mē) development of an anastomosis of a vein to a vein.

ventral (vĕn′-trăl) pertaining to the front, anterior.

ventricle (vĕn′-trĭk-l) the lower and larger chamber of the heart.

ventriculostomy (vĕn-trĭk″-ū-lŏs′-tō-mē) surgical procedure to correct hydrocephalus.

venule (vĕn′-ūl) small vein.

vermiform (vĕr′-mĭ-form) **appendix** a long narrow worm-shaped tube attached to the cecum.

verruca (vĕr-roo′-kă) (pl. verrucae) wart; a epidermal growth caused by a virus.

verrucous (vĕr-roo′-kŭs) resembling a wart-like growth.

vertebra (vĕr′-tē-bră) a bone of the spinal column.

vertebral (vĕr′-tē-brăl) pertaining to the vertebrae or the vertebral column.

vertebral column the spinal column.

vertebral foramen a hollow cavity enclosed by the vertebral notch.

vertical mattress sutures stitches which pass beneath and over the surface of the wound in both deep and shallow bites.

vertigo (vĕr′-tĭ-gō) the sensation of a whirling motion either of oneself or of external objects.

vesicle (vĕs′-ĭ-kl) small lesion filled with clear fluid; blister.

vesicosigmoidostomy (vĕs″-ĭ-kō-sĭg″-moy-dŏs′-tō-mē) the surgical creation of a new opening between the bladder and the sigmoid colon.

vesicoureteral (vĕs″-ĭ-kō-ū-rē′-tĕr-ăl) **reflux** backward flow of the urine from the bladder into the ureters.

vestibulocochlear (vĕs-tĭb″-ū-lō-kŏk′-lē-ăr) pertaining to the vestibulum and cochlea of the ear.

vestibulocochlear nerve emerges from the brain behind the facial nerve between the pons and medulla oblongata; the eighth cranial nerve.

villi (vĭl′-ī) tiny microscopic projections in the walls of the small intestine through which nutrients are absorbed into the bloodstream.

viral (vī′-răl) **hepatitis** inflammation of the liver caused by a virus.

virus (vī′-rŭs) infectious agent that reproduces by entering a host cell and using the host's genetic material to make copies of itself.

viscera (vĭs′-ĕr-ă) internal organs.

visceral (vĭs′-ĕr-ăl) pertaining to a viscus.

visceral muscle smooth muscle.

visceromegaly (vĭs″-ĕr-ō-mĕq′-ă-lē) enlargement of a visceral organ.

viscous (vĭs′-kŭs) thick or sticky.

visual acuity clarity of vision.

visual field examination measures the area within which objects may be seen when the eye is fixed, looking straight ahead.

vitamin supplement an aid in the maintenance of health in cases of dietary deficiency or in cases of impaired absorption of nutrients.

vitiligo (vĭt-ĭl-ī′-gō) loss of pigment in areas of the skin.

vitrectomy (vĭ-trĕk′-tō-mē) removal of the vitreous humor and its replacement with a clear solution. This is necessary when blood and scar tissue accumulate in the vitreous humor.

vitreous (vĭt′-rē-ŭs) pertaining to the vitreous body of the eye.

vitreous chamber the area behind the lens of the eye which contains vitreous humor.

vitreous humor the soft, jelly-like material that fills the large, inner, vitreous chamber of the eye.

VLDL very low-density lipoprotein.

VMA vanillylmandelic acid.

void (voyd) to expel urine (micturate).

voiding cystourethrography (VCUG) an x-ray is taken of the bladder and urethra as a patient is expelling urine.

Volkmann's (fōlk′-mănz) **contracture** muscular atrophy and degeneration due to an injury to its blood supply (ischemia).

volvulus (vŏl′-vū-lŭs) the twisting of the intestine upon itself.

vomer (vō′-mĕr) a thin, single, flat bone forming the lower portion of the nasal septum.

vomit (vŏm′-ĭt-ĭng) to forcibly expel gastric contents through the mouth.

voyeurism (voy′-yĕr-ĭzm) a psychosexual disorder characterized by an intense desire to watch unsuspecting people disrobe or engage in the sex act.

vulva (vŭl′-vă) the external genitalia of the female including the labia and clitoris.

vulvitis (vŭl-vī′-tĭs) inflammation of the vulva.

wart (wort) (**verruca**) an epidermal growth caused by a virus.

WBC white blood cell.

Weber test compares bone conduction in the two ears; a vibrating tuning fork is placed on the center of the forehead.

wedge resection removal of a part of an organ or structure in the shape of a wedge.

Western blot antibody detection test.

wheal (hwēl) smooth, slightly elevated, edematous (swollen) area that is redder or paler than the surrounding skin; hive.

wheeze (hwēz) abnormal musical sound heard during inspiration or expiration caused by trapped air.

white blood cell leukocyte.

white blood cell count (WBC) laboratory measurment of the number of white blood cells by volume. If elevated, can provide an indication of the presence of infection.

white blood cell differential the microscopic examination of the proportion of different white blood cell types.

Wilms' (vĭlmz) tumor a malignant neoplasm of the kidney usually occurring in children.

wryneck (rī′-nĕk) torticollis. An abnormal position of the head, caused by contracted state of one or more muscles in the neck.

X chromosome the chromosome which determines female sex characteristics.

x-ray high energy radiation which is useful in the diagnosis and treatment of disease.

xenograft (zĕn′-ō-grăft) surgical graft of tissue from one species to another.

xeroderma (zē″-rō-dĕr′-mă) condition of dry, rough, discolored state of the skin.

xeroradiography (zē″-rō-rā″-dē-ŏg′-ră-fē) technique in which an x-ray image is made on a charged plate and then subsequently reproduced by a dry process on specially treated paper.

xiphoid (zĭf′-oyd) **process** the lower, narrow portion of the sternum.

Y chromosome the chromosome which determines male sex characteristics.

yellow bone marrow fatty tissue found in the diaphyses of long bones.

ZDV or AZT zidovudine or azidothymidine (a drug used to treat AIDS).

Ziehl-Neelsen (zēl-nēl′-sĕn) **(ZN) stain** a special stain used to detect the prescence of Mycobacteria and other acid fast organisms.

zona-pellucida (zō′-nă) the solid, inner, thick, membrane envelope of the ovum.

zygoma one of two bones on each side of the face which forms the prominence of the cheek.

zygomatic (zī″-gō-măt′-ĭk) pertaining to the zygoma.

zygomatic arch arch formed on each side of the cheek by the zygomatic process.

zygomatic process of temporal bone thin projection from the temporal bone which articulates with the zygomatic bone.

zygote (zī′-gōt) fertilized ovum.

INDEX

-ary, 15
Arytenoid cartilage, 403
Asbestosis, 411
Ascending colon, 291
Ascending tract, 197
Ascites, 311
Asepsis, 621
Aspermatogenesis, 491
Asphyxia, 415
Aspiration pneumonia, 412
Aspirin, 585
-assay, 544
-asthenia, 167
Asthma, 410
Astigmatism, 250, 251
Astrocytes, 195
Astrocytomas, 221
Ataxia, 201, 222
Ataxic cerebral palsy, 214
Ataxic gait, 222
Ataxic respiration, 415
Atelectasis, 410
Atherosclerosis, 374
Athetoid cerebral palsy, 214
Athlete's foot, 88, 95
Atonic, 180
Atopic dermatitis, 89, 97
Atopic rhinitis, 408
Atria
    blood flow through, 367
    contraction of, 364
    explanation of, 360
Atri/o, 359
Atriocentrivular valve, 360
Atrioventricular bundle (AV bundle),
        363
Atrioventricular node (AV node), 363
Atrophy, 95, 180
Attention-deficit hyperactivity disorder
        (ADHD), 577
Audi/o, 239
Audiogram, 264
Audiometry, 266
Auditory, 264
Auditory ossicles, 261
Auditory process, 263
Auerbach's plexus, 283
Aural, 264
Auricle, 261
Auricul/o, 239
Auriculotemporal, 264
Aur/o, 239
Auscultation, 64, 65, 310, 380
Auto-, 35
Autograft, 84, 99
Autoimmune, 454
Autoimmune diseases, 455
Automatic implantable cardioverter-
        defibrillator (AICD), 384
Autonomic nervous system (ANS), 194,
        205, 210
Avascular, 84

Avascularity, 76
Avoidant disorder, 578
Axial, 561
Axial skeleton
    hyoid bone in, 118
    skull in, 115–118
    thoracic cage in, 122–123
    vertebrae in, 118–122
Axillary, 58
Axill/o, 23, 48
Axi/o, 544
Axons, 196, 197
Azidothymidine (AZT), 455

B
Babcock forceps, 608
Babinski's reflex, 209, 224
Bacilli, 593
Bacillus, 6
Back
    divisions of, 57
    muscles of, 174
Bacteria, 97, 593
Bacterial infections, 87, 98
Bacteriuria, 481
Balance, 259
Balanitis, 491
Balan/o, 50
Baldness, 90
Bandages, 619
Barbiturates, 588
Barium enema (BE), 312, 548
Barotitis media, 264
Bartholin's glands, 509
Basal cell carcinoma, 91, 98
Basal ganglia, 200
Basal nuclei, 200
Basal pneumonia, 412
Basement cells, 472
Bas/o, 435
Basophil, 436, 437
Bedsores, 77–78
Bell's palsy, 217
Bence Jones protein, 151
Benign neoplasms, 91
Benign prostatic hypertrophy (BPH),
        492
Beta blockers, 387
Beta cells, 294
Beta particles, 560
Bi-, 36
Biceps muscle, 170, 171
Bicuspids, 285
Bicuspid valve, 360, 367
Bile, 289
Biliary system, 294
Biliary tract
    abnormal conditions of, 307, 308
    x-rays of, 548
Bilirubin/o, 281
Bil/l, 281
Binocular vision, 244

Bio-, 35
Bi/o, 600
Biopsy
    aspiration of, 153
    explanation of, 97, 184, 621
    punch, 494, 520, 623
    surgical incision, 494
Bipolar disorders, 572
Birthmarks, 91
Blackheads, 89
Black lung disease, 411
Bladder
    abnormal conditions of, 481
    explanation of, 469–470
Blast-, 505
-blast, 14, 74
Blastocyst, 526
Blastomeres, 526, 527
Bleb, 411
Bleeding time, 443
Blephar/o, 49
Blepharochalasis, 247
Blepharopexy, 61
Blepharoptosis, 247
Blepharospasm, 247
Blind spot, 242
Blister, 94
Blood, 45
    abbreviations for, 446
    explanation of, 435–437
    term analysis for, 437–440
Blood abnormalities
    anemias, 440–441
    diagnosis of, 443–446
    leukemias, 442
Blood-brain barrier, 204, 205, 553, 556
Blood cells, 43, 435, 436
Blood pressure, 366
Blood transfusion, 446
Blood urea nitrogen (BUN), 482
Blood vessels
    description of, 365–366
    terms related to, 374–375
B-lymphocytes, 451–453
Body cavities
    description of, 50
    illustration of, 51
    summary of, 52
Body dysmorphic disorder, 575
Body planes, 55, 56
Body systems. *See also specific systems*
    anatomical roots for, 48–50
    anatomical terminology for, 61–64
    organs in various, 44–48
Bolus, 287
Bone, 44. *See also* Skeletal system;
        Skeleton; Vertebrae
    classification of, 110–112
    explanation of, 110
    marks on, 112, 113
    microscopic and macroscopic
        structure of, 110

Bone cutters, 606
Bone grafting, 155
Bone marrow, 46, 451
Bone marrow aspiration, 153, 445
Bone marrow biopsy, 445
Bone marrow transplant, 446
Bone scans, 152, 558, 559
Bony labyrinth, 261
Book-Walter retractors, 609
Borborygmi, 310
Borderline personality disorder, 577
Borrelia burgdorferi, 88
Bowman's capsule, 472
Brachial, 136
Brachial plexus, 208
Brachial pulse, 379
Brachi/o, 109
Brady-, 35
Bradycardia, 373
Bradykinesia, 180, 223
Bradypnea, 415
Brain, 45
    function of, 193
    protective covering of, 204–205
    structure of, 198–201
Brain scan, 225, 553–556
Brain stem, 198, 201
Breast
    abnormal conditions of, 514
    explanation of, 510
    surgery of, 620
Breech position, 528–529
Bronchi, 46, 401, 404
Bronchial tree, 404
Bronchiectasis, 407, 410
Bronchi/o, 49
Bronchioles, 46
Bronchiolitis, 407
Bronchiol/o, 49
Bronchitis, 61
    acute, 408
    chronic, 410
    explanation of, 407
Bronch/o, 49
Bronchodilators, 420
Bronchography, 417, 546, 561
Bronchopneumonia, 412
Bronchoscopy, 419
Bronchospasm, 415
Bronchus, 6
Bruit, 380
Brunner's gland, 290
Buccal cavity. See Oral cavity
Buccal mucosa, 300
Buccinator, 172, 173
Bucc/o, 281
Bulbar conjunctiva, 243
Bulbourethral gland, 47, 489
Bulimia nervosa, 578
Bulla, 94, 411
Bundle branches, 363, 378
Bundle of His, 363

Bunion, 143
Burn terminology, 78–79
Bursae, 130
Bursitis, 140
Butterfly rash, 89
Buttocks muscles, 177

C
Café au lait spots, 89
Calcaneal, 136
Calcaneus, 128
Calcitonin, 334
Calcium
    abnormal values of, 151
    stored in bone, 110
Calcium blockers, 387
Calculus, 6
Caldwell-Luc technique, 421
Caliceal, 478
Calix, 6
Candida albicans, 304
Canine teeth, 285
Canker sores, 304
Capillaries, 45, 365, 366
Capitulum, 6
Carbuncle, 87
Carbunculosis, 87
Carcinoma, 6, 61
    basal cell, 91
    squamous cell, 91
Carcinoma in-situ, 514
Cardia, 288
Cardiac arrest, 378
Cardiac catherization, 382
Cardiac cycle, 363–364
Cardiac disease, 481
Cardiac enzymes, 381
Cardiac monitor, 610
Cardiac muscle, 167, 168
Cardiac pacemaker, 378, 386
Cardiac sphincter, 288
Cardi/o, 359
Card/i/o, 4, 5, 24, 49
Cardioangiography, 381
Cardiography, 14
Cardiology, 4
Cardiomegaly, 380
Cardiopathy, 4
Cardiopulmonary bypass, 387
Cardiotonics, 387
Cardiovascular abnormalities
    description of, 375–378
    laboratory tests to diagnose, 381–383
    physical examination to detect, 379–380
    signs and symptoms of, 380–381
    treatment of, 383–387, 620
Cardiovascular system. See also
        Circulatory system; Heart
    abbreviations related to, 388
    blood vessels and circulatory roots of, 365–370

components of, 359
    heart as component of, 359–364
    term analysis of, 373–375
    word elements related to, 359
Cardioversion, 384
Carditis, 4, 378
Carotene, 81
Carotenemia, 84
Carotenodermia, 84
Carotid pulse, 379
Carpal, 125, 126, 136
Carpal tunnel, 217
Carpal tunnel syndrome (CTS), 217
Carp/o, 109
Cartilage, 44
Cartilaginous joints, 130
Caseation, 413
Catabolism, 48, 58
Cataracts, 252, 253
Catherization, 485
CAT scan, 561
Cauda equina, 201
Caudal, 53, 54, 58
Caudate lobe, 294
Cautery, 610, 621
Cec/o, 281
Cecopexy, 300, 316
Cecum, 291
-cele, 11
Celiac disease, 305
Celiac sprue, 305
Cellac, 300
Cell body, 196
Cell-mediated immune response, 452
Cell/o, 281
Cells, 41–43
Cementum, 285
Centesis, 384
-centesis, 12, 600
Central endocrine glands, 329. See also
        Hypothalamus; Pituitary gland
Central nervous system (CNS). See also
        Nervous system
    brain, 45, 193, 198–201
    disorders of, 213–216, 455
    explanation of, 193, 194
    protective coverings in, 204–205
    spinal cord, 45, 193, 201–204
Central sulcus, 200
Cephal/o, 23, 48
Cephalopelvic disproportion, 532
Cerebellitis, 211
Cerebell/o, 193
Cerebellum
    explanation of, 198, 199
    function of, 201
Cerebral, 211
Cerebral cortex, 198, 199
Cerebral palsy, 214
Cerebr/o, 24, 49, 193
Cerebroangiography, 381
Cerebrospinal, 211

Condyloma acuminatum, 87
Cone biopsy, 621
Congenital disease, 525
Congenital dislocation of the hip (CDH), 147
Congenital megacolon, 305
Congestive heart failure (CHF), 378
Conization, 621
Conjunctival membrane, 242, 243
Conjunctivitis, 248, 254
Conjunctiv/o, 239
Connective tissue
  explanation of, 43
  in skin, 77, 78
Consent forms, 604, 605
Constipation, 311
Contact dermatitis, 89, 98
Continuous positive airway pressure (CPAP), 420
Continuous suture, 617
Contra-, 35
Contraception, 526
Contracture, 182
Contrast medium, 546
Contusion, 96
Conus medullaris, 201
Convergence, 244, 246
Conversion disorder, 575
Convolutions, 199
Coombs' test, 443
Core/o, 239
Coreometer, 248
Corium, 76. See also Dermis
Cornea, 240
Corneal, 248
Corneal transplant, 258
Corne/o, 239
Corniculate cartilage, 403
Coronal suture, 116
Coronary, 373
Coronary artery bypass graft (CABG), 385
Coronary artery disease (CAD), 376
Corpus callosum, 199
Corpus luteum, 508
Cortef (hydrocortisone), 350
Cortical, 211, 478
Cortic/o, 193, 329
Corticosteroids, 154, 258
Corticotrophin-releasing hormone (CRH), 331
Cortisol, 294, 335, 350
Coryza, 409
Costal, 136
Costal cartilage, 122
Cost/o, 24, 48, 109
Costochondral, 136
Costovertebral, 136
Cowper's glands, 489
Coxal bone, 124
Coxa valga, 145
Coxa vara, 145

Cradle cap, 89
Cranial, 53, 54, 58
Cranial bones, 115–116
Cranial cavity, 50–52
Cranial nerves
  explanation of, 205–207
  illustration of, 208
  physical examination of, 222
Crani/o, 23, 48, 109
Craniotomy, 136
Cranium, 115
Creatine kinase (CK), 183
Creatinine, 474
Creatinine clearance, 482
Crest, 113
Cretinism, 348
Crib death, 413
Cricoid cartilage, 403
-crine, 329
Crohn's disease, 305
Croup, 408
Crown, 285
Crust (skin), 95
Cry/o, 600
Cryotherapy, 98
Cryptorchidism, 491, 492
Crypts of Lieberkuhn, 290
Cuboid, 128
Cul-de-sac of Douglas, 512
Culd/o, 505
Culdocentesis, 520
Culdoscope, 512
Culdoscopy, 520, 522
Culture and sensitivity test, 418
Cultures, 97, 151
Cuneiform cartilage, 403
Curettes, 606
Cushing's syndrome, 346
Cuspids, 285
Cutane/o, 5, 23
Cuticle, 80
Cyan/o, 74
Cyanosis, 84, 92, 380, 415
Cycl/o, 239
Cyclopegics, 587
Cyclophotocoagulation, 258
Cycloplegic, 248
Cyclothymia, 572
-cyesis, 505
Cyst, 93
Cystica, 220
Cystic duct, 294
Cystic fibrosis (CF), 413
Cystitis, 481
Cyst/o, 24, 49
Cystocele, 515
Cystojejunostomy, 478
Cystoscopy, 384
Cystourethrography, 483
-cyte, 14
Cyt/o, 24, 48
Cytomegalovirus antibody, 457

Cytoplasm, 42, 58
-cytosis, 435
Cytotoxic T-lymphocytes, 452

D

Dacry/o, 239
Dacryoadenitis, 248
Dacryoaden/o, 239
Dacryocyst/o, 239
Dacryocystorhinostomy, 248
Dacryorrhea, 248
Dactyl/o, 109
Dandruff, 89, 96, 98
Day surgery, 621
Deafness, 265
Deaver retractors, 609
Decending tracts, nerve, 197
Deciduous teeth, 285
Decompression, 621
Decongestants, 420
Decubitus ulcers, 77–78
Deep, 53, 54
Deep fascia, 169
Deep tendon reflexes, 209
Defecation, 292
Defense systems
  illustration of, 453
  nonspecific, 451
  specific, 451–453
Defibrillation, 384
Deficiency anemia, 440
Deglutition, 287
Dehiscence, 96, 617, 621
Delayed images, 552
Demyelination, 211, 215
Dendrites, 196–197
Dens, 120
Dental caries, 304
Dentin, 285
Dent/o, 281
Deoxyribonucleic acid (DNA), 43, 523
Dependent disorder, 578
Depersonalization disorder, 573
Depersonalization neurosis, 573
Depressive disorders, 572
Dermatitis, 84, 89, 95
Dermat/o, 23, 48, 74
Dermatology, 84
Dermatome, 84
Dermatomes, 610
Dermatomycosis, 84, 88
Dermatophyte, 84, 88
Dermatophytosis, 84, 88
Dermis
  anatomy and physiology of, 77–78
  characteristics of, 76
  illustration of, 75
Derm/o, 23, 48, 74
Descending colon, 291
-desis, 12, 600
Desquamation, 92

Esotropia, 248, 255
Esthesi/o, 600
Estr/o, 329
Estrogen
    explanation of, 341, 508
    secretion of, 335, 527
Ethm/o, 109
Ethmoid, 136
Ethmoidal sinuses, 116
Etiology, 59, 64, 65
Eupnea, 407
Eustachian tubes, 261, 265
Euthyroid, 341
Euthyroid goiter, 348
Evisceration, 258, 622
Evoked potentials, 216
Evoked responses, 225
Ewing's tumor, 150
Ex-, 34, 601
Excoriation, 95
Excretory urogram, 483, 547, 548
Exercise test, 382
Exertional dyspnea, 380
Exfoliation, 92
Exfoliative cytology, 519
Exhibitionism, 574
Exo-, 34
Exocrine, 341
Exocrine secretions, 329
Exophthalmia, 254, 341
Exophthalmos, 341
Exostosis, 143
Exotropia, 248, 255
Expectorants, 420
Expiration, 401, 402
Explosive disorder, 576
External acoustic meatus, 261
External canthus, 243
External ear, 261
External genitalia, 47
External nares, 402
External respiration, 401
External sphincter, 292
External urethral sphincter, 470
Extracapsular cataract extraction
        (ECCE), 252, 253
Extracorporeal, 478
Extracorporeal shock wave lithotripsy
        (ESWL), 484
Extradural hemorrhage, 221
Extraocular, 248
Extravasation, 374
Extremities
    lower, 127–129
    upper, 125–126
Extrinsic ocular muscles, 242–243
Eye
    abbreviations related to, 259
    anatomy of inner, 240–242
    anatomy outer, 242–244
    physiology of vision, 244–247
    surgery of, 620

term analysis for, 247–250
word elements related to, 239
Eye abnormalities
    description of, 250–256
    diagnosis of, 256
    diagnostic procedures for, 257
    medical treatment for, 258
    signs and symptoms of, 256–257
    surgical treatment for, 258–259
Eyelids, 242, 243

F
Facets, 112, 113
Facial bones, 117–118
Fallopian tubes
    abnormalities of, 517
    explanation of, 506, 508
    insufflation of, 520
False ribs, 122–123
False vocal cords, 403
Fascial, 180
Fasciculations, 222
Fasciculi, 169
Fasciectomy, 180
Fasci/o, 167
Fasciorrhaphy, 180
Fascitis, 180
Fasting blood sugar (FBS), 344, 350
Feces, 292
Female reproductive system
    abbreviations related to, 523
    anatomical roots for, 50
    anatomy and physiology of, 506–510
    concept map of, 511
    illustration of, 47
    term analysis for, 512–514
    word elements related to, 505
Female reproductive system
        abnormalities
    of breast, 514
    diagnosis of, 518–520
    of menstruation, 517–518
    treatment of, 521–522, 620
    of uterus, tubes, ovaries, and other
            adnexae, 514–517
    of vagina and external genitalia, 517
Femoral, 136
Femoral hernia, 309
Femoral pulse, 379
Femor/o, 109
Femur, 110, 127, 134
Fertilization, 526
Fetal period, 527–528
Fetishism, 574
Fetoscopy, 533
Fetus, 527–528
Fibrillation, 378
Fibrinogen, 436
Fibroadenoma, 514
Fibroblast, 76, 85
Fibroids, 515
Fibroma, 6

Fibromyomas, 515
Fibrous joints, 130
Fibrous tunic, 240
Fibula, 128
Fibular, 136
Fibul/o, 109
Filiform, 85
Filiform papillae, 284, 285
Filiform warts, 87
Filtrate, 472
Filament/o, 601
Filum terminale, 204
Fimbriae, 508
Finger clubbing, 416
First cuneiform, 128
First degree burns, 78
Fissure
    in ano, 304–305
    brain, 199, 200
    explanation of, 95
Fistula in ano, 305
Flaccid, 222
Flagellum, 488
Flashes (eye), 257
Flat plate of abdomen, 312
Flatulence, 311
Flatus, 311
Flexor digitorum superficialis, 171
Floaters (eye), 257
Floating ribs, 123
Fluorescein staining, 257
Fluor/o, 544
Fluoroscopy, 312, 546, 548, 562
Flutter, 378
Follicle-stimulating hormone (FSH),
        333, 508
Follicular, 85
Follicular cysts, 517
Follicul/o, 74
Fontanels, 116
Foot
    bones of, 128, 129
    directional terminology for, 55
Foot cells, 472
Foot processes, 472
Foramen, 112, 113, 116
Foramen of Monro, 200
Forceps delivery, 533
Foreskin, 489
Formal thought disorder, 575
Fossa, 112, 113
Fourth degree burns, 78
Fovea centralis, 242
Fowler position, 612
Fractures
    classification of, 148–149
    explanation of, 148
    immobilization of, 155
    reduction of, 155
Fraternal twins, 527
Free tie, 617
Frontal, 136

Jock itch, 88
Joints, 44
    abnormal conditions of, 141–142
    categories of, 130
    in knee, 134, 142, 153
    movements made by, 131–133
    names of, 131
    terms related to, 139–140
Juxtaglomerular apparatus, 474
Juxtaglomerular cells, 474

K
Kaposi's sarcoma, 455, 456
Karyoplasm, 43
Karyotype, 526
Keratin, 76
Keratinized cells, 76
Keratinocyte, 76, 85
Kerat/o, 75, 239
Keratoconjunctivitis, 249
Keratoconus, 249
Keratolytics, 98
Keratomycosis, 249
Keratoplasty, 258
Keratosis, 85, 92
Kernig's sign, 223
Ketoacidosis, 343, 344
Kidney, ureters, and bladder (KUB)
        study, 483
Kidneys, 45, 47
    abnormal conditions affecting,
            479–481
    description of, 468–469
    nuclear medicine studies of, 560
Killer T-lymphocytes, 452
Kimmelstiel-Wilson syndrome, 481
-kinesia, 167
Kinesimeter, 181
Kinesi/o, 167
Kinesiology, 180
-kinesis, 167
Kleptomania, 576
Knee jerk, 210
Knee joint
    arthroscopy of, 153
    explanation of, 134
    internal derangement of, 142
Kocher forceps, 608
Kraurosis, 517
Kyphosis, 146, 220

L
Label, 562
Labial, 512
Labial frenulum, 284
Labia majora, 509
Labia minora, 509
Labi/o, 505
Labioglossopharyneal, 302
Labl/o, 281
Labor
    explanation of, 526
    stages of, 528–529

Laboratory studies
    abbreviations related to, 596
    clinical chemistry, 594, 595
    clinical microbiology, 593, 595
    hematology, 594, 595
    histopathology, 593, 595
    immunohematology, 594, 595
Labyrinthitis, 264
Labyrinth/o, 239
Laceration, 96, 622
Lachman and Drawer, 150
Lacrimal, 249
Lacrimal apparatus, 242, 244
Lacrimal duct probes, 609
Lacrimal ducts, 244
Lacrimal gland, 244
Lacrimation, 257
Lacrim/o, 239
Lactation, 510, 530
Lacteals, 448
Lactic acid, 88
Lactiferous duct, 510
Lactiferous sinuses, 510
Lact/o, 505
Lactogenesis, 512
Lactogenic, 343
Lambdoidal suture, 116
Laminectomy, 137, 211
Lapar/o, 49, 281
Laparoscope, 302
Laparoscopic-assisted vaginal
        hysterectomy, 521
Laparoscopic cholecystectomy,
        307
Laparoscopic hysterectomy, 521
Laparoscopic laser endometriosis
        vaporization, 522
Laparoscopic surgery, 317
Laparoscopy, 315, 520, 522
Large intestine, 46
    abnormal conditions of, 304–306
    explanation of, 281, 291
    function of, 292
Laryngeal prominence, 403
Laryngitis, 62
Laryng/o, 49
Laryngopharynx, 287, 402
Laryngotracheobronchitis, 407, 408
Larynx, 7, 46, 401–403
Laser angioplasty, 384
Laser photocoagulation, 255
Lasers, 610
Laser surgery, 622
Laser therapy, 98
Lateral, 53, 54, 59
Lateral collateral ligaments, 134
Lateral decubitus, 612
Lateral fissure, 200
Lateral malleolus, 128
Lateral rectus, 242–243
Lateral semilunar cartilage, 134
Lateral sulcus, 200

Lateral ventricles, 200
Latex fixation test, 141, 151
Lavage, 316
Lead pipe rigidity, 216
Left atrium
    blood flow through, 367
    explanation of, 360
Left bundle branch, 363
Left bundle branch block (LBBB),
        378
Left ventricle, 360, 367
Leg
    bones of, 127, 128
    muscles of, 177
Leiomyoma, 181, 515
Leiomyosarcoma, 181
Lens, 242
Lens accommodation, 244–246
Lept/o, 193
Leptomeningeal, 212
Leptomeninges, 204
Lesser curvature, 288
Lesser omentum, 297
Leuc/o, 435
Leukemia, 438, 442
Leuk/o, 435
Leukocyte, 435, 436, 438
Leukocytosis, 438
Leukoderma, 89
Leukopenia, 438
Leukoplakia, 302, 518
Leukorrhea, 518
Levodopa, 216, 226
Lice, 88, 98
Lichenification, 95
Ligament/o, 167
Ligamentous, 181
Ligaments, 170
Ligate, 617
Ligation and stripping, 386, 622
Ligature, 617
Lingual frenulum, 284
Lingual tonsils, 402, 451
Lingu/o, 24, 49, 281
Lipid lowering agents, 445
Lipid/o, 435
Lipid profile, 443
Lip/o, 48
Lipoma
    explanation of, 85
    removal of, 98, 99
Lipoprotein electrophoresis, 443
Lipoproteins, 437, 443
Liposuction, 98
Liquid nitrogen, 88, 98
-lith, 11
Litholytic agent, 316
Lithotomy, 612
Lithotripsy, 307, 317, 478, 484
Liver, 45, 46
    abnormal conditions of, 307, 308
    functions of, 294

Neo-, 35
Neonatal, 530
Neoplasms. *See also* Malignant
    neoplasms
  benign, 150
  explanation of, 91
  malignant, 91, 150
  types of, 91
Neostigmine, 217
Nephr/o, 25, 49
Nephroblastoma, 479
Nephrolithiasis, 478, 480
Nephrolithotomy, 484
Nephrons, 470–472
Nephropathy, 344
Nephropexy, 478
Nephroptosis, 478
Nerve cell fiber, 197
Nerve cell fibers, 196
Nerve cells, 195–196
Nerves, 43, 45
  arrangement of, 197
  explanation of, 193
Nerve tissue
  cells that make up, 195–196
  explanation of, 43
Nervous system. *See also* Neurological
    abnormalities
  abbreviations related to, 227
  anatomical roots for, 49
  central, 198–205
  divisions of, 193–194
  functions of, 194
  illustration of, 45
  peripheral, 205–210
  term analysis for, 211–213
  word elements related to, 193
Neurasthenia, 223
Neurilemma, 197
Neurilemma sheath, 195
Neuritis, 212
Neur/o, 25, 49, 193
Neurofibromas, 221
Neurogenic bladder, 481
Neuroglia, 195
Neurohypophysis, 332, 338
Neurological abnormalities. *See also*
    Nervous system
  brain hemorrhage, 220–221
  of central nervous system, 213–216
  congenital, 219–220
  diagnostic procedures for, 224–225
  infectious, 218
  inflammatory, 218–219
  of peripheral nervous system,
    217–218
  physical examination for, 222
  signs and symptoms of, 223–224
  treatment of, 226–227
  tumors, 221
Neurolysis, 212, 227

Neuromuscular, 212
Neurons
  explanation of, 194, 195
  types of, 196
Neurosis, 6
Neurotripsy, 212
Neutr/o, 435
Neutrons, 551
Neutrophil, 436, 439
Nevi flammeus, 91
Nevus, 91
Nipple, 510
Nocturia, 482
Nodes of Ranvier, 197
Nodule, 93
Nonabsorbable sutures, 615
Non-Hodgkin's lymphoma, 456
Noninsulin dependent diabetes mellitus
    (NIDDM), 344
Nonspecific defense system, 451
Nonsteroidal anti-inflammatory drugs
    (NSAIDs), 141, 154
Nontoothed forceps, 608
Nonviral hepatitis, 308
Noradrenaline, 335
Norepinephrine, 198
  explanation of, 335
  testing levels of, 350
Normochromia, 439
Nose, 401, 402, 620
Nuclear magnetic resonance (NMR). *See*
    Magnetic resonance imaging
    (MRI)
Nuclear medicine
  cardiac applications of, 556
  diagnostic applications of, 552–556
  explanation of, 551–552
  gastrointestinal tract applications of,
    558
  genitourinary system applications of,
    560
  respiratory system applications of,
    556, 557
  skeletal system applications of, 558,
    559
  therapeutic applications of, 560
  tumor and infection applications of,
    560
Nuclear membrane, 43
Nuclear radiation, 545. *See also* Imaging
Nucle/o, 544
Nucleolus, 43
Nucleoplasm, 59
Nucleus, 42, 551
Nuclide, 551, 562
Nulli-, 505
Nulligravida, 431
Nullipara, 431
Nutrient artery, 110, 111
Nutritional supplements, 588
Nystagmus, 257

O
Oblique, 242, 243
Oblique popliteal ligament, 134
Obsessive compulsive disorder, 578
Obstetrical forceps, 608
Obstetrics. *See also* Childbirth;
    Pregnancy
  abbreviations related to, 534
  abnormal conditions related to,
    531–532
  clinical procedures used in, 533
  explanation of, 526
  term analysis for, 530–531
  word elements related to, 505
Obturator foramen, 124
Occipital, 137
Occipital bone, 115
Occipital lobe, 200
Occipit/o, 109
Ocul/o, 49, 239
Odontalgia, 62, 302
Odont/o, 49, 281
Odontoid process, 120
Oil glands, 44
-ole, 15
Olecranal, 137
Olecran/o, 109
Olecranon process, 125
Oligodendroglia, 195
Oligomenorrhea, 517
Oligopnea, 415
Oligospermia, 491
Oliguria, 482
-oma, 11
Onchyomycosis, 88
Onych/o, 48, 75
Onychomalacia, 62
Onychomycosis, 86
O/o, 505
Oocyte, 513
Oogenesis, 508
Oogonia, 524
Oophoralgia, 513
Oophorectomy, 62
Oophor/o, 25, 50, 505
-opaque, 544
Open fracture, 148
Open (skin), 96
Operating room surgery, 622
Operating room theater, 622
Operative cholangiogram, 313
Ophthalmia neonatorum, 254
Ophthalm/o, 23, 49
Ophthalmologist, 249
Ophthalmopathy, 249
Ophthalmoscopy, 257
-opsy, 13, 601
Opthalm/o, 239
Optic, 249
Optic chiasm, 246
Optic disc, 242

Pedophilia, 574
Pedunculated polyp, 93
Pedunculated warts, 87
Pelvic, 59, 138
Pelvic cavity, 50–52
Pelvic floor muscles, 178
Pelvic girdle, 124
Pelvic inflammatory disease (PID), 517
Pelvis, 6
Pelv/o, 109
Penetration (skin), 96
-penia, 11
Penis, 47, 489
Pepsinogen, 289
Peptic ulcers, 304
Per-, 34
Percussion, 64, 65, 380, 414
Percutaneous lithotripsy, 484
Percutaneous liver biopsy, 316
Percutaneous needle biopsy of pleura, 419
Percutaneous transhepatic cholangiography (PTC), 313, 547
Percutaneous transluminal coronary angioplasty (PTCA), 383
Perforation, 96
Peri-, 5, 34, 601
Perianal, 302
Periarthritis, 140
Pericardial, 5, 60
Pericardial cavity, 52, 362
Pericardial centesis, 384
Pericardial tamponade, 381
Pericarditis, 373
Pericardium, 362
Perimetrium, 509, 513
Perimysium, 169
Perine/o, 505
Perineorrhaphy, 513
Perinephric fat, 468
Periodic Table, 551
Periodontal ligament, 285
Periodontitis, 303
Perioperative, 623
Perioperative care, 601
Periosteum, 110–112
Peripheral, 53
Peripheral endocrine glands, 329–330.
    See also specific glands
Peripheral nerves, 208
Peripheral nervous system (PNS). *See also* Nervous system
    autonomic nervous system as part of, 210
    cranial nerves in, 206–207
    disorders of, 217–218
    explanation of, 193, 194, 205
    reflexes of, 110, 209
    spinal nerves in, 208
Peripheral vascular disease, 376
Perirenal fat, 468
Peristalsis, 287, 469

Peristaltic waves, 283
Peritoneal, 60
Peritoneal cavity, 296
Peritoneal dialysis, 485
Peritone/o, 281
Peritoneum, 295–297
Peritonitis, 292, 303
Peritubular capillaries, 470, 473
Periungual, 86
Pernicious anemia, 440
Personality disorders, 576–578
Petechia, 92, 94, 381
Petit mal seizures, 214
-pexy, 13, 601
Peyer's patches, 448, 451
Phac/o, 239
Phacoemulsification, 252
Phacomalacia, 250
-phagia, 14
Phagocytes, 448, 451, 454
Phagocytosis, 76, 448, 451, 452
Phak/o, 239
Phalangeal, 138
Phalanges, 125–128
Phalang/o, 109
Phalanx, 7
Phall/o, 50
Pharmacists, 584
Pharmacologists, 584
Pharmacology. *See also specific types of drugs*
    classifications used in, 585–588
    explanation of, 585
    overview of, 584
Pharnygoesophageal sphincter, 288
Pharyngeal tonsils, 402, 451
Pharyngitis, 63
Pharyng/o, 49, 281
Pharynx, 46
    explanation of, 281, 287, 402
    function of, 401
Phenolsulfonphthalein (PSP), 482
Phenytoin, 218
-phil, 435
Phimosis, 493
Phleb/o, 25, 49, 359
Phlebothrombosis, 374
-phobia, 11, 570
Phobias, 572
-phoresis, 435
Phospholipids, 436
Phosphorus
    abnormal values of, 151
    stored in bone, 110
Phot/o, 239
Photodermatitis, 89
Photophobia, 257
Photorefractive keratectomy (PRK), 259
Phrenic, 60, 407
Phrenoplegia, 407
Phrenotomy, 421

Phyechromocytoma, 347
Physical examination, 64
Physical therapy, 154
Physiotherapy, 154, 227
-phyte, 75
Pia mater, 204
Pica, 578
Piezoceramic materials, 549
Piezoelectricity, 549, 562
Pigmented hair nevus, 91
Piles, 305
Pill-rolling tremor, 216
Pil/o, 48, 75
Pilonidal cyst, 93
Pilosebaceous, 86
Pinealectomy, 351
Pineal gland, 45
    abnormalities of, 337
    function of, 329, 337, 338
Pinna, 261
Pituitar/o, 49, 329
Pituitary, 45
Pituitary gland
    abnormalities caused by, 345, 347
    anterior, 332–334
    explanation of, 329, 332
    hypothalamus and, 331
    influence of melanocytic activity by, 81
    laboratory tests for, 349
    posterior, 332
Pituitary neoplasms, 347
Pityriasis rosea, 90
Placenta, 45, 527, 528, 531
Placental delivery, 528
Placenta previa, 532
Plantar, 55
Plantar reflex, 209
Plantar warts, 87
-plasia, 14
Plasma, 435–437
Plasma cell myeloma, 150
Plasma cells, 76
Plasma membrane, 42
-plasty, 13, 601
Platelet count, 443
Platelet plug, 436
Platelets, 435
-plegia, 12
Pleural, 60
Pleural cavities, 52
Pleural effusion, 409
Pleurisy, 409
Plexus, 208
Plez/o, 544
Plicae circulares, 289
Plurals, formation of, 6–7
-pnea, 14
Pneumoconiosis, 411
Pneumocystis carinii, 412
Pneumocystis carinii parasite, 456
Pneumonectomy, 421

Pneumonia
  etiological agents in, 412
  explanation of, 408, 412
  site of infection of, 412
Pneumonitis, 408
Pneumon/o, 25, 49
Pneumothorax, 409
Podocytes, 472
Poikil/o, 435
Poikilocytosis, 439
Poliomyelitis, 212
Poly-, 36
Polychromia, 439
Polycystic kidneys, 480
Polycystic ovaries, 517
Polycythemia vera, 442
Polydipsia, 343, 344
Polymorphonuclear, 439
Polymyositis, 181
Polyneuropathy, 213
Polyps
  cervical, 514
  explanation of, 306
  pedunculated, 93
  sessile, 93
Polythelia, 513
Polyuria, 344, 482
Pons
  explanation of, 198, 199
  function of, 201
Pont/o, 193
Pontocerebellar, 213
Popliteal, 138
Popliteal pulse, 379
Positive end-expiratory pressure (PEEP), 420
Positron emission tomography (PET), 225
Post-, 34, 601
Posterior, 53, 54, 60
Posterior abdominal muscles, 174
Posterior cruciate ligaments, 134
Posterior pituitary, 332, 338
Posterior synechiae, 256
Posteroanterior, 562
Posteroanterior/lateral chest x-ray, 381
Postnatal, 431
Postoperative, 623
Postoperative care, 601
Postpartum, 431, 530
Postprandial (PP) test, 344, 350
Post-traumatic stress disorder, 573
Postural sense, 222
Posture, 169
Pott's fracture, 148, 149
Pre-, 34, 601
Prednisone, 350
Preeclampsia, 532
Prefixes
  denoting direction and position, 33–34
  denoting number, 36

explanation of, 2, 3
meaning of, 5
of negation, 35–36
Pregnancy. *See also* Childbirth;
  Obstetrics
conception phase of, 526–527
ectopic, 532
embryonic development phase of, 527
fetal development phase of, 527–528
Premenstrual syndrome (PMS), 518
Premolars, 285
Prenatal, 431
Preoperative care, 601
Preoperative checklist, 602, 603
Preoperative reception, 604
Prepuce, 489
Presbycusis, 264
Prescription drugs, 585. *See also*
  Pharmacology
Primary bronchi, 404
Primary follicles, 508
Primary osteoporosis, 144
Primary suture line, 617
Primi-, 505
Primigravida, 431, 530
Primipara, 431
Pro-, 34
Probes, 606, 609
Proct/o, 281
Proctoclysis, 303
Progesterone, 508, 527
Prognosis, 60, 64, 66
Prolactin, 334, 530
Prolactin-inhibiting hormone (PIH), 331
Prolactin-releasing hormone (PRH), 331
Prone, 54
Prone position, 612
Propylthioracil, 351
Prostatectomy, 63
Prostate gland, 47
  explanation of, 489
  transurethral resection of prostate, 494
Prostate specific antigen (PSA), 494
Prostatitis, 491
Prostat/o, 50
Prosthetic devices, 610
Proteinuria, 478
Prothrombin time (PT), 444
Protons, 551
Proximal, 53, 54, 60
Proximal convoluted tubule, 472
Proximal epiphysis, 111
Pruritus, 92
Pruritus ani, 312
Pruritus vulvae, 517
P-R waves, 364
Pseudocyesis, 431
Pseudophakia, 250
Psoralens ultraviolet light (PUVA), 90, 97

Psoriasis
  explanation of, 90, 96
  treatment of, 97, 98
Psychiatric disorders
  affective, 572
  anxiety, 572–573
  dissociative, 573
  eating, 578
  impulse control, 576
  multiaxial system of coding, 571
  personality, 576–578
  psychoactive substance abuse, 576
  psychosexual, 573–575
  schizophrenic, 575
  somatoform, 575—576
Psychiatry
  abbreviations related to, 579
  overview of, 571
  word elements related to, 570
Psych/o, 570
Psychoactive substance abuse disorders, 576
Psychoactive substance dependence, 576
Psychogenic amnesia, 573
Psychogenic fugue, 573
Psychological examination, 222
Psychosexual disorders, 573–575
Ptal/o, 281
Pterygium, 254
Ptosis, 254
-ptosis, 12
Ptyalism, 303
-ptysis, 12
Pubis, 124
Public, 138
Pulmonary, 408
Pulmonary angiography, 417
Pulmonary arteries, 359
Pulmonary circulation, 368
Pulmonary function tests, 418–419
Pulmonary semilumar valve, 361
Pulmonary tuberculosis (TB), 413
Pulmonary veins, 359
Pulmon/o, 25
Pulp cavity, 285
Pulse, 367
Punch biopsy, 494, 520, 623
Punctae, 244
Punctal stenosis, 254
Puncture, 96
Pupil, 240
Pupillary, 250
Pupillary accommodation, 244, 246
Pupillary reflex, 210
Pupill/o, 239
Purkinje fibers, 363
Purpura, 94, 381
Purse-string sutures, 619
Purulent otitis media, 265
Pustule, 94
P waves, 364
Pyelogram, 478

Pyelography, 562
Pyelonephritis, 480
Pyloric sphincter, 288
Pylor/o, 281
Pyloromyotomy, 303, 317
Pylorospasm, 303
Pyoderma, 86
Pyogenic, 86
Pyosalpinx, 513
Pyothorax, 409
Pyramids, 201
Pyromania, 576
Pyuria, 482

Q
QRS waves, 364
Quadrate lobe, 294
Quadri-, 36
Quadriplegia, 222

R
Rachi/o, 109
Rachischisis, 220
Rachitis, 138
Radial, 138
Radial pulse, 379
Radiation therapy, 227
Radiculitis, 213
Radicul/o, 193
Radiculopathy, 213
Radi/o, 14, 109, 544
Radioactivity, 551
Radiogram, 562
Radiography, 14, 563
Radioimmunoassay (RIA), 553, 563
Radioisotope, 563
Radiology, 563
Radiolucent, 546
Radionuclide, 563
Radionuclide scanning, 417
Radiopaque, 546, 563
Radiopharmaceuticals, 552, 558, 563
Radius, 125
Rake retractors, 609
Range of motion (ROM), 150
Raspatories, 606, 607
Raynaud's disease, 376
Re-, 601
Rebound tenderness, 310
Recessive alleles, 524
Rect/o, 281
Rectocele, 515
Rectum, 291, 292
Rectus, 242
Rectus femoris muscle, 171
Red blood cell count, 443, 594
Red blood cell indices, 444
Red blood cell morphology, 444
Red blood cells (RBC), 110, 289
Red bone marrow, 112, 451
Reduction division, 523

Reflexes, 209, 210
Refraction
    errors of, 250, 251
    explanation of, 244
Regional enteritis, 305
Regional nerve block, 612
Relaxin, 527
Renal angiography, 483
Renal artery, 473
Renal biopsy, 485
Renal calculi, 480
Renal capsule, 468
Renal columns, 469
Renal failure, 479
Renal fascia, 468
Renal hypoplasia, 478
Renal papilla, 469
Renal pelvis, 469
Renal tubule, 472
Ren/o, 25, 49
Reproductive systems. *See* Female
    reproductive system; Male
    reproductive system
Resection, 155, 623
Resectoscope, 491
Respiration, 401
Respiratory abnormalities
    acute infections, 408–409
    affecting lungs, 410–413
    diagnosis of, 417–419, 556, 557
    miscellaneous, 413
    physical examination to diagnose,
        414–416
    treatment of, 420–421
    upper respiratory tract, 409
Respiratory acidosis, 413
Respiratory alkalosis, 413
Respiratory bronchioles, 404
Respiratory distress syndrome (RDS),
    411
Respiratory excursion, 414
Respiratory failure, 416
Respiratory insufficiency, 416
Respiratory system
    abbreviations related to, 422
    anatomical roots for, 49
    anatomy and physiology of, 401–402
    bronchi, 404
    concept map of, 406
    illustration of, 46
    larynx, 402–403
    lungs, 405
    nose and nasal cavities, 402
    pharynx, 402
    term analysis for, 407–408
    trachea, 404
    word elements related to, 400
Resting tremors, 222
Retention sutures, 617
Reticulocyte, 439
Reticulocyte count, 444

Retina
    explanation of, 241
    process of vision on, 244–247
Retinal detachment, 255
Retinal photocoagulation, 259
Retinal tears, 255
Retin/o, 239
Retinopathy, 250
Retinopexy, 250, 258
Retinoschisis, 250
Retractors, 606, 608–609
Retrograde pyelogram, 483
Retrograde urography, 483, 547, 548
Retroperitoneal, 296, 303, 468
Reye's syndrome, 216
Rhabdomyolysis, 181
Rhabdomyoma, 181
Rhabdomyosarcoma, 181
Rheumatic fever, 378
Rheumatic heart disease, 378
Rheumatoid arthritis (RA), 141, 455
Rheumatoid factors (RF), 141, 151
Rhin/o, 23, 49
Rhinoplasty, 421
Rhinorrhea, 408, 415
Rhiz/o, 193
Rhizolysis, 218
Rhizotomy, 227
Rhodopin, 242
RhoGam, 441
Rhythm/o, 359
Ribonucleic acid (RNA), 43
Ribosomes, 42
Ribs, 110, 122–123
Richardson retractors, 609
Rickets, 143
Right atrium, 360, 367
Right bundle branch, 363
Right bundle branch block (RBBB), 378
Right ventricle, 360
Ringer's lactate solution, 79
Ringworm, 88
Rinne test, 266
Roentgen/o, 544
Roentgenography, 545. *See also*
    Imaging; X-rays
Roentgenology, 563
Romberg's sign, 222, 224
Rongeurs, 606, 607
Root canal, 285
Roots (word)
    anatomical, 48–50
    explanation of, 2
    means of, 4
    pertaining to external anatomy, 23
    pertaining to internal anatomy, 24–25
    vowels at end of, 4–5
-rrhage, 12
-rrhagia, 12
-rrhaphy, 13, 601
-rrhea, 12

Tibia, 110, 127, 128, 134
Tibial, 139
Tibialis anterior muscle, 171
Tibial tuberosity, 128
Tibi/o, 109
Tic douloureux, 218
Ticks, diseases caused by, 88
Tinea
   diagnostic tests for, 97
   explanation of, 88
   treatment of, 98
Tinea barbae, 88
Tinea capitis, 88
Tinea corporis, 88
Tinea cruris, 88
Tinea pedis, 88
Tinea unguium, 88
Tinnitus, 265
Tissue, 41, 43
Tissue plasminogen activator (TPA), 377
T-lymphocytes
   explanation of, 448, 451–453
   impact of AIDS on, 455
-tocia, 505
Toe
   acquired deformities of, 144
   bones of, 129
Tolbutamide (Orinase), 351
-tome, 13, 601
Tom/o, 545
Tomography, 546, 563
-tomy, 13, 601
Tongue, 284, 285
Tonic, 182
Tonic-clonic seizures, 214
Tonic spasms, 222
Tonometry, 257
Tonsilitis, 408
Tonsillectomy, 63, 408
Tonsill/o, 49
Tonsils, 46, 402, 451
Tophi, 141
Topical application, 90
Topical medication, 98
Torticollis, 182
Total serum bilirubin, 314
Tourniquets, 610
Toxemia, 532
Toxic alopecia, 90
Trabecula, 242
Trabeculectomy, 258
Trabeculoplasty, 259
Trabeculotomy, 258
Trachea, 46, 401, 404
Trache/o, 49
Tracheoesophageal fistula, 409
Tracheostomy, 63, 421
Tracheotomy, 63, 421
Trachoma, 256
Tracts, nerve, 197
Tranquilizers, 226
Trans-, 5, 34, 545, 601

Transcervical fracture, 149
Transducer, 548, 563
Transduction, 259
Transection, 623
Transient ischemic attacks, 377
Transplants, 620
Transurethral resection of prostate, 492,
   494
Transverse colon, 291
Transverse fracture, 148, 149
Transverse incision, 615
Transverse mesocolon, 297
Transverse plane, 55, 56
Transversus abdominis, 171
Transvesical, 5
Transvestic fetishism, 574
Trauma, skin lesions due to, 96
Treatment, 66
Tremor assessment, 222
Trendelenburg position, 612
Tri-, 36
Triceps muscle, 171
Trichotillomania, 576
Tricuspid valve, 360, 367
Trigeminal neuralgia, 218
Triglycerides, 436
Trigone, 469–470
Trigonitis, 478
Triiodothyronine, 332
Trilinear Chart, 563
Trimesters, 527
-tripsy, 601
Trocars, 606
Trochanter, 112, 113
-trohic, 329
Trophic hormones, 333
-trophin, 329
-trophy, 15
-tropic, 329
Tropic hormones, 331, 332
-tropin, 329
True ribs, 122
True vocal cords, 403
Tryroxine, 334
T-tube cholangiogram, 313
Tubal ligation, 522
Tubercle, 112, 113, 413
Tuberculin skin test, 418
Tuberculosis, 97, 456
Tuberculosis bacteria, 413
Tuberosity, 112, 113
Tubular reabsorption, 473, 474
Tubular secretion, 473, 474
Tumors
   Ewing's, 150
   giant cell, 150
   intracranial, 221
   of melanocytes, 91
   nuclear medicine studies of, 560
Tunica adventitia, 365
Tunica intima, 365
Tunica media, 365

Tuning fork tests, 266
Turbinates, 117
T waves, 364
Twins, 527
2-point discrimination test, 222
Tympanic membrane, 261, 266
Tympan/o, 239
Tympanoplasty, 265
Tympany, 310, 414
Type I diabetes mellitus, 344
Type II diabetes mellitus, 344

U
Uin/o, 109
Ulcers, decubitus, 77–78
-ule, 15
Ulna, 125
Ulnar, 139
Ultra-, 34, 545
Ultrasound. *See also* Imaging; X-rays
   to examine digestive system
      abnormalities, 313
   explanation of, 545, 549–550, 564
Ultraviolet (UV) light, 81, 90
Umbilical cord, 527
Umbilical hernia, 309
Undifferentiated somatoform disorder,
   576
Ungu/o, 48
Uni-, 36
Unmyelinated axons, 197
Upper arm muscles, 174
Upper gastrointestinal series (UGI), 313,
   547
Upper respiratory infection (URI), 409
Urea, 474
Uremia, 482
Ureter, 469, 480
Ureteral, 63, 478
Ureteral stricture, 480
Ureter/o, 50
Ureterocystostomy, 484
Uretero-ileostomy, 484
Ureterolith, 478
Ureters, 47
Urethra, 47, 469, 470, 488
Urethral, 64
Urethr/o, 50
Urethrorrhagia, 479
Urethrostenosis, 479
Urge incontinence, 482
Urgent admission, 601
7-uria, 15
Uric acid, 483
Urinalysis, 482
Urinary, 479
Urinary abnormalities
   description of, 479–481
   signs and symptoms of, 481–482
   tests to diagnose, 482–483, 548
   treatment of, 483–486
Urinary bladder, 47

Photo Credits

Chapter 1

Part one opening photo, page 1: © Peter Angelo Simon/Phototake.

Chapter 5

Figure 5–1, page 41: Sandra McMahon/Precision Graphics; Figure 5–2, page 42: Elizabeth Morales-Denney/Precision Graphics; Figure 5–3, pages 44–47: Sandra McMahon/Precision Graphics; Figure 5–4, page 51: Sandra McMahon/Precision Graphics; Figure 5–5, page 51: Sandra McMahon/Precision Graphics; Figure 5–6, page 54: Sandra McMahon/Precision Graphics; Figure 5–7, page 55: Sandra McMahon/Precision Graphics; Figure 5–8, page 56: Sandra McMahon/Precision Graphics; Figure 5–9, page 57: Sandra McMahon/Precision Graphics. Adapted by Tech-Graphics.

Chapter 6

Part two opening photo, page 73: © Peter Angelo Simon/Phototake; Figure 6–1, page 75: Laurie O'Keefe/Precision Graphics; Figure 6–2, page 76 (a): David M. Phillips/Visuals Unlimited, (b) (including inset) Cyndie C.H. Wooley/Precision Graphics; Figure 6–3, page 79: Laurie O'Keefe/Precision Graphics; Figure 6–4, page 80: Cyndie C.H. Wooley/Precision Graphics; Figure 6–5, page 80 (a): Cyndie C.H. Wooley/Precision Graphics, (b), John D. Cunningham/Visuals Unlimited; Figure 6–6, page 81: Joe McDonald/Visuals Unlimited; Concept map 6–1, page 83: Randy Miyake. Adapted by Tech-Graphics; Table figure alopecia, page 90: Ron Spomer/Visuals Unlimited; Table figure macule, page 93: Julie Horan/Radiant Illustration and Design; Table figure papule, page 93: Julie Horan/Radiant Illustration and Design; Table figure purpura, page 94: Julie Horan/Radiant Illustration and Design; Table figure pustule, page 94: Julie Horan/Radiant Illustration and Design; Table figure wheal, page 94: Julie Horan/Radiant Illustration and Design; Table figure vesicle, page 94: Julie Horan/Radiant Illustration and Design; Table figure atrophy, page 95: Julie Horan/Radiant Illustration and Design; Table figure cicatrix, page 95: Julie Horan/Radiant Illustration and Design; Table figure crust, page 95: Julie Horan/Radiant Illustration and Design; Table figure erosion, page 95: Julie Horan/Radiant Illustration and Design; Table figure fissure, page 95: Julie Horan/Radiant Illustration and Design; Table figure lichenification, page 95: Julie Horan/Radiant Illustration and Design; Table figure scale, page 96: Julie Horan/Radiant Illustration and Design; Table figure liposuction, page 98: J. Boliver/Custom Medical Stock Photo.

Chapter 7

Figure 7–1, page 111: Sandra McMahon/Precision Graphics; Figure 7–2, page 111: Sandra McMahon/Precision Graphics; Figure 7–3, page 114: Darwen and Vally Hennings; Figure 7–4, page 115: Sandra McMahon/Precision Graphics; Figure 7–5, page 116: Sandra McMahon/Precision Graphics; Figure 7–6, page 117: Sandra McMahon/Precision Graphics; Figure 7–7, page 118: Sandra McMahon/Precision Graphics; Figure 7–8, page 119: Sandra McMahon/Precision Graphics; Figure 7–9, page 120: Sandra McMahon/Precision Graphics; Figure 7–10, page 121: Sandra McMahon/Precision Graphics; Figure 7–11, page 122: Sandra McMahon/Precision Graphics; Figure 7–12, page 122: Sandra McMahon/Precision Graphics; Figure 7–13, page 123: Sandra McMahon/Precision Graphics; Figure 7–14, page 124: Sandra McMahon/Precision Graphics; Figure 7–15, page 125: Sandra McMahon/Precision Graphics; Figure 7–16, page 126: Sandra McMahon/Precision Graphics; Figure 7–17, page 127: Sandra McMahon/Precision Graphics; Figure 7–18, page 128: Sandra McMahon/Precision Graphics; Figure 7–19, page 129: Sandra McMahon/Precision Graphics; Figure 7–20, page 129: Sandra McMahon/Precision Graphics; Figure 7–21, page 130: Sandra McMahon/Precision Graphics; Figure 7–22, pages 132–133: Sandra McMahon/Precision Graphics; Figure 7–23, page 134: Sandra McMahon/Precision Graphics; Concept Map 7–1, page 135: Randy Miyake. Adapted by Tech-Graphics; Table figure rheumatoid arthritis, page 141: SIU/Visuals Unlimited; Table figure herniated disc, page 142: Sandra McMahon/Precision Graphics; Table figure bunion, page 143: Julie Horan/Radiant Illustration and Design; Table figure ganglion, page 143: Julie Horan/Radiant Illustration and Design; Table figure osteoporosis, page 144: Lester V. Bergman & Associates, Cold Spring, NY 10516; Table figure genu valgum, page 145: Julie Horan/Radiant Illustration and Design; Table figure genu varum, page 145: Julie Horan/Radiant Illustration and Design; Table figure kyphosis, page 146: Julie Horan/Radiant Illustration and Design; Table figure lordosis, page 146: Julie Horan/Radiant Illustration and Design; Table figure scoliosis, page 146: SIU/Visuals Unlimited; Table figure spondylolisthesis, page 147: Julie Horan/Radiant Illustration and Design; Table figure talipes equinovarus, page 147: Julie Horan/Radiant Illustration and Design; **Table figure talipes equinus, page 147:** Julie Horan/Radiant Illustration and Design; **Table figure talipes valgus, page 148:** Julie Horan/Radiant Illustration and Design; **Table figure talipes varus, page 148:** Julie Horan/Radiant Illustration and Design; **Table figure fractures, page 149:** Julie Horan/Radiant Illustration and Design; **Table figure arthroscopy, page 153 (top and bottom):** SIU/Visuals Unlimited; **Table figure arthroplasty, page 154 (left and right):** SIU/Visuals Unlimited.

Chapter 8

Figure 8–1, page 167: Cyndie C.H. Wooley/Precision Graphics; **Figure 8–2, page 168:** Cyndie C.H. Wooley/Precision Graphics; **Figure 8–3, page 168:** John D. Cunningham/Visuals Unlimited; **Figure 8–4, page 169:** Sandra McMahon/Precision Graphics; **Figure 8–5, page 170:** Sandra McMahon/Precision Graphics; **Figure 8–6, page 170:** Sandra McMahon/Precision Graphics; **Figure 8–7, page 172:** Sandra McMahon/Precision Graphics; **Figure 8–8, page 173:** Sandra McMahon/Precision Graphics; **Figure 8–9, page 175:** Sandra McMahon/Precision Graphics; **Figure 8–10, page 176:** Sandra McMahon/Precision Graphics; **Figure 8–11, page 178:** Sandra McMahon/Precision Graphics; **Concept map 8–1, page 179:** Randy Miyake. Adapted by Tech-Graphics; **Table figure muscular dystrophy, page 182:** Custom Medical Stock Photo.

Chapter 9

Figure 9–1, page 194: Precision Graphics; **Figure 9–2, page 195:** Teri J. McDermott/Precision Graphics; **Figure 9–3, page 196:** Teri J. McDermott/Precision Graphics; **Figure 9–4, page 197:** Julie Horan/Radiant Illustration and Design; **Figure 9–5, page 198:** John and Judy Waller; **Figure 9–6, page 199:** Teri J. McDermott/Precision Graphics; **Figure 9–7, page 199:** Fred Hossler/Visuals Unlimited; **Figure 9–8, page 200:** Teri J. McDermott/Precision Graphics; **Figure 9–9, page 202:** Teri J. McDermott/Precision Graphics; **Figure 9–10, page 203:** Sandra McMahon/Precision Graphics; **Figure 9–11, page 204:** Laurie O'Keefe/Precision Graphics; **Figure 9–12, page 205:** Carlyn Iverson; **Figure 9–13, page 206:** Sandra McMahon/Precision Graphics; **Figure 9–14, page 208:** Julie Horan/Radiant Illustration and Design; **Table figure plantar reflex, page 209:** Julie Horan/Radiant Illustration and Design; **Table figure knee jerk, page 210:** Julie Horan/Radiant Illustration and Design; **Table figure Alzheimer's disease, page 213:** Martin/Custom Medical Stock Photo; **Table figure seizure disorders, page 214:** The StockShop Inc./Medichrome; **Table figure multiple sclerosis, page 215:** Julie Horan/Radiant Illustration and Design; **Table figure Parkinson's disease, page 216:** The StockShop Inc./Medichrome; **Table figure Bell's palsy, page 217:** Julie Horan/Radiant Illustration and Design; **Table figure trigeminal neuralgia, page 218:** Julie Horan/Radiant Illustration and Design; **Table figure hydrocephalus, page 219:** SIU/Visuals Unlimited; **Table figure spina bifida occulta, page 219:** Julie Horan/Radiant Illustration and Design; **Table figure spina bifida cystica, page 220:** Julie Horan/Radiant Illustration and Design; **Table figure intracranial tumors, page 221 (left):** Custom Medical Stock Photo, **(right)** English/Custom Medical Stock Photo; **Table figure Kernig's sign, page 223:** Julie Horan/Radiant Illustration and Design; **Table figure Brudzinski's sign, page 224:** Julie Horan/Radiant Illustration and Design; **Table figure myelography, page 225:** Julie Horan/Radiant Illustration and Design.

Chapter 10

Figure 10–1, page 240: Sandra McMahon/Precision Graphics; **Figure 10–2, page 241:** Elizabeth Morales-Denney/Precision Graphics; **Figure 10–3, page 241:** A.L. Blum/Visuals Unlimited; **Figure 10–4, page 243:** Elizabeth Morales-Denney/Precision Graphics; **Figure 10–5, page 244:** Bill Beatty/Visuals Unlimited; **Figure 10–6, page 245:** Elizabeth Morales-Denney/Precision Graphics; **Figure 10–7, page 245:** Elizabeth Morales-Denney/Precision Graphics; **Figure 10–8, page 246:** Elizabeth Morales-Denney/Precision Graphics; **Figure 10–9, page 247:** Julie Horan/Radiant Illustration and Design; **Figure 10–10, page 251:** Elizabeth Morales-Denney/Precision Graphics; **Figure 10–12, page 252:** Julie Horan/Radiant Illustration and Design; **Figure 10–13, page 253:** Julie Horan/Radiant Illustration and Design; **Figure 10–14, page 253:** G. D. Heggie, RT(NM), M.Ed. Electronically prepared by Julie Horan/Radiant Illustration and Design; **Table figure acute conjunctivitis, page 254:** Julie Horan/Radiant Illustration and Design; **Table figure hordeolum, page 254:** Julie Horan/Radiant Illustration and Design; **Table figure pterygium, page 254:** Julie Horan/Radiant Illustration and Design; **Table figure retinal tears, page 255:** G. D. Heggie, RT(NM), M.Ed. Electronically prepared by Julie Horan/Radiant Illustration and Design; **Table figure strabismus, page 255:** Julie Horan/Radiant Illustration and Design; **Figure 10–15, page 260:** Elizabeth Morales-Denney/Precision Graphics; **Table 10–17, page 262:** Darwen and Vally Hennings/Precision Graphics; **Figure 10–16, page 262:** Elizabeth Morales-Denney/Precision Graphics; **Figure 10–18, page 263:** Precision Graphics; **Table figure hearing aids, page 267:** Photo courtesy of Beltone Electronics Corporation.

Chapter 11

Figure 11–1, page 282: Sandra McMahon/Precision Graphics; **Figure 11–2, page 283:** Sandra McMahon/Precision Graphics; **Figure 11–3, page 284:** Laurie O'Keefe/Precision Graphics; **Figure 11–4, page 285:** Julie Horan/Radiant Illustration and Design; **Figure 11–5, page 286:** Cyndie C.H. Wooley/Precision Graphics;

Figure 11–6, page 287: Cecile Duray-Bito/Precision Graphics; Figure 11–7, page 288: Carlyn Iverson; Figure 11–8, page 289: Julie Horan/Radiant Illustration and Design; Figure 11–9, page 290 (a–d): Sandra McMahon/Precision Graphics, (e) G. Shih-R. Kessel/Visuals Unlimited; Figure 11–10, page 291: Carlyn Iverson; Figure 11–11, page 292: Laurie O'Keefe/Precision Graphics; Figure 11–12, page 293: Carlyn Iverson; Figure 11–13, page 295: Carlyn Iverson; Figure 11–14, page 296: Carlyn Iverson/Todd Buck; Figure 11–15, page 297: Cecile Duray-Bito/Precision Graphics; Concept map 11–1, page 298: Randy Miyake. Adapted by Tech-Graphics; Concept map 11–2, page 299: Randy Miyake. Adapted by Tech-Graphics; Table figure peptic ulcers, page 304: Lester V. Bergman & Associates, Cold Spring, NY 10516; Table figure diverticulum, page 305: Lester V. Bergman & Associates, Cold Spring, NY 10516; Table figure intussuception, page 306: Julie Horan/Radiant Illustration and Design; Table figure volvulus, page 306: Julie Horan/Radiant Illustration and Design; Table figure cholelithiasis, page 307: Julie Horan/ Radiant Illustration and Design; Table figure hepatitis, page 308: The StockShop Inc./Medichrome; Table figure hernia, page 308 (left): Biophoto Associates/Photo Researchers, (right) Lester V. Bergman & Associates, Cold Spring, NY 10516; Table figure inguinal hernia, page 309: Carlyn Iverson; Table figure emaciation, page 311: AP/Wide World Photos; Table figure endoscopy, page 315 (endoscopy, laparoscopy, sigmoidoscopy): Julie Horan/Radiant Illustration and Design; Table figure gastrojejunostomy, page 317: Julie Horan/Radiant Illustration and Design.

Chapter 12

Figure 12–1, page 330: Laurie O'Keefe/Precision Graphics; Figure 12–2, page 331: Carlyn Iverson; Figure 12–3, page 332: Cecile Duray-Bito/Precision Graphics; Figure 12–4, page 333: Julie Horan/Radiant Illustration and Design; Figure 12–5, page 334: Laurie O'Keefe/Precision Graphics; Figure 12–6, page 335: Cyndie C.H. Wooley/Precision Graphics; Figure 12–7, page 336: Cyndie C.H. Wooley/Precision Graphics; Figure 12–8, page 337: Sandra McMahon/Precision Graphics; Concept map 12–1, page 339: Randy Miyake. Adapted by Tech-Graphics; Concept map 12–3, page 340: Randy Miyake. Adapted by Tech-Graphics; Table figure acromegaly, page 345 (all photos): Reprinted with permission from *American Journal of Medicine*, 20 (1956).; Table figure giantism, page 345: AP/Wide World Photos; Table figure thyroid gland, page 346 (left): Ken Greer/Visuals Unlimited, (right) Custom Medical Stock Photo; Table figure Cushing's syndrome, page 346: Science VU/Visuals Unlimited; Table figure dwarfism, page 347: AP/Wide World Photos; Table figure cretinism, page 348: Lester V. Bergman & Associates, Cold Spring, NY 10516.

Chapter 13

Figure 13–1, page 360: Elizabeth Morales-Denney/Precision Graphics; Figure 13–2, page 361 (a and c): Darwen and Vally Hennings, (b) Philippe Plailly/Photo Researchers, (d) Science Photo Library/Photo Researchers; Figure 13–3, page 362: Laurie O'Keefe/Precision Graphics; Figure 13–4, page 362: Matthew Thiessen; Figure 13–5, page 363: Cyndie C.H. Wooley/Precision Graphics; Figure 13–6, page 364 (a): Ken Sherman/The StockShop Inc./Medichrome, (b) John and Judy Waller; Figure 13–7, page 365: Elizabeth Morales-Denney/Precision Graphics; Figure 13–8, page 366: Cyndie C.H. Wooley/Precision Graphics; Figure 13–9, page 367: Elizabeth Morales-Denney/Cyndi C.H. Wooley/Precision Graphics; Figure 13–10, page 368: Cyndie C.H. Wooley/Precision Graphics; Figure 13–11, page 369: Elizabeth Morales-Denney/ Precision Graphics; Figure 13–12, page 370: Elizabeth Morales-Denney/Precision Graphics; Concept map 13–1, page 371: Randy Miyake. Adapted by Tech-Graphics; Concept map 13–2, page 372: Randy Miyake. Adapted by Tech-Graphics; Table figure aneurysm, page 375: CNRI/Photo Researchers; Table figure coronary artery disease, page 376 (left): Cabisco/Visuals Unlimited, (right) William Ober/Visuals Unlimited; Table figure varicose veins, page 377: Julie Horan/Radiant Illustration and Design; Table figure myocardial infarction, page 377: Julie Horan/Radiant Illustration and Design; Figure 13–13, page 379: Julie Horan/Radiant Illustration and Design; Table figure cardiac catheterization, page 382: Julie Horan, Radiant Illustration and Design; Table figure angioplasty, page 383: Julie Horan/Radiant Illustration and Design; Table figure defibrillation, page 384: SIU/Visuals Unlimited; Table figure coronary artery bypass graft, page 385: Darwen and Vally Hennings; Table figure insertion of cardiac pacemaker, page 386: Julie Horan/Radiant Illustration and Design; Table figure ligation, page 386: Julie Horan/Radiant Illustration and Design; Exercise figure 13–5, page 393: Elizabeth Morales-Denney/Precision Graphics. Adapted by Tech-Graphics; Exercise figure 13–5, page 394: Elizabeth Morales-Denney/Precision Graphics. Adapted by Tech-Graphics.

Chapter 14

Figure 14–1, page 401: Laurie O'Keefe/Precision Graphics; Figure 14–2, page 403: Custom Medical Stock Photo; Figure 14–3, page 403: Laurie O'Keefe/Carlyn Iverson; Figure 14–4, page 404: Cyndie C.H. Wooley/Precision Graphics; Figure 14–5, page 405: Cyndie C.H. Wooley/Precision Graphics; Concept map 14–1, page 406: Randy Miyake. Adapted by Tech-Graphics; Table figure tracheoesophageal fistula, page 409: Julie Horan/Radiant Illustration and Design; Table figure bronchiectasis, page 410: Julie Horan/ Radiant Illustration and Design; Table figure emphysema, page 411: Julie Horan/Radiant Illustration and Design; Table figure pneumonia, page 412: Julie Horan/Radiant Illustration and Design; Table figure cystic fibrosis, page 413: Jeffrey Reed/The StockShop Inc./Medichrome; **Table figure finger clubbing, page 416:** Julie Horan/Radiant Illustration and Design; **Table figure pulmonary function tests, page 418 (a):** SIU/ Visuals Unlimited, **(b)** John and Judy Waller; **Table figure bronchodilators, page 420:** SIU/Visuals Unlimited; **Table figure tracheotomy, page 421:** Julie Horan/Radiant Illustration and Design; **Exercise figure 14–5, page 429:** Laurie O'Keefe/Precision Graphics. Adapted by Tech-Graphics.

Chapter 15

Figure 15–1, page 436: Julie Horan/Radiant Illustration and Design; **Table figure sickle cell anemia, page 440 (left and right):** Stanley Flegler/Visuals Unlimited; **Table figure acquired hemolytic anemia, page 441:** Cyndie C.H. Wooley/Precision Graphics; **Table figure rouleaux, page 444:** Julie Horan/Radiant Illustration and Design; **Figure 15–2, page 447:** Laurie O'Keefe/Precision Graphics; **Figure 15–3, page 449:** Cyndie C.H. Wooley/Precision Graphics; **Figure 15–4, page 450:** Cyndie C.H. Wooley/Precision Graphics; **Figure 15–5, page 453:** Publication Services; **Table figure Kaposi's sarcoma, page 456:** Science VU-AFIF/Visuals Unlimited.

Chapter 16

Figure 16–1, page 468: Laurie O'Keefe/Precision Graphics; **Figure 16–2, page 469:** Carlyn Iverson; **Figure 16–3, page 470:** Carlyn Iverson/Todd Buck; **Figure 16–4, page 471:** Cyndie C.H. Wooley/Precision Graphics; **Figure 16–6, page 472:** Cyndie C.H. Wooley/Precision Graphics; **Figure 16–7, page 473:** Cyndie C.H. Wooley/Precision Graphics; **Figure 16–8, page 473:** Cecile Duray-Bitol/Precision Graphics; **Figure 16–9, page 475:** Wayne Clark/Precision Graphics; **Concept map 16–1, page 476:** Randy Miyake. Adapted by Tech-Graphics; **Concept map 16–2, page 477:** Randy Miyake. Adapted by Tech-Graphics; **Table figure nephrolithiasis, page 480:** Julie Horan/Radiant Illustration and Design; **Table figure polycystic kidneys, page 480:** Julie Horan/Radiant Illustration and Design; **Table figure lithotripsy, page 484:** SIU/Photo Researchers; **Table figure dialysis, page 485:** SIU/Visuals Unlimited; **Table figure cystoscopy, page 486:** Julie Horan/Radiant Illustration and Design; **Figure 16–10, page 487:** Laurie O'Keefe/Precision Graphics; **Figure 16–11, page 488:** John and Judy Waller; **Concept map 16–3, page 490:** Randy Miyake. Adapted by Tech-Graphics; **Table figure epispadias, page 492:** Julie Horan/Radiant Illustration and Design; **Table figure hydrocele, page 492:** Julie Horan/Radiant Illustration and Design; **Table figure hypospadias, page 493:** Julie Horan/Radiant Illustration and Design; **Table figure testicular torsion, page 493:** Julie Horan/ Radiant Illustration and Design; **Table figure varicocele, page 493:** Julie Horan/Radiant Illustration and Design; **Table figure vasectomy, page 495:** Julie Horan/Radiant Illustration and Design.

Chapter 17

Figure 17-1, page 506 (a): Carlyn Iverson, **(b and c)** Carlyn Iverson/Gerrity; **Figure 17-2, page 509:** Carlyn Iverson; **Figure 17-3, page 510:** Carlyn Iverson; **Concept map 17–1, page 511:** Randy Miyake. Adapted by Tech-Graphics; **Table figure cervical polyps, page 514:** Julie Horan/Radiant Illustration and Design; **Table figure cystocele and rectocele, page 515:** Julie Horan/Radiant Illustration and Design; **Table figure malposition of uterus, page 516:** Julie Horan/Radiant Illustration and Design; **Table figure uterine prolapse, page 517:** Julie Horan/Radiant Illustration and Design; **Table figure laparoscopy, page 520:** Julie Horan/Radiant Illustration and Design; **Table figure sterilization, page 522:** Julie Horan/Radiant Illustration and Design; **Figure 17–4 page 524:** Cecile Duray-Bito/Precision Graphics; **Figure 17–5, page 525 (left):** Science VU/Valerie Lindgren/Visuals Unlimited, **(right)** Bernd Wittich/Visuals Unlimited; **Figure 17–6, page 528:** Cabisco/Visuals Unlimited; **Figure 17–7, page 529:** Cyndie C.H. Wooley/Precision Graphics; **Table figure amniocentesis, page 533 (a):** SIU/Visuals Unlimited, **(b)** Carlyn Iverson.

Chapter 18

Part three opening photo, page 543: © Peter Angelo Simon/Phototake; **Figure 18–1, page 550:** Julie Horan/ Radiant Illustration and Design; **Figure 18–2, pages 554–555:** G. D. Heggie, RT(NM), M.Ed.; **Figure 18–3, page 557:** G. D. Heggie, RT(NM), M.Ed.; **Figure 18–4, page 559:** G. D. Heggie, RT(NM), M.Ed.

Chapter 22

Figure 22–1, page 602–603: Julie Horan/Radiant Illustration and Design; **Figure 22–2, page 605:** Julie Horan/Radiant Illustration and Design; **Figure 22–3, page 607:** Julie Horan/Radiant Illustration and Design; **Figure 22–4, page 608:** Julie Horan/Radiant Illustration and Design; **Figure 22–5, page 608–609:** Julie Horan/Radiant Illustration and Design; **Figure 22–6, page 609:** Julie Horan/Radiant Illustration and Design; **Table figure Fowler, page 612:** Julie Horan/Radiant Illustration and Design; **Table figure lateral decubitus, page 612:** Julie Horan/Radiant Illustration and Design; **Table figure lithotomy, page 613:** Julie Horan/Radiant Illustration and Design; **Table figure prone position, page 613:** Julie Horan/Radiant

Illustration and Design; **Table figure supine position, page 613:** Julie Horan/Radiant Illustration and Design; **Table figure Trendelenburg, page 613:** Julie Horan/Radiant Illustration and Design; **Figure 22–7, page 614:** Julie Horan/Radiant Illustration and Design; **Table 22–8, page 614:** Julie Horan/Radiant Illustration and Design; **Figure 22–9, page 616:** Julie Horan/Radiant Illustration and Design; **Figure 22–10, page 617:** Julie Horan/Radiant Illustration and Design; **Figure 22–11, page 618:** Julie Horan/Radiant Illustration and Design; **Figure 22–12, page 618:** Julie Horan/Radiant Illustration and Design; **Figure 22–13, page 618:** Julie Horan/Radiant Illustration and Design; **Figure 22–14, page 619:** Julie Horan/Radiant Illustration and Design.

Appendices

Appendix opening photo, page 633: © Peter Angelo Simon/Phototake.

A set of 500 Activity Cards
(ISBN 0–314–08925–X) can be
shrinkwrapped with the text.

Chapter 2

2B

infestation by itch mites

127B

Medical
Suffixes

2

SCABIES

127